The Tr
of The Massachusetts
General Hospital

The Trauma Handbook of The Massachusetts General Hospital

Editor

Robert L. Sheridan, M.D.

Clinical Director
Division of Trauma and Burns
Massachusetts General Hospital
Shriners Hospital for Children

Associate Professor of Surgery
Harvard Medical School
Boston, Massachusetts

Illustrations by:

Laurel C. Lhowe
Medical Illustrator
Boston, Massachusetts

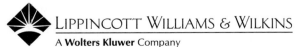

LIPPINCOTT WILLIAMS & WILKINS
A **Wolters Kluwer** Company
Philadelphia · Baltimore · New York · London
Buenos Aires · Hong Kong · Sydney · Tokyo

Acquisitions Editor: Brian Brown
Developmental Editor: Alyson Forbes/Tanya Lazar
Production Editor: Jeff Somers
Manufacturing Manager: Colin Warnock
Cover Designer:
Compositor: Circle Graphics
Printer: RR Donnelley Crawfordsville

JUL 2 3 2004
JUL 2 9 2004

© 2004 by LIPPINCOTT WILLIAMS & WILKINS
530 Walnut Street
Philadelphia, PA 19106 USA
LWW.com

Printed in the USA

Library of Congress Cataloging-in-Publication Data

The trauma handbook of the Massachusetts General Hospital / editor, Robert L.
  Sheridan ; illustrations by Laurel C. Lhowe.
    p. ; cm.
  Includes bibliographical references and index.
  ISBN 0-7817-4596-9 (alk. paper)
  1. Traumatology—Handbooks, manuals, etc. 2. Wounds and injuries—
Handbooks, manuals, etc. 3. Emergency medical services—Handbooks, manuals,
etc. I. Sheridan, Robert L. (Robert Leo), 1955- II. Massachusetts General
Hospital.
  [DNLM: 1. Wounds and Injuries—therapy. 2. Emergencies. 3. Emergency
Medical Services. WO 700 T775658 2004]
  RD93.T6877 2004
  617.1—dc22
                                                                    2003061928

*To Martha, for 30 years
of friendship and support.*

Contents

Contributing Authors xi

Preface xvii

Acknowledgments xix

I. ORGANIZATIONAL ISSUES

1. A Brief History of Trauma Surgery.............. 1
   Andrew M. Cameron

2. Trauma Systems and Injury Severity Scoring..... 10
   Alasdair Conn and Laurie S. Petrovik

3. Prehospital Care and Transport 29
   Paul D. Biddinger and Stephen H. Thomas

4. Organization of the Emergency Department and
   Trauma Team 50
   David A. Peak and Alice A. Gervasini

5. Disaster Planning............................ 58
   Adrian A. Maung and Susan M. Briggs

II. IMMEDIATE CARE

6. Initial Evaluation and Resuscitation:
   Primary Survey and Immediate Resuscitation 71
   Shaun M. Kunisaki and Charles J. McCabe

7. The Trauma Airway 89
   Harish S. Lecamwasam, Ruben Peralta,
   and Peter F. Dunn

8. Secondary Survey Evaluation of the Trauma
   Patient 108
   Vicki E. Noble and David A. Peak

9. Unique Critical Care Issues Related to Trauma ... 120
   Ruben Peralta, Alexander Iribarne,
   Oscar J. Manrique, and Horatio Hojman

10. Transfusion and Coagulation Issues in Trauma ... 128
    Walter H. Dzik and Christopher P. Stowell

11. Initial Evaluation and Management of the
    Burn Patient 148
    Robert L. Sheridan, John T. Schulz III,
    Colleen M. Ryan, and Mary Elizabeth Bilodeau

12. Trauma Anesthesia   174
     Kristopher R. Davignon and Keith Baker

13. Prevention Strategies: Thromboembolic
     Complications, Alcohol Withdrawal, Infection and
     Gastrointestinal Bleeding   195
     *Ruben Peralta, Alexander Iribarne,
     Oscar J. Manrique, and Robert L. Sheridan*

III. EVALUATION AND MANAGEMENT OF SPECIFIC INJURIES

14. Nervous System 1: Head Injury   213
     Yogish D. Kamath and Lawrence F. Borges

15. Nervous System 2: Spinal Cord and Peripheral
     Nerve Injuries   224
     Yogish D. Kamath and Lawrence F. Borges

16. Evaluation and Acute Management of
     Maxillofacial Trauma   239
     *Jeffrey A. Hammoudeh, Leonard B. Kaban, and
     Thomas B. Dodson*

17. Ocular and Adnexal Trauma   258
     Nicoletta Fynn-Thompson and Lynnette Watkins

18. Neck Injuries   284
     Ruben Peralta and Oscar J. Manrique

19. Chest Trauma 1: Chest Wall, Pleural Space,
     and Lung Parenchyma   296
     Christopher R. Morse and James S. Allan

20. Chest Trauma 2: Tracheobronchial and
     Esophageal Injuries   314
     Frances Fynn-Thompson and James S. Allan

21. Chest Trauma 3: Blunt and Penetrating Injuries
     to the Heart and Central Vessels   328
     David Tom Cooke and Thomas MacGillivary

22. Vascular Trauma 1:
     Cervicothoracic Vascular Trauma   342
     Luke Marone and Richard Cambria

23. Vascular Trauma 2:
     Abdominal Vascular Injuries   351
     Carrie Sims and David Berger

24. Vascular Trauma 3:
     Peripheral Vascular Injuries   372
     Susan M. Briggs and Steven M. Abbate

25. Abdominal Trauma 1: Diagnostic Techniques   385
     Ara J. Feinstein and Charles M. Ferguson

26. Abdominal Trauma 2: Diaphragm and
     Abdominal Wall   402
     Sharon L. Stein and John T. Schulz III

27. Abdominal Trauma 3: Hepatic and Biliary
     Tract Injuries   413
     *Jennifer A. Wargo, Ruben Peralta, and
     Robert L. Sheridan*

28. Abdominal Trauma 4: Splenic Injuries.   433
     Douglas R. Johnston and Robert L. Sheridan

29. Abdominal Trauma 5: Injuries to the Pancreas
     and Duodenum   446
     Matthew M. Hutter and Andrew L. Warshaw

30. Abdominal Trauma 6: Hollow Viscus Injuries   462
     *Ruben Peralta, Alexander Iribarne, and
     Oscar J. Manrique*

31. Abdominal Trauma 7: Damage Control and the
     Abdominal Compartment Syndrome   475
     *Glenn Egrie, Ruben Peralta, and
     Robert L. Sheridan*

32. Genitourinary Trauma.   484
     *Adam S. Feldman, Patricio C. Gargolo, and
     Joseph A. Grocela*

33. Orthopedic Trauma 1: Spine Fractures   509
     Raymond Malcolm Smith

34. Orthopedic Trauma 2: Pelvic Fractures   518
     Mark S. Vrahas and David Joseph

35. Orthopedic Trauma 3: Extremity Fractures   526
     David W. Lhowe

36. Hand Injuries   540
     *J. Alejandro Conejero, David A. Lickstein, and
     Jonathan M. Winograd*

37. Techniques of Soft Tissue Reconstruction   558
     Bohdan Pomahac and Jonathan M. Winograd

IV. SPECIAL CONSIDERATIONS

38. Pediatric Trauma 1: Resuscitation and
     Initial Evaluation   571
     Rashni Dasgupta and Daniel P. Ryan

39. Pediatric Trauma 2: Definitive Care.   580
    Akemi L. Kawaguchi, David Lawlor, and
    Jay J. Schnitzer

40. Considerations in the Pregnant Woman   592
    Larry Rand and Kevin C. Dennehy

41. Geriatric Trauma   608
    Kari Rosenkrantz and Robert L. Sheridan

42. Trauma Radiology   619
    Thomas Ptak and Andrew Hines-Peralta

43. Organ and Tissue Procurement in Trauma   655
    Andrew M. Cameron and Francis L. Delmonico

44. Psychiatric Issues in Trauma   662
    John K. Findley and Lawrence Park

45. Rehabilitation of the Trauma Patient.   682
    Ricardo Knight

46. Medicolegal Considerations and Duties   710
    Brett D. Pangburn, Laura L. Stephens,
    Carolyn V. Wood, and Robert L. Sheridan

Subject Index   733

Contributing Authors

Steven M. Abbate, M.D. *General Surgery Service, Massachusetts General Hospital, Boston, Massachusetts*

James S. Allan, M.D. *Assistant Professor of Surgery, Department of Surgery, Harvard Medical School; Thoracic Surgeon, Department of Surgery, Massachusetts General Hospital, Boston, Massachusetts*

Keith Baker, M.D., Ph.D. *Assistant Professor of Anesthesia, Department of Anesthesia and Critical Care, Harvard Medical School; Assistant Anesthetist, Department of Anesthesia and Critical Care, Massachusetts General Hospital, Boston, Massachusetts*

David Berger, M.D. *Assistant Professor of Surgery, Harvard Medical School; Associate Visiting Surgeon, Massachusetts General Hospital, Boston, Massachusetts*

Paul D. Biddinger, M.D. *Director of Prehospital Care, Massachusetts General Hospital; Instructor in Surgery, Harvard Medical School, Boston, Massachusetts*

Mary Elizabeth Bilodeau, RN, BSN. *Burn Unit Nurse Practitioner, Massachusetts General Hospital, Boston, Massachusetts*

Lawrence F. Borges, M.D., FACS *Associate Professor of Surgery, Harvard Medical School; Visiting Neurosurgeon, Department of Neurosurgery, Massachusetts General Hospital, Boston, Massachusetts*

Susan M. Briggs M.D., MPH, FACS *Associate Director of Trauma, Massachusetts General Hospital; Director, Harvard Medical International Trauma and Disaster Institute; Assistant Professor of Surgery, Harvard Medical School; Supervising Officer, NDMS Specialty Medical Teams, Boston, Massachusetts*

Richard Cambria, M.D. *Professor of Surgery, Harvard Medical School; Chief, Division of Vascular and Endovascular Surgery, Massachusetts General Hospital, Boston, Massachusetts*

Andrew M. Cameron, M.D., Ph.D. *Resident, Department of Surgery, Massachusetts General Hospital, Boston, Massachusetts*

J. Alejandro Conejero, M.D. *General Surgery Resident, Massachusetts General Hospital; Clinical Fellow in Surgery, Harvard Medical School, Boston, Massachusetts*

Alasdair Conn, M.D. *Chief, Emergency Services, WHT 1, Boston, Massachusetts*

David Tom Cooke, M.D. *Clinical Fellow in Surgery, Harvard Medical School; Resident in General Surgery, Department of Surgery, Massachusetts General Hospital, Boston, Massachusetts*

Rashni Dasgupta, M.D. *Resident, Department of General Surgery, Harvard Medical School; Resident, General Surgery, Massachusetts General Hospital, Boston, Massachusetts*

Kristopher R. Davignon, M.D. *Clinical Fellow Harvard Medical School, Critical Care Fellow, Department of Anesthesia and Critical Care, Massachussetts General Hospital, Boston, Massachusetts*

Francis L. Delmonico, M.D. *Professor of Surgery, Harvard Medical School; Director, Renal Transplantation, Massachusetts General Hospital, Boston, Massachusetts*

Kevin C. Dennehy, MB, BCh, FFARCSI *Department of Anesthesia and Critical Care, Massachusetts General Hospital, Boston, Massachusetts*

Thomas B. Dodson, DMD, MPH *Associate Professor, Oral and Maxillofacial Surgery, Harvard School of Dental Medicine; Visiting Oral and Maxillofacial Surgeon, Director of Resident Training, Department of Oral and Maxillofacial Surgery, Massachusetts General Hospital, Boston, Massachusetts*

Peter F. Dunn, M.D. *Instructor, Department of Anesthesia and Critical Care, Massachusetts General Hospital, Boston, Massachusetts*

Walter H. Dzik, M.D. *Blood Transfusion Service, Massachusetts General Hospital, Boston, Massachusetts*

Glenn Egrie, M.D. *Senior Resident, Department of Surgery, Massachusetts General Hospital, Boston, Massachusetts*

Ara J. Feinstein, M.D. *Resident in General Surgery, Massachusetts General Hospital, Boston, Massachusetts*

Adam S. Feldman, M.D. *Resident, Department of Urology, Massachusetts General Hospital, Boston, Massachusetts*

Charles M. Ferguson, M.D. *General Surgery Program Director, Massachusetts General Hospital, Boston, Massachusetts*

John K. Findley, M.D. *Clinical Instructor, Department of Psychiatry, Harvard Medical School, Massachusetts General Hospital, Boston, Massachusetts*

Frances Fynn-Thompson, M.D. *Cardiothoracic Surgery Fellow, Harvard Medical School; Cardiothoracic Surgery Fellow, Massachusetts General Hospital, Boston, Massachusetts*

Nicoletta Fynn-Thompson, M.D.   *Resident, Department of Ophthalmology, Harvard Medical School; Resident, Department of Ophthalmology, Massachusetts Eye & Ear Infirmary, Boston, Massachusetts*

Patricio C. Gargolo, M.D.   *Resident, Department of Urology, Massachusetts General Hospital, Boston, Massachusetts*

Alice A. Gervasini, Ph.D., RN.   *Trauma Program Nurse Manager, Massachusetts General Hospital, Boston, Massachusetts*

Joseph A. Grocela, M.D.   *Instructor in Urology, Department of Urology, Harvard Medical School; Urologist, Department of Urology, Massachusetts General Hospital, Boston, Massachusetts*

Jeffrey A. Hammoudeh, DDS, M.D.   *Chief Resident, Harvard Oral and Maxillofacial Surgery, Massachusetts General Hospital, Boston, Massachusetts*

Andrew Hines-Peralta, M.D.   *Department of Radiology, Beth Israel Deaconess Medical Center, Boston, Massachusetts*

Horatio Hojman, M.D.   *Attending Surgeon, Yale-New Haven Hospital, New Haven, Connecticut*

Matthew M. Hutter, M.D.   *Instructor in Surgery, Harvard Medical School, Chief Surgical Resident, Assistant in Surgery, Department of Surgery, Massachusetts General Hospital, Boston, Massachusetts*

Alexander Iribarne, M.D.   *Harvard Medical School, Boston, Massachusetts*

Douglas R. Johnston, M.D.   *Clinical Fellow in Surgery, Department of Surgery, Harvard Medical School, Surgical Resident, Department of Surgery, Massachusetts General Hospital, Boston, Massachusetts*

David Joseph, M.D.   *Clinical Instructor, Elmhurst Hospital, Elmhurst, New York*

Leonard B. Kaban, DMD, M.D.   *Walter C. Guralnick Professor and Chairman, Department of Oral and Maxillofacial Surgery, Harvard School of Dental Medicine, Boston, Massachusetts*

Yogish D. Kamath, M.D.   *Staff Neurosurgeon, Massachusetts General Hospital, Boston Massachusetts*

Akemi L. Kawaguchi, M.D.   *Resident in General Surgery, Massachusetts General Hospital, Boston, Massachusetts*

Ricardo Knight, M.D.   *Instructor, Physical Medicine & Rehabilitation, Harvard Medical School; Assistant Physiatrist, Physical Medicine & Rehabilitation, Massachusetts General Hospital, Boston, Massachusetts*

Shaun M. Kunisaki, M.D., MSc *Clinical Fellow, Department of Surgery, Harvard Medical School; Resident, Department of Surgery, Massachusetts General Hospital, Boston, Massachusetts*

David Lawlor, M.D. *Department of Pediatric Surgery, Massachusetts General Hospital, Boston, Massachusetts*

Harish S. Lecamwasam, M.D., MSc *Clinical Fellow, Anesthesia and Critical Care, Massachusetts General Hospital, Harvard Medical School, Boston, Massachusetts*

David A. Lickstein, M.D. *Department of Surgery, Albany Medical Center, Albany, New York*

Thomas MacGillivary, M.D. *Attending Cardiac Surgeon, Massachusetts General Hospital, Harvard Medical School, Boston, Massachusetts*

Oscar J. Manrique, M.D. *Research Fellow, Department of Surgery, Harvard Medical School, Universidad Militar "Neuva Granada"; Research Fellow, Department of Surgery, Massachusetts General Hospital, Boston, Massachusetts*

Luke Marone, M.D. *Fellow in Vascular Surgery, Massachusetts General Hospital, Boston, Massachusetts*

Adrian A. Maung, M.D. *Clinical Fellow in Surgery, Department of Surgery, Harvard Medical School; Resident, Department of General Surgery, Massachusetts General Hospital, Boston, Massachusetts*

Charles J. McCabe, M.D. *Associate Professor, Department of Surgery, Harvard Medical School; Associate Chief, Emergency Services, Massachusetts General Hospital, Boston, Massachusetts*

Christopher R. Morse, M.D. *Clinical Fellow in Surgery, Department of Surgery, Harvard University; Resident in Surgery, Department of Surgery, Massachusetts General Hospital, Boston, Massachusetts*

Vicki E. Noble, M.D. *Resident in Emergency Medicine, Massachusetts General Hospital, Boston Massachusetts*

Brett D. Pangburn, Esq. *Office of the General Counsel, Partners Healthcare System, Inc., Boston, Massachusetts*

Lawrence Park, M.D. *Attending Psychiatrist, Massachusetts General Hospital, Boston, Massachusetts*

David A. Peak, M.D. *Attending in Emergency Medicine, Massachusetts General Hospital / Harvard Medical School, Boston Massachusetts*

Ruben Peralta, M.D.   *General Surgery, Trauma and Surgical Critical Care, Massachusetts General Hospital, Harvard Medical School, Boston, Massachusetts*

Laurie S. Petrovik, MS   *Administrative Coordinator, Biostatistics and Performance Improvement, Division of Burn, Trauma, and Critical Care, Department of Surgery, Massachusetts General Hospital, Boston, Massachusetts*

Bohdan Pomahac, M.D.   *Fellow in Plastic Surgery, Massachusetts General Hospital, Boston, Massachusetts*

Tom Ptak, M.D., Ph.D., MPh   *Assistant Professor, Department of Radiology, Harvard University; Emergency / Trauma Neuroradiologist, Division of Emergency Radiology, Massachusetts General Hospital, Boston, Massachusetts*

Larry Rand, M.D.   *Chief Resident, Department of Obstetrics, Massachusetts General Hospital, Boston, Massachusetts*

Kari Rosenkrantz, M.D.   *Trauma Research Fellow, Massachusetts General Hospital, Boston, Massachusetts*

Colleen M. Ryan, M.D.   *Co-Director, Sumner Redstone Burn Center, Massachusetts General Hospital; Staff Surgeon, Shriners Hospital for Children; Associate Professor of Surgery, Harvard Medical School, Boston, Massachusetts*

Daniel P. Ryan, M.D.   *Visiting Surgeon, Massachusetts General Hospital; Associate Professor of Surgery, Harvard Medical School, Boston, Massachusetts*

Jay J. Schnitzer, M.D., Ph.D.   *Associate Professor of Surgery, Department of Surgery, Harvard Medical School; Associate Visiting Surgeon, Pediatric Surgery, Massachusetts General Hospital, Boston, Massachusetts*

John T. Schulz III, M.D., Ph.D.   *Instructor in Surgery, Department of Surgery, Harvard Medical School; Assistant in Surgery, Department of Surgery, Massachusetts General Hospital, Boston, Massachusetts*

Robert L. Sheridan, M.D.   *Clinical Director, Division of Burns and Trauma, Massachusetts General Hospital; Assistant Chief of Staff, Shriners Hospital for Children; Associate Professor of Surgery, Harvard Medical School, Boston, Massachusetts*

Carrie Sims, M.D.   *General Surgery Service, Massachusetts General Hospital, Boston, Massachusetts*

Raymond Malcolm Smith, M.D.   *Chief Othopaedic Trauma Service, Massachusetts General Hospital, Boston, Massachusetts*

Sharon L. Stein, M.D.   *Resident, General Surgery, Department of Surgery, Massachusetts General Hospital, Boston, Massachusetts*

Laura L. Stephens, Esq.   *Office of the General Counsel, Partners Healthcare System, Inc., Boston, Massachusetts*

Christopher P. Stowell, M.D., Ph.D.   *Assistant Professor, Department of Pathology, Harvard Medical School; Director, Blood Transfusion Service, Massachusetts General Hospital, Boston, Massachusetts*

Stephen H. Thomas, M.D., MPH   *Assistant Professor, Surgery, Harvard Medical School; Director of Undergraduate Medical Education, Emergency Services, Massachusetts General Hospital, Boston, Massachusetts*

Mark S. Vrahas, M.D.   *Assistant Professor, Department of Orthopaedic Surgery, Harvard Medical School; Partners Chief of Orthopaedic Trauma Services, Department of Orthopaedic Trauma, Massachusetts General Hospital, Brigham & Women's Hospital, Boston, Massachusetts*

Jennifer A. Wargo, M.D.   *Resident in General Surgery, The Massachusetts General Hospital, Boston, Massachusetts*

Andrew L. Warshaw, M.D.   *W. Gerard Austen Professor of Surgery, Department of Surgery, Harvard Medical School; Surgeon-in-Chief and Chairman, Department of Surgery, Massachusetts General Hospital, Boston, Massachusetts*

Lynnette Watkins, M.D.   *Instructor, Department of Ophthalmology, Harvard Medical School; Director, Emergency Ophthalmology Services, Massachusetts Eye & Ear Infirmary, Boston, Massachusetts*

Jonathan M. Winograd, M.D.   *Division of Plastic and Reconstructive Surgery, Massachusetts General Hospital, Boston, Massachusetts*

Carolyn V. Wood, Esq   *Partners Healthcare System, Boston Bar Association / HIPAA State Law Task Force, Boston, Massachusetts*

Preface

Successful trauma care requires a high degree of coordination among multiple disciplines. Those providing this care need a common core of knowledge that crosses all disciplines. No single specialty can competently manage these complex patients in isolation. In this handbook we attempt to present the common knowledge base of one successful program.

We wanted to emphasize the practical clinical art of trauma care. This book is written for practitioners and trainees in the emergency department, intensive care unit or operating room. The book aims to provide the multidisciplinary base of knowledge that is required to function in a system of comprehensive trauma care.

The book is organized so that systems and immediate care issues are discussed first. This is followed by details on the evaluation and management of specific injuries, listed by body system. Following this are special clinical problems. The book closes with a detailed discussion of the medicolegal duties and processes that are such a prominent part of care of the injured patient.

Each of the 46 chapters is authored by a team, generally consisting of a senior trainee in the specific area and an established active practitioner with special expertise in the specialty. With this authorship strategy, we hoped to create chapters that reliably and concisely present the practical information needed to deliver quality multidisciplinary trauma care.

It is an honor to be a small part of the long tradition of injury care at the MGH. All of us who participated in the writing of this book want to thank our families for their love and understanding, our institution for its unwavering support of trauma and burn care, and the editorial staff at Lippincott Williams and Wilkins for their patience and skill.

Acknowledgments

Editorial and Administrative Assistance
Ruben Peralta, MD
Kathryn S. Young, BA
Monica Toledo, BA

Trauma Program Support
Alasdair K. Conn, MD
Alice M. Gervasini, RN PhD
Ronald G. Tompkins, MD ScD
Andrew L. Warshaw, MD

Organizational Issues

1

A Brief History of Trauma Surgery

Andrew M. Cameron, MD, PhD

I. Introduction

The study of the history of medicine aims to put our current daily efforts in context, explain how we got where we are, inspire those who would learn of past triumphs, and warn those who might learn from past mistakes. The history of trauma surgery is as filled with interesting and informative tales as any other in medicine. This chapter briefly reviews some events important in the history of trauma surgery, focusing on the experience in the United States, both military and civilian. It also examines how modern trauma surgery arrived at its current state, both in terms of its scientific tenets and its system of delivery.

II. Trauma Surgery in the United States: Military Chronology

The development of trauma surgery in the United States has been synonymous with its military medical history. Major events that shaped the development of the field of surgery over the 200-year history of the United States (e.g., the discovery of surgical anesthesia and aseptic principles) shaped trauma surgery as well. This review begins with a brief overview of developments in trauma surgery made during wartime.

A. The Revolutionary War

At the time of the birth of the United States, trauma care was based on the European principles espoused by the teachings in the Scottish and London schools. During the War for Independence, trauma care was limited to symptomatic and topical care of minor and moderate soft tissue injuries; amputation was the most commonly performed procedure. American surgeon John Jones authored "Plain Concise, Practical remarks on the Treatment of Wounds and Fracture" in 1775, which became the guide for surgeons during the Revolutionary War. It is considered the first surgical work written by an American and published in North America.

Other notable American surgeons at that time included William Shippen, who had studied in London and replaced John Morgan as chief physician of the Continental Army in 1777. Another prominent physician, Dr. Joseph Warren, was killed in the Battle of Bunker Hill; his brother John (1753–1815) served in the Continental army as hospital surgeon from 1775 to 1782. It was his son, John Collins Warren, who cofounded the Massachusetts General Hospital (MGH) in 1811, the third American hospital and also performed the famous ether operation in 1846. Serving under John Warren during the Revolutionary War was Barnstable native James Thacher. Thacher's military journal kept during this war leaves us a vivid account of trauma surgery at that time:

We have about thirty surgeons, and mates; and all are constantly employed. I am obliged to devote the whole of my time from eight o'clock in the morning to a late hour in the evening, to the care of our patients. Here is a fine field for professional improvement. Amputating limbs, trepanning fractured skulls, and dressing the most formidable wounds, have familiarized my mind to scenes of woe. . . . If I turn from beholding mutilated bodies, mangled limbs, and bleeding, incurable wounds, a spectacle no less revolting is presented of miserable objects, languishing under afflicting diseases of every description . . . awful harbingers of approaching dissolution . . . emaciated bodies and ghastly visage.

—*Dr. James Thatcher, October 1777*

B.   The Civil War

During the Civil War began the development of systems of trauma care delivery. This was born out of necessity because of the shear magnitude of the number injured (approximately 110,070 northern soldiers and 94,000 southern soldiers died from military trauma). A second major change in trauma surgery during this war was the use of anesthesia (mostly chloroform and, occasionally, ether), which had been demonstrated just 20 years prior.

Surgeon General William A. Hammond (1828–1900) contributed to the knowledge of trauma care delivery by studying the mortality rate of various types of wounds. The Union Army's mortality rate from gunshot wound to the chest was 62%, and for abdominal wounds was 87%. Union medical officers published studies showing the efficacy of antiseptics: bromine or nitric acid for gangrene reduced the mortality rate from 43% to 2%. Other accomplishments involving wound care were brought about by The Sanitary Commission of the US Army, which issued a directive stating "it is good practice to leave the wounds open to heal by granulation." The Sanitary Commission also sought the provision of shelter, clean bedding, and food, as well as nursing care. A leader in these efforts was Clara Barton, who later founded the Red Cross. Secretary of war Stanton directed Hammond to form an ambulance corps. Nursing care introduced during the Civil War was modeled after that established by Florence Nightingale in the Crimean war.

Between 30,000 and 60,000 amputations were performed on Union soldiers during the Civil War under the mantra: "save life, not limb." The mortality associated with these procedures was inversely proportional to the distance from the amputation to the patient's trunk:

Finger amputation: 0.5% mortality
Arm: 23%
Below the knee amputation: 50%
Midthigh above the knee amputation: 55%
Upper thigh amputation: 86%
Hip disarticulation: fatal

An excerpt from his manual for military surgeons describes the manner in which Dr. John Julian Chisolm managed gun shot wounds. A similar strategy from the prominent Philadelphia surgeon Dr. Samuel Gross reveals progress since colonial times, but still little hope existed for much beyond survival with amputation. Even this was far from guaranteed.

The indications for treatment, in all gunshot wounds, are, first, to control hemorrhage; second, to cleanse the wound by removing all foreign bodies; and, third, to apply such dressings and pursue such rational course of treatment as will establish cicatrisation.
—*Dr. John Julian Chisolm, 1861*

Firstly to relieve shock; secondly to arrest hemorrhage, thirdly to remove foreign matter; fourthly to approximate and retain the parts; and fifthly, to limit the resulting inflammation.
—*Dr. Samuel D. Gross, 1861*

C.   World War I
World War I saw several significant advances in the care of trauma patients. Blood was used to treat injured combatants and the open treatment of contaminated wounds with delayed closure was accepted. Motorized ambulances were used regularly, reducing the time from injury to definitive care. As this was still the era before antibiotics, wound treatment was topical, often with Dakin's solution. The research of Alexis Carrel (1873–1943) and George Crile (1864–1943) led to a better understanding of the pathophysiology of traumatic injuries and refinements in the treatment of wounds. Technical advancements in reconstructive maxillofacial surgery led to the beginnings of plastic surgery as a bona fide surgical specialty. The misery of many who contributed to these advancements in the craft of surgery were summarized by Lewis Pilcher (1845–1934) president of the American Surgical Association in 1919.

The traumatic surgery of this war has constituted a tremendous vivisection experimental laboratory in which not mice, nor rabbits, nor guinea pigs, nor dogs have been the subjects of experiments, but human beings, the choicest young men of the civilized world.
—*Dr. Lewis Pilcher, 1919*

D.   World War II
Between World Wars I and II, blood banking became routine. In 1929, Alexander Fleming discovered penicillin and, therefore, antibiotics were used in WW II. British General W. H. Ogilvie directed that all soldiers with colon injuries have a colostomy. Evacuation to a definitive care facility was routinely accomplished within 4 to 6 hours, but inadequately treated shock was still a major unsolved problem, with high rates of acute renal failure and attendant mortality.

E.   Korean War
Mobile Army Surgical Hospital (MASH) units and air ambulances, including helicopters, reduced the time delay

for definitive care 2 to 4 hours. These forward surgical hospitals were forever immortalized in Robert Hooker's novel, Robert Altman's movie, and Alan Alda's TV show, all titled *M*A*S*H*. The latter perhaps portrayed the Columbia transplant surgeon, Keith Reemstma, as Hawkeye Pierce and MGH thoracic surgeon, Hermes Grillo, as Charles Emerson Winchester III. Now, vascular injuries were being repaired, reducing the number of amputations performed. Blood was used extensively but shock and renal failure remained a problem because the physiology of resuscitation was still incompletely understood.

F. Viet Nam War

Major advancements in the understanding of hemorrhagic shock and renal failure were accomplished during the Viet Nam War, with crystalloid being added to resuscitation with blood. Helicopters reduced time from injury to definitive care to less than 1 hour. Captain Ellis Jones, a cardiac surgeon from Johns Hopkins reporting from the Second MASH in the Republic of South Viet Nam made these points matter of factly and his comments stand in remarkable contrast to the statements of the military surgeons who came before him:

Advances in helicopter evacuation directly from the site of injury, and availability of whole blood have given us an opportunity to treat and salvage patients who would have previously never reached a medical facility. Air transport of supplies and medical equipment has greatly facilitated our job . . . The wounds resulting from high velocity missiles are extremely destructive and require through examination, debridement, and repair . . .

When resuscitation has begun in the field at the battalion aid or clearing station the patient usually arrives at the hospital receiving normal saline, Ringer's lactate, or low titer O-positive blood . . . Upon arrival at the hospital, the resuscitative process is continued in preparation for emergency operative treatment. Vital signs are restored to as near normal as possible; appropriate radiographic studies are performed, and the patient is taken to the operating room.

—*Dr. Ellis L. Jones, 1968*

III. Trauma Surgery in the United States: Civilian Events

A. Demonstration of Surgical Anesthesia

A major event in the history of medicine and surgery, the discovery of anesthesia by William Morton in 1846, dramatically changed trauma surgery. This was clearly shown by the almost routine use of anesthesia in the impending War Between the States. The significance of this specific event was its role in bringing about acceptance of the practice. Certainly, others had successfully used anesthesia before 1846: Crawford Williamson Long, a surgeon in Jefferson, Georgia, had used ether to perform toe amputations, having witnessed the drug's recreational use during ether frolics while an undergraduate at the University of Pennsylvania. Horace Wells, a Connecticut dentist, had used nitrous oxide to assist in tooth extractions. Neither, however, had parlayed these inconsistent successes into a publicly accepted proof of the value and safety of surgical anesthesia.

October 16, 1846 William Thomas Green Morton, a Boston dentist, convinced MGH surgeon John Collins Warren to allow him to attempt to give anesthesia to one of Warren's patients. Warren was scheduled to operate that day in the Bulfinch amphitheater. His patient was Gilbert Abbott, a young man with a vascular tumor of the jaw— probably a venous malformation. With the help of Charles Jackson, a Harvard chemistry professor, Morton had prepared ether and planned to deliver it using a globelike inhalation sphere, which had been designed by Dr. A. A. Gould and made by an instrument maker on Charles Street. As Warren prepared to begin the procedure, the patient inhaled vapor from the globe in which an ether-soaked sponge had been placed (dyed red to conceal its identity, from which Morton had hoped to profit.) The patient breathed the fumes, lost consciousness, and Dr. Warren performed the operation. Several more times the ether orb was used. The patient was motionless throughout. Toward the end of the procedure, no more ether was given and the patient gradually awoke. Dr. Warren then asked the patient if he had felt any pain during the procedure and he replied that he had felt none at all, only an occasional feeling like that of a garden hoe scraping his neck. Warren looked at Morton and then addressing those present declared: "Gentlemen, this is no Humbug."

Before October 16th, 1846 surgical anesthesia did not exist; within a few months, it became a worldwide procedure: and the full credit for its introduction must be given to William Thomas Green Morton, who, on the date mentioned, demonstrated at the Massachusetts General Hospital the simplicity and safety of ether anesthesia.
—*Sir William Osler*

B. The Cocoanut Grove Nightclub Fire

November 28, 1942, fire destroyed Boston's Cocoanut Grove nightclub, killing 491 people and sending hundreds more to area hospitals. It was the second worst building fire in American history (the most deadly was the fire at the Iroquois Theater in Chicago in 1903, which killed 591). This disaster came at a unique time in the history of burn care. It resulted in a number of important advances, including the first comprehensive description of inhalation injury, improvement in the topical treatment of burn wounds, resuscitation of shock, the use of antibiotics, and understanding of the metabolic response to injury. The fire also stimulated the organization of burn care facilities, public safety legislation, and efforts toward burn prevention.

C. R Adams Cowley and "The Golden Hour"

R Adams Cowley was a US Army surgeon, who just after WW II developed ideas from his military experience about the quick treatment of seriously injured people. He coined the phrase "golden hour" to describe the period just after a serious injury during which prompt and coordinated medical care could save lives. Cowley began a two-bed research unit at the University of Maryland in 1961 and lived to see the opening in 1989 of the eight-story Shock Trauma Center in Baltimore that bore his name. Cowley was a leader in the scientific study of shock and trauma, a leader in use of civilian helicopters for medical evacuation, and a pioneer in the use of hyperbaric medicine as well as open-heart surgery. He is considered by many to be the father of modern trauma care.

D.   Trauma Centers

The first two civilian trauma centers in the United States opened in 1966: one at the San Francisco General Hospital under William Blaisdell and the other at Cook County Hospital in Chicago under Robert Freeark. These centers arose in response to the increasing urban violence that accompanied dramatically increased drug use at that time. Shortly thereafter, Cowley established the Maryland system of trauma care, which later became a statewide system. In 1976, the American College of Surgeons (ACS) Committee on Trauma developed a formal outline of injury care, which is updated periodically. The components of this system as it has matured now include leadership, system development, legislation, finance, public information, education, injury prevention; prehospital care with communication, medical direction, triage, and transport; definitive care; interfacility transfer; and rehabilitation. Two other contributions from the ACS include advanced trauma life support (ATLS) courses and the establishment of a National Trauma Registry (National Trauma Data Bank). Most states now have mature trauma systems. Studies have documented the efficacy of trauma systems in reducing unnecessary morbidity and mortality. Much of this progress is owed to the leadership of R Adams Cowley.

E.   September 11, 2001

September 11, 2001 a jet aircraft crashed into the north tower of the World Trade Center (WTC) in lower Manhattan. Minutes later, a second aircraft crashed into the south tower. The impact, fires, and subsequent collapse of the buildings resulted in the deaths of thousands of persons.

The New York City Department of Health conducted a review of the emergency department medical records of the four hospitals closest to the crash site and a fifth hospital that served as a burn referral center. Arrival of injured persons began within minutes and peaked 2 to 3 hours later. These hospitals received 790 injured patients within 48 hours, 71% who were civilian survivors and the remaining 29% injured rescue workers. The injury pattern among rescue workers was different from that seen in civilian survivors. Rescue workers suffered a higher percentage of ocular injuries than civilians: 39 *vs.* 19%, and fewer burns: 2 *vs.* 6%. Similar to injured survivors from other terrorist attacks on buildings, most civilian survivors of the WTC tragedy sustained injuries treated on an outpatient basis.

For example, the hospitalization rate among survivors of the Murrah Federal Building bombing in Oklahoma City was only 20%. In most such multicasualty disasters, there is typically a first wave of survivors with minor injuries, a second wave of more severely injured survivors, and subsequent waves of survivors rescued during extrication from the disaster site. The WTC attacks, however, generated only one large wave of survivors and a second wave the next day largely composed of rescue workers. Few survivors were extricated from the WTC, however, because of the overwhelming force of the collapse of the 110-story towers and the heat of the fire.

SELECTED READING

Boyd DR, Cowley RA. Comprehensive regional trauma/emergency medical services (EMS) delivery systems: the United States experience. *World J Surg* 1983;7(1):149–157.

Flint L. Who is Hawkeye? *Surgery* 2002;131:357–358.

Franchetti MA. Trauma surgery during the Civil War. *South Med J* 1993;86:553–556.

Jones EL, Peters AF, Gasior RM. Early management of battle casualties in Vietnam. *Arch Surg* 1968;97:1–15.

Moore FD. John Collins Warren and his act of conscience. *Ann Surg* 1999;229:187–196.

Moore FD. Teaching the two faces of medical history. *Surg Clin North Am* 1987;67:1121–1126.

Rapid assessment of injuries among survivors of the terrorist attack on the World Trade Center—New York City, September 2001. *JAMA* 2002;287:835–838.

Rutkow IM. James Thacher and his military journal during the American revolutionary war. *Arch Surg* 2001;136:837.

Rutkow IM. The value of surgical history. *Arch Surg* 1991;126: 953–956.

Rutkow IM. World War I surgery. *Arch Surg* 2001;136:1328.

Saffle JR. The 1942 fire at Boston's Cocoanut Grove Nightclub. *Am J Surg* 1993;166:581–591.

Trunkey DD. History and development of trauma care in the United States. *Clin Orthop* 2000;374:36–46.

2

Trauma Systems and Injury Severity Scoring

Alasdair Conn, MD,
and Laurie S. Petrovick, MS

I. Introduction

A number of states have developed trauma systems that require not only the prehospital identification of multiply traumatized patients and the designation of certain hospitals as trauma centers, but also an evaluation system by which trauma outcomes can be determined and monitored. Not all trauma patients are identical, and an attempt is made to normalize coding and adjust for severity of illness by injury severity scoring. The development of trauma systems and their evaluation through injury severity scoring are discussed in this chapter.

II. Epidemiology of Trauma

Death from traumatic injury in people up to the age of 44 is the number one cause of death in the United States. A trauma patient occupies one of every eight beds in US hospitals. Injuries requiring hospitalization affect approximately 2.3 million persons in the United States every year. Approximately 140,000 fatalities occur annually: 21% are suicides; 14% are homicides; and unintentional fatalities (e.g., industrial injuries and highway crashes) comprise the remainder.

In 1966, the National Research Council produced a report entitled, "Accidental Death and Disability: The Neglected Disease of Modern Society," showing that little progress has been made in understanding the scientific aspects of injury control. A follow-up study entitled, "Injury in America," was published in 1985, which, however, documented little progress over the prior 20 years. The report, published by the National Research Council and the Institute of Medicine, showed that injury was still the most expensive of all major health problems, costing between $75 and $100 billion dollars per year, and that support for injury research was minimal. The authors advocated several approaches in the prevention of injury: more research to provide a clearer understanding of injury mechanisms; advocating for established trauma systems with designated trauma centers; and full integration of rehabilitation into the trauma management process. Injury costs approximately 4.1 million years of lives lost in the United States; cancer costs 1.7 million years of lives lost; and heart disease and stroke costs 2.1 million years of lives lost.

III. Development of American Trauma Systems

In the United States, individual states have legal authority for oversight of healthcare delivery. Each state licenses health practitioners—including physicians, nurses, paramedics, and emergency medical technicians (EMT). Most states have a Certificate of Need process for hospitals and other components of hospitals, such as magnetic resonance (MRI) scanners. Thus, states control hospital licensure and, under most circumstances, they do not allow hospitals to develop trauma programs unless it is in the public interest. Many components must be in place to have a fully functioning statewide system for trauma. Although the earliest state trauma systems were developed without knowledge of these essential components, later development has used the guidelines for successful trauma system implementation. In 1988, Donald Trunkey and others described the development of such state systems. At that time, however, only two states, Maryland and Virginia, had all of the components in place. A follow-up study published in 1992 indicated that, although many trauma systems were in development, only five states had achieved implementation of all essential components at the time. To assist in this process, the National Highway Traffic Safety Administration developed two programs. The first was the "Development of Trauma Systems" course, a 1-day course advising states on the required essential components of such systems and how they could be successfully achieved. The second program established the Technical Advisory Task Forces, which would evaluate individual states on a consulting basis against ten fixed criteria. In the late 1980s and early 1990s, many states volunteered to go through this process using their own state's evaluation against the ten criteria as a guideline for further development (Table 2.1). Almost all states have completed this independent evaluation and approximately five states now have had a 10-year reevaluation process using the same criteria. Although "Development of Trauma Systems" has received much attention, implementation at the local level often raises specific issues. The two most prevalent are funding—particularly for the indigent traumatized patient—and the perception that with implementation of such trauma systems an excessive number of patients will be transferred into large urban centers to the financial detriment of community hospitals.

IV. Trauma Center Verification

Most states with successful trauma systems have implemented an independent review of trauma centers to ensure that they are in compliance with trauma center standards. The American College of Surgeons' Committee on Trauma (ACSCOT) promulgates the essential components that should be in place for levels I, II, III, and

Table 2-1. General emergency medical services overview of system components

1. Regulation and Policy
2. Resource Management
3. Human Resources and Training
4. Transportation
5. Facilities
6. Communications
7. Trauma Systems
8. Public Information and Education
9. Medical irection
10. Evaluation

IV trauma centers, and these are continually updated. For the latest version of the document, contact the American College of Surgeons (see references). Although many states have adopted these standards verbatim, others have modified them to meet local and regional needs. The Verification Committee of the ACS, on a voluntary basis, will inspect a hospital and determine if it meets the College's criteria to be a trauma center. Several states have adopted this mechanism and require verification by the ACS before a hospital can apply to the state to be a designated trauma center. Other states have adopted or modified the criteria but use independent reviewers. An example of the latter approach would be Pennsylvania, which has the Pennsylvania Trauma Systems Foundation that will send a team (consisting of a surgeon, an administrator, a nurse, and an emergency physician) to independently evaluate Pennsylvania hospitals according to their own criteria.

The process of *verification* is different from that of *designation*. A particular urban area may have several hospitals that can independently choose to undergo verification as a trauma center by the ACS. The state, however, may determine that only one or two of these hospitals should be designated as trauma centers, because the volume of trauma patients does not justify multiple trauma centers for optimal patient outcome. As the controlling authority, the state can develop triage criteria for the prehospital providers, determine what constitutes a trauma patient by regulation, and then direct trauma patients to only those trauma centers designated by the state and not just verified by ACSCOT. A new program in the latter stages of development by the ACSCOT can be used for system verification, which would assist in this process.

Implicit in a state's ability to designate trauma centers is to remove that designation as well as to evaluate outcome. Trauma system legislation generally includes methods to monitor performance and designate participating centers. In the trauma verification and designation process, the two most difficult issues are continued funding of the trauma system and the ability of hospitals and appropriate medical professionals to oversee medical information and determine patient outcome in a confidential, peer-review environment. Confidentiality statutes may need to be updated as part of the trauma systems development.

V.   Data Supporting Efficacy of Trauma Systems

Currently, approximately 40 preventable death studies are found in the trauma literature. These studies examine autopsy data looking for deaths that in an ideal system should have been preventable. Indeed, the ACS verification process mandates that all deaths in a trauma center must be categorized as (a) clearly not preventable deaths (b) potentially preventable deaths; and (c) clearly preventable deaths. An example of a not preventable death would be a patient who has sustained a high velocity gunshot wound through the central nervous system and is found asystolic at the scene. In many cases before trauma system implementation, patients died from injuries that would not normally be expected to be fatal. This was because of inadequate prehospital care and triage; delayed recognition of injuries or delay in management (e.g., the patient exsanguinating from internal injuries having to wait several hours for an operating room). In the 40 preventable deaths in the literature, preventable death before system implementation varies from 20% to 40%. In one preventable death study in pediatric patients, a preventable death rate of 50% was recorded. Following implementation of trauma systems, the preventable death rate should rapidly decrease to below 5%, with the goal of less than 2%. This has been achieved in relatively new systems on a statewide basis. All systems that have published data before system implementation and compared them with data after implementation, however, have reported a decrease in reportable death rates. Data on mortality are much easier to obtain than that on morbidity. The data supporting cost-effectiveness of trauma systems are much more difficult to evaluate owing to the confusion of hospital data where charges by the hospital for trauma care bear little relationship to the actual cost of that care.

VI. Designing and Financing a Trauma System

Implementation of a successful trauma system means adherence to certain standards and the monitoring of patient outcome. Many national guidelines exist for prehospital identification of a trauma patient, published by the ACS, as well as the American College of Emergency Physicians (ACEP). Numerous guidelines issued by ACS, ACEP and the National Association of EMS Physicians (NAEMSP) detail which patients should be transported by helicopter. As noted above, standards exist for both trauma systems and trauma registries.

Exact design of a trauma system is dependent on needs at the local level. In more rural environments, it may be most appropriate for patients to be transported to the closest medical facility where resuscitation and evaluation can be performed. Patients can then be transferred into a trauma center for tertiary care. This pattern of patient flow as a component of a trauma system is often used for patients with severe burns. Severe burns are usually assessed and patients resuscitated at the local level and then transferred—often several hundred miles—to an appropriate pediatric or adult burn center for further management. In more urban areas, a local system design often requires paramedics and EMT to bypass smaller facilities and take the major trauma patients to designated facilities. Under these circumstances, the implementation of an appropriately designed trauma system can be involved in a political process.

Funding is required both for the governmental infrastructure to evaluate the trauma system and for the provision of trauma care. Many states have built financing into their trauma system legislation to cover the statewide trauma registry, the verification and designation teams, and the appropriate oversight personnel. This funding should then be placed in the annual budget of the state's Department of Health. Other states have been creative in their approach; Florida has an additional fine on moving traffic violations to support their trauma systems, under the assumption that individuals who speed are more likely to require trauma care than the general populace. Virginia has developed first a "One for Life" and then a "Two for Life," by which a portion of the fee for a vehicle license plate is allocated to the state's Emergency Medical Services for financing the trauma system. Other innovative approaches have been taxes on liquor sales and firearms.

Financing for hospital care and medical care is more complex. Several states have set up financial pools for indigent care; others e.g., California) have set up pools specifically for the management of trauma. In these cases and under certain circumstances, hospitals can apply for either partial or full reimbursement for the costs of delivering care to indigent trauma patient in the interest of citizens.

VII.   Trauma Scoring

  A.   History

  The first attempt to classify injuries occurred in the 1950s, but it was not until the 1970s when real progress occurred with the development of trauma scoring. As trauma systems became more organized and it was apparent that trauma was an epidemic, it became increasingly important to have a uniform method of measurement and specific vocabulary to assess and compare trauma treatments and outcomes. This led to the development of sophisticated trauma scoring systems for field triage, assessment of trauma care, and quantification of expected and unexpected outcomes. Due to the tremendous number and degree of possible injuries a trauma patient could have (International classification of diseases [ICD]-9 has >2000 trauma injuries) and the complex physiologic derangement, development of trauma scoring was and still is difficult.

  B.   Purpose

  Trauma scoring has many applications. Getting the appropriate trauma patient to the appropriate facility in a timely manner is of utmost importance for that patient's survival. Field triage scores assist prehospital personnel in making the proper decision and transport the patient to the appropriate level of care. Trauma scoring allows trauma personnel to treat a severely injured patient with a poor prognosis aggressively and creatively and help them to make appropriate referral decisions. Trauma scoring can also assess the response to therapy. Performance improvement programs benefit greatly from trauma scoring by using objective data to make or change policies and set priorities. Through trauma scoring, patients can be objectively analyzed for unexpected outcomes and further review of these cases can lead to performance improvement audits. Trauma scoring assists with research efforts by grouping patients for comparison, and can be used as inclusion or exclusion criteria for a study.

  C.   Criteria

    1.   Validity

    A trauma score should correlate with other similar scoring systems and have a high correlation with outcomes such as mortality and morbidity.

    2.   Stability and Reliability

    Repeated measurements should produce the same results and, if more than one individual is collecting the data and scoring, they should produce the same result.

    3.   Utility

    The system should be user friendly and reasonable for everyone involved. It should use similar language to describe clinical injuries and severity. The score should be universally used.

D. Scoring Methods
    1. Trauma Triage Systems—Physiologic (Table 2-2)
        a. Glasgow Coma Scale (GCS)
        b. Trauma Score (TS)
        c. Revised Trauma Score (RTS)
        d. Circulation, Respiration, Abdominal/ Thoracis, Motor, and Speech Scale (CRAMS)
    2. Definitive Trauma Scoring Systems— Anatomic (Table 2-3)
        a. Abbreviated Injury Score (AIS)
        b. Injury Severity Score (ISS)
        c. Pediatric Trauma Score (PTS)
    3. Outcome Scoring Systems (Table 2-4)
        a. Trauma and ISS (TRISS)
        b. A Severity Characterization of Trauma (ASCOT)
E. Future Scores (Table 2-5)
    1. Harborview Assessment of Mortality (HARM)
    2. New Injury Severity Score (NISS)
F. Summary
The different trauma scoring tools are helpful to trauma personnel in a variety of ways. One of the most important functions of trauma scoring is that it allows trauma teams and centers to have a uniform way of measuring the outcomes of the program. All of the scores are affected by inaccurate and incomplete data. While acknowledging the usefulness of trauma scoring, it is important to realize that there are limitations to all of the scoring systems and that they are not the absolute predictors of outcome.

VIII. Trauma Registry
  A. Definition
Data collected, stored, and reported on basic demographics, injury events; prehospital and clinical information (including trauma scores); and performance improvement on trauma patients who meet specific criteria, the trauma registry becomes the primary tool used for the systematic evaluation of the quality of care provided by trauma services. By relying on objective data extrapolated from the registry, instead of subjective opinions, administrators can make valid decisions regarding the quality of care rendered and the resources used.
  B. Criteria
    1. Reliability
The program should be able to procure all cases to be included in the registry and exclude all the cases not meeting the inclusion criteria. The registry information should be inspected for incomplete or missing data.
    2. Validity
The registry must be monitored for inaccurate data entry. A system must be set up for methodic review and comparison of data entered in the registry with that in the medical record. Data sets must be defined (what each data element means and from where the information comes) and all personnel collecting data

(*text continues on page 22*)

Table 2-2. Trauma triage systems—physiologic

Scoring Methods—Triage/Physiologic	Definition	Advantage	Disadvantage
GCS	Developed in 1974 to quantify the level of consciousness and degree of head injury. It is the sum of three coded values representing verbal, motor and eye response. Scores range from 3 to 15; the higher the score, the better CNS function.	Easy to use Important for triage—good prognostic indicator Used in other trauma triage systems Widely used in prehospital environment and can be used to reevaluate in the hospital Important to measure CNS injury to determine outcome	Is only an indicator for head injury Alcohol and drugs interfere with scoring Intubation will interfere with scoring Does not take into account focal or lateralizing signs
TS	Assesses patient severity using GCS and four physiologic parameters: –respiratory rate –respiratory effort –systolic blood pressure –capillary refill Scores range 0 to 16, with lowest values denote poor prognoses	Is a simple and quick method of assessment Important prehospital indicator for severity of injury Accurately predicts outcome Good interrater reliability	Physiologic compensation will cause undertriage Hypovolemia, hypoxia or cerebral injury will overtriage the severity of the patient Intubation, alcohol, and drugs interfere with the scoring of GCS Respiratory effort and capillary refill are hard to measure in the field Physiological rates change frequently

RTS	RTS is the result of the coded values (0–4, 4 being normal) for systolic blood pressure, GCS, RR RTS used in the hospital is the weighted sum of GCS, RR, and SBP (score 0–7.84) High values equal better prognosis	Standard of physiologic injury measurement—most widely used field triage tool Efficient scoring method that can predict outcome, better than TS Easier to calculate than TS because elements are easily measured in the field Head injuries better evaluated because more weight is given to GCS in the equation	Intubation, alcohol, and drugs will interfere with the scoring of GCS Calculation can be awkward because measured values require conversion for quantification Physiologic rates change frequently
CRAMS	Used for field triage; uses five values: –Circulation impairment –Respiratory disruption –Abdominal wall tenderness –Motor disruption –Speech impairment Each value receives a score of 0–2	Easy to use in the field Separates major trauma with scores of <8 and minor trauma with scores of 9 or 10	CRAMS is less sophisticated than TS or RTS Values are less definitive and more subjective than trauma score or RTS Thoracic or abdominal fields have not been documented for reliability

GCS, Glasgow Coma Score; CNS, central nervous system; TS, trauma score; RTS, revised trauma score; SBP, systolic blood pressure; RR, respiratory rate; CRAMS, circulation, respiratory, abdominal or thoracic, motor, and speech (scale).

Table 2-3.   Definitive trauma scoring systems—anatomic

Scoring Methods	Definition	Advantage	Disadvantage
AIS	Establishes a standard language and systematic format to describe anatomic injury and severity Severity is ranked from 1 to 6, with 1 being minor, 5 critical, and 6 being almost always fatal Injuries are categorized in six regions: –Head/neck –Face –Thorax –Abdomen –Extremities –External	Includes both blunt and penetrating trauma Includes >1300 injury descriptions Most commonly used anatomic measures of injury severity To an extent, will predict outcome	Does not include physiologic measures Time consuming to score all trauma injuries and extensive training is required Only single injuries considered
ISS	An extension of the AIS, the ISS is the sum of the squares of the three highest AIS scores from injuries to three different body regions An AIS of 6 is automatically calculated to 75.	National standard for injury severity assessment and anatomic injury scoring system Robust predictor of mortality Considers multiple injures Uses both anatomic indices and severity indices	Does not account for multiple injuries in the same body region Penetrating injuries can be under-scored because injury can be localized in one body region Each body region has the same weight in the score

| PTS (physiologic and anatomic) | Customized pediatric scoring system
Six variables:
–Size
–Airway
–SBP
–CNS
–Open wound
–Skeletal
Scored using values from 1,2,–1.
The six values are summed to yield the PTS, which ranges from –6 to –12, –6 being the most critical | Can be assessed and calculated quickly
Good triage tool that indicates injury severity | No statistical advantage over RTS
No upper age limit has been defined |

AIS, Abbreviated Injury Scale; ISS, Injury Severity Scale; PTS, Pediatric Trauma Score; CNS, central nervous system; RTS, Revised Trauma Score; SBP, systolic blood pressure.

Table 2-4.   Outcome scoring systems

Scoring Methods— Outcome	Definition	Advantage	Disadvantage
TRISS	Estimates the probability of patient survival. Based on a regression equation using ISS, TS, RTS, type of injury, and patient age. Two methods for TRISS: –PRE (patient outcomes verses baseline database) –DEF (two patient groups are compared)	Endorsed by the ACS Good outcome predictor used for performance improvement	Same limitations for the ISS, TS, and RTS Age is split dichotomously No preexisting medical history
ASCOT	Combines the emergency department values for GCS, SBP, RR, AIS severity scores (square root), and age. Four body regions are weighted in the equation to reflect serious injuries	Better for multiple single body area injuries Good reliability in predicting outcome for both blunt and penetrating trauma Age is divided into five groups	All disadvantages for AIS scores and GCS Requires complex computer system

TRISS, Trauma Injury Severity Score; ASCOT, A Severity Characterization of Trauma; TS, Trauma Score; RTS, Revised Trauma Score; ACS, American College of Surgeons; SBP, systolic blood pressure; RR, respiratory rate; AIS, Abbreviated Injury Scale; GCS, Glasgow Coma Scale.

Table 2-5. Future scores

Scoring Methods	Definition	Advantage	Disadvantage
HARM	Uses ICD9 codes (reclassified to 109 categories), mechanism (16 categories from Ecodes), intent (5), and age Is a probability, between 0–1 of hospital mortality	Effectively predicts outcome Does not use physiologic parameters Multiple injuries can be used	Incorrect or missed injuries when coding Needs to be tested against an independent heterogeneous data set
NISS	Takes the patient's three most severe injuries, regardless of body region	Better predictor of mortality than ISS Uses multiple injuries	Needs more evaluation Research performed on blunt trauma
ICISS	Is the product of all survival risk ratios for each injury for an individual patient (uses traumatic ICD9 scores). Can add age, mechanism, and RTS to get a probability of survival model.	Powerful predictor Uses all injuries, regardless of region Does not use AIS, which can be time consuming	Needs more evaluation Assumes injuries are independent (some injuries in combination are more severe)

HARM, Harborview Assessment of Mortality; NISS, New Injury Severity Score; ISS, Injury Severity Score; RTS, Revised Trauma Score; AIS, Abbreviated Injury Scale; ICISS, *International Classification of Diseases*, 9th ed. and ISS.

should abide by the definitions. Consistency in data collection helps ensure meaningful data.

3.   Utility

The registry enhances the trauma program by contributing to changes in practice, treatment, and policies. The registry should identify areas for trauma education and prevention. It should also be cost effective, user friendly, and have easily accessible information in report format.

C.   Purpose

1.   Performance Improvement

After specific indicators and complications are selected, the trauma registry assists the program by tracking and identifying patients for further peer review. The results of the peer review are recorded in the registry so that trends and variations in systems can be further analyzed. The registry allows for a systems-wide approach to improving trauma care.

2.   Public Health

The registry can provide information on high-risk groups, changing patterns of injuries or mechanisms, cost of care, and outcomes. Public health agencies can use this information to direct resources to the appropriate outreach and prevention programs or create new ones.

3.   Outcomes Research

Because trauma is one of the leading causes of death and disability, it is imperative to evaluate the quality of care and outcomes to improve interventions and treatment strategies.

4.   Resource Utilization

The registry can also provide information on resources that are used and costs that occur for trauma patients. These data justify funding for the program.

5.   Research

The trauma registry has a vast amount of information available for research activities.

D.   Common Reports

1.   Patient Log

The patient log usually contains demographic, prehospital, and injury data, which give a snapshot of the trauma service at a specific time. The log can be generated for a specific period of time and updated on a daily basis.

2.   Administrative Summaries

Administrative summaries monitor trauma service activity, acuity, outcome, and resources

3.   Performance Improvement Report

Performance improvement reports can be for individual peer review or a trending report for specific filters or performance improvement issues.

E.   Patient Confidentiality

The trauma registry program must have strict procedures in place to maintain patient confidentiality and that all Health Insurance Portability and Accountability Act of 1996 (HIPAA) regulations are painstakingly followed at all times.

F.   Oversight of the Registry Data
The trauma registry program should have a manager who is responsible for maintaining the accuracy of the data and deciding who will have access to the information. This person should know the bias and the accuracy in the data set to prevent its misuse and erroneous research efforts. This position should also deal with Internal Review Board issues that can arise from the use of the trauma registry.

G.   Limitations
The trauma registry program can be an expensive endeavor. Personnel must be hired and trained and computers and software must be purchased. The system must be flexible to avoid becoming obsolete. Generally, the trauma registry is not a population-based data set, and patients who have injuries not requiring hospital admissions are generally not included in the trauma registry.

H.   Summary
The registry is a powerful tool used to help the trauma service by collecting, organizing, and reporting critical data used for clinical and administrative decision-making.

IX.   Performance Improvement (PI)

A.   Introduction
Performance improvement is imperative in today's healthcare environment because organizations are now demanding higher quality of care provided by healthcare facilities. The purchaser of healthcare is now an informed consumer demanding better quality care and services. It has been determined that the cost of poor quality care represents 20% to 30% of healthcare expenses and revenues decrease by 10% because of problems in quality of care. Dissatisfied customers will tell at least nine people about their experience, whereas satisfied customers will tell four or five people about their positive experience. Many accreditation agencies and government bodies also mandate PI.

B.   History
The terms, concepts, and philosophy of quality management have changed dramatically over the last 30 years. Over the years, quality assurance has evolved to quality improvement, continuous quality improvement, total quality management, and, lastly but not finally, performance improvement. It has matured from a concept of identifying and then punishing individuals into an organized process of analyzing systems and making improvements. Quality assurance relies on inspections after the output is produced, whereas performance improvement evaluates systems before producing the output. Most of the concepts have been derived from industry and healthcare struggles to apply these techniques and principles to improve their operations.

C.   Performance Improvement Concepts

1.   Expectations
Internal and external customers (in healthcare, the patients) are the driving force behind performance improvement. The customer's expectations, as well as professional and national standards, must be met and exceeded.

2.   Empowering Employees
Shifting the blame from employees to the system allows employees to feel more valued and less defensive. Employees are a valued asset in an organization and should be brought into the PI process. Satisfied employees will do better at their job and, therefore, increase their work performance.

3.   Quality Management
Administration must embrace PI concepts and welcome change. The quality manager should value each employee's contribution to the PI process and should encourage team building with employees to solve PI issues.

4.   Plan-Do-Check-Act (PDCA) Cycle
Continuously look for ways to improve processes.

Plan: measure process, identify improvement opportunity, and generate solutions
Do: map out and implement plan for improvement.
Check: evaluate the results and draw conclusions (was objective achieved?)
Act: monitor the changes, then standardize the method if it was successful; otherwise, start the cycle again

5.   Statistics
Data are collected and analyzed using statistical methods. Using statistics allows decisions to be made objectively and not on a whim.

D.   Trauma Performance Improvement Program
1.   Trauma Service Performance Improvement Plan
Trauma services must have a well-documented and detailed plan, which includes an overview of the process, key personnel involved, committees, link to a hospital-wide program, list of indicators, collection methods, reports, and confidentiality provision. This plan should be approved by the hospital administration and should be inclusive of all aspects of trauma care.

2.   Accountability
Because trauma crosses multiple departments, the program must be able to address issues involving other services. The program must have a director who is responsible for the overall program and reports PI findings to the hospital administration.

3.   Indicators and Issues to Monitor
Data are collected on the indicators, which then can trigger an audit to analyze for issues associated with clinical practice or trauma systems.

    a.   Process. Examples of potential processes to measure include, but are not limited to; compliance with protocols and pathways, appropriate prehospital and emergency department triage, Delay in treatment or diagnosis, error in judgment, timeliness of subspecialties response, timeliness of reports, and outpatient follow-up (American College of Surgeons [ACS] recommendations).

b. Outcome. Examples of potential outcomes to measure include, but are not limited to; mortality, morbidity, intensive care unit (ICU) length of stay, hospital length of stay, cost, functional independence measure and quality of life (FIM), and patient satisfaction (ACS recommendations).

c. Sentinel Events. Joint Commison on Accreditation of Health Organization (JACHO) describes a sentinel event as any event that has an unexpected outcome that results in death or disability or has a significant chance for an adverse outcome.

4. Data Collection

a. Data Entry. Data collected can be entered into the trauma registry, which serves to control the monitoring and analyzing of PI.

b. Information Sources. Sources of information that can be collected and used as the indicators for data include concurrent chart review, prehospital run sheets, trauma flow sheets, and retrospective review of medical records, which includes physician documentation, operating room reports, laboratory and radiology department reports, and nurses notes.

5. Evaluation

Each occurrence that has been identified as a PI opportunity should be reviewed in one of the committees listed below and all reviews should be multidisciplinary. Corrective actions should be generated from these meetings.

a. Trauma Program Performance Committee or Trauma Executive Committee. The trauma program performance committee or trauma executive committee reviews system-related occurrences.

b. Trauma Peer Review. The trauma peer review committee reviews mortality and morbidity.

6. Corrective Action

If the monitoring and evaluation generate a variation in expected outcome, then corrective actions must be taken. Corrective actions should create an improvement in the quality of patient care. Some corrective actions include (a) change or development of new protocols; (b) policies or procedures; (c) heightened policy enforcement; (d) education of staff; (e) enhancement of resources; (f) creation of a clinical pathway; and (g) formation of a PI team to analyze the issue further (ACS recommendations). Trauma rounds is an educational format used for corrective action.

7. Closing the Loop

The corrective action must be monitored to ensure that the improvements implemented have increased the quality of care. Otherwise, a new corrective action must be created and evaluated.

E.   **Major Tools of the Trade**
   1.   **Collecting and Displaying Data**
      a.   **Surveys.** Written questionnaires are used to collect quantitative data to identify patterns.
      b.   **Check Sheets.** Recording the frequency of events, either prospective or retrospective, over a period of time, shows patterns.
      c.   **Scatter Diagram.** Scatter diagrams identify relationships between the changes observed in two different sets of variables.
      d.   **Histogram.** A bar graph, the histogram shows the frequency distribution of data points from a process.
      e.   **Run and Control Charts.** The run chart is used to improve process performance over time by studying variation and its source. The control chart is virtually the same as the run chart, but has statistically derived upper and lower limits.
   2.   **Major Tools for Targeting Improvement**
      a.   **Flowcharts.** A flowchart is a picture of a process depicting the way the process is, not how it should be.
      b.   **Brainstorming and Affinity Chart.** A session to elicit many ideas, solutions, questions, causes, and opportunities without judgment or decisions typifies brainstorming. These ideas can then be put on an affinity chart that groups together related items for analysis.
      c.   **Cause and Effect Diagrams (Fishbone Diagram).** The Fishbone diagram illustrates the relationship between a problem and the factors that contributes to it.
      d.   **Activity Network.** Activity network is a graph that includes time and tasks and depicts the most efficient path and practical schedule for the completion of any project.
      e.   **Storyboard.** Storyboard shows a plan to implement the improvement idea and turn it into a reality. The most often used one is the PDCA model.

F.   **Patient Confidentiality**
Confidentiality must be meticulously followed at all times during PI activities and throughout the committee reviews. All government and hospital policies must be followed. Special attention must be made to ensure that all documents are clearly marked with "confidential, for peer review only." All documentation after a meeting should be collected and destroyed. All paperwork should be shredded.

G.   **Summary**
A good PI plan will increase the quality of care provided to the trauma patient and help to further improvements in systems and clinical care.

X.   **Common Traps**
   A.   Should all severely traumatized patients be taken to the trauma center? Answer: No.

A patient can be triaged to a smaller community hospital after evaluation by the paramedics has shown a fractured femur at scene. After evaluation, the patient might be shown to have a type 1 laceration to the spleen and a very small pneumothorax on computed tomography (CT) scanning that does not require a chest tube. Under these circumstances, the ISS would be 34, which seemingly suggests more appropriate management at a trauma center. If the patient is appropriately managed at the local level, however, this may not be required.

B. With the existing methodologies, not all trauma patients are the same. A patient who is severely injured but hemodynamically stable (e.g., a patient with a contained aortic rupture and a major subdural, thus having an ISS of 50) is expected to survive for several hours with appropriate management but without operative care. Although the probability of survival attempts to correct for these discrepancies, comparisons of survival between different centers having a different mix of blunt versus penetrating or patients transferred versus those not transferred make it difficult to obtain a scientific comparison.

C. Missed injuries. With improved imaging techniques, injuries can be reported that are of doubtful clinical significance. A patient in an outlying hospital may have a clinically insignificant pneumothorax, but this is not identified by plain x-ray study. In a more sophisticated center, such a small pneumothorax may be identified by helical CT scanning and, hence, a higher ISS may be ascribed to that particular patient. This could then be purportedly used to demonstrate improved survival at centers that have the ability to identify these clinically insignificant injuries by "ISS creep."

D. All cost data ascribed to trauma patients should be viewed with skepticism. Hospitals and physicians have a charge structure that may be independent of the cost of delivering the care and, although computerized methodologies exist in individual institutions for ascribing the cost to patients, these are not universally accepted and no common methodology exists.

E. Determination of survival may be dependent on pre-existing medical conditions that currently are not scientifically ascribed into the trauma severity scoring process. For example, a patient with impaired renal function, which can vary from a slightly elevated creatinine level to being on hemodialysis, may have a different outcome from trauma dependent on the severity of his or her renal condition. Add to this mix, a patient with diabetes, hypertension, and known vascular disease and then the patients are difficult to compare. Particularly in geriatric trauma, the family may determine at some stage, based on a living will or other such living entity, that aggressive lifesaving mechanisms may be stopped. This makes it more difficult to determine whether the death was caused by underlying disease or should be judged as a potentially preventable death.

SELECTED READING

American College of Surgeons, Committee on Trauma. *Resources for Optimal Care of the Injured Patient.* Chicago: American College of Surgeons, 1999.

Brenneman FD, Boulanger BR, Mclellan BA, et al. Measuring injury severity: a time for a change. *J Trauma* 1998;44(4):580–582.

Butler, S. Module 3: Recording and Using Trauma Data. In: A Comprehensive Curriculum for Trauma Nursing. Bayley, EW, Turcke, SA. Eds. Boston: Jones and Barlett Oublishers, 1992:25–39.

Champion, HR, Sacco, WJ, Copes, WS. Trauma Scoring. In: Feliciano DV, More EE, Mattox KL, eds. Trauma, 3rd ed. Stamford, CT: Appleton and Lange, 1996:53–67.

FitzPatrick, M.K., McMaster, J. Performance Improvement in Trauma Care. In: Trauma Nursing: From Resuscitation Through Rehabilitation. McQuillan K, Von Rueden K, Hartsock R. eds., 3rd ed. New York: WB Saunders, 2002:34–47.

Leebov W, Ersoz CJ. The Health Care Manager's Guide to Continuous Quality Improvement. Chicago: American Hospital Publishing, 1991.

Olser T. Injury Severity Scoring: Perspectives in Development and Future Directions. *Am J Surg* 1993;165(2A Suppl.):43S–51S.

Pollock DA, McClain PW. Trauma Registries: Current Status and Future Prospects. *JAMA* 1990: 263(14):1913–1914.

Rutledge R. The Goals, Development and Use of Trauma Registries and Trauma Data Sources in Decision Making in Injury. *Surg Clin North Am* 1995;75(2):305–326.

Senkowski CK, McKenney MG. Trauma Scoring Systems: A Review. *J Am Coll Surg* 1999;189(5):491–503.

West TA, Rivara FP, Cummings P, et al. Harborview Assessment for Risk of Mortality: an Improved Measure of Injury Severity on the Basis of ICD-9-CM. *J Trauma* 2000;49(3):530–541.

Wisner DH. History and Current Status of Trauma Scoring Systems. *Arch Surg* 1992;127(1):117.

3

Prehospital Care and Transport

Paul D. Biddinger, MD,
and Stephen H. Thomas, MD, MPH

I. Introduction

Over the past four decades, prehospital care and emergency medical services (EMS) in the United States have evolved rapidly from nearly nonexistent to key links in the chain of survival in trauma care. In the mid-1960s, after a landmark report titled *Accidental Death and Disability: The Neglected Disease of Modern Society* detailed serious deficiencies in prehospital care, state and federal lawmakers began to enact new standards for personnel, equipment, and oversight in EMS systems. The concept of the "golden hour," the first hour after injury when acute medical intervention can be of most necessity and benefit, has further motivated prehospital care providers to try to improve response times and expedite transport of patients to a trauma center. Today's prehospital care providers are well trained to assess victims of trauma for life-threatening injuries, safely remove patients from the scene, and provide certain life-saving interventions, when needed. All providers of acute trauma care must be familiar with the capabilities and limitations of EMS to ensure a seamless transition from the prehospital setting to the emergency department and beyond.

II. Prehospital Systems

Each municipality or rural area has several options with regard to the administration of their emergency medical services. EMS can be administered directly by the local government, either as a stand-alone agency or under the command of the fire department. Prehospital care can also be provided by a local hospital or private ambulance company under contract by the city or county; in most rural areas, it can be provided by volunteers on call from home. The optimal structure of an emergency medical system is frequently debated, but it certainly varies depending on the setting. The most important factors that influence the choice of system include population size and density, municipal budget, and political considerations. Air medical systems are typically administered by a hospital (or hospital consortium) or state agency to provide care for a large region.

III. Personnel Training and Qualifications

A. Ground Transport

1. *First Responders*

First responders are trained in basic first aid measures (e.g., bandaging, splinting, hemorrhage control, and cardiopulmonary resuscitation [CPR]). Generally, those trained at this level are police, firefighters, and others who may be the first to arrive at an accident scene before an ambulance. First responders usually do not transport patients.

2. **Emergency Medical Technician Levels and Capabilities**

   a. **The EMT-Basic.** The EMT-basic (EMT-B) is trained to assess signs and symptoms; safely extricate, immobilize, and transport the patient; and administer certain noninvasive therapies (e.g., oxygen). Although not trained in cardiac rhythm interpretation, many EMT can defibrillate through use of automatic external defibrillators (AED). Transport by basic EMT is termed "basic life support" (BLS). Most EMT-B courses consist of approximately 120 to 160 hours of clinical instruction and several hours of observation in emergency departments and obstetric units.

   b. **The EMT-Intermediate.** The EMT-Intermediate (EMT-I) is additionally trained to obtain peripheral intravenous (i.v.) access, administer i.v. fluids, and use airway adjuncts (e.g., laryngeal mask airway [LMA] or pharyngotracheal lumen airway [PTLA]). The EMT-I generally does not administer medications. Most systems that employ EMT-I are in rural areas that cannot afford or recruit full paramedic coverage.

   c. **The EMT-Paramedic.** The EMT-Paramedic (EMT-P) is trained in advanced airway management, including endotracheal intubation, cardiac rhythm interpretation and, defibrillation (advanced cardiac life support, or ACLS), and parenteral medication administration. Additionally, many paramedics are trained in cricothyroidotomy and needle chest decompression when state and regional protocols allow. Transport by paramedics is termed "advanced life support" (ALS). Paramedic training programs consist of at least 500 hours of classroom instruction as well as mandatory supervised hospital and field internships.

3. **Advanced Scope of Practice**
   Many states now allow for paramedics with specialized additional training and supervision to function at a level beyond standard protocols. Such paramedics are frequently paired with a nurse and, for purposes of ground transport, are most likely to be encountered in services providing ground critical care transport.

B. **Air Transport**

   1. **Crew Configuration**

      a. **Physicians.** Physicians are standard members of the air medical crew in most non-US settings. In programs in the United States, however, most crews (>90%) are staffed by nonphysicians.

      b. **Nurses.** Nurses staffing air transport programs preferably have experience in both emergency and critical care settings, with additional experience (e.g., pediatric or obstetric), depending on the characteristics of the flight program's patient population.

  c. **Paramedics.** Paramedics working on air
transport programs traditionally have been part of
the flight crew to provide expertise relative to
trauma scene care.

  d. **Other Crew Members.** Other crew members (e.g., neonatal nurse practitioners, balloon
pump specialists) can be used, depending on local
preferences and specific patient needs.

 2. **Advanced Scope of Practice**

An advanced scope of practice is present for most nonphysician air medical crew. This implies that nonphysicians working in air medical transport have an
extended level of training and medical care capability. For example, nurses and paramedics have for
years used neuromuscular blockade-facilitated endotracheal intubation with backup surgical cricothyroidotomy. Additionally, because of the relative isolation
and high patient acuity, nonphysician flight crews
must be trained and empowered to recognize and treat
many types of medical and surgical complications (e.g.,
hypotension requiring adjustment of infused fluids or
vasopressors, tension pneumothorax requiring needle
decompression) that can occur in flight.

C. **Critical Care Transport Specialists**

With increasing regionalization of specialized medical and
surgical services, critical care transport, by air or ground,
is increasingly recognized as an area of expertise. Currently, no consistent national standards exist for critical
care transport, but at least one nongovernmental accreditation agency (the Commission on Accreditation of Medical Transport Systems) has recognized that the level of
care, rather than the transport vehicle, should be a prime
focus for evaluation of critical care transport services.

IV. **Access to the Patient**

A. **Activation of Emergency Medical Services**

Approximately 96% of the US population currently has
access to emergency care via the 911 telephone system.
Enhanced 911 systems use computer databases to display
the address of the caller activating the 911 system in the
event the caller is unable to speak.

B. **Scene Safety**

The first priority of rescuers in any emergency is to ensure
scene safety. Rescuers have a duty to themselves, to bystanders, and to the people they have been sent to assist
that they will be able to leave the scene with their patients
and not become patients themselves.

 1. **Highway**

Many rescuers are injured or killed each year by surrounding traffic on the scene of motor vehicle collisions.
When approaching an accident, the rescuers must survey the scene for potential hazards (e.g., passing traffic, hazardous materials, electrical wires). Whenever
possible, the ambulance should be parked at an angle
between traffic and the accident to create a safety zone
for both the patient and rescuers.

2. Violent Crime

Violent crimes often occur in scenes that remain unsafe after the initial injury. Despite the temptation to arrive and aid the victim as soon as possible, rescuers must not enter a violent crime scene until the police or others have first secured it.

3. Hazardous Materials Exposures

Rescuers must arrive at a safe distance uphill and upwind of any incident with the potential for exposure to hazardous materials. Whenever possible, the materials should be identified before personnel enter the scene, and the highest level of appropriate personal protective equipment must be worn. Scenes are generally divided into three zones: the **hot zone** being the area of maximal danger; the **warm zone,** an area to which patients are removed for emergency stabilization; and the **cold zone,** an area where vehicles are parked and patients have final pretransport stabilization before being loaded for transport. Specialized teams may need to be activated before the patient can be reached. In all cases, victims must be adequately decontaminated before arrival at the hospital to avoid further spread of toxins to other patients and healthcare providers.

4. Specialized Rescue

Certain circumstances require mobilization of additional resources before the patient can be safely reached. These include water rescue, trench and confined space rescue, and high angle (high elevation) rescue. These resources may be beyond the training of local authorities and additional personnel may need to be summoned from state or larger community units.

C. Extrication

Extrication is the technique of removing the patient from an entrapment. Because significant force using hydraulic or air pressure must often be used to manipulate the debris, carefully trained rescuers are critical to minimize the risk of further injury to the patient either from the debris or from unnecessary movement. Although certain therapies (e.g., oxygen administration, i.v. therapy, parenteral analgesia, needle decompression of the thorax, and occasionally intubation) can be started before the patient is free of the entrapment, the time delay in transport to a hospital while extrication occurs is generally associated with worse outcome. Prolonged extrication time (>20 minutes) is considered a marker of potentially severe injury and warrants triage directly to a trauma center, when possible.

V. Field Airway Management

A. Airway Adjuncts

All EMS providers are trained in the use of oropharyngeal airways (OPA), nasopharyngeal airways (NPA), and bag-valve-mask (BVM) ventilation. Additionally, multiple devices are designed to assist in the prehospital management of the airway of a comatose or apneic trauma patient.

These devices are used by rescuers not trained in endotracheal intubation, or for rescuers unable to achieve endotracheal intubation.

1. Esophageal Obturator Airway

The esophageal obturator airway (EOA) is a cuffed tube with a closed tip that is inserted blindly into the mouth and designed to enter and occlude the esophagus. A mask is attached to the tube at the mouth after placement to facilitate ventilation. The device carries the risks of unrecognized tracheal occlusion, vomiting (especially on removal), and esophageal injury. The EOA is now rarely used since newer devices have become available.

2. Pharyngotracheal Lumen Airway and Combitube

The pharyngotracheal lumen airway (PTLA) and Combitube (Tyco-Healthcare-Kendall USA, Mansfield, Massachusetts) are similar devices with multiple attached tubes designed for blind insertion. Their success in use depends on the operator being able to identify correctly which of the blindly inserted tubes is in the esophagus, and which tube can adequately ventilate the trachea. Rescuers not trained in endotracheal intubation generally use these devices.

3. Laryngeal Mask Airway

The laryngeal mask airway (LMA) was first introduced in the operative setting in the late 1980s as an alternative to endotracheal intubation for selected patients. The device has increasingly been used in the emergency department and prehospital setting as a rescue alternative when endotracheal intubation cannot be achieved. The LMA consists of an inflatable V-shaped mask at the end of a large-bore tube that is placed blindly into the larynx. It is relatively easy to use and minimizes the risk of gastric insufflation during assisted ventilation. It does not, however, protect the trachea from aspiration of blood or vomitus. A variation of the standard LMA, the intubating LMA (ILMA), has a guide at the distal portion of the mask to facilitate passage of a smaller sized endotracheal tube through the LMA into the trachea to secure the airway. Given the reluctance of many ground EMS agencies to incorporate neuromuscular blockade-facilitated intubation into their prehospital care protocols, the LMA is assuming a prominent place as both a primary and a rescue airway.

B. Endotracheal Intubation

1. Oral Endotracheal Intubation

Orotracheal endotracheal intubation (ETI) intubation remains the gold standard of airway protection, although this technique is most dependent on operator skill and patient factors. Generally, a Miller (straight) or MacIntosh (curved) laryngoscope blade with a light at the tip is inserted into the mouth and the tongue and supraglottic structures are elevated anteriorly. Once the vocal cords are visualized, the endotracheal tube (ETT) is passed into the trachea. Many factors can make oral ETI difficult or impossible: operator inexperience, inadequate patient sedation or relaxation, blood or vomitus in the airway, and anatomic variables (e.g., anterior larynx or expanding neck hematoma). Outside of investigational protocols, oral ETI is attempted in the prehospital setting only by rescuers with paramedic training or air medical crews.

2.   Nasal Endotracheal Intubation

Nasotracheal intubation (NETI) can be attempted for patients who still have some spontaneous respiratory effort, but need definitive airway control. The technique is of greatest use when orotracheal intubation is either not possible or unlikely to succeed because of anatomic or traumatic reasons. The nasal ETI technique which, in fact, is uncommonly used at the receiving trauma center setting, is encountered more frequently in the prehospital setting when neuromuscular blockade is not available (and jaw clenching prevents oral intubation). Success rates range from 48% to 84% in the prehospital setting. ETT placement must be confirmed using the usual methods. Nasal ETI is contraindicated in patients with midface fractures.

3.   Neuromuscular Blockade

Neuromuscular blocking agents (paralytics) are an integral component of rapid sequence intubation in the hospital. Historically, however, concern has existed about their use by prehospital personnel who only infrequently intubate and, if unable to intubate or ventilate a previously spontaneously breathing patient, have severely limited or no access to backup or rescue techniques. Many helicopter transport services have reported high rates of successful intubations (>96%) using paralytics; in general, however, they use a select and experienced group of practitioners. Some ground transport services have also reported high success rates (>94%) using paralytics, but most frequently this is in high-volume urban areas under very close medical direction. Currently, use of paralytics (and concomitant induction agents) to facilitate intubation should only be allowed in systems with highly trained and highly experienced providers operating under tight medical control; sufficient backup or rescue techniques must be available in the event of failed ETI.

C.   Advanced Rescue Airway Techniques

   1.   Cricothyrotomy

Approximately 70% of US ground paramedics are allowed to perform some form of surgical airway access. Skills range from needle cricothyrotomy with jet ventilation to use of percutaneous kits that employ the Seldinger technique (e.g., the Melker kit [Cook, Inc., Bloomington, Indiana]) to open cricothyrotomy. The need for cricothyrotomy in the field, however, is very low. Surprisingly, for such lack of experience, reported success rates with the procedures in the field are high (82% to 100%). All systems using paralytics must equip and train their providers in a surgical airway technique in the event of failed intubation and ventilation.

2. Digital Endotracheal Intubation

A method of last resort for the completely comatose patient, digital ETI involves placing one's fingers along the base of the tongue into the vallecula epiglottica and lifting anteriorly to facilitate passage of the ETT into the trachea. This technique carries a high risk of operator injury but can be an optimal means of establishing an airway when laryngoscopy is physically difficult or impossible (e.g., entrapped patient upside-down).

VI. Other Medical Field Care

A. Needle Decompression

Most paramedics are permitted to perform chest decompression in the patient with suspected tension pneumothorax. Signs suggestive of tension pneumothorax include tachypnea, hypoxia, unilateral decreased or hyperresonant breath sounds, jugular venous distention, and deviation of the trachea away from the affected side. For the patient in severe distress with these signs or in cardiac arrest following trauma, the rescuer should place a long (2 inch) 14-gauge or 16-gauge needle just above the second rib in the midclavicular line on the suspected side (on both sides in cardiac arrest). Generally, the needle can be removed and the catheter left in place, but providers must be observant for the possibility that the catheter can kink, necessitating repeat decompression.

B. Vascular Access

When possible, every trauma patient should have two large-bore (e.g., 14- or 16-gauge) i.v. catheters placed in the field. Attempts at cannulation, however, have been reported to add as much as 12 minutes to on-scene times. Rescuers must not waste time when adequate access has not been obtained. For most patients, the appropriate rule of thumb is two attempts per provider, ideally during transport of the patient.

C. Hemodynamic Support

1. Fluid Choice

All trauma patients should initially receive isotonic crystalloid i.v. fluids. The current advanced trauma life support (ATLS) manual recommends lactated Ringer's (LR) solution over normal saline as the fluid of choice to avoid the hyperchloremic acidosis associated with infusion of large volumes of saline. Because LR has lower osmolality than plasma, infusion of large volumes of LR can contribute to an increase in cerebral edema in the head-injured patient.

2. Fluid Volume

In the 1990s, a Houston study group found that aggressive prehospital fluid resuscitation of hypotensive victims of penetrating trauma did not improve survival and actually increased total blood loss when compared with delayed resuscitation in the hospital. The results of this study, and its applicability to other settings, are still debated. This is an area of ongoing research interest, however, and prehospital providers (and physicians writing their protocols) should be cognizant of the need to avoid over resuscitation (with concomitant risk of increased hemorrhage) and under resuscitation (with attendant risk of hypoperfusion). Times for transport and definitive control of suspected hemorrhage are important factors to consider when choosing to delay prehospital fluid resuscitation. This practice should be undertaken only after careful consideration of the issues. Suggested guidelines for prehospital fluid resuscitation of the patient with uncontrolled hemorrhage are listed in **Table 3-1**. Obviously, not all parameters will be consistently improved by fluid administration (e.g., altered mental status in the head-injured patient) and providers must exercise judgment to the adequacy of their resuscitation (**Table 3-1**).

Patients with controlled hemorrhage in the field (e.g., from an isolated extremity injury with adequate pressure applied) should be fully resuscitated with i.v. fluids.

3. Blood Product Administration

Most ground ambulance systems are not able to administer blood products in the field. In rare cases, however, EMS systems have the capability to administer blood products. For the patient transported from the scene, crews should follow the ATLS guidelines and administer untyped, not crossmatched O-negative (in women of childbearing age) or O-positive blood after an initial infusion of 2 L of crystalloid has failed to correct hemodynamic instability.

D. Spinal Immobilization

1. Cervical Collar

An appropriately sized, rigid cervical collar should be placed on every victim of trauma with neck pain or

Table 3-1. Suggested clinical targets for prehospital fluid resuscitation of the trauma patient with uncontrolled potential hemorrhage

Parameter	Goal
Blood pressure	SBP > 80 or MAP > 50–60 mm Hg
Heart rate	<120 beats/min
Oxygen saturation	>96%
Mentation	Able to follow commands

SBP, systolic blood pressure; MAP, mean arterial pressure.
Adapted from McCunn M, Dutton R. End-points of resuscitation: how much is enough? *Current Opinion in Anaesthesiology* 1999;46:216–223, with permission.

tenderness in the prehospital setting. Furthermore, a cervical collar should be placed on patients whose mechanism of injury is such that cervical injury might have occurred, even in the absence of pain or tenderness, if they have any of the following: (a) altered mental status; (b) evidence of intoxication; (c) a coincident distracting injury (e.g., a long bone fracture or burn); or (d) any subjective or objective neurologic deficit. Because the cervical collar alone does not provide adequate immobilization for transport, patients should always be additionally stabilized with a rigid backboard and some form of lateral stabilization (e.g., foam blocks) secured with straps or tape. Special steps (e.g., use of a towel roll under the shoulders) may need to be taken to maximize head position (i.e., prevent flexion) in pediatric patients. Currently, some EMS systems are undertaking investigation of the safety of enabling prehospital providers to "clear the C-spine" and, thus, decrease the incidence of unnecessary cervical spine (C-spine) immobilization. The impetus for this is the discomfort of the collar and that the accompanying backboard can cause discomfort and pressure trauma (see below).

2. Backboard

Every victim of trauma requiring a cervical collar or with midline spinal tenderness along the thoracic or lumbar spine should be placed on a long, rigid backboard and adequately secured for transport to the hospital. As with suspected C-spine injuries, patients whose mechanism of injury is such that thoracic or lumbar spinal injury might have occurred, even in the absence of pain or tenderness, should be placed on a backboard if they have any of the following: (a) altered mental status; (b) evidence of intoxication; (c) a coincident distracting injury (e.g., a long bone fracture or burn); or (d) any subjective or objective neurologic deficit. Pregnant patients should have the right side of the backboard elevated 30 degrees to keep the uterus off of the inferior vena cava and avoid hypotension and fetal hypoperfusion. Patients with gunshot wounds to the neck, thorax, or abdomen not meeting the criteria outlined above are not at increased risk for occult spinal injury and, therefore, do not need full immobilization on a backboard. Placing a patient on a backboard is not innocuous: studies have shown that pressure-mediated skin damage can begin to develop after as little as 30 minutes on a backboard.

3. Kendrick Extrication Device

The Kendrick extrication device (KED) is made up of a series of parallel splints longitudinally bound together in a vestlike device that provides assistance with spinal stabilization during the extrication of a traumatized patient from an enclosed space (e.g., a motor vehicle). It does not provide full spinal immobilization and, therefore, cannot be used *in lieu* of a backboard for adults. Because of its wrap-around nature, however, it can be useful for pediatric patients who cannot or will not lie still on a standard backboard.

E.   Pneumatic Antishock Garment and Military Antishock Trousers

Developed during the Vietnam War to treat exsanguinating soldiers in the field, the pneumatic antishock garment (PASG) (formerly known as the military antishock trousers [MAST]) was a mainstay of prehospital trauma care for nearly 20 years until its use was called into question by two outcome studies in the 1990s. The device consists of a set of nylon pants with separately inflatable leg and abdominal sections that attach to a manual pump with pressure gauge. Currently, the literature does not support the use of the PASG in penetrating trauma. Some reason exists to believe MAST can be a useful immobilization device for pelvic or femur fractures. Indications for use in blunt trauma patients with severe hypotension are still debated, but the MAST are used in some regions for this indication.

F.   Exposure of the Patient

All victims of major trauma should be completely exposed to identify all major injuries. Whereas exposure of the patient should ideally be completed as soon as possible, care must also be taken not to cause further problems (e.g., hypothermia outdoors, privacy in crowded public areas).

G.   Extremity Immobilization

Patients with unstable vital signs should have only the injured extremities immobilized because of the potential for further hemorrhage if moved (e.g., pelvis [see MAST above] and long bones, especially suspected femur fractures). Angulated extremity fractures should be carefully evaluated for distal neurovascular status. Currently, most prehospital jurisdictions call for traction splinting of suspected femur fractures, but this is subject to debate as these devices require precious time for application, are of debatable benefit in the field, and have contraindications (e.g., pelvic fracture) that may be inapparent in the field. Any patient with an angulated fracture (of any extremity) with absent distal pulses should have in-line traction applied and be splinted. All other suspected fractures should be immobilized in the position of greatest comfort for transport.

H.   Wound Care

External hemorrhage is best controlled with direct pressure and elevation above the heart. Bandages that become soaked through with blood should not be removed, but rather reinforced with further gauze. Tourniquets are indicated only for limb-threatening or life-threatening hemorrhage that cannot be controlled with continuous direct pressure, elevation, and bandaging. If tourniquets are applied in the field, they should not be removed by EMS providers.

I.   Analgesia

All victims of trauma with significant painful injuries (e.g., displaced fractures, dislocations, burns) should receive analgesia with short-acting parenteral agents as early as feasible. The suboptimal provision of analgesia, which characterizes most of acute care medicine, is also an issue in the field. In providing improved field analgesia, however, prehospital providers should be cognizant of the risks of hypotension, alterations in mental status, and obscuration of examination findings.

J. Other Considerations

1. Pediatric Trauma

Trauma is the leading cause of death for children between ages 1 and 15 years. Because such trauma still represents a relatively small proportion of the overall trauma volume within an EMS system, providers may not feel adequately trained or comfortable with the special issues that arise in pediatric trauma. The most significant differences between adult and pediatric trauma are (a) vital sign abnormalities indicating significant injury may be delayed as compared with adult patients and the age-specific nature of normal pediatric vital signs can lead practitioners to misinterpret absolute vital signs; (b) procedures, including i.v. access and intubation, are more technically challenging in children; and (c) children may be unable to give adequate histories or cooperate with procedures (e.g., immobilization) and require additional restraint for safe transport. Recent data demonstrate that well-trained paramedics can deliver equally high-quality care to both adult and pediatric trauma patients. Such care, however, requires both intensive education and periodic review of skills. The importance of ongoing training is emphasized by the relative infrequency with which severely injured pediatric patients are encountered in most EMS systems.

2. Burns

Prehospital priorities for care of burned patients include (a) protection of the airway, breathing, and C-spine, when appropriate; (b) obtaining i.v. access; (c) removal of any substances causing ongoing injury (e.g., tar); (d) local wound care with saline solution and either sterile gauze or sterile sheets; and (e) analgesia. Patients meeting appropriate triage criteria (**Table 3-2**) should be transported directly to a designated burn center, when feasible.

3. Mass Casualty Incidents or Disasters

A mass casualty incident (MCI) is any event that produces multiple casualties (injuries or illness). A disaster is any event that overwhelms the capabilities of the local emergency response system and facilities. Although the two concepts are different, the principles of triage and care often overlap.

    a. Principles of Triage. Rescuers must be able to perform a very brief (<60 second) evaluation of each patient in an MCI, focusing on ventilation, perfusion, and mental status and triage each patient according to severity of injury. In large incidents, a color-coded tag is attached to each

Table 3-2.   Criteria for transport directly to a designated burn center

1. Partial thickness burns greater than 10% total body surface area
2. Burns that involve the face, hands, feet, genitalia, perineum, or major joints
3. Third-degree burns in any age group
4. Electrical burns, including lightning injury
5. Chemical burns
6. Inhalation injury
7. Burn injury in patients with preexisting medical disorders that could complicate management, prolong recovery, or affect mortality. Burns in any patients with concomitant trauma (e.g., fractures) in which the burn injury poses the greatest risk of morbidity or mortality. In such cases, if the trauma poses a greater immediate risk than the burns, it may be necessary to stabilize the patient in a trauma center before transfer to a burn unit. Physician judgment is necessary in such situations and should be in concert with the regional medical control plan and triage protocols.
8. Burns in children being cared for in hospitals without qualified personnel or equipment for the care of children
9. Burn injury in patients who will require special social, emotional, or long-term rehabilitative intervention.

victim to aid in efficient triage and transport. A sample METTAG system is shown in **Table 3-3**.

b.   Incident Command. Incident command is generally the responsibility of the ranking fire service officer on scene. EMS officials and, occasionally, an on-site physician are responsible for coordinating the medical activities and care with the incident commander.

c.   Community-wide Disaster Systems. Planning and preparation before a disaster or MCI is critical to a successful response. Preparations should include plans for field response; staging and transportation; documentation of available local hospital resources; communications plans and backup; documentation; and debriefing and counseling after events and recovery. Regular practice and drills are vital to train rescuers and test the system.

VII.   Techniques of Transport
A.   Ground Vehicle
  1.   Standard Ambulances
  Standard ambulances come in various types, which are characterized by different vehicle designs. Type I ambulances are conventional vehicles that lack a passageway between the driver's and patient care compartments. Type II vehicles are van-type trucks. Type III vehicles are larger units with a forward cab and a walk-through passageway to the patient care area.

Table 3-3. METTAG system of field triage in a mass casualty incident, defining treatment priorities

Zero Priority (BLACK)	First Priority (RED)	Second Priority (YELLOW)	Third Priority (GREEN)
Deceased or live patients with obvious fatal and non-resuscitatable injuries	Severely injured patients requiring immediate care and transport (e.g., respiratory distress, thoracoabdominal injury, severe head or maxillofacial injuries, shock or severe bleeding, severe burns)	Patients with injuries that are determined not to be immediately life threatening. (e.g., abdominal injury without shock, thoracic injury without respiratory compromise, major fractures without shock, head injury/cervical spine injury, and minor burns)	Patients with minor injuries that do not require immediate stabilization. (e.g., soft tissue injuries, extremity fractures and dislocations, maxillofacial injuries without airway compromise and psychological emergencies)

METTAG, Medical Emergency Triage Tag.

Some units may require special equipment to provide electrical power to medical devices.

2.   Critical Care Ambulances

Critical care ambulances are generally type III vehicles, but in reality the level of care, rather than the physical characteristics, are what define a critical care ambulance.

B.   Air Transport
1.   Helicopters

Helicopters of many types are used for patient transport. Depending on the resources and needs of a particular region, helicopters of particular sizes, speeds, and physical characteristics may be chosen. Most helicopters in use now (at least in the United States) are twin-engine models, which have improved safety margin because of the redundancy afforded by the extra engine. Helicopter transports usually involve one patient only, unless patients are of lesser acuity; in which case, two-patient transports can be performed in many helicopter models. Much variation is seen between helicopter models with respect to size and speed; slower aircraft travel at little >100 to 110 mph, whereas faster helicopters cruise nearly double that speed.

2.   Fixed-wing Aircraft

Fixed-wing aircraft vary just as helicopters do, with a myriad of propeller-powered and jet-powered vehicles in use. Again, the needs and resources of a particular region (and program) dictate the choice of aircraft. In general, jet aircraft provide a smoother ride, faster speed, and are more likely to be able to pressurize to sea level (especially when flying at higher altitudes). Because of the isolation of patient care in a fixed-wing aircraft, patients should be relatively stable before fixed-wing transport is undertaken.

VIII.   Issues in Transport
A.   Moving Patients

It is not uncommon for i.v. catheters to become dislodged, ETT tubes to move, and so forth during patient transport. Every possible care should be taken to fix medical access devices securely and transfer patients slowly and deliberately. Optimally, one prehospital provider should have the sole responsibility of assuring the maintenance of ETT placement during patient transfers. Additionally, reconfirmation of ETT placement (e.g., by monitoring lip line) is warranted each time an intubated patient is transferred from one surface to another.

B.   Communication Issues

Communication between prehospital providers and hospital personnel has generally occurred with simplex (one-way) radio systems using either ultrahigh frequency (UHF) or very high frequency (VHF). Increasingly, cellular technology allows EMS providers to receive dispatch and scene information by computer and to speak with dispatch or hospital personnel in a duplex (two-way) fashion, either with paired radio frequencies or cellular telephones.

Whenever possible, prehospital personnel should have backup to their primary means of communication.

Prehospital providers deliver most medical care by pre-written protocols and standing orders (so-called "off-line" medical control) that do not require the direct communication with a physician. In these systems, cases are reviewed retrospectively through standard processes (e.g., CQI). In certain instances, however, (e.g., the administration of i.v. opiates) paramedics must usually contact a physician directly by radio or telephone for on-line medical control. In such cases, the orders given by the physician must still conform to the state guidelines and not exceed the paramedic's scope of practice. Rescuers can also use the on-line system to obtain a "field-consultation" from the physician, when necessary, in cases of refusal to transport or other questions.

C. Destination Guidelines

Severely injured patients in trauma should be transported directly to a designated level I or II trauma center, bypassing smaller hospitals when transport times are not excessive. One study revealed that patients who must be secondarily transferred from a local hospital to a trauma center had a 30% increase in risk of mortality compared with those who were transported directly from the scene to the trauma center. Further, for similarly injured patients, the risk of dying in tertiary trauma centers was 54% lower than in secondary centers and 75% lower than in primary centers. Rescuers should follow state protocols regarding indications for transport directly to a trauma center, but most protocols are similar to those in Figure 3-1 taken from the American College of Surgeons Field Triage Algorithm.

D. Transporting the Patient in Arrest

A victim of trauma in cardiac arrest should be transported directly to the nearest available emergency department, regardless of its trauma center designation. Such victims have a dismal prognosis, but warrant the immediate application of hospital resources to treat potentially reversible causes of death.

IX. Special Considerations in Air Transport

A. Scene Response Triage

Scene response triage remains an inexact science. Experienced sources acknowledge that the judgment of the prehospital personnel at the scene is of primary importance, but the decision to use helicopter transport can be bolstered by criteria such as that listed below and in **Table 3-4**.

1. **Mechanism of Injury**
2. **Physiologic Variables**
3. **Anatomic Variables**
4. **Time and Logistics**

B. Aircraft Issues

1. **Space**

Space constraints are a major issue in providing intra-transport care in any aircraft. Both the actual space (i.e., cubic feet) and the arrangement of the space (i.e.,

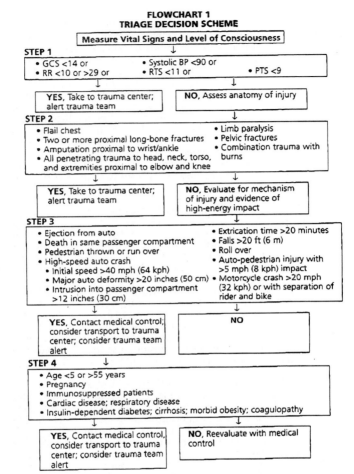

FLOWCHART 1
TRIAGE DECISION SCHEME

Measure Vital Signs and Level of Consciousness

STEP 1

- GCS <14 or   • Systolic BP <90 or
- RR <10 or >29 or   • RTS <11 or   • PTS <9

| YES, Take to trauma center; alert trauma team | NO, Assess anatomy of injury |

STEP 2

- Flail chest
- Two or more proximal long-bone fractures
- Amputation proximal to wrist/ankle
- All penetrating trauma to head, neck, torso, and extremities proximal to elbow and knee
- Limb paralysis
- Pelvic fractures
- Combination trauma with burns

| YES, Take to trauma center; alert trauma team | NO, Evaluate for mechanism of injury and evidence of high-energy impact |

STEP 3

- Ejection from auto
- Death in same passenger compartment
- Pedestrian thrown or run over
- High-speed auto crash
  - Initial speed >40 mph (64 kph)
  - Major auto deformity >20 inches (50 cm)
  - Intrusion into passenger compartment >12 inches (30 cm)
- Extrication time >20 minutes
- Falls >20 ft (6 m)
- Roll over
- Auto-pedestrian injury with >5 mph (8 kph) impact
- Motorcycle crash >20 mph (32 kph) or with separation of rider and bike

| YES, Contact medical control; consider transport to trauma center; consider trauma team alert | NO |

STEP 4

- Age <5 or >55 years
- Pregnancy
- Immunosuppressed patients
- Cardiac disease; respiratory disease
- Insulin-dependent diabetes; cirrhosis; morbid obesity; coagulopathy

| YES, Contact medical control, consider transport to trauma center; consider trauma team alert | NO, Reevaluate with medical control |

When in Doubt, Take to a Trauma Center!

Figure 3-1.   American College of Surgeons field triage algorithm.

cabin configuration) can have profound effects on the ability of the air medical crew to perform interventions such as intubation. This translates into a need for the air medical crew to sometimes adjust care provision accordingly; for example, intubating patients before flight if a significant chance of airway deterioration exists while en route. Some interventions (e.g., provision of chest compressions) are extremely difficult to provide effectively in the air medical setting.

Table 3-4. NAEMSP guidelines for dispatching a helicopter to an emergency scene

CLINICAL
General
–Trauma victims need to delivered as soon as possible to a regional trauma center.
–Stable patients who are accessible to ground vehicles probably are best transported by ground.

Specific
Patients with critical injuries resulting in unstable vital signs require the fastest, most direct route of transport to a regional trauma center in a vehicle staffed with a team capable of offering critical care enroute. Often this is the case in the following situations:

–Trauma Score <12
–Glasgow Coma Scale score <10
–Penetrating trauma to the abdomen, pelvis, chest, neck, or head
–Spinal cord of spinal column injury or any injury producing paralysis of any extremity if any lateralizing signs
–Partial of total amputation of an extremity (excluding digits)
–Two of more long bone fractures or a major pelvic fracture
–Crushing injuries to the abdomen, chest, or head
–Major burns of the body surface area; burns involving the face, hands, feet or perineum; or burns with significant respiratory involvement or major electrical or chemical burns
–Patients involved in a serious traumatic event who are <2 or >55 years of age
–Patients with near-drowning injuries, with or without existing hypothermia
–Adult patients with any of the following vital sign abnormalities:
  —Systolic blood press <90 mm Hg
  —Respiratory rate <10 or >35/min
  —Heart rate <60 or >120/min
  —Unresponsive to verbal stimuli

OPERATIONAL SITUATIONS IN WHICH HELICOPTER USE SHOULD BE CONSIDERED
Mechanism of injury
–Vehicle roll-over with unbelted passengers
–Vehicle striking pedestrian at >10 mph
–Falls from >15 feet
–Motorcycle victim ejected at >20 mph
–Multiple victims

Difficult access situations
–Wilderness rescue
–Ambulance egress or access impeded at the scene by road conditions, weather, or traffic

Time and distance factors
–Transportation time to the trauma center >15 minutes by ground ambulance
–Transport time to local hospital by ground greater than transport time to trauma center by helicopter
–Patient extrication time >20 minutes
–Utilization of local ground ambulance leaves local community without ground ambulance coverage

2. Noise
Noise is of a sufficient degree to preclude reliable aus-cultation and monitoring of aural alarms (e.g., on a ven-tilator). The flight crew must learn to use other means of patient assessment and equipment monitoring.

3. Vibration
Vibration is a theoretic problem for aircraft. High-frequency vibrations have been shown to induce fatigue; in general, however, the ride in a helicopter (or fixed-wing aircraft) can often be much smoother than a ride in a ground ambulance.

4. Lighting
Lighting in an aircraft and, to a lesser extent in a ground ambulance, is different from that normally available in a well-lit hospital resuscitation area. Some helicopters, for instance, have patient care cabins that are contiguous with (and not separated from) the pilot seat; in such situations, the medical crew must work in red, blue, or dimmed lighting.

5. Altitude
Altitude issues relate to hypoxemia, pressure-volume changes, temperature, and humidity.

    a.   Altitude-related Hypoxemia. Altitude-related hypoxemia is usually not an issue, because patients customarily receive oxygen therapy and the altitude is not sufficiently high for the crew to require supplemental oxygen. Exceptions to this general rule occur, however, with both patients (e.g., premature neonates with narrow therapeu-tic windows for oxygen administration) and crew (e.g., crew in programs based at higher altitudes, who wear oxygen masks to prevent hypoxemic symptoms).

    b.   Ambient Pressure and Gas Volume. Boyle's law dictates the inverse relationship be-tween ambient pressure and gas volume. It comes into play with respect to both equipment (e.g., ventilator, intraaortic balloon pump, Minnesota tubes for upper gastrointestinal (GI) hemorrhage tamponade) and patients (e.g., need for preflight placement of a gastric tube to prevent vomiting in unconscious patients).

    c.   Temperature. High altitude is associated with decreased ambient temperature. Especially in colder climates (where the patient may be hypo-thermic before loading onto the aircraft) and with suboptimal heating systems in most aircraft, hypo-thermia can be a risk during helicopter transport.

    d.   Altitude and Temperature. Higher alti-tude and lower temperature are associated with decreased humidity. This can result in hardening of secretions (e.g., as in the ETT). The air medical crew should monitor (and suction) potential oc-currences, as indicated.

    e.   Aircraft and Flying Altitude. Helicopters generally transport patients at altitudes of 500 to

2000 feet above ground level. Therefore, unless transports occur at geographic locations where ground level is significantly elevated, altitude issues are a relatively minor concern for most helicopter transports. On the other hand, fixed-wing transports occur at much higher altitudes, which bring into play issues of cabin pressurization (and risks of sudden decompression).

6. Safety

Safety is the paramount consideration for any air transport service. At any time, in any mission, the pilot or medical crew should be empowered to halt the transport if safety considerations become a concern. Direct comparison between air and ground vehicle safety is difficult, because crashes involving medical helicopters (or less commonly, fixed-wing aircraft) are both more reliably tracked and more widely publicized than crashes of ground vehicles.

C. Preflight Versus In-flight

Preflight versus in-flight medical management decision-making balances the generally diminished ability to perform interventions in a moving vehicle with the cost of extra time delay associated with performance of procedures before loading patients onto the aircraft. Sometimes, considerable judgment must be exercised in determining whether to perform a critical procedure (e.g., intubation) before or after transport commences.

D. Fixed-wing Transport

Fixed-wing transport has been mentioned in many sections above, but adequate coverage of this topic is beyond the scope of this chapter. Except in cases where a fixed-wing aircraft is used solely because critical patients cannot be evacuated by air (e.g., fog precludes helicopter operations but a fixed-wing aircraft can safely operate in a remote area), patients transported by airplane have less acuity and greater stability than those transported by ground.

X. Common Traps and Decision Dilemmas

A. "Scoop and Run" Versus "Stay and Play"

Proponents of the "scoop and run" paradigm believe that the priority of the EMS system is to get patients rapidly to the hospital where definitive care can be provided. On the other hand, to "stay and play" is to perform interventions at the scene, which translate into earlier supportive care for patients. The "correct" approach is actually quite dependent on the patient. A patient with a gunshot wound to the abdomen needs to get to the hospital as quickly as possible, whereas a patient with an isolated angulated extremity fracture would benefit from EMS providers taking the time to provide good splinting and start an i.v. for analgesia purposes. As is usually the case with medical decision-making, healthcare provider judgment is critical.

B. Delays at the Scene

Common causes of delay at the scene include extrication, need for scene safety or crowd control, and need for patient decontamination. Such delays can best be minimized by careful cooperation among the various responsible agencies (e.g., EMS, fire, police) practiced before scenes of major trauma occur.

C.   Transport to Community Versus Tertiary Care Hospital

Is a trauma patient better off getting to a small community hospital near the scene of injury, or is patient outcome improved by helicopter transport directly from the scene to a level I trauma center? The literature on this question is mixed, although overall suggestion is that direct transport to a level I center is best for at least some patients. Given that logistics issues differ among various areas of the country, the best method to approach the hospital triage controversy is for all interested parties to come to agreement for a protocol that guides triage, yet is sufficiently flexible to allow judgment to be exercised by individual prehospital providers.

D.   Medical Control

Recent studies have uncovered a significant problem with EMS: inconsistent medical oversight and training. Further research is needed to address the optimal means of airway training and skills retention, and also the wider questions surrounding the need for stricter, more consistent, medical control (both on-line and off-line) in the United States.

SELECTED READINGS

Ali J, Adam RU, Gana TJ, et al. Effect of the prehospital trauma life support program (PHTLS) on prehospital trauma care. *J Trauma* 1997;42:786–790.

Bond RJ, Kortbeek JB, Preshaw RM. Field trauma triage: combining mechanism of injury with the prehospital index for an improved trauma triage tool. *J Trauma* 1997;43:283–287.

Cone DC, Wydro GC, Mininger CM. Current practice in clinical cervical spinal clearance: implication for EMS. *Prehosp Emerg Care* 1999; 3:42–46.

DeVellis P, Thomas SH, Wedel SK. Prehospital and ED analgesia for air transported patients with fractures. *Prehosp Emerg Care* 1998;2:293–296.

DeVellis P, Thomas SH, Wedel SK. Prehospital fentanyl analgesia in air-transported pediatric trauma patients. *Pediatr Emerg Care* 1998; 14:321–323.

Dieckmann RA, Athey J, Bailey B, et al. A pediatric survey for the National Highway Traffic Safety Administration: emergency medical services system re-assessments. *Prehosp Emerg Care* 2001;5: 231–236.

Domeier RM. Indications for prehospital spinal immobilization. National Association of EMS Physicians Standards and Clinical Practice Committee. *Prehosp Emerg Care* 1999;3:251–253.

Eckstein M, Chan L, Schneir A, et al. Effect of prehospital advanced life support on outcomes of major trauma patients. *J Trauma* 2000; 48(4):643–648.

Engum SA, Mitchell MK, Scherer LR, et al. Prehospital triage in the injured pediatric patient. *J Pediatr Surg* 2000;35:82–87.

Gerich TG, Schmidt U, Hubrich V, et al. Prehospital airway management in the acutely injured patient: the role of surgical cricothyrotomy revisited. *J Trauma* 1998;45:312–314.

Liberman M, Mulder D, Sampalis J. Advanced or basic life support for trauma: meta-analysis and critical review of the literature. *J Trauma* 2000;49:584–599.

Marson AC, Thomson JC. The influence of prehospital trauma care on motor vehicle crash mortality. *J Trauma* 2001;50:917–920; discussion 920–921.

Novak L, Shackford SR, Bourguignon P, et al. Comparison of standard and alternative prehospital resuscitation in uncontrolled hemorrhagic shock and head injury. *J Trauma* 1999;47:834–844.

Orf J, Thomas SH, Ahmed W, et al. Appropriateness of endotracheal tube size and insertion depth in children undergoing air medical transport. *Pediatr Emerg Care* 2000;16:321–327.

Paul TR, Marias M, Pons PT, et al. Adult versus pediatric prehospital trauma care: is there a difference?. *J Trauma* 1999;47:455–459.

Thomas SH, Cheema F, Wedel SK, et al. Helicopter EMS trauma transport: Annotated review of selected outcomes-related literature. *Prehosp Emerg Care* 2002;6:359–371.

Thomas SH, Harrison T, Wedel SK, et al. Helicopter EMS roles in disaster operations. *Prehosp Emerg Care* 2000;4:338–344.

Thomas SH, Harrison T, Wedel SK. Flight crew airway management in four settings: a six-year review. *Prehosp Emerg Care* 1999;3:310–315.

Thomas SH, Harrison TH, Buras WR, et al: Helicopter transport and blunt trauma outcome. *J Trauma* 2002;52:136–145.

Wayne MA, Friedland E. Prehospital use of succinylcholine—a 20-year review. *Prehosp Emerg Care* 1999;3(2):107–109.

Organization of the Emergency Department and Trauma Team

David A. Peak, MD and Alice A. Gervasini, PhD, RN

I. Introduction

The initial management of a trauma patient is a complex task necessitating coordinated activities from multiple providers. The initial care delivered to trauma victims clearly influences patient outcomes. Early recognition of severe injuries, coupled with appropriate treatment, results in better survival and less morbidity.

Challenges facing the trauma team include multiple concurrent tasks, changing plans, a heavy workload, a compressed work environment, and the complexity of the patient. Additionally, the care of the trauma patient often requires the team to deviate from a traditional or usual task cadence and skip certain tasks in favor of more critical ones. The systematic approach to trauma patients ensures that priorities of management are executed in a logical and orderly fashion.

Communication between trauma team personnel is simplified because each member knows his or her role and task priorities, can function independently in the initial time-critical period, and knows which member will provide further direction. This structured approach ensures that multiple concurrent tasks requiring access to the patient by many caregivers in a limited working area can be coordinated in an efficient manner.

II. Personnel

Certain basic criteria must be met for the care of trauma patients. Trauma team members should be present or immediately available to receive trauma patients. Optimal available experts should be used to fill each team role, which requires sourcing from throughout the hospital. An experienced trauma surgeon with an available operating room must be immediately available and is considered crucial to the optimal care of the injured patient in all phases of management by the American College of Surgeons Committee on Trauma. Prehospital staff are important members of the patient care team and should be appropriately qualified. The basic core personnel of a trauma team meeting the trauma patient should include the following: team leader, airway expert, procedural team members, at least one nurse, a scribe, and an x-ray technician. In addition to the roles discussed below, in most tertiary care trauma centers, a senior surgery resident provides addition supervisory support in the role of a trauma senior.

A. Team Leader

The team leader is responsible for ensuring the team is appropriately staffed and available and the trauma area is appropriately supplied before patient arrival. This person should activate the appropriate trauma response before patient arrival to ensure the availability of necessary resources according to prehospital ambulance communication and preset standards and advise any referring hospital at time of referral. Preplanning is imperative such that anticipated needs for specialty equipment or medications is shared with the nurses and can be readily available. Once the patient arrives, the team leader must prioritize the assessment, investigation, and management of the trauma patient and effectively communicate this to the trauma team. This person is also responsible for obtaining information on the mechanism of injury, allergies, time of last meal, and significant past medical history of the trauma patient. The team leader should perform the primary and secondary surveys, and is initially responsible for all phases of the resuscitation, including the decision to perform, supervise, or assist in major procedures or intubation. The team leader is responsible for patient comfort and appropriate communication to alert patients. This person must make appropriate and timely referrals and arrange for the transfer of the patient to a place for definitive care. The team leader should relieve team members from duty when they are no longer needed. Finally, the team leader is ultimately the point person for communication with family members, caregivers, and the media. The team leader generally will stand at the head of the bed or off to one side of the patient in a preselected site and should be the only voice heard during the initial evaluation and resuscitation to ensure adequate communication to the rest of the team.

B.   Airway Expert
A person skilled at trauma airway techniques must be part of the trauma team. This can be addressed in a number of ways with personnel from anesthesia, surgery, or emergency medicine at the head of the bed on patient arrival. In many institutions, the team leader will also serve as the airway expert. Some institutions use a different team member to handle airway management that may include both the decision to intubate and the medications used. No well-controlled studies prove that one system is superior. It must be clear from the onset if someone other than the team leader will make the decision to intubate (and determine the medications to be used). When a separate airway expert person is used, that person must work in concert with the team leader's overall plan and communication scheme and must be skilled at all methods of airway management and confirmation of tube placement or ventilation.

C.   Procedural Person (s)
Severely traumatized patients may need a number of nearly concurrent diagnostic tests and procedures completed by skilled providers on arrival to the trauma center. Routinely, these tasks include intravenous (i.v.) access and procurement of blood; focused abdominal sonogram for trauma (FAST); bladder catheterization; and can include chest thoracostomy, chest thoracotomy, diagnostic peritoneal lavage, fracture reduction or splinting, and procurement of surgical airway at the discretion of the team

leader. For severely traumatized patients, these tasks are better handled concurrently by multiple procedural experts. Procedural persons are allocated preselected space on one or both sides of the patient bed.

D. Nursing

Skilled trauma nursing care is a key ingredient for successful care of the trauma patient. As a member of the resuscitation team, the nurse will have varying responsibilities based on the type of hospital, size, and design. These include pre-planning and good communication with the team leader to ensure that the designed approach to the resuscitation is well coordinated. The number and available procedural personnel will dictate the number of nurses that need to be at the bedside during the initial resuscitation. At least one nurse needs to be positioned at the bedside as a direct caregiver. Resuscitation nurses are actively involved in exposing the patient, establishing hemodynamic monitoring, initiating and maintaining fluid resuscitation, patient warming techniques, and any procedures arising from the primary and secondary survey. The nurse is also involved in patient identification and family notification. Ongoing patient monitoring is an essential component of the initial evaluation and resuscitation to assess the patient's condition and judge the effect of treatment delivered. Nursing requires preselected space on one side of the patient bed to allow access to the patient.

E. Scribe

A scribe is required to document accurately the assessment (primary and secondary survey called out by the team leader), patient clinical data (vital signs), and interventions to the patient. The documentation needs to be clear, concise and accurate. It should also reflect the patients' emergency experience beyond the initial resuscitation to include response to medications, changes in assessment and hemodynamic parameters, presence of specialty team members, changes in the plan of care, and general condition upon transfer to another location (OR, ICU, Floor). Ideally, this role is filled by a nurse skilled in trauma care who is allocated preselected space to the side or near the foot of the patient bed.

F. X-ray Technician

An experienced x-ray technician must be immediately available with appropriate cassettes to obtain a trauma series or necessary portable x-rays as directed by the team leader.

G. Senior Traumatologist

As mentioned, according to the American College of Surgeons Committee on Trauma, a senior traumatologist is considered an essential component of optimal care of the trauma patient throughout the entire evaluation of the severely ill patient. That person should be available immediately to assist in the management decisions of the critically ill trauma patient and have the resources available to deliver prompt care in the operating theatre, if necessary. The senior traumatologist should be present to meet the severely injured patient based on preset standards and available to the team leader in a timely manner for advise on all trauma patients. When present, the senior traumatologist has the ultimate responsibility of patient care and either advises the team leader concerning the care of the patient or, at his or her discretion, assumes the team leadership role.

H. Patient Care Support Personnel

Ancillary support for the trauma team will vary based on patient and family needs, and the degree of profile the incident might be generating in the department or community. Ideally, there should be personnel available to assist the team with crisis intervention, religious or spiritual needs, psycho/social needs of the patient and/or family, and communication to outside agencies and media. Consideration for team membership include: psychiatric clinical nurse specialist, trauma nurse coordinator, chaplain, social workers, public relations staff, and in some communities volunteer networks.

III. Facility Design Considerations

Facility design is an important consideration for the optimal care of the trauma patient. Optimal design will ensure (a) smooth and rapid transfer of the patient from the prehospital setting; (b) adequate space for team members to perform necessary evaluation and procedures; (c) and necessary supplies, appropriate monitor devices, and adequate lighting. Additional requirements include a means to communicate with prehospital providers and consultants, as well as easy access to the stat laboratory, blood bank, and operating theatre. The trauma bay must have easy access to both portable radiologic equipment and to additional radiologic areas (e.g., computed tomography [CT] scan). Additionally, the receiving trauma area should be adequately equipped to prevent or reverse hypothermia, including the ability to warm the room. Level I trauma centers require the presence of cardiopulmonary capability and an operating microscope within the trauma system.

IV. Equipment

Necessary equipment must be prestocked and immediately available for use. Equipment necessary for the trauma area includes oxygen and suction, defibrillator/pacer, airway management equipment (laryngoscopes, endotracheal tubes, cricothyroidotomy and tracheostomy trays, mechanical ventilator, end-tidal CO_2 detectors, oral airways); i.v. fluid supplies (including central venous catheters and methods to deliver warm fluids rapidly); skeletal tongs, and operating trays (including peritoneal lavage, venous cut-down, tube thoracostomy, thoracotomy, intracranial burr hole, and minor surgery with suture supplies). Additional requirements include nasogastric tubes, laboratory supplies, urinary catheters, warming blankets or passive warmers; and a means to monitor adequately the critically ill patient (electrocardiogram and continuous cardiac monitor device, blood pressure or invasive blood pressure capabilities, pulse oximetry, core temperature recorders, and, possibly, intracranial pressure recorders and central venous pressure recorders).

V.   Liaison and Communication with Prehospital Providers

Prehospital care is under the purview of the emergency medical services (EMS) and functions in coordination within the larger health community to ensure continuity of care from the time of the trauma incident through the transfer to the trauma center. An EMS system for trauma care must include a qualified EMS director, trauma-educated prehospital staff; triage, treatment, and transfer protocols for trauma integrated into the EMS system; and policies and means for communication with receiving trauma centers. Each level must employ a means for continuous education, quality assessment and improvement. Inadequate prehospital care decreases the risks for a successful recovery and increases the requirements of the hospital trauma team. The trauma center should have an EMS liaison to function as the interface between the prehospital system and the intrahospital trauma team to ensure a smooth transition of quality care delivered and a means of open communication between providers. Some uniformity should exist between the prehospital trauma triage protocol and the intrahospital trauma activation protocol. Trauma team members should understand the basic tenets of the prehospital system, prehospital care, personnel, triage protocols, and treatment protocols, including any need for prehospital medical control. Communication with prehospital providers is paramount for two reasons: first, it allows the trauma team initially to prepare for the incoming trauma; second, it provides essential knowledge to the kinematics of the trauma, the response time, on-scene time, transport time, and response to prehospital treatment. Knowledge of the kinematics of the trauma mechanism cannot be overstated and the prehospital providers may be the only resource for this information.

VI.   The Trauma Team Concept

The trauma team concept has evolved to address the unique challenges that severely injured patients present, including the need for multiple concurrent tasks, the complexity of the patient, and a compressed work environment in terms of both time and space. The use of a highly functioning team with clear leadership and team roles with protocols speed decision-making and optimize resource management with the goal of matching patient injury acuity with hospital resources. Effective trauma team training requires special instruction in effective communication methods, team hierarchy, treatment protocols, and the flexibility to effectively change treatment plans as well as to expand or decrease personnel appropriately.

VII.   Team Activation Issues

Great debate and ongoing research exist regarding what criteria should be used to activate the hospital trauma response. Most centers use a combination of physiologic factors and certain types of anatomic site of injury or trauma mechanisms to activate the trauma team. Optimal trauma team activation should limit the potentially deadly undertriage of seriously injured patients and limit unnecessary activation in patients who will not benefit from the commitment of significant hospital resources. No current standards exist for acceptable undertriage or overtriage. The American College of Surgeons has suggested that an overtriage rate of

50% may be necessary to achieve an undertriage rate of 10%. It is additionally unclear what measurable outcomes (Injury Severity Score [ISS], intensive care unit [ICU] admissions, fluid resuscitation, early surgery, morbidity, death) correctly define those patients who truly benefit from the resources of trauma team activation. According to the *American College of Surgeons Trauma Programs: Resources for Optimal Care of the Injured Patient* document, the minimal criteria for the definition of major trauma resuscitation include:

1. Confirmed blood pressure of <90 systolic in adults and age-specific hypotension for children
2. Respiratory compromise, obstruction, or intubation
3. Transfer patients from other hospitals receiving blood to maintain vital signs
4. **Emergency** physician's discretion
5. Gunshot wounds to the abdomen, neck, or chest
6. **Glasgow Coma Score (GCS) <8** with mechanism attributed to trauma

At Massachusetts General Hospital (MGH), a full trauma response (trauma stat) is activated by the above criteria in addition to any mass casualty incidents and, at the request of the MedFlight helicopter crew, a specialized transfer team of prehospital providers experienced with the severely injured. Literature suggests that certain patient parameters (e.g., elderly, significant comorbidity) might help to address the realization that such patients have much higher mortality, complication rates, and longer hospital stays compared with other patients with similar injuries. Many centers use a two-, three-, or even four-tiered response based on physiologic factors combined with certain types of anatomic site or trauma mechanisms. At MGH, we use a two-tiered response to trauma, with the second response (trauma alert) activated by the following:

1. Depressed or open skull fracture
2. Injury induced altered mentation, GCS ≤13, or significant neurologic deficit
3. Extensive maxillofacial injury
4. Penetrating (not a gunshot wound) injury to the neck or torso
5. Major pelvic fracture
6. Multiple long bone fractures
7. Air transport of a multisystem trauma patient
8. Interfacility transfer of a multisystem trauma patient

The second response differs from the first in the number of resources that are automatically generated (e.g., operating room availability) and the response times of the personnel who respond from outside the emergency department (within minutes as opposed to immediately in a trauma stat). Literature suggests that a GCS ≤14 accurately predicts the need for patient hospitalization and may be a reasonable addition above.

VIII. Training Issues

More than any other hospital program, the hospital response to trauma requires a coordinated commitment from multiple surgical and medical specialties, nursing services, and administration personnel who work together as a team. The trauma team requires education in trauma pathophysiology, procedural techniques, and critical care resuscitation as well as special education and practice with team dynamics, communication, and leadership to deliver optimal care. Whereas team training is common in other fields, it is not necessarily commonplace in medicine. Optimal training includes case- or scenario-based or simulator-driven practice sessions with team members to go over communication, protocols, team member roles, and expectations and to practice transition to contingency plans. Such training appears to enhance both individual team member performances as well as overall team performance, which leads to more effective care and should be considered an integral part of trauma team training (**Figure 4-1**).

IX.   Common Traps and Decision Dilemmas

Common traps can be broken down into coordination issues or direct patient care decisions. Coordination issues include, but are

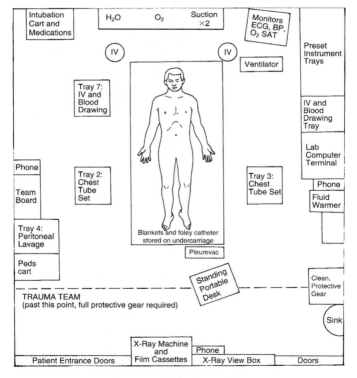

Figure 4-1.   An organized and rehearsed approach to resuscitation of the seriously injured patients facilitates logical and efficient evaluation and interventions. (Adapted from American College of Surgeons Committee on Trauma. *Resources for optimal care of the injured patient.* Chicago: American College of Surgeons, 1999;15:170, with permission.)

not limited to, the following: inappropriate reception by staff, delayed arrival of senior traumatologist or other team members, delay in initiation or arrival of consultation, inappropriate prioritization of critical tasks, inadequate documentation, delay in dispatch to the operating room, inefficient trauma team coordination and communication, and failure to switch to contingency plans effectively. Potential errors in patient care decisions include, but are not limited to, the following: delayed or inadequate fluid or blood resuscitation, inadequate external hemorrhage control, delay in appropriate investigation techniques (e.g., CT scan), inadequate management of hypothermia, infrequent or inadequate respiratory or ventilation monitoring, inappropriate drugs or dosing, delayed chest decompression, and failure to change to appropriate contingency plans.

SELECTED READING

American College of Surgeons Committee on Trauma. *Resources for optimal care of the injured patient.* Chicago: American College of Surgeons, 1999:15.

American College of Surgeons Committee on Trauma. *Resources for optimal care of the injured patient,* revised edition. Chicago: American College of Surgeons, 2000.

Demetriades D, Sava J, Alo S, et al. Old age as a criterion for trauma team activation. *J Trauma* 2001;51:754–757.

Driscoll PA, Vincent CA. Variation in trauma resuscitation and its effect on patient outcome. *Injury* 1992;23:107–110.

Holcomb JB, Dumire RD, Crommett JW, et al. Evaluation of trauma team performance using an advanced human patient simulator for resuscitation training. *J Trauma* 2002;52:1078–1086.

Mackenzie CF, Lippert FK. Emergency department management of trauma. *Anesthesiol Clin North Am* 1999;17:45–61.

McQuillan KA, Von Rueden KT, Hartstock RN, Flynn MB, Whalen E. Trauma Nursing: From resuscitation through rehabilitation, 3rd ed. Philadelphia: W.B. Saunders, 2002.

Norwood SH, McAuley CE, Berne JD, et al. A prehospital Glasgow coma scale score ≤14 accurately predicts the need for full trauma team activation and patient hospitalization after motor vehicle collisions. *J Trauma* 2002;53:503–507.

Sava J, Alo K, Velmahos GC, et al. All patients with truncal gunshot wounds deserve trauma team activation. *J Trauma* 2002;52: 276–279.

Sheehy SB, Blansfield JS, Danis DM, Gervasini AA. Manual of Clinical Trauma Care: The first hour. St. Louis: Mosby, 1999.

Xiao Y, Hunter WA, Mackenzie CF, et al. Task complexity on emergency medical care and its implication for team coordination. *Hum Factors* 1996;38:636–645.

5

Disaster Planning

Adrian A. Maung, MD,
and Susan M. Briggs, MD, MPH

I. Introduction

Disasters follow no rules. No one can predict the complexity, time, or location of the next disaster. Traditionally, medical providers have held the erroneous belief that all disasters are different. Thus, one of the most significant problems in mass casualty management is that medical providers do not *prepare* for disasters, they *respond* to them. In reality, all disasters, regardless of cause, have similar medical and nonmedical consequences. Disasters differ only in the degree to which these consequences occur and disrupt the normal medical and nonmedical infrastructure of the disaster scene.

II. Principles of Mass Casualty Management

Disaster medical care is significantly different from the care medical providers deliver on a day-to-day basis. The key principle of disaster medical care is to do the *greatest good for the greatest number of patients,* whereas the objective of conventional medical care is to do the *greatest good for the individual patient.*

A consistent medical approach to mass casualty incidents (MCI), based on an understanding of their common features and the response expertise they require, is becoming the accepted practice in the United States. This strategy, called the *Mass Casualty Incident Response,* has the primary objective of reducing the mortality caused by the disaster.

In general, mass casualty incidents involve a limited geographic and demographic scope and assume a positive balance between needs and resources. The complexity of today's disasters, especially disasters involving weapons of mass destruction, increasingly challenges the validity of this concept. Currently, complex disasters often exceed the ability of the local community to cope with them and require specialized medical resources from outside of the community.

Natural disasters, man-made disasters, and terrorism encompass the spectrum of possible disaster threats. Weapons of mass destruction (e.g., chemical, biological, nuclear weapons) can create "contaminated environments" and provide the greatest challenge of all. No longer will emergency medical responders be able to bring victims into hospitals for fear of further contaminating medical facilities. Medical providers, therefore, must be equipped to triage, deliver initial stabilization, and possibly provide definitive care at staging areas outside the hospital facility.

III. ABCs of Disaster Response

Similar to the fundamentals of trauma care, a mass casualty incident can be approached in a uniformed manner with four basic elements of medical response.

1. Search and rescue
2. Triage and initial stabilization

3. Definitive medical care
4. Evacuation

A. Search and Rescue

Rescue of victims is often initiated by relatives and other survivors of the event followed by the local emergency medical service (EMS) and fire department. These resources, however, can be quickly overwhelmed and specialized equipment and personnel may be required, which can include the following

- Urban search and rescue teams
- Heavy construction equipment
- Canine units

During the extrication process, these patients may require stabilization and treatment beyond the capabilities of the paramedics. Physicians may be called on to provide critical care in the field. Critical interventions include:

- Airway protection, including intubation under difficult conditions
- Vascular access for rapid fluid resuscitation with cut-down, central, or intraosseous lines
- Pain control in unstable patients
- Hypothermia care
- Immobilization
- Amputation of injured or trapped extremities

These life-saving procedures often must be done under difficult conditions with limited resources. Physicians with field experience are skilled in "austere" medicine. In a wide scale disaster, however, any physician can be called on to perform these critical interventions at the disaster site.

B. Triage and Initial Stabilization

Triage is often the most important aspect of any disaster medical response. It is also most often the point at which physicians initially encounter the patients. In a mass casualty response, triage is a dynamic process with frequent reassessment as additional resources become available. It is based on the assumption of a potential imbalance between the need for and availability of resources. Two general categories of disaster triage exist.

1. Conventional Triage

In triage scenarios that physicians use every day, patients are quickly assessed for the level of injury and assigned a priority level. Immediate critical interventions are then implemented and patients transferred to appropriate medical care. This is the model on which the trauma level care system is based. The objective is to *do the greatest good for the individual patient.* This model is valid only if sufficient resources are available to take care of all the victims.

2. Field Triage

In a MCI, the scope of the disaster may be large enough to invalidate the previous model. The availability of resources might become a crucial factor affecting the survival of victims. The objective now shifts to *doing the greatest good for the greatest number of people.*

a.   Field Triage Goals

- Prioritize and categorize casualties so that patients can receive timely rescue, treatment, and evacuation in an orderly fashion
- Optimize the use of available medical, nursing, and emergency personnel at the disaster site
- Optimize the use of available logistic support and equipment.

b.   Levels of Field Triage.

Field triage is conducted on three levels.

(1)   Level 1: On-site Triage

- Rapid categorization of victims with severe injuries needing immediate care
- Patients categorized as "acute" or "nonacute"
- Triage carried out by the first responders to the disaster site, usually the local population

(2)   Level 2: Medical Triage

- Rapid categorization of victims at a casualty site done by the most experienced medical personnel available
- The casualty collection or triage sites should be located close to the disaster site and be visible for disaster victims, but provide safety from climactic conditions and hazards and be upwind from potentially contaminated environments.

Victims can be categorized with color-coding.

RED < Urgent: Patients who require immediate life-saving interventions (airway, breathing, circulation)

YELLOW < Delayed or expectant

- Patients who do not require immediate life-saving interventions for whom treatment may be delayed
- Patients who are not expected to survive because of injury severity complicated by the conditions and lack of resources at the site

GREEN < Minor: Individuals who require minimal or no medical care

BLACK < Deceased

(3)   Level 3: Evacuation Triage

- Assigns priorities to disaster victims for transfer
- Goal is to transfer victims to the most appropriate facility by the most efficient and appropriate route
- Same medical personnel as level 2 triage

C. Definitive Medical Care

Depending on the magnitude and cause of the disaster, the requirements for definitive medical care will vary. Many disasters will likely utilize the remaining local resources as well as nearby regional facilities outside the disaster area. Large-scale disasters, on the other hand, may require the mobilization of specialty medical teams, including mobile surgical teams. Medical providers must be prepared with equipment and supplies to deliver definitive medical care in the field as hospital infrastructures and facilities may be contaminated or destroyed. Lightweight, flexible, and mobile equipment is essential.

D. Evacuation

Disaster victims can be evacuated by air, land, or sea to remaining facilities. As part of the predisaster planning process, hospitals and officials should identify what resources are available or lacking within their facility or location. This allows for the development of transportation options for evacuation of specific injuries (e.g., burn patients transported to a regional burn center).

IV. Medical Consequences of Weapons of Mass Destruction

A. Terrorism

Terrorism is the unlawful use of force or violence against persons or property to intimidate or coerce a government, civilian population or any segment thereof, in a furtherance of political or social objectives (Federal Bureau of Investigation). This most often takes the form of blast injuries from a variety of explosive devices. It can also involve the use of weapons of mass destruction.

B. Nuclear

Nuclear attacks can cause injury from either radiation exposure or the blast of the nuclear device. Possible disaster scenarios include dispersal of radioactive substances with or without an explosive device, attacks on nuclear reactors, or detonation of nuclear weapons. The radiation exposure can occur in many types: localized or whole-body exposure, internal or external contamination. Basic principle of minimizing injury is to reduce the exposure time and maximize the distance and shielding from the radiation source. Most radiation injuries do not constitute medical emergencies from a MCI viewpoint; management consists of supportive care and treatment of symptoms.

C. Biological

Biological warfare has been in existence since at least the classical Greek and Roman times. During medieval sieges, diseased cattle or human bodies would be catapulted into the besieged towns or dropped into water supplies. During World War II, Germany and Japan both attempted to use biological agents and tested them on prisoners of war. In more recent times, a number of countries have been actively developing their biological stockpiles. It is also of concern that these agents can be obtained and used by terrorist groups. Possible indications of a biological attack include:

- Disease entity that is unusual or that does not occur naturally in a given geographic area
- Data suggestive of a massive point-source outbreak
- Apparent aerosol or oral route of infection
- High morbidity and mortality relative to the number of personnel at risk
- Illness limited to a geographical area or site
- Sentinel dead animals of multiple species
- Absence of a competent natural vector in the area of outbreak
- Low attack rates in personnel who work in areas with filtered air supplies or closed ventilation systems

The Centers for Disease Control (CDC) currently classifies certain agents as "Category A." These agents are felt to be those most likely to be used in a biological attack. Healthcare providers should be aware of these agents, their common presentations, and treatments for exposure to them. They include anthrax, plague, botulism, tularemia, and smallpox.

1. Anthrax

Anthrax is caused by a gram-positive, spore-forming *Bacillus anthracis*. It creates a toxin that affects neutrophils and macrophages. It inhibits bacterial phagocytosis and prevents the oxidative burst of neutrophils. The spores are hardy and resistant to some disinfectants, and to sun and heat. Most officials believe that the most likely attack would be in form of aerosolized spores; however, anthrax can also be acquired from cutaneous contact or ingestion of contaminated foods.

The disease has three clinical forms: cutaneous, pulmonary, and gastrointestinal. The cutaneous form starts as a painless pruritic papule that can resemble an insect bite. It is occasionally surrounded by vesicles and eventually develops into an ulcer with a necrotic center. Lymphadenopathy with systemic signs of malaise, fever, and headache can occur. The lesions usually start on the extremities and then spread to head and neck. If untreated, the fatality rate is 20%. The pulmonary form has a biphasic presentation. Early on, it can mimic an upper respiratory infection with dry cough, low-grade fever, and malaise. The onset of symptoms usually occurs between 1 and 6 days after exposure, although it can vary substantially. After the initial symptoms, the spores invade hilar and mediastinal lymph nodes, causing substernal pain, bloody pleural effusions, and a widened mediastinum (hemorrhagic mediastinitis is considered to be a pathognomonic sign). Fulminant acute phase then develops with meningitis, high fever, severe respiratory distress, and fatal shock. This form is essentially fatal in 100% if untreated and in 80% of patients treated after the onset of symptoms. Gastrointestinal anthrax often presents with nonspecific symptoms. Abdominal pain, fever, nausea, and vomiting predominate but upper or lower gastrointestinal bleeding or peritonitis can occur.

Diagnosis is made with cultures of the affected body fluids. Treatment consists of antibiotics and supportive care for the involved organ systems. Intravenous penicillin, ciprofloxacin, or doxycycline should be used. The duration of therapy should be 60 days. For high-risk exposure, a 60-day course with ciprofloxacin or doxycycline should be given along with vaccination.

2. Plague

The plague, caused by a gram-negative bacterium *Yersinia pestis* is naturally transmitted by fleas. In the naturally occurring disease (bubonic plague), the bacteria migrate after the initial fleabite to the regional lymphatics (cervical, groin or maxillary) where a large, painful infected lymph node (bubo) develops. Two to eight days later, patients experience a sudden onset of chills, fevers, and sweats. The patient can then develop septicemia, disseminated intravascular coagulation (DIC) or focal areas of gangrene. In a biological warfare scenario, the likely presentation will be with a pneumonic plague. Patients would present 2 to 6 days after exposure with fever, dyspnea, and productive or bloody cough. The chest x-ray study may show bilateral infiltrates or consolidation. Buboes are usually absent in the pneumonic plague. Diagnosis is made with cultures of affected fluid, although more rapid techniques are available at state laboratories. Treatment is with streptomycin, doxycycline, or gentamicin. Ciprofloxacin and chloramphenicol can also have some efficacy. The untreated plague has a mortality rate of 55%.

3. Botulism

Clostridium botulinum, a spore-forming, gram-positive anaerobic bacillus found in the soil, makes a highly poisonous toxin. An estimate has been made that 1 g of this toxin could kill a million individuals. It functions as a neurotoxin that binds presynaptic nerve endings, inhibiting the release of acetylcholine. Four clinical types of botulism have been described: food-borne, wound, infant intestinal, and adult intestinal. Most adult botulism is characterized by muscular weakness about 12 to 72 hours after initial exposure. Symmetric descending paralysis follows, starting in the cranial nerves and spreading to involve the respiratory muscles and extremities. Neurologic signs can develop with symmetric cranial nerve palsies leading to dysarthria, dysphonia, and dysphagia. Death usually occurs from respiratory muscle paralysis, unless respiratory support is given. Treatment is usually supportive but an antitoxin is available from the CDC that diminishes the length of ventilatory support greatly. In most cases, several weeks of mechanical ventilation are needed.

4. Tularemia

Tularemia is normally a disease caused by *Francisella tularensis,* an aerobic, catalase-positive, gram-negative coccobacillus found in rural areas. Transmission occurs usually via insect bites or contact with contaminated animal products. Aerosolized cases can occur and present after a 3- to 5-day incubation with sudden onset of fevers, chills, pneumonia, and hilar lymphadenopathy. Headaches, backaches, chills, rigors, and pharyngitis can also occur. Treatment is usually with streptomycin and gentamicin. Doxycycline and ciprofloxacin are recommended in large-scale outbreaks.

5. Smallpox

Smallpox, a disease caused by a DNA virus, is the only disease on the category A list with a significant potential for human-to-human transmission. It is transmitted via droplets or aerosols during early clinical stages. In this form, the virus can survive up to 24 hours. The incubation period is about 1 to 2 weeks. Fevers, malaise, severe headaches, backaches, and abdominal pain can develop. A maculopapular rash then appears on the mucosa of the mouth, pharynx, face, and forearms and spreads later to the lower extremities and trunk. Vesicles usually develop within 1 to 2 days after the rash and become pustular. One week after the eruption, crust forms and scabs develop. Smallpox can be distinguished from chicken pox by several criteria. Smallpox lesions can occur on palms and soles; chickenpox usually does not. In addition, small pox lesions are usually in the same stage, whereas chickenpox can have lesions of various stages in close proximity to each other. Treatment is largely supportive. Diagnosis can be made by electron microscopic examination of the vesicle fluid or by polymerase chain reaction (PCR) techniques. Vaccination within 4 days has been shown to improve the course. Fatality rates approach about 30% with supportive care. Death occurs from severe toxemia, septic shock from bacterial superinfection, or DIC.

D. Chemical

Over the years, various countries have developed a number of chemical agents for use in unconventional warfare. The most potential agents in a MCI can be divided into four categories: nerve agents (tabun [GA], sarin [GB], soman [GD], GF, VX); blood agents (hydrogen cyanide, cyanogen chloride); blistering agents (lewisite, nitrogen and sulfur mustards, phosgene oxime); and pulmonary agents (phosgene, chlorine, vinyl chloride).

1. Nerve Agents

Nerve agents work by irreversibly binding and inhibiting acetylcholinesterase, thus increasing the amount of acetylcholine at neuromuscular junctions. This initially leads to an overstimulation of the end neurons, but then progresses to paralysis. This initial overstimulation or cholinergic crisis is marked by central nervous system (CNS) symptoms: agitation, confusion, delirium, hallucinations, seizures, and coma. Over-stimulation of muscarinic receptors leads to bradycardia, bronchospasm, bronchorrhea, and miosis. Nicotinic effects are usually tachycardia, hypertension, muscle fasciculation, pain, and weakness. Death usually occurs from respiratory failure, either from muscle weakness itself, airway loss, or bronchorrhea.

Besides supportive treatment, large amounts of atropine should be given. Atropine, however, only treats the muscarinic effects—not the nicotinic ones. In addition to atropine, pralidoxime, an antidote to organophosphates, should be given as soon as possible. It works by reversing the binding of organophosphates to acetylcholinesterase but only if "aging" (permanent covalent bonding) has not occurred. Various agents age at different rates. For example, soman ages in 2 minutes, whereas sarin ages in 5 hours. Providers taking care of affected patients should take special precautions by wearing isolation suits and butyl rubber gloves because nerve agents can penetrate latex gloves.

2. Blistering or Mustard Agents

Blistering or mustard agents affect mostly skin, mucous membranes, and the respiratory tract by causing burns and blisters. They bind to nucleic acids and sulfur or sulfhydryl groups in proteins and act as alkylating agents. Usually, no immediate symptoms are noted; in 2 to 20 hours, however, eye irritation, lacrimation, hoarseness, and burning sensation on the skin develop. The skin damage begins with generalized, painful inflammation and progresses to blistering and desquamation. Death usually occurs, either from sepsis or direct lung injury causing pulmonary edema and respiratory failure. Effects can occur in the immune system and bone marrow, with increased risk of neoplasm in survivors. Treatment is usually supportive with no specific antidote. Care preferably should be administered in burn units because the initial symptoms and complications are similar to common burn injuries.

3. Blood Agents

Blood agents are most dangerous if inhaled. They bind to cytochrome aa3 in the electron transport chain and interrupt cellular respiration. This leads to tissue hypoxia and lactic acidosis. At high concentrations, death is almost instantaneous. At lower doses, patients experience tachypnea, restlessness, headache, and palpitations and then seizures, coma, and death. The diagnosis is usually made on clinical grounds but a high venous PO_2 relative to arterial PO_2 should raise suspicion. Treatment is with intravenous sodium nitrite because it converts hemoglobin to methemoglobin, which has higher affinity for cyanide. Sodium thiosulfate should then be given because the conversion of cyanomethemoglobin to thiocyanate via rhodanese requires a sulfur substance.

4. Ricin

Ricin, extracted from castor beans, is a potent cytotoxin that inhibits protein synthesis. It is toxic, either by ingestion or inhalation. Ingestion can lead to hemorrhagic gastroenteritis, shock, and death. Inhalation causes cough, chest tightness, dyspnea, and fever. Over a course of 2 to 3 days, it then develops into airway necrosis and lung injury manifested by hemoptysis and pulmonary edema. No specific treatment exists, except support of the affected organs.

E.   Blast Injuries

With the recent worldwide events, blast injuries, once considered unique to the military, are now in the realm of civilian physicians. Explosion is caused by the rapid conversion of a chemical (solid or liquid) into a gas, along with the resultant energy release. Propellants (e.g., gunpowder) release energy relatively slowly. On the other hand, high explosives (e.g., C4) can cause almost an instantaneous transformation under extremely high pressures. Trauma after a blast has traditionally been divided into the following:

- Primary: Damage from shock wave
- Secondary: Damage from projectiles
- Tertiary: Damage from victim being thrown against solid surface

1.   Primary Blast Injury

Primary blast injury (PBI) occurs as a direct effect of changes in atmospheric pressure caused by the blast wave. The force of the blast wave is proportional to the size of the charge and the proximity of the victim, but can also be modified by the environment. Detonation in a closed environment will lead to an increase in both the magnitude and duration of the wave. The shock wave can also be reflected from a solid boundary. Underwater explosions result in an increase in overpressure from reflection from the air water interface. The incompressibility of water also results in the blast waves traveling further.

New research indicates that most of the PBI results from the consequences of extreme pressure differentials developed at body surface. It is generally confined to air-containing organs and manifests with certain patterns of injury (**Table 5-1**).

2.   Secondary Blast Injury

Secondary blast injury occurs when objects accelerated by the energy of the explosion strike the victim. These objects are either primary projectiles liberated by the bomb casing (mostly found in military munitions) or secondary projectiles from environmental debris (most terrorist bombs.) The pattern of injury is in the form of penetrating wounds or traumatic amputations.

3.   Tertiary Blast Injuries

Tertiary blast injuries occur when the victim's body is thrown against a solid object. The pattern of injury

Table 5-1.   Consequences of primary blast injury

Organ System	Injury
Lung	Pulmonary contusion
	Hemopneumothorax
	Pneumothorax
	Traumatic emphysema
	Alveolovenous or bronchopulmonary fistulas
	Arterial air emboli
Gastrointestinal Tract (colon, most commonly)	Hemorrhages ranging from petechiae to large hematomas
	Rupture
Tympanic membranes	Rupture[a]

[a]Sensitive marker of significant primary blast injury unless ear protection is worn.

is similar to trauma from motor vehicle accidents or falls.

a.   Treatment of Blast Injuries. Primary blast injury is the most difficult to treat. Secondary and tertiary injuries are more obvious and present injuries similar to other trauma scenarios. Victims should be assessed for airway compromise and possible pneumothorax. Spontaneous respiration is preferred because it decreases the likelihood of arterial air emboli (AAE); however, positive pressure ventilation may be needed if respiratory compromise occurs. PBI behaves similar to pulmonary contusions. Therefore, victims should be given the highest FIO_2 possible. Blast injured lungs should be managed with techniques used for pulmonary contusion or acute respiratory distress syndrome (ARDS) with pressure-controlled ventilation and permissive hypercapnia. In evaluating different causes for shock, also consider cardiogenic shock from AAE. This is managed initially with 100% oxygen and maintaining preload. Fowler or Trendelenburg positions may increase the likelihood of cerebral or coronary AAE and should be avoided. Fluid resuscitation should be just enough to restore tissue perfusion. Abdominal evaluation is similar as performed for all trauma patients.

Older data indicate that patients with PBI have poorer outcomes if operative procedures are required within the first 24 hours. This is presumably secondary to unrecognized pneumothorax (PTX), bronchopleural fistulas, and AAE. Local, regional, or spinal anesthesia is preferred, if possible.

Observation duration for delayed complications of thoracic and abdominal PBI is unknown.

Patients without chest complaints with normal chest x-ray study and arterial blood gas are candidates for discharge after 6 hours of observation for delayed presentation for PTX and AAE. Patients who are rendered unconscious or physically felt the blast wave should be admitted for 1 to 2 days. Patients with pain, tenderness, or other indication for abdominal injury should be watched 48 to 72 hours.

F.   Decontamination

Decontamination is the process by which a chemical, biological, or radiation agent is removed or the amount is decreased so it is no longer of a threat. Two major goals of decontamination are:

- Prevent or reduce further injury to the victim
- Prevent secondary contamination of rescue personnel

SELECTED READING

Briggs SM, Brinsfield KH. Advanced Disaster Medical Response: Manual for Providers. Boston: Harvard Medical International, 2003.

Briggs SM, Leong M. Classic concepts in disaster medical response. In: Leaning J, Briggs SM, Chen LC, eds. *Humanitarian crises: the medical and public health response.* Cambridge, MA: Harvard University Press, 1999:69–79.

CDC Emergency Preparedness and Response Website: www.bt.cdc.gov

Eachempati SR, et al. Biological warfare: current concerns for the health care provider. *Journal of Trauma: Injury, Infection and Critical Care* 2002;52:179–186.

Emergency Medicine Clinics of North America 1996;14(2). (Entire issue)

Feliciano DV, et al. Management of casualties from the bombing at the centennial Olympics. *Am J Surg* 1998;176(6):538–543.

Hirshberg A, Holcomb JB, Mattox KL. Hospital trauma care in multiple-casualty incidents: a critical view. *Ann Emerg Med* 2001; 37(6):647–652.

Mettler FA, et al. Major radiation exposure—what to expect and how to respond. *N Engl J Med* 2002;346:1554–1561.

Slater MS, Trunkey DD. Terrorism in America: an evolving threat. *Arch Surg* 1997;132(10):1059–1066.

Stein M, Hirshberg A. Medical consequences of terrorism: the conventional weapon threat. *Surg Clin North Am* 1999;79(6):1537–1552.

Wightman JM et al. Explosions and blast injuries. *Ann Emerg Med* 2001;37:664–678.

Immediate Care

6

Initial Evaluation and Resuscitation: Primary Survey and Immediate Resuscitation

Shaun M. Kunisaki, MD, MSc,
and Charles J. McCabe, MD

I. **Introduction**
   A. **Background**
   The primary survey of the trauma patient follows an orderly and stepwise sequence consistent with the guidelines of Advanced Trauma Life Support (ATLS), which was first piloted and established by the American College of Surgeons (ACS) during the years 1978–1983. The popular mnemonic of airway with cervical spine (C-spine) control, breathing, circulation, disability (ABCD) serves as a practical roadmap for the initial evaluation of the injured patient. The primary survey is perhaps the most useful skill that any emergency physician or surgeon needs to master. The principles of the primary survey and resuscitation are the same regardless of whether the patient is being treated at a level I trauma center or at a small community hospital. Strict adherence to the principles of a comprehensive initial evaluation and resuscitation will avoid missing occult, but serious injuries that are associated with high morbidity and mortality.
   B. **Life-threatening Conditions**
   Successful management during the initial evaluation and resuscitation requires knowledge of the commonly identified life-threatening injuries that can occur.

   1. Airway obstruction
   2. Inadequate ventilation
      • Tension pneumothorax
      • Open pneumothorax
      • Massive hemothorax
      • Flail chest
   3. Inadequate circulation
      • Hemorrhage
      • Cardiac tamponade

   All emergency physicians and surgeons who are directing trauma resuscitations should be able to recognize these problems clinically to treat these injuries in a prompt and timely manner.
II. **Equipment and Personnel Issues**
   A. **Equipment**
   Preparation is essential to a successful trauma resuscitation. All emergency departments, regardless of their size, should dedicate a specific area within the department for most trauma resuscitations. A path should be defined from

the trauma resuscitation area to radiology, the operating suite, the intensive care unit, and the helipad. The trauma bay should have all the basic equipment necessary for successful performance of the primary survey and resuscitation. Inventory should be routinely checked to avoid not having the appropriate equipment available in an acute and life-threatening situation. Control of the airway requires that suction devices and airway adjuncts be immediately available. Suction with a large bore tonsil (Yankauer) tip allows for the clearance of blood, vomitus, and secretions that may be obstructing the airway. Magill forceps can be used to remove foreign bodies. A nasopharyngeal (NP) or oropharyngeal (OP) airway should be readily available as a temporizing measure in patients who may have problems maintaining their airway when simple maneuvers such as the chin lift or jaw thrust have failed. Cervical collars in a variety of sizes will help to ensure proper control of the C-spine if patients are brought in by paramedics with no (or a poorly fitted) collar.

Basic emergency intubation equipment and medications for a definitive airway should be readily available in case of acute respiratory decompensation. A bag-valve-mask should be at the head of the bed to preoxygenate and ventilate the patient before intubation. Laryngoscopes should be tested before patient arrival. The Macintosh no. 3 blade is a popular laryngoscope blade for orotracheal intubation. Some physicians prefer the Miller blade for orotracheal intubation because it allows an anterior or floppy epiglottis to be lifted out of the way for easier visualization of the vocal cords. Endotracheal tubes (ETT) in the appropriate sizes (i.e., 7.0, 7.5, 8.0) should always be available. Devices such as an end-tidal carbon dioxide detectors are useful to confirm endotracheal intubation. Intubation medications, including a neuroprotective agent (e.g., lidocaine), an induction agent (e.g., etomidate), and a neuromuscular blocker (e.g., succinylcholine), should be readied before patient arrival if prehospital data suggest that a definitive airway may be required. The laryngeal mask airway (LMA) can be useful as a temporizing measure following a failed intubation in a difficult airway situation.

Tension pneumothorax can lead to rapid decompensation of the trauma patient; a 14-gauge angiocatheter should be immediately available in these instances to decompress the pleural space. Thoracostomy tubes (e.g., 28F), sterile thoracostomy tube trays, and lidocaine local anesthetic should be near the bedside and ready for use.

Hemorrhage is the leading cause of shock in the trauma patient. Establishing venous access quickly is of essence. Short, large-bore intravenous (i.v.) catheters (e.g., 14 gauge or 16 gauge) are the lines of choice, given their ability to infuse fluids expeditiously. An alternative line that can be used if standard i.v. lines cannot be established is a large bore percutaneous catheter (e.g., 8.5F), which can be inserted quickly into the femoral or subclavian vein using the Seldinger technique. Warm lactated Ringer's solution should be available, given the potentially large fluid requirements needed for these patients.

B. Personnel

The trauma resuscitation team is composed of physicians, nurses, and other personnel who offer complementary skills. Ideally, the trauma team should be composed of at least three people who act as a well-organized unit. All members should be present by the time the patient arrives in the trauma bay. The horizontal approach, which involves multiple tasks being performed simultaneously as opposed to sequentially, works well in the university setting. For example, the team leader can be assessing the patient's airway while the intravenous lines are established. At the same time, another person can insert a chest tube or Foley catheter. Obviously, smaller hospital emergency departments may not have the luxury of having multiple individuals available to perform simultaneous care. In such cases, the physician is left to perform the initial evaluation and resuscitation in a sequential manner in accordance with the protocols outlined in this chapter.

One often forgotten but important aspect of trauma resuscitations is strict compliance with universal precautions. Standard barrier protection should include gown, gloves, and facial protection. Accidental exposure represents a real risk to the trauma resuscitation team, given the high incidence of hepatitis and human immunodeficiency virus (HIV) present in the population affected by trauma.

III. Preparation for Patient Arrival

A. Designated Team Leader

A trauma team should be available 24 hours a day within the hospital. An experienced team leader is critical to an efficient resuscitation. The leader stands at the head of the bed and sets the tone for the rest of the team. This person assumes ultimate responsibility and authority for all management decisions. At larger teaching hospitals, a senior resident from emergency medicine or surgery will typically be delegated the role as the team leader. At the Massachusetts General Hospital, the responsibilities of the team leader during the initial resuscitation include, but are not limited to, the following.

1. Obtaining prehospital history (including allergies, medications, medical history)
2. Assuming control of the airway, if necessary
3. Performing the primary survey and calling out examination findings to the nurse recorder
4. Proceeding with the secondary survey only after the primary survey has been completed
5. Designating individuals to perform specific procedures (e.g., venous access, chest tube, rectal exam, bladder catheterization, abdominal ultrasound)
6. Making all initial management decisions
7. Communicating directly with the trauma chief resident and attending physician

B.   Transition from Prehospital to Hospital Care

At the Massachusetts General Hospital, trauma cases are initially graded based on the acuity of injury. The three grades are (a) trauma stat, (b) trauma alert, and (c) trauma consult. *Trauma stat* cases have a high index of suspicion for requiring immediate operative management and, therefore, each case mandates maximal mobilization of hospital personnel for availability as the patient arrives in the trauma bay. *Trauma alert* cases raise concern for possible immediate operative management and, therefore, each requires mobilization of members of the in-house trauma service when the patient arrives in the bay. Examples of injuries warranting a trauma alert grading include stab wounds to the neck, chest, or abdomen; major pelvic fractures; multiple long bone fractures; Glasgow Coma Scale (GCS) score of less than 13; extensive maxillofacial trauma; and transfers of multisystem trauma. All less life-threatening injuries are given the *trauma consult* grading.

Obtaining an accurate and concise account of the events of the trauma and the prehospital course are important components to initiating a successful primary survey and resuscitation. This exchange of information, which can be valuable to the trauma resuscitation team, takes only 30 to 60 seconds to obtain. To avoid pandemonium, all team members should be quiet while emergency medical service (EMS) personnel are speaking directly to the designated trauma team leader.

The EMS presentation typically begins with the patient age, sex, and the mechanism of injury. If the patient was involved in a motor vehicle event, details of the crash can give insight into increased risks for significant injury. High-speed collision, rollover, ejection from the vehicle, prolonged extrication time, and death of a passenger heighten concern for serious injury. Significant vehicular body damage and a bent steering wheel, which also imply high-energy mechanisms, are associated with an increased risk for severe injury. EMS personnel give information to whether the patient was restrained or whether airbags were deployed. Relevant details regarding gunshot or stab wounds include the anatomic location of the injury as well as the exact weapon used.

The patient's complaints while in the field are presented. Hemodynamics (blood pressure, pulse, respiratory rate) and neurologic status (loss of consciousness, GCS score) at the scene and on route to the hospital are then described. A brief report of the physical examination highlighting any significant findings is given. Finally, any EMS interventions on route are relayed to the trauma team. Typically, this includes any sizes of i.v. catheters placed and amounts of fluids infused, which are important data. If the patient was intubated on route or at an outside facility, the trauma team needs to be informed of the size of the ETT as well as the names and times of any medications (e.g. sedatives, paralytics) that were given. All lines and tubes should be assessed for *position* and *patency* during the resuscitation. Tubes should be *pluralized*.

Finally, a brief history known by the mnemonic, AMPLE, developed at Cook County Hospital is obtained: **a**llergies, **m**edications (especially, use of anticoagulants such as warfarin [Coumadin; Dupont, Wilmington, DE], beta-blockers), **p**ast medical history (e.g., coronary artery disease, asthma, diabetes), **l**ast meal, and **e**vents leading to the accident (e.g., antecedent alcohol/drug use) are all useful information to know when conducting the primary survey.

IV. Primary Survey
   A. Basic Framework
   The primary survey represents the first of the four major phases in the management of the trauma patient.

   1. Primary survey
   2. Resuscitation
   3. Secondary survey
   4. Definitive care

   The four-phase progression affords the trauma team the opportunity to conceptualize and prioritize the myriad tasks required in a successful resuscitation. In actuality, primary survey and resuscitation occur in parallel or simultaneously. As outlined by the ATLS, the secondary survey does not begin until the primary survey is completed, resuscitative efforts are well established, and the patient is demonstrating normalization of vital functions. Admission for observation, intensive care monitoring, operative procedures, and transfers to a specialized trauma center for further management all fall under definitive care.

   The sequence of the initial evaluation is commonly referred to as the "ABCD" of trauma care:

   • **A**irway with C-spine control
   • **B**reathing
   • **C**irculation with hemorrhage control
   • **D**isability

   If done correctly, the primary survey will take as little as 1 to 2 minutes to perform in most uncomplicated trauma patients. Strict adherence to a memorized algorithm for the initial assessment will help to avoid errors.

   B. Airway Evaluation and Immediate Interventions
      1. Initial Assessment and Management
      A severely injured patient with airway compromise can deteriorate rapidly. Identifying airway obstruction is always the first task of the trauma team during the primary survey. The team leader should know the maneuvers to maintain a patent airway. This includes recognizing the need for endotracheal intubation, performance of a rapid sequence intubation (RSI), and indications for a surgical airway.

      Initial resuscitation begins by looking at basic signs of a possibly obstructed airway (e.g., gasping and stridor). Gasping implies oropharyngeal airway obstruction, whereas stridor suggests partial occlusion of the trachea. Getting the patient to speak by asking a simple question (e.g., What is your name? What hurts right now?) is a useful first step. Good phonation suggests that the patent's airway is clear. Blood and vomitus can be cleared from the oropharynx with suctioning. Foreign bodies can be removed with forceps or two fingers.

Lethargic patients may have posterior displacement of the tongue, leading to airway obstruction. In these cases, simple maneuvers (e.g., chin lift or jaw thrust) will alleviate the situation. The chin lift is performed by placing the fingertips beneath the patient's chin and lifting the chin forward. The jaw thrust involves placing the thumb on the mandibular rami and pushing the jaw forward. Airway adjuncts are temporizing measures in maintaining an airway if immediate intubation is not required. The NP is better tolerated in an awake patient.

The LMA can be a valuable adjunct as a temporary airway until a more definitive airway is established. This device consists of an irregular silicone mask with an inflatable rim that provides a seal over the larynx. The LMA, thus, allows ventilation of the trachea with minimal gastric distention.

Extensive maxillofacial trauma, facial burns, and inhalation injuries can lead to edema of the upper airway. In these cases, early establishment of a definitive airway through intubation may be the only reasonable therapeutic option.

2. Definitive Airways

Besides airway obstruction, four other absolute indications for emergent intubation of the trauma patient during the primary survey exist.

a. Apnea
b. Inadequate oxygenation and ventilation
c. Inability to protect the airway (usually, GCS score of ≤8)
d. Need to perform necessary diagnostic studies in an uncooperative or unattended patient

The details of intubation are discussed elsewhere in this book. Orotracheal intubation is the definitive airway of choice in the emergency department, because it is the most widely practiced procedure and has minimal morbidity. Orotracheal intubation, however, is not successful in managing all airway problems in the trauma setting. Thus, it is essential to be familiar with alternative airways because they can be life saving.

Blind nasotracheal intubation has many advocates and is supported as a method for endotracheal intubation by ATLS. It allows for the least manipulation of the C-spine and is successful in experienced hands. Nasotracheal intubation is best tolerated in conscious patients who are spontaneously breathing. Major contraindications to nasotracheal intubation are apnea, coagulation defects, and the presence of midface or basilar skull fractures.

If intubation is not successful and the patient cannot be adequately mask ventilated, an emergent surgical airway must be established. Cricothyroidotomy is preferable to tracheostomy because the landmarks are more clearly defined. In addition, cricothyroidotomy takes less time to perform and is associated with less bleeding. Nevertheless, all surgical airways can be challenging to perform because of the often difficult anatomy (in the setting of the inability to extend the patient's possibly injured C-spine) and high stress conditions. An assistant can be helpful when conducting these procedures.

Cricothyroidotomy can be accomplished by either needle or surgical approaches. The neck is prepared and local anesthetic is given, if the patient is conscious. The needle technique is performed by placing a 12- or 14-gauge needle catheter attached to a syringe through the cricothyroid membrane into the trachea at a 45-degree caudal direction. Once air is aspirated, the cannula is advanced and connected to 15 L of oxygen under 15 parts per square inch (PSI) of pressure using a Y-connecter. Exhalation occurs through the normal route. Needle cricothyroidotomy, however, is only temporary. In the best scenario, ventilation is inadequate and hypercarbia is inevitable after 30 to 40 minutes. Thus, all needle cricothyroidotomies need to be urgently converted to a more definite airway. Jet insufflation is contraindicated in complete airway obstruction because no means exists for exhalation and barotrauma can result in a tension pneumothorax.

Adequate oxygenation and ventilation can be accomplished with a surgical cricothyroidotomy. This technique involves making a horizontal or vertical incision that exposes the cricothyroid membrane. A scalpel handle, curved hemostat, or tracheal spreader is then used to perforate the membrane. A no. 6 cuffed ETT or tracheostomy tube is placed into the trachea and secured in place. The major contraindications to surgical cricothyroidotomy occur with younger children (the cricoid is the sole support of the upper airway in children) and patients with complete laryngotracheal disruption. The role for emergent tracheostomy in the trauma patient is somewhat controversial. Tracheostomy may be indicated in laryngeal fractures, suggested by the triad of hoarseness, subcutaneous emphysema, and a palpable fracture.

3. Cervical Spine Control

All patients should be considered to have spine fracture until proved otherwise. Prehospital personnel usually immobilize the C-spine with a hard collar. C-spine protection should always be maintained to prevent further injury to a potentially fractured spine during manipulation of the airway. In-line cervical immobilization by an assistant with the collar off is essential during all airway maneuvers, including orotracheal intubation and cricothyroidotomy.

C. Breathing Evaluation and Immediate Interventions

1.   Initial Assessment and Management

After the airway is deemed to be patent, the primary survey shifts to the evaluation of the chest to ensure the adequacy of breathing and ventilation. Oxygen saturation should be monitored. The chest should be exposed and its movement observed. Four potentially life-threatening mechanical chest wall injuries should be identified during this phase of the evaluation.

1.   Tension pneumothorax
2.   Open pneumothorax
3.   Massive hemothorax
4.   Flail chest

All four of these injuries should be identified clinically and addressed promptly *before* radiographs are taken of the unstable patient. Chest wall inspection for penetrating chest wounds may reveal an open pneumothorax. Auscultation for equal axillary breath sounds bilaterally is useful and should always be performed. Absent or diminished breath sounds should raise the possibility for a pneumothorax or hemothorax on the ipsilateral side. In the intubated patient, absent left axillary breath sounds may denote a right mainstem intubation. Percussion of the chest wall may demonstrate hyperresonance or dullness, suggestive of tension pneumothorax or massive hemothorax, respectively. Palpation of the chest wall, paying attention to asymmetric chest wall expansion, fractures, crepitus, and unstable rib segments (i.e., flail chest), may suggest significant underlying chest pathology. Inspection of the neck for a deviated trachea and jugular venous distention can be seen in tension pneumothorax. Oxygen saturation should be monitored. A normal physical examination, combined with good oxygen saturation on the pulse oximeter, are reassuring that breathing is adequate in the trauma patient.

2.   Four Life-threatening Chest Injuries

Tension pneumothorax occurs when there is a laceration of the pleura from penetrating trauma or fractured ribs. It can also be caused by a ruptured bronchus or alveolus from the high intrathoracic pressure against a closed glottis. On inspiration, air enters the pleural cavity, but the one-way valve effect of the injury does not allow expiration of the intrapleural gas. The tension ultimately leads to shifting of the mediastinum to the contralateral side and kinking of the vena cava. Venous return is impaired and cardiovascular collapse ensues. Tension pneumothorax is a clinical diagnosis. The classic signs of tension pneumothorax are cyanosis, hypotension, tracheal deviation, jugular venous distention, subcutaneous emphysema, absent breath sounds, and tympany on percussion. Do not wait for a chest radiograph if adequate clinical evidence exists for a tension pneumothorax and the patient is in shock or respiratory distress.

Treatment of a tension pneumothorax in an unstable patient always starts with initial conversion to an open pneumothorax using a 14-gauge angiocatheter in the second intercostal space along the midclavicular line. In both stable and unstable patients, tension pneumothorax requires tube thoracostomy. First, the chest wall is inspected and any chest scars are recognized. The physician should then infiltrate with 1% lidocaine over the 5th and 6th ribs along the midaxillary line. A transverse incision is made with a scalpel over the 6th rib, and a tunnel is created superiorly and posteriorly with a Kelly clamp over the 5th rib to avoid the neurovascular bundle. The pleural space is entered and digitally explored to assure entrance into the thoracic cavity. A large-bore chest tube is guided into the hole and aimed at the posterior apex. The chest tube is sutured in place with heavy suture and connected to suction. Positive-pressure ventilation can convert a simple pneumothorax to a tension pneumothorax

Open pneumothorax occurs with a penetrating chest wound into the thoracic cavity. On inspiration, air enters the pleural cavity through the chest wound, leading to collapse of the ipsilateral lung. An upright end-expiratory chest radiograph may reveal an otherwise occult pneumothorax in the stable patient. Immediate treatment of an open pneumothorax includes sealing the defect with Vaseline gauze and sterile dressing taped on three sides to allow air to be evacuated through the wound. A chest tube should urgently be placed at a remote site on the ipsilateral side to avoid tension pneumothorax. Large wounds may require formal closure in the operating room.

The third life-threatening chest injury, massive hemothorax, is defined by blood in the pleural cavity. Minor hemothoraces are caused by trauma to the lung parenchyma, whereas massive hemothoraces are usually secondary to lacerations of intrathoracic vessels (e.g., the intercostal, internal mammary, or pulmonary artery). The patient may present may be hypotension and no breath sounds and dullness to percussion on physical examination. Treatment of a hemothorax includes emergent placement of a large-bore chest tube into the fifth or sixth intercostal space in the midaxillary line. A pleurovacuum should be connected to an autotransfuser, given the potential for significant blood loss. All blood needs to be evacuated from the pleural space to prevent formation of fibrinous material in the pleural space with entrapment of adjacent lung. Consideration for emergent thoracotomy is given if the initial output is greater than 1500 mL or more than 200 mL/h output occurs for 4 consecutive hours. Beware that no output or an abrupt decrease in output may mean an occluded chest tube.

The final life-threatening chest injury, flail chest, is defined as a freely moving segment of chest wall. Blunt chest trauma causes fractures of at least three sequential ribs, with fractures occurring in two places along the same rib creating a free floating chest wall. Many flail chests can be difficult to detect clinically because of splinting by the patient. The fundamental problem with a flail chest is the high likelihood of significant underlying pulmonary contusion. Respiratory compromise from the often-described paradoxical (inward) movement of the chest wall on inspiration. Immediate management of a flail chest is required only in cases of significant respiratory distress. Such cases may require intubation with positive pressure ventilation, which is required in about half of all patients. All patients will ultimately require aggressive pain control (e.g., rib blocks, epidural anesthesia) and aggressive pulmonary toilet on admission to the hospital.

D. Circulatory Evaluation and Immediate Interventions

1. Initial Assessment and Management

After the airway and breathing are evaluated and secured, the primary survey shifts to an evaluation of the circulatory system. The major goal of this phase of the primary survey is to identify and treat shock, defined as inadequate tissue perfusion. The last potentially life-threatening injury, pericardial tamponade, is also addressed. As a general rule, if the patient has a normal neurologic status and has warm extremities, perfusion is probably adequate. A patient who is cool and tachycardic is in shock until proved otherwise. Nurses should obtain a blood pressure and heart rate at the earliest possible time during the resuscitation. A more formal assessment of circulation includes checking for palpable pulses. Palpable carotid, femoral, and radial pulses suggest systolic blood pressures of at least 60, 70, and 80 mm Hg, respectively. Muffled heart sounds may signify pericardial tamponade. Although tachycardia is neither a sensitive nor specific indicator of shock, any heart rate greater than 120 bpm should be considered hypovolemic shock until proved otherwise. All external bleeding sites should be identified by cutting off all clothing. External bleeding should be controlled to the greatest extent possible using firm pressure.

If possible, someone should always be designated to obtain venous access as soon as the patient arrives in the trauma bay. The trauma patient needs at least two short, large-bore (14 or 16 gauge) peripheral i.v. catheters. Poiseuille's law dictates that flow is inversely related to length and proportional to the fourth power of the radius of the cannula. The antecubital veins are the most reliable sites for prompt venous access. Cannulation into an obviously fractured extremity should be avoided. If adequate peripheral access is unobtainable in an expedient manner, access should be obtained via the modified Seldinger technique using a percutaneous, single lumen 8.5F introducer line into the subclavian, internal jugular, or femoral vein. Subclavian or internal jugular access is useful in many cases of penetrating chest trauma. The Massachusetts General Hospital favors the femoral vein in circumstances in which exist space constraints at the head of the bed and a risk of pneumothoraces associated with lines placed into the neck or chest in an emergent fashion. Potential abdominal injury is not a contraindication to lower extremity access. Many institutions favor saphenous vein cutdowns. Ultimately, the choice of venous access is dependent on the skill and experience of the physician.

Few laboratory tests change the initial management of the trauma patient. Nevertheless, blood work should be taken quickly once access is obtained and sent to the laboratory for analysis. Hematocrit is not sensitive for acute blood loss. The blood bank sample is perhaps the most critical tube because of the potential desire to transfuse type-specific blood in the hemorrhaging trauma patient. Stat blood work, including the hematocrit level, coagulation parameters, toxicology panel, human chorionic gonadotrophin ([hCG] for all women of childbearing age), and glucose, should also be sent because they may help to guide management after the primary survey.

All patients suspected of being in shock should be given a fluid challenge of 2 L of warm crystalloid as a bolus immediately after i.v. access is obtained. This maneuver will improve the hemodynamics of patients who had bleeding that had since ceased. Those who have no response or a transient response may have ongoing blood loss or cardiac tamponade. As a general rule, 3 mL of isotonic crystalloid is required to replace 1 mL of whole blood loss. Continued hypotension or tachycardia raises the issue of hemorrhagic shock, missed tension pneumothorax, or pericardial tamponade.

2. Hemorrhagic Shock

The most common cause of shock in the trauma patient is hemorrhagic (hypovolemic) shock. This state results from the loss of whole blood or of plasma and extracellular fluid, as is seen in the burn or crush injury patient. Significant internal hemorrhaging can occur in a variety of places in the trauma patient. Lethal internal spaces for exsanguination are in the abdomen cavity, retroperitoneum (4000 mL), hemithorax (2500 mL), femur (1500 mL), and tibia or humerus (750 mL). Abdominal ultrasound is becoming the standard for bedside evaluation of hemoperitoneum and hemothorax.

Major bleeding from scalp lacerations can require rapid suturing or stapling for control. Bleeding reduces intravascular volume, leading to decreased preload and stroke volume. Tissue perfusion becomes inadequate once the body's compensatory mechanisms are overwhelmed and cardiac output decreases. The treatment of hemorrhagic shock is restoration of intravascular volume and control of ongoing hemorrhage. Use of vasopressors in an effort to improve blood pressure is contraindicated in hemorrhagic shock. Vasopressors merely increase peripheral vascular resistance and aggravate the cellular derangement of cellular hypoperfusion.

The magnitude of the physiologic insult is directly proportional to the volume of blood that is shed. The American College of Surgeons (ACS) has developed a shock classification system to help identify and manage patients in hemorrhagic shock. Most individuals can easily compensate for a 15% or less reduction in blood volume by baroreceptor-mediated reflex vasoconstriction and tachycardia and increased levels of norepinephrine. Signs or symptoms on physical examination may be minimal. These individuals are categorized as class I hemorrhagic shock. Isotonic crystalloid (2 L) is usually sufficient for these patients.

Patients with a 15% to 30% reduction in blood volume can sustain a normal perfusion pressure if they remain supine, but cardiac output is reduced and postural hypotension develops if they stand suddenly. They may be tachycardic and have a narrow pulse pressure. Blood flow to the heart and brain remains preserved, whereas visceral blood flow is reduced. These individuals are categorized as class II hemorrhagic shock. Blood transfusions are considered for these patients, although 4 L of isotonic crystalloid may be sufficient for resuscitation of these patients. Additional i.v. access may be required.

The response to a substantial blood loss (30% to 40% of blood volume) is class III hemorrhagic shock. Patients have frank hypotension, diaphoresis, and confusion. Pressure bags and rapid infusers should be set up to deliver up to 1500 mL/minute of fluid. The blood bank should be notified emergently for blood transfusion of O(–) packed red blood cells. Rh(–) cells are preferred for women of childbearing age.

Those who have lost more than 40% of blood volume (class IV hemorrhagic shock) are at imminent risk of death. They are usually obtunded and experience precipitous death if intravascular volume is not quickly restored with volume and blood products. Massive blood transfusion into patients who sustained great blood loss may be required until control of hemorrhage is accomplished. In circumstances of massive transfusion, adjunctive infusion of other blood products (e.g., fresh frozen plasma, platelets) and calcium may be required. Operative intervention to stop blood loss is likely in this setting.

The role of colloid in the resuscitation of the hemorrhaging trauma patient remains somewhat controversial. Colloid-containing solutions (e.g., albumin, hetastarch, and dextrans) have long been advocated for volume expansion. Supporters of colloid argue that larger solutes are better retained in the intravascular space. They also believe that crystalloids can cause hemodilution of serum proteins and reduce plasma oncotic pressure, resulting in extravasation of fluid into the pulmonary interstitium.

Nevertheless, despite decades of scrutiny, crystalloid continues to be the fluid of choice at most institutions because it is readily available, inexpensive, and has low infectious risk. Although colloid solutions can achieve, with less volume of infusate, an equivalent expansion of intravascular volume than a substantially larger volume of infused crystalloids, several randomized controlled trials, analyzed in a meta-analysis, do not support the conclusion that colloids achieve superior outcome, including survival, as a resuscitation fluid. Hemoglobin-based red blood cell substitutes remain an active area of investigation.

Lactated Ringer's solution is favored over normal saline (0.9%) as the isotonic fluid of choice because the higher chloride in normal saline has the potential to cause hyperchloremic metabolic acidosis. Other crystalloid products, particularly hypertonic saline (7.5%, 4 mL/kg) with or without dextran, continue to be investigated as potentially better resuscitative agents. One concern with conventional isotonic crystalloids is that infusion of large volumes increases cerebral edema and intracranial pressure in patients with traumatic brain injury. Small volume infusions of hypertonic saline have been shown in laboratory studies to produce rapid volume expansion and improve cerebral hemodynamics after hemorrhagic shock. To date, however, no human study has documented the superiority of hypertonic saline in trauma patients.

3.   Other Causes of Shock in the Emergency Department

Although hemorrhagic shock is the most common cause of shock in the trauma patient, other causes of shock can be encountered during the primary survey. The other common causes identified in the emergency department are:

1.   Cardiogenic shock
2.   Obstructive shock
3.   Neurogenic shock
4.   Septic shock

Cardiogenic shock is defined as the inability of the heart to maintain adequate tissue perfusion, because of intrinsic pump failure. Cardiogenic shock is most readily recognized by chest discomfort, pulmonary edema, and electrocardiogram abnormalities. This form of shock most commonly occurs in the elderly patient with an acute myocardial infarction or ventricular arrhythmia that either precipitated or resulted from the trauma. Shock can also occur via blunt chest trauma, leading to a myocardial contusion. Penetrating trauma to the heart can lead to cardiogenic shock from laceration of the heart into a chamber (usually the right ventricle) or transection of a coronary artery. Emergency bedside echocardiography may help to confirm the presence of cardiogenic shock. Initial therapy for cardiogenic shock, which depends on the underlying cause of the pump dysfunction, can include use of inotropic agents (e.g., dopamine, dobutamine, and norepinephrine) in an intensive care unit setting.

Obstructive shock includes tension pneumothorax and pericardial tamponade. This form of shock is an important, often under-recognized, form of shock in the trauma patient who arrives into the emergency department. Intrinsic pump function is preserved and intravascular volume may be normal in obstructive shock. Nonetheless, the heart is unable to generate adequate cardiac output because of mechanical obstruction. Tension pneumothorax leads to shifting of the mediastinum to the contralateral side, kinking of the venae cavae, and impaired venous return. This problem can only be recognized quickly with a high index of suspicion for tension pneumothorax in anyone who presents with shock.

Pericardial tamponade is a common cause of obstructive shock that typically occurs after penetrating chest trauma within the "precordial box," defined as the area between the midclavicular lines, the clavicles, and the costal margin. Blood in the pericardial space leads to poor ventricular filling and, therefore, reduced stroke volume. Tamponade can be recognized clinically by Beck's triad, which consists of distended neck veins, hypotension (especially, narrowed pulse pressure), and distant heart sounds. Beck's triad, however, is only about 40% sensitive. Heart sounds can be difficult to hear in a noisy trauma bay, and distended neck veins may not be present if the patient is hypovolemic. Suspected cases can now be confirmed using bedside ultrasound by placing the probe in the subxiphoid position. Transient improvement in hemodynamics can be provided in the unstable patient by aspirating fluid via subxiphoid pericardiocentesis using a 30- to 60-mL syringe and a long 18-gauge needle directed toward the left shoulder at a 45-degree angle.

This procedure, however, is usually unsuccessful in draining blood. Further treatment of pericardial tamponade may require a subxiphoid pericardial window or emergency thoracotomy and pericardiotomy, ideally performed in the operating room.

Neurogenic shock in the setting of acute spinal cord injuries results in hypotension because of decreased sympathetic tone. Isolated head injuries do not cause neurogenic shock. Bradycardia, as opposed to tachycardia, is a unique cardiovascular manifestation of neurogenic shock. Paraplegia and loss of the bulbocavernous (S5) reflex (observed by loss of rectal tone while squeezing the glans of the penis or tugging on the Foley catheter) support the diagnosis of neurogenic shock. Initial treatment of neurogenic shock is fluid resuscitation because of the relative hypovolemic state. Further therapy includes the use of vasopressors, atropine, and cardiac pacing.

The last form of shock, septic shock, consists of the triad of leaky capillaries, low systemic vascular resistance, and myocardial dysfunction. This form of shock is caused by the systemic release of inflammatory mediators (e.g., endotoxin, tumor necrosis factor [TNF], interleukin IL-1, and IL-2. The net result is a hyperdynamic states characterized by peripheral vasodilatation and third spacing of fluids. Septic shock is not a common cause of shock in the trauma patient resuscitated in the emergency department. Nevertheless, it can be seen in patients having delayed resuscitation. Treatment of septic shock consists of fluid resuscitation, vasopressors (e.g., phenylephrine or norepinephrine), and treatment of the underlying cause. Antibiotics and surgical drainage can also be helpful.

4.   Emergency Department Thoracotomy

The precise role of an emergency department thoracotomy in the resuscitation of the trauma patient continues to undergo evolution. Currently, a clear role exists for emergency thoracotomy in penetrating chest trauma with signs of life (i.e., agonal respirations, cardiac electrical activity, reactive pupils) within 5 minutes before arrival to the emergency department. These patients often present with pulseless electrical activity without evidence of pneumothorax. The chest is rapidly opened through a left anterolateral approach (inferior nipple to posterior axillary line), with minimal skin preparation. For isolated injuries to the right chest, a right thoracotomy or median sternotomy is an acceptable alternative incision. Other team members simultaneously secure the airway and achieve venous access. In a recent meta-analysis, the overall survival rate in all patients having emergency department thoracotomy after blunt or penetrating trauma was only 7.4%.

After the chest is opened, the physician has the opportunity to perform the following:

1. Occlusion of the descending aorta to increase perfusion to the heart and brain and possibly decrease distal hemorrhage
2. Longitudinal pericardiotomy anterior to the phrenic nerve, with delivery of the heart from the pericardial sac
3. Internal cardiac massage
4. Control of thoracic hemorrhage

Cardiac wounds can be digitally controlled en route to the operating room. Stab wounds have the best outcomes.

The survival rate can be as high as 50% for those who arrive with signs of life and then have cardiac arrest in the hospital after a single stab wound to the left chest.

More controversial is the role of thoracotomy in blunt injury with loss of vital signs in the trauma bay. Survival of patients without signs of life after multiple injuries resulting from blunt trauma have been reported, but is extremely rare even in the best of hands. In addition, the high costs associated with the procedure, including loss of patient dignity, infectious risks to healthcare providers, and waste of hospital resources, make it difficult to justify performing the procedure on a liberal basis. Patients sustaining blunt injuries with loss of signs of life before arrival in the trauma bay are not candidates for thoracotomy.

E. Disability Evaluation and Immediate Interventions

One of the final components to the initial evaluation and resuscitation of the trauma patient is the brief neurologic examination. An abbreviated neurologic examination as part of the primary assessment will identify significant intracranial injuries that may require an emergent neurosurgical intervention. The examiner should ask the patient to "open your eyes". The GCS score is then calculated by determining the patient's verbal response and gross motor function. The three components to the GCS are as follows:

1. Eye opening
   - Spontaneous (E4)
   - To speech (E3)
   - To pain (E2)
   - None (E1)
2. Best motor response
   - Obeys: moves limb to command (M6)
   - Localizes to painful stimulus (M5)
   - Withdraws away from pain (M4)
   - Decorticate (M3)
   - Decerebrate (M2)
   - No movement (M1)

3. Verbal response
    - Oriented (V5)
    - Confused conversation (V4)
    - Inappropriate or random words (V3)
    - Incomprehensible sounds (V2)
    - None (V1)

All patients with a GCS score of ≤8 require immediate intubation to protect the airway. Intubation in these patients can also be helpful in the treatment of secondary brain injury from hypoxia and allows for mild hyperventilation to decrease intracranial pressure. Patients who arrive to the hospital already intubated obviously cannot have a verbal response. Thus, these patients have a best possible score of T11.

Pupils should be checked in all patients for symmetry and responsiveness. An ipsilateral fixed and dilated pupil, contralateral hemiparesis, and decerebrate posturing are indicative of tentorial herniation. Signs of impending central herniation are seen with the findings of hypertension, bradycardia, and irregular respirations (Cushing's triad). An emergent neurosurgery consult should be obtained at this point in the trauma evaluation for any GCS score <12, localizing signs, or other evidence for brain herniation.

V. **Common Traps in Conducting the Primary Survey**
    A. **Airway**
    - Failure to manage the airway early
    - "There is no shambles like an airway shambles"— failure to have a back-up plan with an anticipated difficult airway
    - Failure to enlist the help of anesthesia, when needed
    - Failure to immobilize the C-spine during airway procedures
    B. **Breathing**
    - Failure to identify tension pneumothorax on clinical examination
    - Failure to use a large-bore chest tube in cases of hemothorax
    C. **Circulation**
    - Inadequate i.v. access
    - Inadequate fluid resuscitation
    - Failure to notify the blood bank early
    - Failure to appreciate penetrating abdominal trauma and hemoperitoneum
    - Failure to look for an injury in the axilla or perineum
    - Injudicious use of the emergency thoracotomy
    D. **Disability**
    - Attributing a change in mental status to drug or alcohol use
    - Failure to involve neurosurgery early in the case
    E. **General**
    - Lack of leadership during the trauma resuscitation
    - Delay in transferring a patient to a trauma center
    - Failure to involve a surgeon early in the case

- Failure to appreciate the low physiologic reserves of the elderly
- Proceeding with the secondary survey without completing the primary survey
- "Death begins in x-ray"—sending an unstable patient to radiology

SELECTED READING

American College of Surgeon Committee on Trauma. *Advanced trauma life support for doctors,* 6th ed. Chicago: American College of Surgeons, 1997.

Nolan J. Fluid resuscitation for the trauma patient. *Resuscitation* 2001;48:57–69.

Rhee PM, Acosta J, Bridgeman A, et al. Survival after emergency department thoracotomy: review of published data from the past 25 years. *J Am Coll Surg* 2000;190:288–298.

Sims CA, Wattanasirichaingoon S, Menconi MJ, et al. Ringer's ethyl pyruvate solution ameliorates ischemia/reperfusion-induced intestinal mucosal injury in rates. *Crit Care Med* 2001;29:1513–1518.

Wade CE, Kramer CG, Grady JJ, et al. Efficacy of hypertonic 7.5% saline and 6% dextran-70 in treating trauma: a meta-analysis of controlled studies. *Surgery* 1997;122:609–616.

Younes RN, Aun F, Accioly CQ, et al. Hypertonic solutions in the treatment of hypovolemic shock: a prospective, randomized study in patients admitted to the emergency room. *Surgery* 1992;111:380–385.

The Trauma Airway

Harish S. Lecamwasam, MD, MSc,
Ruben Peralta, MD, and Peter F. Dunn, MD

I. Introduction

The specific technique used for airway management depends on the type and degree of trauma suffered. For example, the presence of a basilar skull fracture precludes the use of nasotracheal intubation. Extensive facial trauma may preclude orotracheal intubation, necessitating cricothyroidotomy or tracheostomy (section VI.B.). Neck trauma (blunt or penetrating) may necessitate the use of an awake fiberoptic technique for the placement of an endotracheal tube (ETT) (section VI.A.1.).

Regardless of the specific trauma incurred, the initial step in the management of an airway is the administration of supplemental oxygen and, if indicated, ventilatory support.

II. Evaluation of the Trauma Airway

    A. History

        1. The Trauma

        Nature of Trauma, e.g. a motor vehicle collision, restrained versus unrestrained, frontal collision, loss of consciousness, scope of injuries, and so on before encountering the patient (see Chapter 6, *Initial Evaluation and Resuscitation*).

        2. Difficulties Managing the Patient's Airway En-route to the Hospital

        3. Pertinent Medical Information

    B. Initial Assessment

        1. Vital Signs

        Evaluate vital signs, and airway, breathing, circulation, and neurologic status (ABCN).

        2. Airway Management Devices

        Note presence of any airway management devices (e.g., ETT, cuffed oropharyngeal airway) and their adequate function.

        3. Points of Intravenous Access

    C. Examination

        1. A trauma patient should be carefully inspected for signs of evidence of facial fractures, bleeding and soft tissue swelling, all of which can make mask ventilation and orotracheal intubation challenging.

        2. If cervical spine (C-spine) injury has not been ruled out, care must be taken to maintain C-spine stability during this examination.

        3. Establishing an adequate airway can be difficult in the presence of the following:

            1. Facial fractures (see Chapter 16, *Evaluation and Acute Management of Maxillofacial Trauma*)

            2. Blood, vomitus, secretions, or foreign bodies in the oropharynx or larynx

3. Disruption of laryngeal, glottic, or tracheal anatomy
4. C-spine injury
   - Positioning the patient to optimize laryngoscopy (the "sniffing position" [see section V.C.1.e) can be difficult or impossible with cervical spine immobilization (cervical collar, traction).
   - Distortion of anatomy from hematoma or disruption of an unstable cervical spine.

4. Specific findings in addition to factors associated with the trauma that can predispose to a difficult airway include:

1. Inability to open the mouth
2. C-spine immobility caused by preexisting disease (e.g., cervical fusion)
3. Short thyromental distance (distance from the notch of the thyroid cartilage to the mentum with the neck maximally extended. A normal thyromental distance is considered to be 6 cm (approximately four fingerbreadths).
4. Receding chin (micrognathia)
5. Large tongue (macroglossia)
6. Prominent incisors
7. Short, muscular neck
8. Morbid obesity

5. The Mallampati classification can be used to predict the difficulty of visualizing the glottis during direct laryngoscopy. This classification is based on the finding that glottic visualization is impaired when the base of the tongue is disproportionately large compared with the mouth opening. Assess with the patient sitting upright, with the head in a neutral position, the mouth open as wide as possible, and the tongue protruded maximally without phonation. The modified Mallampati classification includes four categories.

1. Class I: Faucial pillars, soft palate, and uvula are visible.
2. Class II: Faucial pillars and soft palate may be seen, but uvula is masked by the base of the tongue.
3. Class III: Only soft palate is visible; intubation is predicted to be difficult.
4. Class IV: Soft palate not visible; intubation predicted to be difficult.

6. Poor dentition can increase the risk of tooth injury or loss during airway manipulation. If time permits, identify loose teeth and protect or remove them before initiation of airway management.
7. Assess the mobility of laryngeal structures. The trachea should be palpable in the midline above the sternal notch.
8. Look for scars from previous neck surgery, an enlarged thyroid, or other paratracheal masses.

9. If a patient's C-spine has been medically cleared of fracture, assess the patient's cervical mobility. Patients should be able to touch their chin to their chest and extend their neck posteriorly. Lateral rotation should not produce pain or paresthesia.

D. Laboratory Assessment

Typically, a history and physical examination are sufficient for the initial assessment of most airways. However, useful adjuncts may include:

1. Radiographs (chest and C-spine series) or computerized tomograms may reveal tracheal injury or deviation.

2. Arterial blood gas assessments may reveal patients who are hypoxemic (especially in cold or vasocontricted patients in whom pulse oxymetry may be unreliable) or hypercarbic.

III. Airway Management

Delayed gastric emptying and the absence of fasting place trauma patients at high risk for aspiration of gastric contents. Therefore, the definitive control of their airway requires the placement and use of a cuffed ETT.

A. Nonemergent Airway Management

1. A trauma patient who is conscious, able to speak; follow commands; and has adequate respirations and stable vital signs most likely is not in need of emergent airway management.

2. Unconscious patients who are maintaining their airway (adequate respiratory rate and tidal volume, adequate pulse oximetry saturation, and reasonable PO_2, PCO_2 and pH with arterial blood gas assessment) may not need emergent invasive airway management.

B. Urgent Airway Management

1. An airway obstruction must be rapidly ruled out if a patient is conscious and following commands, but unable to speak and has an obstructed breathing pattern stridor (uses accessory muscles of respiration, nasal flaring).

2. Inability to rapidly relieve airway obstruction and respiratory distress can necessitate emergent control of the patient airway.

C. Emergent Airway Management

If a patient is unconscious and without adequate respiratory effort; has airway obstruction that cannot be relieved; or progressive respiratory distress, initiate immediate bag-mask ventilatory support with 100% oxygen as the first step in intubating the trachea and securing the airway.

IV. Mask Ventilation

A. Indications

1. Preoxygenation

Administer 100% oxygen by mask ventilation to provide an oxygen reserve that delays desaturation while endotracheal intubation or another means of definitive airway management is secured.

2. To assist or control ventilation as part of initial resuscitation

B. Technique

1. The technique of mask ventilation involves the placement of a face mask and maintenance of a patent airway.

2. A mask is selected to provide a snug fit around the bridge of the nose, cheeks, and mouth. Clear plastic masks have a less noxious odor and allow for visualization of the lips (for color) and mouth (for secretions or vomitus).

3. In patients with known or suspected C-spine injuries, care must be taken to maintain the neck in neutral position at all times.

4. Mask placement

a. Hold the mask in the left hand so that the little finger is at the angle of the mandible, the third and fourth fingers are along the mandible, and place the index finger and thumb placed on the mask.

b. The right hand is available to control the reservoir bag.

c. If the patient is large, two hands may be required to maintain a good mask fit, necessitating an assistant to control the bag.

d. Head straps can be used to assist mask fit.

5. Patients with facial trauma, or those who are edentulous can present a problem when attempting to achieve an adequate seal with the face mask because of distorted anatomy or collapse of mandible to maxilla distance, usually maintained by teeth.

a. An oral or nasal airway, if appropriate, can be considered to correct this problem.

b. An oral airway may not be well tolerated in a patient whose gag reflex is intact.

c. Complications from use of oral airways include vomiting, laryngospasm, and dental trauma. The wrong size oral airway can worsen obstruction. If the oral airway is too short, it can compress the tongue; if it is too long, it can lie against the epiglottis.

d. Nasal airways are better tolerated by awake or sedated patients with an intact gag reflex. Nasal airways, however, should not be used in the presence of a basilar skull fracture; they can cause epistaxis and are usually avoided in patients who are anticoagulated.

e. If necessary, the cheeks and surrounding tissue can also be compressed against the mask in an attempt to decrease leaks.

f. Because two hands may be required for such maneuvers, an assistant may be needed if the patient's breathing must be assisted or controlled.

6. Airway obstruction during spontaneous ventilation can be recognized by stridor or a "rocking" motion of the chest and abdomen. In addition, no respiratory excursions will be noted in the reservoir bag. Peak airway pressures will be elevated when positive pressure ventilation is attempted. Under such circumstances, airway patency may be restored (as clinically appropriate) by the following:

1. Neck extension
2. Jaw thrust, by placing the fingers under the angles of the mandible and lifting forward
3. Head rotation
4. Insertion of an oral or nasal airway

7. Difficult mask ventilation can be anticipated in patients with facial trauma, or those with a beard, body mass index >26 kg/m^2, lack of teeth, age >55 years, or a history of snoring. Appropriate oral and nasal airways as well as laryngeal mask airway (LMA) should be readily available to assist mask ventilation in these patients.

8. Complications

a. The mask can cause pressure injuries to soft tissues around the mouth, mandible, eyes, or nose and exacerbate preexisting injuries in patients with facial trauma.

b. Loss of the airway can result in laryngospasm or vomiting.

c. Mask ventilation does not protect the airway from aspiration of gastric contents.

d. Airway obstruction from the tonic contraction of the laryngeal and pharyngeal muscles—laryngospasm—may be relieved by jaw thrust and the application of constant positive airway pressure. If this fails, a small dose of succinylcholine (intravenously [i.v.] or intramuscularly [i.m.]) may be required.

V. Endotracheal Intubation

A. Rapid Sequence Intubation

1. Because most trauma patients have consumed food or drink within several hours of their trauma, and because trauma delays gastric emptying, all trauma patients are at high risk for aspiration of their gastric contents. Therefore, endotracheal intubation with a cuffed ETT is preferred when ventilatory support is needed.

2. Given the risk of aspiration, if a difficult airway is not suspected, the ETT should be placed using a rapid sequence induction (RSI).

a. Following preoxygenation with 100% oxygen (3 to 5 minutes with tidal breathing, or four vital capacity breaths when time is of the essence), an induction agent is immediately followed by a rapidly acting neuromuscular blocking (paralytic) agent, and intubation is performed at the earliest possible instant.

   b. Positive pressure ventilation should not attempted at any time before intubation because any gastric distention could further elevate the risk of aspiration.

   c. Cricoid pressure (Sellick maneuver) should be maintained until proper placement of the ETT is confirmed as a further deterrent to aspiration. The clinical utility of the Sellick maneuver or its safety with a possible C-spine injury has not been established, however.

3. If a difficult airway is suspected, an awake fiberoptic intubation (section VI.A.1) should be considered.

B. Indications

   1. Emergency tracheal intubation is indicated in patients with the following:

   1. Airway obstruction
   2. Hypoventilation
   3. Severe hypoxemia
   4. Severe cognitive impairment (Glasgow Coma Scale [GCS] score <8)
   5. Cardiac arrest
   6. Severe hemorrhagic shock

   2. Emergency tracheal intubation is indicated in patients with smoke inhalation and the following:

   1. Airway obstruction
   2. Severe cognitive impairment (GCS score <8)
   3. Major cutaneous burn (>40%)
   4. Prolonged transport time
   5. Impending airway obstruction
      • Moderate to severe facial burn
      • Moderate to severe oropharyngeal burn
      • Moderate to severe airway injury seen on endoscopy

C. Orotracheal Intubation (Preferred)

   1. Technique

   a. Intubation is usually performed with a laryngoscope following the induction of anesthesia (usually, RSI).

   b. The Macintosh and Miller blades are most commonly used.

   c. The Macintosh blade is curved, and the tip is inserted into the vallecula (the space between the base of the tongue and the pharyngeal surface of the epiglottis). It provides a good view of the oropharynx and hypopharynx, thus allowing more room for ETT passage with diminished epiglottic trauma. Size ranges vary from 1 to 4, with most adults requiring a Macintosh no. 3 blade.

   d. The Miller blade is straight, and it is passed so that the tip lies beneath the laryngeal surface of the epiglottis. The epiglottis is then lifted to expose the vocal cords. The Miller blade allows better exposure of the glottic opening but provides a

smaller passageway through the oropharynx and hypopharynx. Size ranges range from 0 to 3, with most adults requiring a Miller no. 2 or no. 3 blade.
e. For optimal ease with laryngoscopy, position the patient in the so-called "sniffing" position—atlantoaxial extension and flexion of the lower C-spine.

(1) The sniffing position attempts to align the oral, pharyngeal, and laryngeal axes so that the pathway from the lips to the glottis is nearly in a straight line.

(2) The sniffing position, however, requires mobility of the C-spine, leading to concerns regarding the safety of direct laryngoscopy with a possible unstable C-spine.

(3) Given that most of the motion in attaining the sniffing position is associated with atlantoaxial movement, it has been argued that direct laryngoscopy with neck stabilization is safe in patients with suspected or known lower C-spine injury.

(4) Studies are, however, retrospective (typically, with an assistant maintaining the neck in neutral position by holding slight traction at the mastoid processes).

(5) Studies are retrospective, however, and the sample sizes have been small, suggesting that caution must be maintained when direct laryngoscopy is attempted.

(6) Also, keep in mind that excessive traction itself has been associated with neurologic deterioration.

(7) Intubation while the patient is awake is the alternative to direct laryngoscopy following the induction of general anesthesia.

(8) Although it is reasonable to assume that any potential neurologic deterioration can be easily determined and thus averted in the awake patient, studies have indicated no advantage to this technique over direct laryngoscopy in patients at risk.

f. Hold the laryngoscope in the left hand near the junction between the handle and blade. After propping the mouth open with a scissoring motion of the right thumb and index finger, insert the laryngoscope into the right side of the patient's mouth to avoid the incisor teeth while sweeping the tongue to the left. The lips should not be pinched between the blade and teeth. Then advance the blade toward the midline until the epiglottis comes into view. Lift t the tongue and pharyngeal soft tissues to expose the glottic opening. Use the laryngoscope to lift rather than act as a lever to prevent damage to the maxillary incisors or gingiva.

g. An appropriate ETT size depends on the patient's age, body habitus, and type of surgery. A 7.0-mm ETT with stylet is used for most women and an 8.0-mm ETT with stylet for most men. Hold the ETT in the dominant hand as one would hold a pencil and advance through the oral cavity from the right corner of the mouth, and then through the vocal cords.

If visualization of the glottic opening in a Macintosh laryngoscope is incomplete, it may be necessary to use the epiglottis as a landmark immediately beneath which an ETT is passed into the trachea. External manipulation of the cricoid or thyroid cartilage, if feasible, also aids in visualization. Once the tip of the ETT is through the vocal cords, remove the stylet, and advance the ETT so that the cuff of the ETT lies just below the cords. Note the markings on the ETT in relation to the patient's incisors (or lips) and record in the patient chart for reference. Inflate the cuff just to the point of obtaining a seal in the presence of 20 to 30 cm H_2O positive airway pressure.

h. Verify proper endotracheal intubation by determining end-tidal carbon dioxide and auscultating over the stomach first and left then right lung fields. If breath sounds are heard on one side of the thorax only, a main stem intubation has likely occurred, and the ETT should be withdrawn until breath sounds are heard bilaterally. Listening for breath sounds high in each axilla will decrease the chances of being misled by transmitted breath sounds from the opposite lung.

i. Securely fasten the endotracheal tube with tape, preferably to taut skin overlying bony structures.

j. Complications of orotracheal intubation include injury to the lips or tongue, teeth, pharynx, or tracheal mucosa. Rarely, avulsion of arytenoid cartilages or damage to vocal cords occurs.

2. **Induction Agents**
    a. Given the hemodynamic instability that can be frequently associated with trauma, choose an induction agent carefully.
    b. Although the skeletal muscles of the neck can preferentially provide stability to an injured C-spine, the administration of paralytic agents to facilitate intubation in trauma patients with C-spine injuries does not appear to worsen neurologic outcomes.
    c. In a hemodynamically stable patient, sodium thiopental (4 mg/kg i.v.) or propofol (2.5 mg/kg i.v.) can be safely used to induce general anesthesia. Because of the vasodilatory and negative inotropic

properties of these agents, significant hypotension can occur at standard induction doses in hypovolemic or hemodynamically unstable patients.

d. Etomidate (0.3 mg/kg i.v.) can offer more cardiovascular stability in hypovolemic patients. Ketamine (1-2 mg/kg i.v.) can maintain hemodynamic stability through its sympathomimetic effects. In those trauma patients whose sympathetic nervous system is maximally stressed, ketamine can cause hypotension at standard induction doses because of its negative inotropic effect.

e. Premedication with a benzodiazepine (e.g., midazolam) and an antisialagogue (e.g., scopolamine) may inhibit some of the undesirable side effects of ketamine (e.g., hallucinations and oral secretions).

f. The neuromuscular blocking agent most often used in a rapid sequence induction is the depolarizing agent, succinylcholine (1 mg/kg i.v.).

   (1) Succinylcholine can be associated with release of intracellular potassium and hyperkalemic cardiac arrest in patients with burns, denervation, or crush injury.

   (2) Succinylcholine can be used within the first 24 hours following a burn injury because the expansion of extra-junctional receptors needed to produce the hyperkalemic response does not occur immediately.

   (3) If succinylcholine is contraindicated, a nondepolarizing agent (no risk of hyperkalemia) must be selected. The only nondepolarizing neuromuscular blocking agent that may produce paralysis with similar rapidity is rocuronium (1.2 mg/kg i.v.). Rocuronium is not associated with any adverse hemodynamic effects at this dose.

D. Nasotracheal Intubation
  1. Indications
   a. Nasotracheal intubation may be required in patients having an intraoral procedure.
   b. The nasotracheal route is now rarely used for long-term intubation because of increased airway resistance and the increased risk of sinusitis.
  2. Contraindications
  Basilar skull fractures, especially of the ethmoid bone; nasal fractures, chronic epistaxis, nasal polyps, coagulopathy, and planned systemic anticoagulation and thrombolysis (i.e., the patient with acute myocardial infarction) are relative contraindications to nasal intubation.
  3. Technique
   a. The nasal mucosa is anesthetized and vasoconstricted with a 4% cocaine solution or a phenylephrine-lidocaine mixture using cotton-tipped pledgets.

b. If both nares are patent, the right naris is preferred because the bevel of most ETT, when introduced through the right naris, will face the flat nasal septum, reducing damage to the turbinates.
c. The inferior turbinates interfere with passage and limit the size of the ETT. Usually an ETT 6.0 to 6.5 mm is used for women and one 7.0 to 7.5 mm for men.
d. Preoxygenation, anesthesia, and paralysis are induced as described in the section on orotracheal intubation.
e. After passage through the nares into the pharynx, advance the tube through the glottic opening. Passage under direct vision using a laryngoscope and assisted by Magill forceps may be required.

4. Complications
Complications are similar to those described for orotracheal intubation. Nasal hemorrhage, submucosal dissection, and dislodgement of enlarged tonsils and adenoids can also occur. Nasal intubation can also be associated with infection of the frontal and maxillary sinuses and bacteremia.

VI. Adjuncts to the Difficult Airway
A difficult airway can be divided into an *anticipated* difficult airway and an *unanticipated* difficult airway. An anticipated difficult airway is an airway that on initial examination appears as though it would provide significant challenges to simple orotracheal intubation on examination (e.g., significant facial trauma, significant neck trauma with gross abnormalities in anatomy). An unanticipated difficult airway can be defined as one in which visualization of the glottis is not possible despite three of more attempts at direct laryngoscopy by an experienced laryngoscopist. When either of these situations are encountered, alternative methods for airway management must be considered. These alternate methods can be divided into nonsurgical methods and surgical methods.

A. Nonsurgical Adjuncts to the Difficult Airway
1. Fiberoptic Intubation
The flexible fiberoptic endoscope consists of glass fibers that are bound together to provide a flexible unit for the transmission of light and images. The fiberoptic bundle is fragile, and excessive bending can result in damage to the visual elements. The working channel can be used to administer topical anesthetics and provide suction. The visual field often becomes limited as the fiberoptic endoscope nears the glottic opening, because secretions, blood, or fogging of the lens can obscure the view. Immersion of the tip of the fiberoptic endoscope in warm water helps to prevent fogging.

a. Standard Equipment for Oral or Nasal Fiberoptic Intubation

1. An oral bite block or Ovassapian airway (Hudson Respiratory Care Inc., Temecula, California)
2. Topical anesthetics and vasoconstrictors

3.   Suction
4.   A sterile fiberoptic endoscope with light source

b.   Indications

(1)   The flexible fiberoptic endoscope can be used in both awake and anesthetized patients to evaluate and intubate their airways. It can be used for both nasal and oral endotracheal intubation and should be considered as a first option in an anticipated difficult airway rather than as a "last resort."

(2)   Whereas initial fiberoptic intubation can be used for patients with known or suspected cervical spine pathology, its advantages over direct laryngoscopy remain indeterminate, as discussed previously. Fiberoptic intubation should always be considered as an initial intervention in a patient with a known history of a difficult airway.

c.   Technique

(1)   If attempting fiberoptic intubation in an awake patient, topical anesthesia of the airway is vital. This would involve the anesthesia of the chorda tympani branch of the facial nerve (sensory innervation to anterior two thirds of the tongue), glossopharyngeal nerve (sensory innervation to posterior one third of tongue), external branch of the superior laryngeal nerve (sensory innervation from base of tongue to glottis), and the recurrent laryngeal nerve (sensory innervation inferior to glottis).

(2)   Although each nerve can be individually blocked, administration of nebulized 4% lidocaine remains the most expeditious and efficacious method of simultaneous blocking of all the nerves.

(3)   Sedation (fentanyl, midazolam) should also be administered judiciously to improve patient tolerance of this technique.

(4)   An ETT is placed over a lubricated fiberoptic endoscope, suction tubing is attached to the suction port, and the control lever is grasped with one hand while the scope is advanced or maneuvered with the other hand.

(5)   An oral airway is helpful and well tolerated for oral laryngoscopy.

(6)   It is important to keep the endoscope in the midline when advancing it to prevent entering the piriform fossa.

(7)   Position the tip of the endoscope anteriorly when in the hypopharynx and advance toward the epiglottis. If mucosa or secretions impair the view, retract the scope or remove it to clean the tip and reinsert it in the midline.

(8)   As the endoscope slides beneath the epiglottis, the vocal cords will be seen.

(9) Advance the endoscope with the tip in a neutral position until tracheal rings are noted.

(10) If topical anesthesia is adequate, the patient will tolerate this procedure with no coughing.

(11) The endoscope is stabilized, and the ETT is advanced over it and into the trachea. If there is resistance to passage, turn the ETT 90 degrees in the counterclockwise direction to avoid resistance against the anterior commissure and allow passage through the vocal cords.

2. **The Laryngeal Mask Airway**
   a. **Indications**

      (1) The LMA is used as an alternate to mask ventilation or as a temporizing measure until endotracheal intubation is possible for airway management. The latter is particularly relevant with trauma patients, because this population can be associated with a higher incidence of a difficult airway for the many of the reasons discussed.

      (2) The LMA does not provide any protection against the aspiration of gastric contents. Therefore, in trauma patients, the LMA should never be considered an alternative to endotracheal intubation, and serves primarily as an adjunct in the management of a difficult airway.

   b. **Use.** Because the LMA come in a variety of pediatric and adult sizes (**Table 7-1**), it is important to select an appropriate LMA size to maximize the probability of appropriate cuff fit. Maneuvers for the appropriate insertion of the LMA are shown in **Figure 7-1**.

Table 7-1. Laryngeal mask airway sizes

Patient Age/Size	LMA Size	Cuff Volume	ETT Size (ID)
Neonates/infants to 5 kg	1	Up to 4 mL	3.5 mm
Infants, 5–10 kg	1.5	Up to 7 mL	4.0 mm
Infants/children, 10–20 kg	2.0	Up to 10 mL	4.5 mm
Children, 20–30 kg	2.5	Up to 14 mL	5.0 mm
Children, 30 kg to small adults	3.0	Up to 20 mL	6.0 cuffed
Average adults	4.0	Up to 30 mL	6.0 cuffed
Large adults	5.0	Up to 40 mL	7.0 cuffed

LMA, laryngeal mask airway; ETT, endotracheal tube; ID, internal diameter.

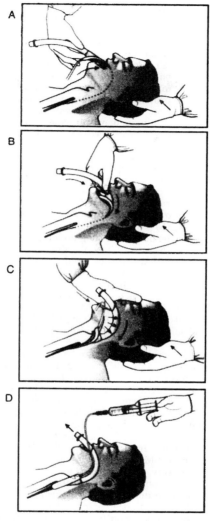

Figure 7-1.   A: With the head extended and the neck flexed, carefully flatten the laryngeal mask airway (LMA) tip against the hard palate. B: With the index finger, push the LMA in a cranial direction following the contours of the hard and soft palate. C: Maintaining pressure with the finger on the tube in the cranial direction, advance the mask until definite resistance is felt at the base of the hypopharynx. D: Inflation without holding the tube allows the mask to seat itself optimally. (From Brain AIJ, Denman WY, Goudsouzian NG. *Laryngeal mask airway instructional manual.* Berkshire, UK: Brain Medical Ltd., 1996:21–25, with permission.)

(1) Ensure correct cuff deflation and lubrication. Lubrication of the LMA inner surface should be avoided because any lubricant dripping into the larynx can precipitate laryngospasm.

(2) Position patient head appropriately as possible; use of the "sniffing" position to optimize endotracheal intubation also typically provides the best positioning for LMA insertion. The constraints in attaining this position have been described previously.

(3) Insert LMA (Fig. 7-1). A soft bite block should be used to protect against a patient biting down on the flexible LMA tube and impairing gas flow.

(4) Inflate the cuff. Typically, a smooth ovoid expansion of the tissues is seen above the thyroid cartilage with adequate inflation of the *appropriately positioned* LMA.

(5) Ensure adequate ventilation as would be done following endotracheal intubation.

(6) After establishing an airway with the LMA, it can be used as a conduit to place an ETT, either blindly or via a fiberoptic endoscope. The caliber of ETT that can be used depends on the size of LMA placed.

3. The Intubating LMA

The intubating LMA (Fastrach) (LMA North America Inc., San Diego, California) includes a curved stainless steel tube (inner diameter 13 mm) covered with silicone, a 15-mm end connector, a handle, cuff, and an epiglottic lifting bar. The tube is of sufficient diameter to accept a cuffed 8-mm ETT, and has a length designed to ensure that the ETT cuff will sit distal to the vocal cords. The primary differences between the Fastrach LMA and the basic LMA are the steel tube, handle, and epiglottic lifting bar.

The Fastrach LMA is inserted similar to the basic LMA. Once inserted and with the cuff inflated, the Fastrach LMA can be used as the sole airway device. Alternately, it can be used as a conduit to intubation.

a. If endotracheal intubation is to be pursued, it can be done either fiberscopically or blindly. If blind intubation is to be attempted, a special ETT with a blunt bullnose tip is used to minimize soft tissue damage.

b. If attempting blind intubation, the Euromedical ILM ETT should be lubricated and gently inserted into the Fastrach tube. At 15 cm, the ETT tip will lie at the epiglottic lifting bar. The ETT should be gently pushed into the trachea while grasping the LMA handle for support. Using the Fastrach handle as a lever while intubating is not recommended. Once the intubation is deemed successful, the tube position should be verified, the cuff inflated, and ETT secured as discussed in Section V. Of note, the inventor of the Fastrach LMA has reported a success rate of 98.5% of blindly intubating patients using the device within two attempts.

c. Once intubated, the Fastrach LMA can either be left in place or removed, leaving the ETT in place. If the Fastrach LMA is left in place, the LMA cuff should be deflated; if it is removed, the LMA cuff should be deflated and the LMA gently removed by manipulating the handle while using an endotracheal tube stabilizer to keep the ETT in place. The ETT stabilizer can be removed once the LMA has cleared the patient's mouth and the ETT stabilized with the operator's other hand or by an assistant.

4. The Light Wand

The light wand consists of a malleable lighted stylet over which an oral ETT can be passed blindly into the trachea. To insert, the room lights are dimmed, and the light wand and ETT are advanced following the curve of the tongue. A glow noted in the lateral neck indicates that the tip of the ETT lies in the piriform fossa. If the tip enters the esophagus, a marked diminution in the brightness of the light occurs. When the tip is correctly positioned in the trachea, a marked glow is noted in the anterior neck. At this point, the ETT is slid off in the same manner as a standard stylet.

B. Surgical Adjuncts to the Difficult Airway

1. Cricothyroidotomy

A cricothyroidotomy can be performed by either a needle technique or a surgical incision.

a. Needle Cricothyroidotomy

(1) **Indication.** The most important indications for needle cricothyroidotomy are emergency airway when endotracheal intubation is unsuccessful and oropharyngeal airway obstruction is caused by trauma or foreign body.

(2) **Technique**

1. Place the patient in a supine position with the neck in neutral position, if cervical injury has not been excluded.
2. Identify the thyroid cartilage, cricothyroid membrane, cricoid cartilage, and suprasternal notch as landmarks and prepare the neck in a sterile fashion.
3. Stabilize the thyroid cartilage between thumb and forefinger.
4. Insert a 12- or 14-gauge angiocatheter attached to a syringe through the cricothyroid membrane in a posterior and slightly caudal direction, with constant aspiration of the syringe (**Fig. 7-2**). Confirm tracheal placement by aspiration of air from the catheter. Stabilize the angio-

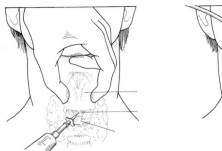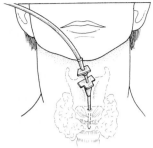

Figure 7-2.   Needle cricothyroidotomy. (From Carrico CJ, Thal ER, Weigelt JA. *Operative trauma management.* **Stamford: Appleton & Lange, 1998, with permission.)**

catheter and remove the needle. Confirm position within the trachea by reaspiration of air from the angiocatheter before connecting to the oxygen source.

5. Connect a 3-mm inner diameter ETT adapter or a 7.5-mm inner diameter ETT adapter inserted into a 3-mL syringe barrel to the angiocatheter.

6. Connect the airway to a high-flow oxygen supply (50 psi, approximately 500 mL/sec) via a jet ventilator or a wall oxygen flow meter opened to its maximal setting.

7. By cyclically interrupting the flow of oxygen, flow is delivered at a 1:2 ratio of inspiration to expiration (1 second on, 2 seconds off). The chest should be seen to rise and fall with each jet.

8. Although jet ventilation can be used as a temporizing method for oxygenation, it may not provide adequate ventilation.

9. Jet ventilation is absolutely contraindicated in cases of complete upper airway obstruction because severe barotraumas can result.

(3) Complications
Serious complications can be associated with misplaced needle cricothyroidotomy catheters; these include airway obstruction, tension pneumothoraces, subcutaneous or mediastinal emphysema, bleeding, hypoxia, and death. Patients with neck trauma, laryngotracheal trauma, and with difficult anatomy (burns, stiff necks) are at greatest risk. Other complications include aspiration of gastric contents, esophageal, tracheal, and thyroid gland injury.

b. **Surgical Cricothyroidotomy.**
    (1) Indications. The indications for surgical cricothyroidotomy are similar to those for

a needle cricothyroidotomy. Surgical cricothyroidotomy is the procedure of choice for an emergency surgical airway.

(2) Technique

The patient is placed in the supine position and the skin is prepared in the standard surgical fashion. If the patient is awake, 1% lidocaine should be used to provide local anesthesia. With a scalpel, perform a transverse incision over the cricothyroid membrane and incise the membrane. A hemostat will enlarge the tract, allowing insertion of a cuffed tracheostomy or ETT (**Fig. 7-3**). If the patient requires long-term intubation, conversion to a tracheostomy is recommended.

(3) Complications

Complications associated with this procedure include aspiration, creation of a false passage in the subcutaneous tissue, subglottic stenosis or edema, laryngeal stenosis, hemorrhage or hematoma formation, laceration of the esophagus or trachea, mediastinal emphysema and vocal cord paralysis. Misplacement of the tube in the paratracheal position can result in airway obstruction, tension pneumothoraces, subcutaneous emphysema, hypoxia, and death.

2. Tracheostomy

    a. Indication. Current indications for emergency tracheostomy are limited. The operating room is the ideal place to perform a tracheostomy. One of the main indications for an emergency tracheostomy is failure of endotracheal intubation or a cricothyroidotomy in a patient with severe

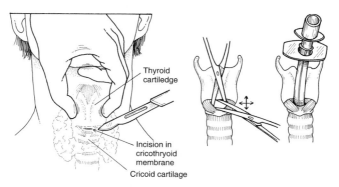

Figure 7-3. Surgical cricothyroidotomy. (From Carrico CJ, Thal ER, Weigelt JA. *Operative trauma management.* Stamford: Appleton & Lange, 1998, with permission.)

facial trauma and blunt or penetrating laryngeal trauma.

b.   Technique

For patients in whom C-spine injury has not been ruled out, the procedure is performed with neck maintained in a neutral position. If the C-spine has been cleared of injury, extension of the neck will facilitate the procedure. Make a transverse incision approximately two fingerbreadths above the suprasternal notch. In-patients whose superficial cervical landmarks are indistinct, a vertical skin incision maybe used. After incising the skin and subcutaneous tissue, cut the platysma and the investing cervical fascia vertically between the medial margins of the sternohyoid and sternothyroid muscles. The thyroid isthmus frequently overlies the intended tracheostomy site and may need to be divided if it cannot be mobilized. Identify the tracheal rings and make a vertical incision through the second ring down onto a portion of the third. Pull back the existing endotracheal tube until the tip is just proximal to the tracheostomy site. Stay sutures can be used to assist in distracting the tracheal walls anteriorly and laterally while passing the tracheostomy tube. These sutures can be left in place postoperatively in patients with (a) difficult neck anatomy; (b) agitation; or (c) a halo in place. After proper inspection and testing of the tube's cuff, push the tracheostomy tube straight into the tracheostomy and, once inside the trachea, direct the tube inferiorly following the natural curve of the tube. Re-inflate the balloon. After confirming proper placement, connect the tracheostomy via sterile tubing to the ventilation system. Confirm proper positioning as described in section V.C.1.h. Secure the flange on the tracheostomy tube to the skin with nylon sutures and apply dressing. Umbilical taped is used to secure the flange around the neck. If used, stay sutures are taped to the anterior chest wall for easy identification. Percutaneous tracheostomy does not have a role in the management of an emergent airway.

c.   Complications. Complications for tracheostomy can be divided into mild, moderate, and serious. Depending on time, tracheostomy complications can also be categorized into early and late complications. Some of the serious early complications are pneumothorax, paratracheal insertion, aspiration, bleeding, subcutaneous emphysema, transient hypoxia, and death. Late complications can include tracheoesophageal fistula, tracheoinominate fistula, and laryngeal or tracheal stenosis.

3.   Retrograde Tracheal Intubation

a.   Indication. A retrograde tracheal intubation is performed when previously described techniques have been unsuccessful. It is performed in a conscious patient who is ventilating with a stable airway.

b. Technique. Identify the cricothyroid membrane and puncture the midline with an 18-gauge i.v. catheter. Introduce an 80-cm, 0.025-inch guidewire and direct it cephalad.

c. Using a laryngoscope, visualize and retrieve the wire.

d. Pass an ETT over the wire, which serves as a guide through the vocal cords.

e. Rigid bronchoscopy may be necessary to support an airway partially obstructed by a foreign body, traumatic disruption, stenosis, or mediastinal mass.

f. General anesthesia will usually be required for insertion. It is important to have a range of scope sizes available (including pediatric sizes). An inhalation induction with spontaneous ventilation is most commonly used.

SELECTED READING

American College of Surgeons Committee on Trauma. *Advanced trauma life support for doctors.* Chicago: American College of Surgeons, 1997.

Carrico CJ, Thal ER, Weigelt JA. *Operative trauma management.* Stamford: Appleton & Lange, 1998.

Checkan E, Weber S. Intubation with and without neuromuscular blockade in trauma patients with cervical spine injury. *Anesth Analg* 1990;70:S54.

Fried L. Cervical spine chord injury during skeletal traction. *JAMA* 1974;229:181–183.

Grande CM, Barton CR, Stene JK. Appropriate techniques for airway management of emergency patients with suspected spinal chord injury. *Anesth Analg* 1988;76:714–715.

Horton WA, Fahy L, Charters P. Disposition of cervical vertebrae, anlanto-axial joint, hyoid and mandible during x-ray laryngoscopy. *Br J Anaesth* 1989;63:435–438.

Langeron O, Masso E, Huraux C, et al. Prediction of difficult mask ventilation. *Anesthesiology* 2000;92:1229–1236.

Mallampati S, et al. A clinical sign to predict difficult tracheal intubation: a prospective study. *Can Anaesth Soc J* 1985; 32:429–434.

Meschino A, Devitt JH, Schwartz ML, et al. The safety of awake tracheal intubation in cervical spine injury. *Can Anaesth Soc J* 1988; 35:S131–132.

Peralta R, Hurford W. Airway trauma. *Int Anesthesiol Clin* 2000; 38:111–127.

Samsoon, GLT, Young JRB. Difficult tracheal intubation: a retrospective study. *Anesthesia* 1987;42;490–497.

Stellin GP, Barker S, Murdock M, et al. Orotracheal intubation in trauma patients with cervical fractures. *Crit Care Med* 1989;17:S37.

Wilson RF, Arden RL. Laryngotracheal trauma. In: Wilson RF, Walt AJ, eds. *Management of trauma pitfalls and practice,* 2nd ed. Baltimore: Williams & Wilkins, 1996:288–313.

Secondary Survey Evaluation of the Trauma Patient

Vicki E. Noble, MD, and David A. Peak, MD

I. Introduction

The secondary survey concept was developed to ensure a methodic and efficient protocol for evaluating the trauma patient once life-threatening injuries have been identified and treated. Without such a protocol, it is possible to miss or overlook injuries that are not immediately life threatening but have the potential to result in severe disability and even delayed mortality. Rates of significant missed injury in adults have been estimated at between 9% to 28%, whereas the rate of pediatric missed injuries is estimated at 20%. Therefore, the importance of attention to detail in that initial trauma workup is essential to ensure that all of the patient's injuries are identified and the patient's condition is well understood. It is important to stress, however, that the secondary survey can only begin after the primary survey has been completed and immediately life-threatening injuries identified and treated. The temptation to focus on the most obvious injuries (e.g., open fractures) must be controlled.

Throughout the secondary survey, the patient must continue to be monitored and have resuscitative measures frequently reassessed. It is not uncommon to have to return to the ABCs at different stages of the trauma evaluation as the patient's condition changes. Once begun, always remember that the goal of the secondary survey is the same as for any other stage of the patient's evaluation: to identify and prioritize injuries and begin further testing or treatment as appropriate. The secondary survey can be separated into patient history, the physical examination, and selective testing.

II. Patient History

AMPLE, meaning allergies, medications, past medical history, last meal, events leading to the accident, is a helpful mnemonic and is used to direct history taking during the secondary survey. Often this information is gathered simultaneously while performing the physical examination described below, but it is important that by the end of the secondary survey, all of the data categories listed below are known and documented. Although these data may not be immediately available in the case of an unresponsive patient, every effort should be made to obtain them.

A. Allergies

It is important to document medication and environmental allergies in trauma patients, as medications can be given and exposures occur during a trauma resuscitation that can lead to secondary injuries. For example, a patient with a latex allergy needs special precautions and a patient with a penicillin allergy may require alternative antibiotics as prophylaxis for open fractures.

B. Medications and Drug Use

Medications and drug use are useful for the physician to know because they can change the physiologic response of a patient to traumatic injuries and can mask the underlying seriousness of the injuries that have been identified. The classic example is the elderly trauma patient who is on a beta-blocker and, therefore, maintains a normal heart rate in the case of hypovolemia. Another example is the trauma patient with a long list of psychiatric medications. This should alert the trauma team to the possibility that the patient's injuries could be self-inflicted. Coumadin or other anticoagulant use should increase the concern for hemorrhage.

C. Past Illness and Medical History

Significant medical problems can have a serious impact on both the patient's response to major trauma and how the trauma team prioritizes injuries or plans resuscitative measures. For example, a trauma patient with a history of coronary artery disease will present additional challenges to the trauma team during resuscitation. An elderly patient with osteoporosis may have orthopedic injuries with a minor mechanism blunt trauma.

D. Last Meal

Knowing the contents of the last meal is important for airway management and to prepare for intubation. In most cases, the trauma resuscitation team should assume that the patient has a full stomach in order to avoid aspiration and secondary injury. Patients, therefore, will require cricoid pressure during intubation. Nasogastric or orogastric emptying should follow every intubation unless contraindicated.

E. Events and Environment of Injury Site

Information on events and the environment of the injury site is often difficult to obtain from patients because they may be unconscious, agitated, or confused. It is important to remember to question family members or friends who have accompanied the patient to the hospital, but most often this information is best obtained from the emergency medical personnel who have transported the patient. They have been trained to notice these details and can provide more objective data.

1. Mechanism of Injury

Proper questioning concerning the mechanism of injury as well as other contributing factors adds invaluable information to the potential for pathology.

a. Blunt Trauma. Important questions regarding blunt trauma include:

1. What was the condition of the car or motor vehicle?
2. Was there significant front end or side damage or intrusion in the motor vehicle?
3. Was there any evidence of the patient hitting the steering wheel, dashboard, windshield, and so forth?
4. Were any safety precautions taken (e.g., helmet wearing or safety belt use)?

5. Did the airbags deploy?
6. Was the patient ambulatory at the scene?
7. Was the patient moving all extremities at the scene?
8. What happened to other passengers or victims?

b. Penetrating Trauma
Important questions to ask include:

1. Was the weapon identified? If so, what are its characteristics?
2. Was there secondary trauma (e.g., patient shot and then fell off balcony)?
3. Was the perpetrator apprehended (important information for ensuring safety of your patient and care providers)?

2. Exposure
The trauma team must know the length of time to extrication and what the environmental conditions were (rain, snow, heat exposure) to evaluate the degree of exposure and risk of hypothermia or hyperthermia.

3. Burns
Important questions to ask include:

1. Was the patient secondarily burned after a collision?
2. Was the patient in a closed environment where smoke inhalation becomes a factor?

4. Hazardous Materials
It is important to know if hazardous materials were involved to protect providers from secondary exposures and indicate the need for decontamination of the patient. In addition, the physician will know to look for toxidromes to explain the patient's complaints or condition.

III. Physical Examination
The physical examination described below is to be undertaken after the primary survey is completed and life-threatening injuries addressed. The key to a secondary examination is consistency in a thorough head-to-toe evaluation, with reassessment when necessary. Once the primary survey is complete and the patient is stabilized, the physician leading the resuscitation should perform the following examination.

A. Head
1. Scalp
The scalp is to be completely examined for lacerations, ecchymoses, depressions, or swelling. Significant bleeding can occur with scalp lacerations and may require sutures or pressure dressings for hemostasis. Bleeding can be especially significant and, therefore, is more urgent to control in children.
2. Eyes
It is important to examine a patient's eyes before significant swelling makes an examination difficult or impossible.

a. Visual acuity should be documented. A rough estimate (e.g., reading the writing on a sponge package) may suffice.

b. Pupil size and reactivity are essential to note, especially in patients with head injuries.

c. Document any observed conjunctival or fundus injuries.

d. If contact lenses are present, remove them if no concern exists for globe rupture or penetration.

e. It is important to look for ocular entrapment or muscle dysfunction, which can indicate significant bony injury to the orbit, compressive hemorrhage, or neurologic injury.

f. Proptosis can indicate globe rupture or retrobulbar hematoma and should be followed up with ophthalmologic evaluation.

g. Always inspect for foreign bodies, including glass, and the potential for corneal injury.

h. Periorbital ecchymoses may indicate a facial or basilar skull fracture.

3. Ears and Nose

a. Always inspect for cerebrospinal fluid (CSF) leak.

b. It is important to look for septal and auricular hematomas because, if missed, they can lead to significant cartilage necrosis and permanent disfiguring outcomes.

4. Maxilla and Facial Bones

a. Facial bones should be palpated for deformity or depression. If any question regarding midface stability arises, perform stomach decompression with an oral gastric tube and take special care if intubation is required.

b. Teeth, mandible, and alveolar membranes should be inspected for signs of fracture. If intubation is required, loose or broken teeth or dentures can prove to be a real hazard, if not identified.

B. Cervical Spine and Neck

1. Spine

Bony and ligamentous injuries are identified by palpating for tenderness or bony step-offs, while maintaining in-line manual stabilization. Injuries to the cervical spine (C-spine) should be assumed in cases of distracting injuries, neurologic symptoms or signs, or any altered level of consciousness, including intoxication. These patients should have continued C-spine stabilization and should all undergo radiologic evaluation.

2. Airway

Airway injuries are identified by inspecting for subcutaneous emphysema or tracheal deviation. If significant, neck swelling or an expanding hematoma is noted, preemptive airway management should be considered to prevent compromise.

3. Vascular Injuries

Suspicion for vascular injuries should be raised by focal neurologic findings, evidence of arterial bleeding, significant abrasions or hematomas in the neck region, identification of carotid bruits, and taking notice of penetrating wounds. Penetrating wounds through the platysma should never be probed because significant hemorrhage may occur (**Table 8-1**).

4. Jugular Venous Distention.

Jugular venous distention (JVD) in trauma is a sign of increased venous pressure secondary to such life-threatening injuries as cardiac tamponade and tension pneumothorax, but can also be noted with over aggressive fluid hydration in patients with cardiac insufficiency. It is frequently absent in hypovolemic patients.

It is important in neck injuries to distinguish between injuries anterior or posterior to the sternocleidomastoid muscle (i.e., the anterior or posterior triangle).

C. Thorax

Usually, the chest will have been evaluated during the primary survey in an attempt to identify any of the life-threatening injuries listed in **Table 8-2**. The secondary survey, however, should include the following as iatrogenic injury can occur during resuscitation and primary injuries can become unmasked as the resuscitation continues.

1. Auscultation

a. Decreased or unilateral breath sounds can suggest pneumothorax, a right main stem bronchus intubation, or hemothorax. It is important to remember that pneumothoraces and hemothoraces can be bilateral.

b. Decreased or "muffled" heart sounds are consistent with cardiac effusion or tamponade, but are often difficult to hear in a busy trauma bay.

2. Inspection

Contusions and hematomas can be signs of underlying injury. A "seat belt sign" over the chest wall is indicative of a significant deceleration injury and raises suspicion for related injuries (e.g., fractured clavicle, blunt aortic injury, pulmonary and cardiac contusion, and rib fractures).

3. Palpation

a. Crepitus, which is an indicator of a hollow viscous perforation, whether it is tracheal, bronchial,

---

Table 8-1. Zones of the neck

Zone I: Level of cricoid cartilage down to level of the clavicle
Zone II: Area above the cricoid cartilage to the angle of the mandible
Zone III: Between the angle of the mandible and the base of the skull

---

**Table 8-2.   Chest trauma—potentially
life-threatening injuries**

Pulmonary contusions or lacerations
Cardiac contusions or lacerations
Ruptured esophagus
Aortic or other major vascular injuries
Diaphragmatic rupture
Tracheal or bronchial rupture

pulmonary, or esophageal, is important to identify
to plan for further evaluation.

b.   Tenderness and deformities over the sternum, ribs (anterior and posterior), and clavicle
are important indicators of potential underlying
injuries to the lung, heart, or major vessels.

D. Abdomen
The goal of the abdominal examination is to divide
patients into those who need emergent laparotomy and
those who can be observed or sent for further radiologic
evaluation (**Table 8-3**).

1. Physical Examination
Inspection for external signs of trauma is similar to
that for chest injuries because hematomas can indicate significant underlying trauma. The lap belt sign
is an important finding that indicates deceleration
and should prompt the physician to think of shearing-
type abdominal injuries as well as hollow viscous perforations. Tenderness to palpation is an important
finding, but the most important element of the abdominal examination is to remember to perform *frequent*

Table 8-3.   Potential indications for emergent laparotomy

Unstable blunt abdominal trauma with positive diagnostic peritoneal lavage or ultrasound

Blunt abdominal trauma with recurrent hypotension despite
adequate resuscitation

Early or subsequent peritonitis

Hypotension with penetrating abdominal wound

Bleeding from the stomach, rectum, or genitourinary tract from
penetrating trauma

Evisceration

Almost all gunshot wounds traversing the peritoneal cavity or
visceral and vascular retroperitoneum

Free air, retroperitoneal air, or ruptured diaphragm after blunt
trauma

Contrast enhanced computed tomography demonstrates ruptured
gastrointestinal tract, intraperitoneal bladder injury, or renal
pedicle injury

reevaluations to identify evolving injuries while waiting for definitive testing. It is important to note that the reliability of the abdominal physical examination can be compromised in patients with intoxication, shock, neurologic injury, or distracting injuries.

2. Radiology

Three mainstays of adjunctive radiologic testing exist in the trauma evaluation. As technology has improved (ultrasound has become more reliable and computed tomographic [CT] scanners have become faster) much debate has ensued regarding the indications for each of the following modes of testing and which to use under what circumstances. This debate will be discussed in further detail in later chapters. Plan to use one or more of the following to identify and prioritize abdominal injuries in all trauma patients.

a. The Focused Abdominal Sonography in Trauma. Focused abdominal sonography in trauma (FAST) examinations should routinely be done at the bedside in conjunction with the secondary survey. It is included in the revised Advanced Trauma Life Support (ATLS) manual as part of a routine secondary survey. It provides rapid, noninvasive information that can show hemoperitoneum, bladder rupture, or pericardial effusions and can impact the next therapeutic intervention for the patient.

b. Diagnostic Peritoneal Lavage. Diagnostic peritoneal lavage (DPL) can also be done at the bedside for patients who are felt to be too unstable to travel to a CT scanner. The DPL is an invasive but highly sensitive test for hemoperitoneum or ruptured viscous injury and may obviate the need for emergent laparotomy. The characteristics that indicate a positive test are listed in **Table 8-4**. DPL has fallen out of favor as a routine test in many centers because of the speed and reliability of CT scanners and the trend toward safe, nonoperative management of many injuries.

c. Computed Tomography Scans. Now available in all trauma centers, CT scans are also often found within the emergency department itself. They are a superior source of information for identification and classification of injuries and can often provide multiple diagnoses. The limiting factor is patients must travel to the radiology suite or CT scanner from the trauma resuscitation bay, which requires that patients be hemodynamically stable because they will have limited monitoring during the time they are being imaged. Attempting to image unstable patients has taught many physicians to respect the oft-quoted phrase "death begins in radiology."

E. Genitourinary

Genitourinary injuries are rarely immediately life threatening but, if missed, can cause significant morbidity,

Table 8-4.   Diagnostic peritoneal lavage numbers for patients with blunt trauma

Frank blood	Positive	Laparotomy
>100,000 RBC/mm³	Positive	Laparotomy
50–100,000 RBC/mm³	Equivocal	Reassess, further investigate
<50,000 RBC/mm³	Negative	2% chance of missed injury
>500 WBC/mm³	Positive	Laparotomy
Bacteria/particulate matter	Equivocal	Reassess, further investigate
Feces	Positive	Laparotomy
Alkaline phosphatase >10	Positive	Laparotomy

(*Note:* Advanced trauma life support only uses counts of >100,000 RBC and >500 WBC as indicators for laparotomy, but other studies have included the following guidelines and so have been compiled here to use as a reference. We use >50,000 RBC for penetrating trauma.)
RBC, red blood cells; WBC, white blood cells.

including incontinence, sexual dysfunction, and chronic pain. They are, therefore, an important part of the secondary survey.

1.   Rectal Examination
The rectal examination should be performed before urinary catheter insertion as an abnormal or "high-riding" prostate can be indicative of pelvic fracture and is associated with urethral injury. Additionally, gross blood or rectal wall defects raise the suspicion of bowel injury that will require further testing. Finally, as noted below, sphincter tone and perianal sensation should be documented as they provide prognostic information for those patients with spinal cord injury.

2.   Genital Examination
Blood noted at the urethral meatus can indicate urethral injury and requires a retrograde urethrogram or other further evaluation before insertion of the urinary catheter. Scrotal swelling or ecchymoses raises suspicion for fracture and should be documented and followed with further investigation. Vaginal bleeding or lacerations also needs to be addressed to prevent fistula formation, urinary complications, or potential for sexual dysfunction.

F.   Musculoskeletal
Often, musculoskeletal injuries are the most dramatic injuries and it is the responsibility of the physician or trauma team not to be distracted by the most obvious injury but to proceed methodically through the secondary survey.

1. Inspection

Inspect for deformity, swelling, ecchymoses, lacerations, and abrasions, which could give clues to underlying bony injury.

2. Palpation

Palpate for tenderness, deformity, foreign bodies, and crepitus.

3. Joint Evaluation

Evaluate range of motion of all joints, both active and passive, to assess tendon and ligament function. In addition, effusions should be noted and further evaluated, which could indicate hemarthroses or further joint injury.

4. Pulse Examination

Documenting extremity pulses is important for two reasons. First, absent pulses can be the first indication of a vascular injury (especially in a patient with altered mental status) and will necessitate further evaluation. Second, many orthopedic injuries cause massive swelling or ecchymoses that can lead to secondary injury, if not identified. Serial examinations are required to rule out delayed compartment syndrome. Skeletal bony deformities, with compromised distal pulses or other signs of ischemia, should be reduced to anatomic position and reassessed and splinted, whenever possible.

5. Back Examination

All secondary surveys must examine the back for midline bony tenderness and deformity. Use spinal (log roll) precautions until the initial assessment is concluded. Concern for spinal stability and compromise must be weighed against concern for the development of decubitus ulcers that can occur quickly in paralyzed or obtunded patients. If there is any concern for injury, clear the patient off the backboard and leave on log roll precautions until radiologic evaluation is complete.

G. Neurologic

Managing complex trauma patients with multiple injuries is challenging. The use of sedating or paralytic agents is often required, but they can compromise the physician's ability to continuously assess and evaluate brain and spinal cord injuries. The trauma team resuscitating the patient must attempt to document neurologic activity before these medications are given, if needed, and to *frequently* reassess the patient. For this reason, short-acting agents are generally preferred during the initial trauma assessment and resuscitation.

1. Glasgow Coma Scale

The Glasgow Coma Scale (GSC) must be performed, scored, and documented (**Table 8-5**).

2. Neurologic Examination

If a patient has any evidence of head or spinal cord injury, the secondary survey is the time to perform a more thorough neurologic examination, including evaluating mental status, and motor, sensory, and cere-

Table 8-5.   Glasgow coma scale

Eye opening
4—open eyes spontaneously
3—open eyes to command
2—open eyes to pain
1—no eye opening

Best motor response
6—obeys commands
5—localizes pain
4—withdraws to pain
3—decorticate posturing (abnormal flexion)
2—decerebrate posturing (abnormal extension)
1—none (flaccid)

Verbal response
5—oriented, fluent speech
4—confused conversation
3—inappropriate words
2—incomprehensible words
1—no speech

Best possible score—15
Worst possible score—3

bellar functions, if possible. Rectal tone and perianal sensation are important physical examination findings because they have prognostic implications for patients with spinal cord injuries. Changes from an initial examination are reliable indicators of progressive injury, (e.g., expanding spinal cord hematomas or intracranial bleeds), thus, initial examination documentation can significantly help those caring for the patient on the floor or in the intensive care unit.

IV.   Studies Tests, and Immediate Treatment
The appropriate evaluation and treatment of injuries for each organ system will be discussed in detail in the subsequent chapters. Following is an overview of what the trauma team will attempt to accomplish by the time the secondary survey is completed.

    A.   Plain x-ray Studies
        1.   Trauma Series
        The traditional trauma series includes the lateral C-spine, portable chest, and anteroposterior (AP) pelvis as the initial radiographic evaluation of all trauma patients.

        2.   Long Bone Films
        Long bone x-rays after reduction of gross deformities can be obtained in the trauma bay during the secondary survey if no other acute interventions are being undertaken. Otherwise, these can be deferred until the patient is stabilized.

    B.   Computed Tomography Scans, Focused Abdominal Sonogram for Trauma Examinations and Diagnostic Peritoneal Lavage
    The order and priority of CT, FAST, and DPL tests for abdominal injury will be discussed in later chapters.

C. Blood Work and Urinalysis

Blood work and urinalysis should be obtained on all trauma patients during the secondary survey. It is important to test all women of childbearing age for pregnancy (either serum or urine) in order to limit radiation to the developing fetus, whenever possible. Blood bank samples should be obtained for a type and screen in case the patient requires blood. Typical blood tests performed on a trauma patient include complete blood counts, chemistries, electrolytes, and urinalysis. Additional tests (e.g., toxicologic evaluation) can help identify causes of a patient's mental or physiologic status.

D. Tetanus Toxoid

Any patients with lacerations, abrasions, or open fractures should be asked about their tetanus status. If any question arises or the information is unknown, tetanus immunization should be given.

E. Antibiotics

Patients with open fractures, significantly contaminated soft tissue injuries, or suspicion of bowel perforation injuries are often given antibiotics during the trauma resuscitation.

F. Analgesia

It is the responsibility of the trauma team and the physician directing the resuscitation to remember that the patient is often experiencing significant pain and stress during the evaluation. Reassurance and calm communication are invaluable in establishing order in any resuscitation. In addition, interventions (e.g., reduction of grossly dislocated fractures) can significantly improve a patient's pain without necessitating additional analgesia. Significant debate has arisen on whether giving systemic pain medication masks important clinical signs and symptoms and obscures changes in the physical examination that can endanger the patient. It is the responsibility of the physician caring for the patient to establish the balance between safety and humane treatment of a patient's pain.

G. Patient Rights

It is additionally the responsibility of the trauma team and the physician directing the resuscitation to maintain a healthy respect for patient rights and to maintain strict professionalism. In addition to the physical stress of the trauma, patients can feel additional emotional stress during a trauma evaluation if the trauma team does not use frequent reassurance and clear communication concerning each part of their assessment, including blood draws, physical examination, and other interventions. Exposure is important to assess for injury, but sensitive areas should be covered immediately, whenever possible. Patient comfort and education should remain a priority.

V. Tertiary Survey and Repeat Vital Examinations and Assessment

The concept of a tertiary survey has been developed to further stress two points. First, the status of the trauma patient can be very dynamic and evolve over time. This requires frequent reassessment and close monitoring in the acute phase. Second, the trauma team should perform a very thorough reevaluation of the entire patient after initial life threats and major injuries are assessed and stabilized. As stated, seemingly minor but potentially important injuries can be easily overlooked when faced with a critical trauma patient with multiple injuries. It is the responsibility of the trauma team to diagnose and treat all of the patient's injuries.

VI. Documentation

Most trauma centers assist the documentation effort by having a dedicated nurse document the initial resuscitation as it is taking place. If this is the case, the physician performing the primary and secondary survey should be sure to call out examination findings in a strong voice and the rest of the trauma team should keep their conversation to a minimum to ensure accurate transfer of information. Documentation of both the physical examination and interventions performed in the trauma bay should be thorough, complete, and include reassessments and significant clinical changes.

VII. Transfer to Definitive Care

Ultimately, transfer to definitive care is the responsibility of the person directing the trauma resuscitation. The burden is on the trauma leader to know the capabilities of his or her facility, but also to recognize when a patient is hemodynamically stable for transfer.

SELECTED READING

Advanced trauma life support student course manual. Chicago: American College of Surgeons, 1997.

Grossman MD. Tertiary survey of the trauma patient in the intensive care unit. *Surg Clin North Am* 2000;80(3):805–824.

Houshian S, Larsen MS, Holm C. Missed injuries in a level I trauma center. *J Trauma* 2002;52(4):715–719.

McCabe C, Warren RL. Trauma: annotated bibliography of recent literature. *Am J Emerg Med* 2001;19(5):437–452.

McCarthy MC. Trauma and critical care. *J Am Coll Surg* 2000;190: 232–243.

Moore EE, Mattax K, Felician D. *Trauma,* 2nd ed. Norwalk: Appleton & Lange, 1991.

Scalea TM, Rodriguez A, et al. Focused assessment with sonography for trauma (FAST): results from an international consensus conference. *J Trauma* 1999;46(3):466–472.

9

Unique Critical Care Issues Related to Trauma

Ruben Peralta, MD, Alexander Iribarne, MS,
Oscar J. Manrique, MD, and Horacio Hojman, MD

I. Role of the Intensive Care Unit in Trauma Care

Trauma is the principal public health problem in most of the countries around the world. The role of the intensive care unit (ICU) enables the resuscitative process to be continually coordinated; and ensures that no details are neglected or overlooked and that the resuscitation is timely and focused. A multidisciplinary team focused on resuscitation, monitoring, and life support most effectively provides trauma care in the ICU. In addition, for patients who have sustained lethal brain injuries, the trauma ICU can play an important role in the support and maintenance of potential organ donors. During the course of management of the seriously injured patient, the major goals of the ICU include early reestablishment and maintenance of tissue oxygenation, diagnosis and treatment of occult injuries, and prevention and treatment of infections and multisystem organ dysfunction syndrome. The Leapfrog Group, which is composed of more than 130 public and private organizations that provide healthcare benefits and work with physicians to improve hospital systems for patient safety, has named three initial methods for improving patient safety: computer physician order entry, evidence-based hospital referral, and ICU physician staffing. This group has shown that these standards would significantly enhance outcomes.

II. Staffing

The importance of predesignated "trauma team" members with assigned duties cannot be overemphasized. The complex trauma patient admitted to our surgical ICU (SICU) is managed in a multidisciplinary approach fashion, with focus on *preventing* a variety of secondary injuries that can occur, including the development of secondary brain injury, barotrauma, sepsis, multiorgan failure, and *managing* pain and agitation.

III. Neurologic Issues

A. Monitoring

Brain injury, either alone or in combination with other injuries, is the major determinant of survival and functional outcome in most cases of trauma. Avoidance of hypotensive and hypoxic episodes is of critical importance in the management of patients with traumatic brain injury. Increased intracranial pressure (ICP) is another major factor that can contribute to secondary brain injury. As a result, monitoring and controlling ICP and cerebral perfusion pressure (CPP) is essential in head trauma patients. The threshold for treatment of elevated ICP is 20 mm Hg. The CPP pressure should be maintained greater than 60 mm Hg. Other factors that can worsen neurologic injury include hypercarbia and increased body temperature. Frequent examination of the critically ill patient, thus, is necessary to detect subtle and newly formed neurologic problems. A complete examination includes an assessment of global function with the Glasgow Coma Scale (**see Chapter 8**), detection of cranial nerve abnormalities, and evaluation for localized motor and sensory deficits. The nature of definitive care depends on the presence or absence of surgically correctable lesions (epidural or subdural hematoma). Patients with such lesions require prompt operative evacuation. The urgency for an early computed tomography (CT) scan of the head is a function of the likelihood of a surgically correctable lesion. A portable CT scanner is part of the armamentarium we use in the management of the unstable patient.

B. Pain Management.

Pain control is a subject that affects most patients in the SICU. The first goal in evaluating the patient with pain or agitation is to determine and eliminate the insult. Pain or agitation that is not adequately treated can have a number of adverse effects on homeostasis that include increased oxygen consumption, increased minute volume demands, impaired lung mechanics with associated pulmonary complications, sleep deprivation, and psychic stress. Many factors can produce agitation (e.g., hypoxia, pain, sepsis, hypercarbia, substance or alcohol abuse withdrawal, delirium). After localizing the cause of the pain, patients may require sedation to allow safe care. Short-acting agents are indicated when brief sedation is required. The most common pharmacologic agents used for sedation are benzodiazepines (e.g., midazolam) and propofol.

Intravenous bolus opioids (e.g. morphine, fentanyl, hydromorphone [Dilaudid]) are the most commonly administered form of analgesia. In addition, other techniques exist for pain control. Regional techniques for pain management include nerve, interpleural, and epidural blocks. Also, patient-controlled analgesia with opiates can be used.

The use of neuromuscular blocking agents in the ICU is indicated to facilitate mechanical ventilation and control increases in intracranial pressure caused by coughing and agitation. Paralytic agents are also used for status epilepticus, tetanus, and muscle spasms and to facilitate procedures. Neuromuscular blocking agents, however, do not have analgesic, sedative, or amnesic properties and their use is associated with numerous side effects (e.g., cardiovascular side effects, myalgias, hyperkalemia).

Persistent paralysis, awareness leading to psychological sequelae, and inadequate ventilation in the event of ventilator disconnection are also problems associated with neuromuscular blockade. They are associated with increased immobility, which causes deep venous thrombosis (DVT), skin breakdown, peripheral nerve injuries, and various myopathies including the acute quadriplegic myopathy syndrome (AQMS). Thus, when administering neuromuscular blocking agents, appropriate sedation and analgesia should also be administered and it should be used only for a brief period. A plan or protocol for sedation should exist in which a frequent evaluation, daily interruption, and decreasing doses of the sedative is recommended.

IV. Pulmonary Issues

A.   Respiratory Failure

One of the most common organs to fail in trauma patients is the lung. As a result, respiratory failure or insufficiency is one of the most common indications for admission of the trauma patient to the ICU. Some of the many causes for respiratory failure include fluid overload, shock, aspiration, fat embolism syndrome, spinal cord injury, post-traumatic acute respiratory distress syndrome, and aspiration. One of the most common causes of respiratory failure in the trauma setting, however, is chest trauma. The recent multicenter trial by the Acute Respiratory Distress Syndrome Network (ARDSnet) suggests that traditional tidal volumes used for mechanical ventilation contribution to stretch-induced lung injury or lung injury by barotrauma. In the ARDSnet study, patients with hypoxemia (PaO_2/FIO_2 <300) and clinical findings consistent with acute lung injury or ARDS were randomized to traditional tidal volumes (10 to 15 mL/Kg) or reduced tidal volume ventilation to limit plateau pressures. This trial was stopped early because of a statistical improvement in survival in the low tidal volume group (31% *vs.* 40%). Assuming other components of DO_2 are optimal (hemoglobin, cardiac output), strategies recommended for the management of respiratory failure include V_T 6 to 10 mL/kg, Pplat <30 to 35, adequate recruitment with positive end-expiratory pressure (PEEP), extended inspiratory time, use of high-frequency ventilation, and selective use of prone positioning. Recent published studies show that placing patients with acute respiratory failure in a prone position improves their oxygenation, but it does not improve survival.

B.   Pulmonary Contusion

Pulmonary contusions are one of the most frequent complications after blunt chest trauma. A pulmonary contusion has been defined as a pathologic state in which hemorrhage and edema of the lung parenchyma occur without parenchyma disruption. This pathology produces decreased lung compliance and the development of ventilation-perfusion mismatch. Respiratory failure occurs more often in patients with large contusions, in the elderly, and in those with underlying chronic lung disease. Clinical diagnosis includes low PaO_2 and radiographic studies showing a well-defined infiltrate underlying the contused area on the chest wall.

Management is directed toward maintaining good oxygenation and preventing barotrauma, as described above. Patients with persistent low PaO_2 levels who do not respond to supplemental oxygen, pulmonary toilet, and pain control should be intubated and mechanically ventilated.

V. Orthopedic Issues

A. Fat Embolism

Fat embolism (FE) and the posttraumatic fat embolism syndrome (FES) are clinical conditions in which pulmonary and/or central nervous system dysfunction is caused by fat microembolism to the lungs, brain, skin, and other organs in patients with fractures of long bones or the pelvis. The syndrome is poorly understood and is clinically manifested with dyspnea and confusion approximately 24 to 48 hours after major trauma. Fracture of bone releases neutral fat, which embolizes in the pulmonary vasculature. Local hydrolysis of fat by lung lipase releases toxic free fatty acids, which generate endothelial injury. Elevated right coronary artery pressures following embolism can help open the foramen ovale, causing severe, even fatal systemic embolism. Many other causes, however, can also produce this syndrome (**Table 9-1**). Because the clinical manifestations are usually mild, FE is often unrecognized. Once the syndrome becomes evident, however, treatment is similar to that for ARDS. Fracture fixation should be attempted to prevent reembolization and supportive management provided with oxygen and ventilatory assistance with PEEP. Maintaining a normal cerebral perfusion with well-oxygenated blood is the best management of neurologic dysfunction.

B. Compartment Pressure Monitoring

Compartment syndrome occurs when pressure in a rigidly enclosed space exceeds capillary perfusion pressure, leading to ischemic damage of the tissues. Diagnosis is made with a high index of suspicion, clinical examination, and adjunctive tests. The symptoms are more important than physical findings in the early diagnosis, yet adjunctive tests can be helpful. Direct measurement of compartment

Table 9-1. Settings for fat embolism syndrome

Blood transfusion
Burns
Cardiopulmonary bypass
Collagen disease
Decompression from altitude
Diabetes mellitus
Hemoglobinopathy
Infections
Medullary reaming
Multiple trauma
Neoplasm
Osteomyelitis
Renal transplantation
Suction lipectomy

pressure, which is a well-accepted and reliable technique, requires only a needle connected to a pressure transducer. A handheld compartment measurement device, using an 18-gauge needle, is commercially available. Pressures less than 20 mm Hg are normal. Pressures over 30 mm Hg are considered abnormal and an indication for compartment release. Treatment consists in releasing the elevated pressure, either by reducing the volume of the compartment contents or by incising the fascia. In the leg, we use a two-incision technique, with generous medial and lateral incisions to completely release all surrounding compartments. The skin incisions are left open to keep intracompartmental pressure low, and delayed closure is performed.

VI. Multiple Organ Failure

A. Cause

Multiple organ failure (MOF) remains the leading cause of death in critically ill patients in SICU. The multiple organ dysfunction syndrome, (MODS) is described as a clinical syndrome characterized by progressive dysfunction of multiple and independent organs, with the lungs, kidneys, and liver serving as the principal target organs. The major risk factors for developing MODS include multiple trauma, soft tissue infections, massive hemorrhage, severe pancreatitis, infection, sepsis and shock. Early onset MODS is often a result of inadequate resuscitation or shock, and late onset MODS is usually caused by severe infections. Although techniques for life support and resuscitation have improved, the incidence of MODS has increased. Moreover, for patients with MODS, mortality still remains high and treatment options are mainly supportive. The association of MODS and outcome is reflected in the almost linear relationship between the number of organs that have failed and mortality.

B. Prevention

Preventing MODS is of great importance because the current therapeutic tools are of limited value. Prevention begins in the field, with rapid transportation to the hospital, rapid volume resuscitation in the emergency department, organized assessment of the patient, early diagnosis and surgical intervention, and complete and meticulous ICU care.

C. Management

Despite medical advances in critical care therapeutics, the morbidity and mortality of MODS remains high. Other than treatment of infection and general ICU supportive care, specific therapy for MODS is limited. Current therapy focuses on metabolic and hemodynamic support until the process reverses itself or death occurs. Prevention of organ dysfunction requires maintaining good tissue oxygenation, appropriate plasma volume maintenance, debridement of devitalized tissue, early fracture fixation and stabilization, nutrition, and nosocomial infection control. Good tissue oxygenation levels prevent postoperative incidence of MODS and improve patient outcome. Early enteral nutrition can be important in maintaining the integrity of the gut mucosal barrier function and preventing the development of MODS. Autoinfection with gut microorganisms can be prevented by selective decontamination of the digestive tract, which prevents bacterial translocation.

VII. Renal Issues

Disorders of the renal system are frequently encountered in critically ill patients. Hospital-acquired acute renal failure occurs in as many as 4% of hospital admissions and 20% of critical care admissions.

A. Renal Failure

Trauma patients are at increased risk for the development of acute renal failure (ARF) secondary to hypotension, sepsis, rhabdomyolysis, abdominal compartment syndrome, use of iodinated contrast for diagnostic tests, use of aminoglycosides, amphotericin B, and preexisting conditions (e.g., diabetes). ARF adds complexity to the overall ICU management of the patient, increases length of stay, and is associated with an average hospital mortality rate of approximately 25% to 50 %. Oliguric ARF, which is observed in 50% of cases of ARF, has a mortality rate of 50% to 80%. Nonoliguric renal failure has a better prognosis with a mortality rate of 15% to 40%.

Important strategies that should be taken into consideration, include avoidance of or monitoring levels of aminoglycosides, saline hydration with administration of amphotericin B and use of liposomal preparation, when clinically indicated. For myoglobinuria, hydration, alkaline diuresis, and mannitol can be used. Nonsteroidal anti-inflammatory drugs (NSAID) should be avoided in the setting of renal dysfunction and hypoperfusion. Oliguric ARF can also result in severely traumatized and burned patients as a result of an increased intraabdominal pressure (IAP) and progression to the development of the abdominal compartment syndrome (ACS). (For detailed management and prevention, **see Chapter 31, Abdominal Trauma**).

Prevention of contrast-induced ARF, which is indicated in patients at high risk, including those with chronic kidney disease (CKD), diabetes mellitus (DM), volume depletion, or congestive heart failure (CHF), includes the use of careful hydration with normal saline to avoid CHF; use of nonionic, low osmolality contrast, and acetylcysteine. For the high-risk patient population, a protocol of hydration and administration of acetylcysteine is recommended.

B. Rhabdomyolysis

Rhabdomyolysis is a syndrome resulting from the release of myoglobin, potassium, phosphate, organic acids, and other muscle contents into the plasma secondary to skeletal muscle injury. This syndrome can accelerate the development of shock, hemoconcentration, and hyperkalemia. Aside from trauma, ischemia, drugs (including alcohol and cocaine), direct electrical shock, extensive burns, hypothermia, heat shock, and metabolic derangements can lead to muscle cell lysis.

Complications of rhabdomyolysis include hemodynamic and metabolic disturbances, ARF, compartment syndrome, and disseminated intravascular coagulation. Early recognition and treatment comprise the major step for preventing ARF. The diagnosis of rhabdomyolysis is made by the measurement of serum creatine phosphokinase and serum and urinary myoglobin. Evaluation of metabolic consequences of muscle destruction includes the measurement of serum and urinary electrolytes, including calcium and phosphorus, and renal function indices. ARF, compartment syndrome, and calcium and phosphate derangement are the most common complications of this syndrome.

Management of rhabdomyolysis consists of early correction of the underlying cause and vigorous intravenous volume replacement. Once the systemic circulation has been stabilized and the presence of adequate urine flow has been confirmed, forced mannitol-alkaline diuresis therapy for prophylaxis against hyperkalemia and ARF should be undertaken. When compartment syndrome is suspected, repeated physical examination and measurement of compartment pressures should be done. Fasciotomies should be considered when intracompartmental pressure exceeds 30 mm Hg.

C. Evaluation of Deteriorating Renal Function

The most common method used to track renal function is measurement of the serum creatinine and blood urea nitrogen (BUN) levels. The kidney is the major organ responsible for the excretion of urea and, under normal conditions, this accounts for approximately 80% to 90% of the total nitrogen excretion. Glomerular filtration rate (GFR), a true index for measuring renal function, is estimated using creatinine clearance. Clearance reflects the net effect of glomerular filtration, tubular reabsorption, and tubular secretion, each of which can be affected by several factors. The clearance of creatinine serves as a marker of the GRF, which is the amount of fluid filtered from the plasma in a given time. Circulating concentrations of BUN and creatinine are determined, not only by how efficiently they are excreted by the kidneys, but also by the rates at which they are produced in the body. These indices, however, become abnormal only after a large portion of kidney function is lost. When significant renal dysfunction is detected, it should be monitored by repeated assessment of creatinine clearance.

D. Renal Replacement Therapies

Some of the excretory functions of the kidney can be replaced by a variety of techniques. Some of the most common techniques used in the acute care setting include hemodialysis, peritoneal dialysis, and continuous hemofiltration. Hemodialysis can be done in those who are hemodynamically stable. Evidence supports the use of hemodialysis every day rather than every other day. The advantages of using continuous techniques are less hemodynamic instability resulting in a controlled gradual correction of fluid and electrolyte abnormalities. Continuous renal replacement therapy (CRRT) requires venous access and trained staff to monitor the rate of fluid replacement. Use of CRRT allows RRT to be delivered to very unstable patients as well as allows for the initiation of nutritional therapy. Early intervention can be beneficial, but the evidence remains inconclusive. Despite the proliferation of continuous therapy in the ICU setting, the evidence that it leads to reduced mortality is lacking.

Indications for acute dialysis include hyperkalemia (>6 mEq/L), uremia, severe acidosis, uremic platelet dysfunction, and hypervolemia. Good control of urea levels can prevent platelet dysfunction and mental status changes.

SELECTED READING

The Acute Respiratory Distress Syndrome Network. Ventilation with lower tidal volumes as compared with traditional tidal volumes for acute lung injury and the acute respiratory distress syndrome. *N Engl J Med* 2000;342(18):1301–1308.

Bergestein JM. Extremity compartment syndrome. In: Cameron JL, ed. *Current surgical therapy,* 7th ed. St. Louis: Mosby, 2001:1140–1144.

Forsythe R, Sambol J, Adams C, et al. Multiple organ failure. In: Cameron JL, ed. *Current surgical therapy,* 7th ed, St. Louis: Mosby, 2001:1354–1360.

Kron IL, Cope JT, et al. Cardiovascular Monitoring and Support. In: Baker RJ, Fisher JE, eds. *Mastery of Surgery,* 4th ed. Philadelphia: Lippincott Williams & Wilkins, 2001:90–106.

Levy M. New management strategies in ARDS. *Crit Care Clin* 2002;18:1–290.

Marvin RG, et al. Critical Care. In: Towsend CM, ed. *Sabiston Textbook of Surgery, The biological Basis of Modern Surgical Practice.* 16th ed. Philadelphia: W.B. Saunders Company, 2001:375–393.

Reichman, J. Brezis M. Acute Renal Failure. In: Webb AR, Shapiro MJ, et al., eds. *Oxford Textbook of Critical Care,* First ed. New York: Oxford University Press Inc., 2000:413–422.

Sapirstein A. Renal Disease. In: Hurford WE, ed. *Critical Care Handbook of the Massachusetts General Hospital,* 3rd ed. Philadelphia: Lippincott Williams & Wilkins, 2000:352–369.

Schmidt GA. Pulmonary Embolic Disorders: Thrombus, Air and Fat. In: Hall JB, Schmidt GA, and Wood LDH, eds. *Principles of Critical Care,* 2nd ed. New York: McGraw-Hill, 1998:427–449.

Wilson RF, Tyburski SW, et al. Sepsis in Trauma. In: Wilson RF, and Walt AJ, eds. *Management of Trauma Pitfalls and Practice,* 2nd ed. Baltimore: Williams & Wilkins, 1996:828–866.

Transfusion and Coagulation Issues in Trauma

Walter H. Dzik, MD, and
Christopher P. Stowell, MD, PhD

I. Introduction

In the 1980s, the advent of the human immunodeficiency virus (HIV) and the awareness of the high incidence of transfusion-transmitted hepatitis forced a reevaluation of the risk benefit balance of transfusion as well as a more critical approach to its use. Numerous studies documented the efficacy of compensatory mechanisms in hemorrhaging and anemic patients, and the ability of patients to tolerate a substantially reduced red blood cell (RBC) mass. Although the risk of HIV and hepatitis C virus infection by transfusion has been reduced to negligible levels, other complications of transfusion remain. **Table 10-1** summarizes some of the significant infectious and noninfectious risks of transfusion. *Note:* The risk of an acute hemolytic transfusion reaction caused by ABO incompatibility, which is of particular concern in emergency situations, is greater than the combined risk of all of the transfusion-transmitted viruses.

A. Organization of Emergency Transfusion Services

The logistics of transfusion therapy for trauma patients must be well organized in advance so that they function efficiently and largely invisibly to the trauma service. Improvising procedures for specimen labeling and transport, patient identification, and other details of transfusion therapy in the midst of resuscitation effort is not in the best interest of the patient. The procedures that must be developed and implemented by the trauma service and the blood bank include proper sample and patient identification, communication, and a protocol for expedited release of blood.

B. Patient and Blood Bank Sample Identification

The most common cause of acute hemolytic transfusion reactions caused by ABO incompatibility is mistransfusion. This occurs almost invariably because of mislabeling of the blood bank sample or failure to identify the patient at the time the transfusion is initiated.

C. Key Elements of Procedures Needed to Assure Safe Transfusions

1. Method to Assign Identification Number to Patient

The identity of many trauma victims is uncertain at the time they arrive in the hospital; therefore, some sort of temporary identification system must be used. The disadvantages of using generic identifiers such as "male trauma 1" are obvious. Many trauma services

Table 10-1. Risks of transfusion

Category	Complication	Frequency (per unit)
Immunologic		
	Allergic reaction	1: 100
	Febrile reaction	1: 100
	Delayed hemolytic reaction	1: 1600
	Acute hemolytic reaction	1: 50,000
	Fatal hemolytic reaction	1: 500,000
Infectious		
	Hepatitis B virus	1: 81,000
	Hepatitis C virus	1: 1,600,000
	Human T-lymphotropic virus-I	1: 642,000
	Human immunodeficiency virus-I	1: 1,900,000

have a system in place to assign standard hospital identification numbers to incoming trauma victims that can be used until the patient's identity can be reliably established. Some trauma services have preassigned identification numbers and assemble a packet that includes arm bracelets, addressograph plates, laboratory and radiology requisitions, and blood sample labels made out and ready to deploy when the patient arrives at the hospital.

2. Proper Identification of Blood Bank Specimen

Even if units that are not crossmatched are to be transfused initially, a specimen should be sent to the blood bank expeditiously. Safe collection of a blood bank specimen can be assured if the tube is labeled as shown in **Table 10-2.**

3. Proper Identification of Patient when Transfusion is Initiated

Before the transfusion is initiated, the patient's arm band should be checked against the information on, or attached to, the unit of blood to verify that it is intended for that patient.

4. Communication with the Blood Bank

Systems for rapidly sending samples and requisitions to the blood bank, communicating orders, and transporting blood components to the trauma service must be devised and tested. In situations where the blood bank and the trauma service are not close to one another, it may be necessary to use hospital transport, designated runners, or a pneumatic tube system. Guidelines should also be established for the trauma service to communicate the need for high priority, expedited support for a trauma victim. The blood bank and the trauma service should agree in advance on terminology (e.g., emergency release) to minimize

---

Table 10-2. Labeling the blood bank specimen

Label the tube:
   –At the bedside
   –Using identification information on arm bracelet
   –With two patient identifiers (e.g., name and number)
   –With date and your name or initials

---

miscommunication. Use of a dedicated phone or fax line can also be helpful.

D. Emergency Release of Red Blood Cells ("Uncrossmatched Blood")

Performing complete pretransfusion testing, including ABO and Rh typing, a screen for unexpected RBC alloantibodies (the type and screen) and a full serologic crossmatch takes at least an hour and potentially much longer if the patient has a significant (i.e., hemolytic) RBC alloantibody. To respond to emergent or massive transfusion, however, blood banks are required to have alternative (i.e., emergency release) procedures in place to expedite the provision of RBC. They are also required to maintain documentation that the need for rapid transfusion warrants abbreviation of routine pretransfusion testing. The blood bank usually sends the clinician a form for waiving routine pretransfusion testing, which should be signed and returned at a convenient moment.

The various options to expedite the provision of blood for the trauma patient are summarized in **Table 10-3** and discussed below.

1. Group O Red Blood Cells

Group O RBC have the advantage of being ABO compatible with patients of all ABO blood groups and, therefore, can be issued before a sample has been sent to the blood bank. All patients cannot be supported indefinitely with group O RBC, however, because only approximately 40% of donor units are group O. Extensive use of group O RBC for non-O patients is wasteful. It is therefore common practice to switch from O RBC to ABO group-specific RBC once the ABO group of the patient has been determined.

The use of group O blood for emergent transfusion is a fairly safe practice and the most rapid way to obtain RBC for transfusion. A risk exists, however, that the emergency release group O RBC may not be compatible with patients who have alloantibodies to non-ABO blood group antigens. Non-ABO blood group alloantibodies are found in 1% to 2 % of hospitalized patients.

2. The Rh Problem

Most blood banks have an established procedure with respect to the Rh type of blood issued for emergent or massive transfusion. A common policy is to issue Rh(+) units to male patients and older women and up

Table 10-3. Expedited provision of RBC

ABO Group	Crossmatch	Preparation Time (min)[a]	Testing Required	Risks of Incompatibility
Group O RBC[b]	None	5	None	RBC alloantibody
ABO Group specific	None	15	ABO/Rh type	RBC alloantibody
ABO Group specific	Abbreviated	30	ABO/Rh type Antibody screen immediate spin or electronic crossmatch	Screen negative—none Screen positive—RBC alloantibody
ABO Group specific	Full	60	ABO/Rh type Antibody screen Full crossmatch	None

[a]Preparation time in the blood bank. Does not include time for delivery of specimen to blood bank or delivery of RBC to trauma service.
[b]Rh (–) units are usually reserved for premenopausal women; Rh (+) units are usually issued for men and older women.
RBC, red blood cell.
(Adapted from Blackall DP. Approach to acute bleeding and massive transfusion. In: Hillyer CD, Hillyer KL, Strobl FJ, et al., eds. *Handbook of transfusion medicine.* Academic Press 2001:191, with permission.)

to a predetermined number (e.g., 4 to 10) of Rh(−) units for women of childbearing potential. The use of Rh(−) blood is not required for the patient's immediate safety.

The reason for giving Rh(−) RBC to younger female patients who are Rh(−) or whose Rh type is not known, is to avoid the future formation of Rh alloantibodies. Rh alloantibodies are responsible for the most severe forms of hemolytic disease of the newborn. Because group O Rh(−) donors only comprise about 6% of the population, these units are typically reserved for younger female patients in the trauma setting.

The consequences for a man or older woman developing an Rh alloantibody in the future are not serious. Although the Rh (or D) antigen is highly immunogenic, Rh(−) patients who eventually make Rh alloantibodies will be transfused with Rh(−) units anyway.

The foregoing discussion of Rh is provided chiefly by way of explanation. The physician treating the hemorrhaging patient should let the blood bank deal with the issue of what Rh type blood to issue.

3. Switching Patients to ABO/Rh Group-Specific Red Blood Cell Support

Once the blood bank has been able to determine the patient's ABO and Rh type, group specific, uncrossmatched blood can be provided. The ABO and Rh typing can often be accomplished while the patient is receiving an initial transfusion of group O RBC. The risks are the same as for the use of group O RBC, namely the possibility that the patient has a RBC alloantibody outside of the ABO system.

If a woman of childbearing potential is found to be Rh(−) (and has not already received Rh(+) units), the blood bank will usually provide up to some predetermined number (typically 4 to 10 units) of Rh(−) RBC. Once that point is reached and it appears that the patient will continue to require a considerable number of RBC, the blood bank may switch to Rh(+) units. Again, the clinician should let the blood bank deal with this issue.

4. ABO/Rh Specific Abbreviated Crossmatch

Once the blood bank has been able to perform a screen for unexpected RBC alloantibodies and found it to be negative (i.e., the patient is not alloimmunized), RBC can be released for transfusion after an abbreviated crossmatch to confirm ABO compatibility. The risk of most unexpected RBC alloantibodies can be eliminated by this approach. One form of the abbreviated crossmatch is the immediate spin technique, which detects ABO incompatibility between the patient and the donor unit. The other option is to use the blood bank information system to verify ABO compatibility (the "electronic" crossmatch).

5. ABO/Rh Specific Full Crossmatch

Managing a hemorrhaging patient with a RBC alloantibody can be difficult. If the patient has an unexpected RBC alloantibody (i.e., the antibody screen is positive), a full serologic crossmatch should be performed, if possible. The clinical condition of the patient, however, can make it necessary to initiate transfusion before the alloantibody is identified or full serologic crossmatching can be performed. A transfusion medicine specialist will be able to estimate the clinical consequences, as well as to expedite the provision of suitable units.

6. "Whole" Blood

Donated blood that has not been fractionated into components, or "whole blood," is essentially no longer available. The term whole blood was always a misnomer. After a day in storage at 4°C, platelets are no longer functional, the granulocytes have disintegrated, and the levels of factors VIII and V have begun to drop. Any contribution of whole blood to hemostasis (other than by elevating the hematocrit) was largely imaginary and certainly not as effective as platelets and plasma components that have been stored under conditions that preserve their hemostatic function.

7. The Viscosity Factor: Know Your Components

Packed RBC have a higher hematocrit than whole blood, hence higher viscosity, which some clinicians cite as an impediment to rapid transfusion. Although this has been an issue with packed RBC stored in older anticoagulant or preservative systems, nearly all of the packed RBC available in the United States are collected using a system in which an additional volume of a nutrient or salt solution is added to the RBC, returning the hematocrit and viscosity to physiologic levels (**Table 10-4**).

II. Red Blood Cell Transfusion in Trauma

Because hemorrhaging patients lose both volume- and oxygen-carrying capacity, fluid resuscitation and RBC transfusion must be coordinated. The following approach is consistent with recommendations in chapter 6: *Initial Evaluation and Resuscitation: Primary Survey and Immediate Resuscitation* where this topic is also discussed in some detail.

Table 10-4. Comparison of RBC components

	Packed RBC	Packed RBC	Whole Blood
Anticoaglulant/ preservative	AS-1 Adsol	CPDA-1	CPD
RBC volume (mL)[a]	203	203	203
Unit volume (mL)	350	263	513
Hematocrit	58%	77%	40%
Availability	Common	Uncommon	Scarce

[a] Based on 450 mL collection from donor with a hematocrit of 45%.
RBC, red blood cells.

A.   Patient Assessment

The first step in managing acute hemorrhage is to assess the hemodynamic status of the patient and estimate the amount of blood loss. Estimating blood loss is notoriously difficult (even in the controlled setting of the operating room), particularly if the injuries are internal. The American College of Surgeons has developed a system for classifying shock, which is based on easily determined criteria and can be used to assess the hemorrhaging patient (**Table 10-5**). Because the system correlates the degree of shock with the volume of blood loss, it is a useful tool for directing therapy.

B.   Therapeutic Goals in Managing Acute Hemorrhage

Three goals are seen for the treatment of acute hemorrhage; reversal of shock, control of bleeding, and restoration of the RBC mass. During the acute phase of resuscitation, most patients will tolerate a hematocrit of 19% to 21% if they are euvolemic. Once bleeding has been controlled, the goal should be to bring the patient who is less than 50 years of age to a hematocrit of 24% to 27% (hemoglobin 8 to 9 g/dL) and the patient who is more than 50 years of age to a hematocrit of 27% to 30% (hemoglobin 9 to 10 g/dL). If rebleeding is likely, this target can be revised upward to allow for a physiologic cushion against further blood loss.

III.   Alternatives and Supplements to Red Blood Cell Transfusion in Trauma

A.   Recovery and Reinfusion of Shed Blood

The recovery and reinfusion of a patient's blood intraoperatively has become a widespread practice for elective surgical procedures where substantial blood loss is incurred (e.g., partial hepatectomy, orthotopic liver transplantation, surgery of the aortic arch and thoracic aorta, hip arthroplasty, especially repeat procedures, and some forms of cardiac surgery). Most commonly, shed blood is aspirated from the operative field with the addition of an anticoagulant (usually citrate, heparin or a mixture). It is then accumulated in a reservoir and processed in a centrifugal device that washes the RBC with normal saline (e.g., the Gambro "BRAT" or the Hemonetics "Cell Saver"). The washed red cells, suspended in normal saline, are transferred to a bag from which they can be transfused to the patient much as is done with a conventional unit of banked RBC. No anticoagulant is required after the washing step because no platelets or plasma are present in the finished product.

The principal advantage of these systems is that the efficient recovery and reinfusion of the patient's own cells reduces exposure to donor blood and demands on the blood bank inventory. In addition, the recovered red cells have no signs of storage-related changes. Among the disadvantages are that the supplies and labor are costly; the equivalent of several units of donor blood must be saved to recoup the expense of using the device. It also requires a trained operator. In hospitals where these devices are already in use for

Table 10-5.   American college of surgeons shock class and blood loss

Assessment Parameter	Class I	Class II	Class III	Class IV
Blood loss (mL)	Up to 750	750–1500	1500–2000	>2000
Blood loss (% blood volume)	Up to 15	15–30	30–40	>40
Pulse (beats/min)	<100	>100	>120	>140
Blood pressure	Normal	Normal	Decreased	Decreased
Pulse pressure (mm Hg)	Normal or increased	Normal	Normal	Normal
Respiratory rate (breath/min)	14–20	20–30	30–40	>40
Urine output (mL/h)	>30	20–30	5–15	Negligible
Mental status	Slightly anxious	Mildly anxious	Anxious, confused	Confused, obtunded
Fluid replacement (3:1 rule)	Crystalloid	Crystalloid	Crystalloid and blood	Crystalloid and blood

elective surgery, the logistics and expenses are less of a deterrent to their use.

Shed blood recovery and reinfusion should be considered in hemorrhaging patients going to the operating room, particularly for thoracic trauma and repair of major vessels. It should probably be avoided in patients with abdominal trauma for fear that the operative field may be contaminated with intestinal contents. Bacteria are not eliminated by the washing procedure and might be reinfused when the RBC are returned to the patient (iatrogenic bacteremia). Although published experience attest to the safety of the use of shed blood recovery in patients with abdominal trauma, we do not recommend it.

Some have had successful experience in thoracic trauma with the use of blood recovered from mediastinal drains, which is typically reinfused through an in-line filter. Because such blood is defibrinated, anticoagulation is not necessary. Filtration systems, however, do not eliminate activated clotting factors, cytokines, and other biologically active molecules from the mediastinal drainage fluid, all of which have been associated with complications in some recipients. The small amount of RBC mass recovered probably does not warrant the routine use of these devices.

B.   Blood Substitutes

Both perfluorocarbon emulsions and solutions of modified hemoglobin have been actively studied for use as blood substitutes. Currently, no blood substitutes are licensed for clinical use in the United States or Europe, although one product has been licensed in South Africa where it is available in limited quantities. Several of the hemoglobin-based substitutes have been studied in trauma where they have been modestly successful in replacing banked RBC. All of them have a short intravascular half-life (12 to 36 hours); however, they persist long enough to be useful in the management of acute hemorrhage. Although this is an exciting area of basic and clinical research, a licensed product is probably still a few years away.

IV.   Blood Component Support of Coagulation During Massive Transfusion

Although not apparent at first, packed RBC comprise the single most important blood component for coagulation support during trauma resuscitation. Without adequate oxygen delivery, lactic acidemia and ischemia of vital organs will result in disseminated intravascular coagulation (DIC), fibrinolysis, uncontrolled bleeding, and death. A fundamental goal in coagulation support of the trauma patient is to prevent the development of a coagulopathic, cold, and acidemic patient. Successful resuscitation depends on adequate tissue perfusion, oxygenation, and normothermia.

Disseminated intravascular coagulation results from production of thrombin that exceeds the body's natural antithrombin mechanism. Under physiologic conditions, thrombin (the key enzyme in coagulation) is activated only locally at the site of injury. Diffuse, circulating thrombin results in DIC and occurs in response to systemic signals for thrombin formation. Tissue factor is the key initiator of the coagulation cascade leading to thrombin formation.

Thus, in any condition that results in diffuse expression of tissue factor is found a risk of DIC. In the setting of trauma, tissue ischemia is the most common cause of tissue factor release. Avoiding DIC is critically important because DIC results not only in depletion of residual circulating clotting factors (and thus impaired clotting from cut surfaces), but also results in microvascular thrombosis and worsened tissue ischemia and acidosis. DIC is a common event among patients with shock and acidemia and avoidance depends on optimization of organ perfusion and tissue oxygenation.

In addition to preventing tissue ischemia, proper and skilled coagulation support with blood components and selected medications are also essential to the overall resuscitation of massively bleeding patients. We present a three-stage approach to the coagulation support of massively bleeding trauma patients.

A. Stage 1: Prevent Dilution Coagulopathy During Resuscitation

Nearly all massively bleeding trauma patients have damaged vasculature and surgical bleeding. Very few patients have generalized, spontaneous bleeding at sites of undamaged tissues. The first consideration in blood coagulation support is to prevent the development of hemodilution during the time required to achieve surgical hemostasis.

1. To Avoid Hemodilution, Transfuse Platelets First

Dilution of adequate numbers of platelets is important, predictable, and often neglected. For each blood volume of resuscitation in the absence of administered platelets or increased consumption, the residual platelet count will fall by approximately half. Thus, the 60-kg woman with an initial platelet count of $150,000/\mu L$ will have a platelet count of $75,000/\mu L$ after 6 to 8 units of RBC are administered and a count of $37,000/\mu L$ after 15 to 18 units of RBC, even in the absence of increased consumption. Because of the greater reserve of coagulation factors in humans, hemostasis is adversely affected by platelet hemodilution before dilution of coagulation factors. Because platelets are essential for primary hemostasis (the formation of the initial platelet plug that stops small-vessel bleeding), attention should be given to prevent dilution thrombocytopenia during trauma resuscitation. A typical adult dose of platelets in most US hospitals is approximately 5 units (range 4 to 8 units). Each unit will raise the platelet count of an average-sized, nonbleeding adult by 5000 to $7000/\mu L$. Thus, without ongoing blood loss, 5 units will increase the count by $20,000$ to $35,000/\mu L$. As a result, the bleeding adult patient who receives a 5-unit platelet dose with every blood volume lost will continue to "lose ground" and undergo progressive platelet hemodilution.

    a. Guideline. A platelet count should be measured with each blood volume of resuscitation. The count, predictably, will halve with each additional blood volume because of dilution alone. A target goal platelet count in a seriously injured bleeding patient is 50,000 to 80,000/μL. Once bleeding is controlled, much lower concentrations of platelets (> 20,000/μL) can be tolerated by many patients.

2. **To Avoid Hemodilution, Target the Fresh Frozen Plasma Dose to the Red Blood Cell Dose** Hemodilution of coagulation factors also occurs during massive transfusion when inadequate doses of fresh frozen plasma (FFP) are used. Humans have a reserve of coagulation factors and only approximately 20% of the normal circulating levels of coagulation factors are needed for normal hemostasis. As a result, hemodilution of clotting factors generally occurs later than hemodilution of platelets. Hypoperfusion and tissue ischemia, however, can result in consumption and fibrinolysis and, as a result hemodilution of coagulation factors, is often less predictable than platelet hemodilution. Although most patients receiving one blood volume of resuscitation require no FFP, many massively injured patients requiring two or more blood volumes of resuscitation will need FFP to avoid hemodilution.

   a. **Guideline.** Measuring the international normalized ratio (INR) (prothrombin time [PT]) after each blood volume of resuscitation can be a useful guide to monitor and prevent hemodilution of factors. In actively bleeding patients who have already received one to two blood volumes of resuscitation and who demonstrate prolonged coagulation test results, infusion of 1 unit of FFP per 2 units of RBC will prevent extreme hemodilution. The "2 RBC and 1 FFP" guideline will result in an adequate prothrombin time (PT) (INR), activated partial thromboplastin time (aPTT), and fibrinogen for most patients. The goal of this approach should not be to achieve coagulation times in the normal range but rather to achieve a PT < 15 to 19 seconds or an INR 1.4 to 1.7.

3. **Interpreting Results of Prothrombin Time and International Normalized Ratio** The PT (INR) tests are very important, but widely misinterpreted in common clinical practice. Many clinicians who transfuse FFP do not appreciate that an abnormal PT result is consistent with normal coagulation. The normal PT range (11 to 13 seconds on most laboratories) represents the result found in normal subjects, but does not define the physiologic range of normal coagulation. Because of the natural reserve in coagulation factors, biologic hemostasis is normal even when the PT is mildly elevated beyond the normal range (**Fig. 10-1**). Although no single threshold value establishes a transition between normal and abnormal, patients with a PT <16.5 to 17 seconds (INR <1.5) have adequate factor levels and little advantage is seen to infusing more factors in an attempt to further "correct" the laboratory value. Such a strategy is akin to correcting a hematocrit value from 37% to 42% in a patient with normal cardiac function—simply because

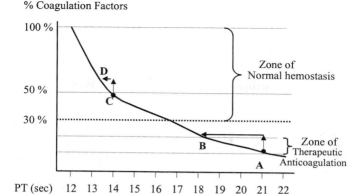

% Coagulation Factors

Figure 10-1.   The nonlinear relationship between levels of coagulation factors and coagulation time results. The zone of normal physiologic hemostasis is shown, as is the zone of coagulation factors corresponding to deliberate anticoagulation with vitamin K antagonists. *Note:* Treating a patient at point *A* with fresh frozen plasma (FFP) to raise the level of factors to point *B* will have a profound effect on the international normalized ratio (INR). The same increase of a patient at point *C*, however, will have a trivial impact on the INR (point *D*).

37% is outside the normal range. Such an approach will not increase oxygen uptake by tissues because a normal cardiac output and a hematocrit of 37% represent more than adequate oxygen supply.

A second reason against infusing large volumes of FFP in an attempt to drive the PT or INR into the "normal" range is shown in **Figure 10-1.** The figure shows that the relationship between coagulation factors and the PT (INR) result is nonlinear. As shown in Figure 10-1, a patient at point "A" will benefit from infusion of FFP to raise coagulation factors to move the patient to point "B." Treatment of a patient at point "C" with the same FFP dose, however, will achieve far less as the patient moves to point "D." Thus, although therapeutic doses of FFP will indeed provide substantial correction of markedly elevated PT values, these same therapeutic doses have a diminishing effect on the PT (INR) result as the patient enters the zone of normal physiologic levels of coagulation factors. As a result, the transfusion of FFP to patients with PT (INR) values in the range of normal coagulation (PT <17; INR <1.5) is both clinically unwarranted and largely ineffectual.

4.   A Limited Role for Cryoprecipitate
Cryoprecipitate represents the cold, insoluble portion of plasma and contains fibrinogen, factor VIII, von

Willebrand factor, and factor XIII. Cryoprecipitate is not a concentrate of FFP. Cryoprecipitate is deficient in multiple essential coagulation factors and lacks prothrombin, thrombin, and factors V, VII, IX, X, and XI. As a result, cryoprecipitate has a limited role in the resuscitation of the trauma patient. Cryoprecipitate, however, can supply additional fibrinogen to the bleeding patient with a low fibrinogen level. Nevertheless, it should be recognized that FFP contains normal concentrations of fibrinogen and that nearly all trauma patients with observed low fibrinogen levels have more wrong with their coagulation system than an isolated deficiency of fibrinogen. Thus, addressing the fibrinogen level alone will not correct the multiple deficiencies in other coagulation factors.

   a.   Guideline. Cryoprecipitate is not a concentrate of FFP. Cryoprecipitate is indicated in the hypofibrinogenemic bleeding patient whose fibrinogen level cannot be sustained with FFP or antifibrinolytic agents. In the actively bleeding patient, a fibrinogen >100 mg/dL should be adequate. Hypofibrinogenemia, despite adequate FFP infusion, suggests the presence of DIC or systemic fibrinogenolysis.

   Cryoprecipitate can also serve a useful role for topical hemostasis in selected patients. When administered topically in conjunction with thrombin, a topical fibrin sealant (fibrin glue) is formed. This form of topical hemostasis is useful in selected instances where electrocautery or suture is not possible.

B.   Stage Two: Look for Fibrinolysis

After surgical hemostasis is achieved, some patients who do not have dilution coagulopathy still demonstrate diffuse bleeding. Clinically, in the operating room may be observed sites rebleeding that had previously been dry. This pattern is typical of accelerated clot lysis and is an under recognized aspect of the physiology of trauma. Fibrinolytic activators (e.g., tissue plasminogen activator) are released from endothelial cells in response to shock and pressors. They produce plasmin, which localizes to and digests the clot. Thus, patients will exhibit clot lysis (fibrinolysis) even before demonstrating any evidence of systemic fibrinogen lysis. These patients improve their clinical hemostasis with the use of fibrinolytic inhibitor therapy. In more extreme cases, excessive plasmin generation spills out into the systemic circulation and lyses multiple circulating coagulation factors, including fibrinogen. This is observed as both a low measured fibrinogen level and as a PT (INR or aPTT) result prolonged beyond the value expected from hemodilution. Clot lysis also results in an elevated D-dimer.

In addition to systemic fibrinolysis and fibrinogenolysis, patients having trauma surgery are subject to local fibrinolysis at the wound site. All wounds that involve serosal surfaces (e.g., peritoneum, pleura, pericardium) can involve local release of plasminogen activators that are found in high concentrations at these surfaces. The local fibrinolysis will dissolve shed blood. This is why blood from wound drainage does not clot. The local fibrinolysis, however, will also dissolve clots in the surgical field surrounding the wound perpetuating bleeding. Although standard treatment involves removing retained blood (by drainage or washout), the use of antifibrinolytic medications can also provide dramatic improvement in hemostasis.

C.   Stage Three: Consider Hypothermia and Platelet Dysfunction

After correcting any dilutional coagulopathy and addressing shock, DIC, and fibrinolysis (if present), the third level of coagulation concern in massive transfusion focuses on hypothermia and platelet dysfunction. Studies have shown that hypothermia impairs coagulation most likely through interference with normal platelet function. In one study, normal subjects placed one arm in a warm water bath and the other arm in a cold water bath. Skin bleeding time measurements (an assay chiefly focused on primary hemostasis) and platelet granule release were impaired in the hypothermic arm. Other studies suggest that hypothermia ($<34°C$) also impairs the rate of fibrin formation by the coagulation cascade. As measured by thromboelastography, trauma patients presenting with hypothermia are initially hypercoagulable unless their core temperature is $<34°C$. Thus, as measured both *in vitro* and *in vivo,* mild hypothermia ($>35°C$) does not likely produce a profound effect on coagulation.

Massively transfused patients frequently demonstrate impaired platelet function resulting from elevated levels of fibrin split products and hypothermia. In addition, a large proportion of circulating platelets in all massively transfused patients represents transfused platelets which, after storage in the blood bank, do not function as well as native circulating platelets. For example, platelet aggregation measurements demonstrate that stored blood bank platelets require much stronger aggregation signals than freshly collected platelets. In addition, the lifespan of transfused, stored platelets is shorter than normal platelets. Massively transfused individuals who reach postoperative intensive care are populated with a cohort of transfused blood bank platelets. Approximately 48 hours after massive transfusion, this cohort of platelets leaves the circulation. Because the patient has not yet generated an adequate number of his or her own platelets, the recipient's platelet count will precipitously decline. If not recognized, this event can be confused as DIC, heparin-induced thrombocytopenia, or other conditions.

V.   Pharmacologic Adjuncts to Blood Components for Coagulation

A.   Antifibrinolytic Agents (Aminocaproic Acid, Aprotinin)

Antifibrinolytic agents are important and potent adjuncts to the coagulation management of selected patients having massive transfusion. Patients who are actively bleeding in the setting of either local or systemic fibrinolysis or fibrinogenolysis (**see Section V.B.**) are candidates for antifibrinolytic therapy. The decision to use these agents should include their potential to induce pathologic thrombosis, which is usually of secondary concern in any massively bleeding patient. Nevertheless, these drugs should not generally be used in patients with thrombotic DIC (ischemic organ beds, blue extremities with laboratory evidence of DIC); patients with upper tract renal hemorrhage as the only bleeding source; or patients with known thrombophilia states. Because aminocaproic acid is less expensive than aprotinin and carries less risk of allergic reaction than aprotinin, it is often preferable to use for antifibrinolytic therapy. A loading dose of 5 to 10 g for a 70-kg adult can be followed by an infusion of up to 1 g/h. The drug requires renal excretion and the dose should be decreased if the patient has renal failure.

B.   Desmopressin

Desmopressin (DDAVP) causes the release of endogenous von Willebrand factor, the most important protein for platelet adhesion. Because physiologic stress and pressors also result in release of endogenous von Willebrand factor, little value is seen to DDAVP use in most severely injured trauma patients.

C.   Clotting Factor Concentrates

Prothrombin complex concentrates (Konyne, Profilnine, Bebulin) are of no proven value in the management of trauma and massive bleeding. These agents are designed for treatment of hemophilia and are not approved for use in trauma. The concentrates are enriched for factor IX; have good levels of coagulation factors II and X; have low levels of factor VII; and are devoid of fibrinogen and factors XIII, XII, XI, VIII, V, and von Willebrand factor. No reason exists to expect them to be superior to FFP. Most actively bleeding patients are not volume restricted and, thus, no rationale is generally seen for a concentrate containing only selected factors (**see section V.A.4**).

D.   Recombinant Activated Factor VII

Recombinant VIIa (NovoSeven Novonordisk, Princeton, New Jersey), a concentrate of activated factor VII, is able to bind directly to tissue factor and initiate coagulation. Although rVIIa is not yet approved for use in trauma patients, it is undergoing experimental use in trauma patients. Because trauma patients often have generalized release of tissue factor, administration of rVIIa risks further exacerbation of DIC. The use of rVIIa in trauma patients risks unintended thrombosis of coronary or cerebral vessels.

VI.   Metabolic Complications of Massive Transfusion: Some Truths, Some Myths

Massive transfusion is associated with several life-threatening metabolic complications. These include hypocalcemia, hypomagnesemia, hypothermia, hyperkalemia, and acidemia. Whereas some of these abnormalities are caused by the infused blood (e.g., hypocalcemia secondary to citrate infusion), others (e.g., hyperkalemia and acidemia) are caused by inadequate tissue perfusion and lactic acidosis. If not addressed during the patient's resuscitation, these complications all contribute to cardiovascular instability with eventual electromechanical dissociation and death. As a result, metabolic disarray during massive transfusion must be anticipated and treated expectantly.

A. Citrate Toxicity

All routine blood components are anticoagulated with tri-sodium citrate. Citrate chelates calcium (and magnesium) and thereby prevents coagulation of blood during storage. On transfusion, the recipient must metabolize and excrete the administered citrate. Citrate metabolism occurs in the tricarboxylic acid cycle (Krebs cycle) in all cells of the body (except erythrocytes). Citrate is also excreted unmetabolized by the kidneys. Patients with decreased glomerular filtration (regardless of the cause) will have impaired citrate excretion and be more at risk for the development of citrate toxicity. Although all organs metabolize citrate, the liver has the highest metabolic rate for citrate based on hepatic blood flow and density of mitochondria (where the Krebs cycle is found). Thus, patients with liver failure, resection, or hepatic ischemia are more likely to demonstrate citrate toxicity.

1. Forget Old Rules Regarding Supplemental Calcium or Bicarbonate.

Old rules of thumb suggesting that supplemental calcium (or bicarbonate) should be given for every "X" number of units of RBC make little sense for two reasons: First, it is not the absolute number of RBC units but rather the rate of blood transfusion per kilogram of the recipient that determines whether citrate toxicity will develop. Second, old rules derive from days before blood component preparation. It is important to recognize that >90% of the citrate in blood components is found in FFP and platelets and very little is found in RBC. This is because the citrate (originally located in the blood bag before blood donation) partitions with the plasma (where it prevents coagulation) and the plasma is separated from the RBC during component preparation before blood storage.

Supplemental calcium is rarely indicated in the patient who is receiving only packed RBC. Supplemental calcium is required, however, when large volumes of FFP (or platelets) are rapidly administered—especially to a patient with impaired renal or hepatic function. The normal individual with good organ perfusion receiving massive blood transfusion can generally receive FFP at a rate of 1 unit every 6 minutes without developing signs of citrate toxicity. Thus, for example, a patient with adequate blood pressure and functioning liver and kidneys who is receiving 4 units per hour should not require any supplemental calcium to address citrate concerns.

2. Measure Ionized Calcium

Citrate toxicity is best assessed by measurement of the ionized calcium (free calcium). The laboratory must have access to an ion-selective electrode to measure ionized calcium. Because citrate binds calcium but does not destroy it, no rationale is see to measure total calcium, which will remain normal despite severe citrate toxicity. Mild depression of the ionized calcium (just below the local normal limits) is of little consequence and is seen in normal asymptomatic individuals having plasmapheresis.

   a.   Guideline. Calcium supplementation should be given if the level of ionized calcium falls to 50% of the lower limit of the normal range.

   The electrocardiogram will become abnormal in cases of severe citrate toxicity. The electrocardiogram, however, is an insensitive guide to citrate toxicity and is not an adequate substitute for direct measurement of the ionized calcium.

3.   Signs and Symptoms of Citrate Toxicity

As the patient's ionized calcium is progressively depressed from unmetabolized and nonexcreted citrate, symptoms are seen in the following progression: neurologic, cardiovascular, hematologic. Awake patients will experience paresthesias and circumoral tingling. Seizures from hypocalcemia as a result of blood transfusion are very rare, and the presence of seizures should not be attributed to transfusion. Unconscious patients or those under anesthesia will develop cardiovascular compromise as their first sign of citrate toxicity, which consists of a prolonged, corrected QT interval; arrhythmias, hypotension, widened QRS complexes, and electromechanical dissociation. Although citrate does chelate magnesium, symptomatic hypomagnesemia is less common. Nevertheless, the observation of torsade de pointes ventricular arrhythmia in the setting of massive transfusion and low ionized calcium levels may reflect critical hypomagnesemia. Citrate toxicity in the patient does not produce coagulopathy. The threshold levels of calcium required to clot are very low and the patient would experience cardiac standstill before the calcium level in the recipient's blood became so low as to inhibit clotting.

B.   Cold Toxicity

Trauma patients can present with hypothermia as a result of environmental exposure before arrival at the hospital or can develop hypothermia as a result of extensive body cavity exposure during surgical interventions. Blood transfusions can further contribute to hypothermia, although this is preventable with the use of modern blood warming devices. Trauma specialists should make arrangements to use only devices approved for blood transfusion use because stored blood is much more sensitive to thermal lysis than blood in the patient. Any novel use of microwave technology or home-fashioned heating elements should not be permitted. Cold lowers the threshold for ventricular irritability in the setting of hyperkalemia or hypocalcemia.

C. Hyperkalemia

Hyperkalemia, a dangerous sign in the setting of massive transfusion, is caused by either extensive tissue injury (hepatic infarction, crush injury, burn) or acidemia resulting from inadequate tissue perfusion and lactic acidosis. Blood transfusion itself does *not* induce hyperkalemia and well-perfused patients without tissue injury can receive enormous quantities of stored blood without becoming hyperkalemic. Confusion over the role of stored blood and potassium arose from measurements of the K+ concentration in the supernatant of stored RBC, which can reach values of 50 mEq/L. Because the volume of this supernatant is so small, the total quantity of K+ delivered by stored blood is typically about 1 to 2 mEq/unit, which is a negligible quantity relative to endogenous stores in the patient. Moreover, after infusion in the patient, stored red cells restore their adenosine triphosphate (ATP)-dependent Na+/K+ pumps and begin to reclaim K+ lost during storage before transfusion. Thus, circulating transfused RBC begin to readsorb K+ from the recipient's plasma. As a result, well-perfused patients who have been massively transfused demonstrate hypokalemia following massive transfusion. The concentration of K+ in FFP and platelets is normal and does not change during storage.

D. Acidemia

As with hyperkalemia, acidemia during massive transfusion is an ominous sign. It is nearly always caused by lactic acidosis from issue ischemia. Blood transfusion itself does not cause acidemia. Awake patients having complete RBC exchange transfusion and well-perfused surgical patients undergoing massive blood transfusion do not develop acidemia as a result of blood infusion. In fact, massively transfused patients develop posttransfusion metabolic alkalosis. This is because transfused citrate is metabolized to CO_2 and H_2O in the Krebs cycle and the net effect of this metabolism is the loss of a H+ (equivalent to the creation of a H_2CO_3).

VII. Putting It All Together

Figure 10-2 shows a four-tier approach for blood component support of the trauma patient who requires massive transfusion. The best results are seen when skill and experience are used to integrate blood support with diagnostic studies, surgical treatments, and the overall life support of the injured patient.

SELECTED READING

American College of Surgeons Committee on Trauma. *Advanced trauma life support for doctors,* 6th ed. Chicago: American College of Surgeons, 1997.

Carson JL, Hébert PC. Anemia and red blood cell transfusion. In: Simon TL, Dzik WH, Snyder EL, et al., eds. *Rossi's principles of transfusion medicine,* 3rd ed. Philadelphia: Lippincott, Williams & Wilkins, 2002:149–164.

Counts R, Haisch C, Simon T, et al. Haemostasis in massively transfused trauma patients. *Ann Surg* 1979;190:91–96.

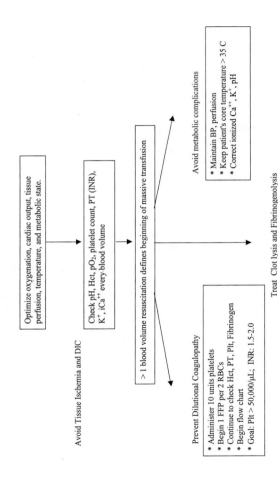

Avoid Tissue Ischemia and DIC

Optimize oxygenation, cardiac output, tissue perfusion, temperature, and metabolic state.

Check pH, Hct, pO₂, platelet count, PT (INR), K⁺, iCa⁺⁺ every blood volume

> 1 blood volume resuscitation defines beginning of massive transfusion

Avoid metabolic complications

* Maintain BP, perfusion
* Keep patient's core temperature > 35 C
* Correct ionized Ca⁺⁺, K⁺, pH

Prevent Dilutional Coagulopathy

* Administer 10 units platelets
* Begin 1 FFP per 2 RBCs
* Continue to check Hct, PT, Plt, Fibrinogen
* Begin flow chart
* Goal: Plt > 50,000/μL; INR: 1.5-2.0

Treat Clot lysis and Fibrinogenolysis

Figure 10-2. Approach to blood component support during massive transfusion.

Dzik WH, Kirkley S. Citrate toxicity in massive transfusion. *Transfus Med Rev* 1988;2:76–94.

Dzik WH. Massive transfusion. In: Churchill WH, Kurtz S, eds. *Transfusion medicine*. Oxford: Blackwell Publications, 1988:211–229.

Hébert PC, Wels G, Blajchman MA, et al. A multicenter, randomized, controlled clinical trial of transfusion requirements in critical care. *N Engl J Med* 1999;340:409–417.

Hippala ST, Myllyla GJ, Vahtera EM. Hemostatic factors and replacement of major blood loss with plasma-poor red cell concentrates. *Anesth Analg* 1995;81:360–365.

Kleinman S. Transfusion-transmitted infection risk from blood components and plasma derivatives. In: Simon TL, Dzik WH, Snyder EL, et al., eds. *Rossi's principles of transfusion medicine,* 3rd ed. Philadelphia: Lippincott, Williams & Wilkins, 2002:703–717.

Kulkarni P, Bhattacharya S, Petros AJ. Torsade de pointes and long QT syndrome following major blood transfusion. *Anaesthesia* 1992;47:125–127.

Leslie SD, Toy PTCY. Laboratory hemostatic abnormalities in massively transfused patients given red blood cells and crystalloid. *Am J Clin Pathol* 1991;96:770–773.

Linko K, Saxelin I. Electrolyte and acid base disturbances caused by blood transfusion. *Acta Anaesthesiol Scand* 1986;30:134–141.

Mannucci P, Federici A, Sirchia G. Hemostasis testing during massive blood replacement. *Vox Sang* 1982;42:113–118.

Michelson AD, Barnard MR, Khuri SF, et al. The effects of aspirin and hypothermia on platelet function in vivo. *Br J Haematol* 1999;104:64–68.

Murray DJ, Pennell BJ, Weinstein SL, et al. Packed red cells in acute blood loss: Dilutional coagulopathy as a cause of surgical bleeding. *Anesth Analg* 1995;80:336–342.

Ozmen V, McSwain NE, Nichols RL, et al. Autotransfusion of potentially culture positive blood (CPB) in abdominal trauma; preliminary data from a prospective study. *J Trauma* 1992;32:36–39.

Reed RI, Bracy AW, Hudson JD, et al. Hypothermia and blood coagulation: dissociation between enzyme activity and clotting factor levels. *Circulatory Shock* 1990;32:141–152.

Spotnitz WD, Welker R. Clinical uses of fibrin sealant. In: Mintz PD, ed. *Transfusion therapy: clinical principles and practice.* Bethesda: AABB Press, 1999:199–222.

Stowell CP, Levin J, Spiess BD, et al. Progress in the development of blood substitutes. *Transfusion* 2001;41:287–299.

Watts D, Trask A, Soeken K, et al. Hypothermic coagulopathy in trauma: effect of varying levels of hypothermia on enzyme speed, platelet function, and fibrinolytic activity. *J Trauma* 1998;44:846–854.

11

Initial Evaluation and Management of the Burn Patient

Robert L. Sheridan, MD, John T. Schulz III, MD, Colleen M. Ryan, MD, and Mary Elizabeth Bilodeau, RN BSN

I. **Introduction**
   A. **Background**
   The prognosis for burn patients, both for survival and for quality of life, has improved dramatically over the past 20 years. This change began with a realization that the natural history of burns can be changed by prompt surgery, the objective of which is to remove deep wounds and achieve immediate biologic closure before the inevitable development of wound sepsis. It is now expected that most people who have serious burns will do well. To meet this expectation, however, requires that burn patients are properly evaluated and managed during the first hours and days after injury. Most such patients initially will be managed within trauma programs before they are transferred to burn units. Many patients with less serious injuries will have all of their management within trauma programs. It is therefore essential that clinicians caring for trauma patients are capable of providing high-quality initial care of adults and children with serious burns.
   B. **Initial Priorities**
   In the first few hours after injury, several priorities must be addressed by the trauma team.
      1. **Primary Survey and Stabilization—Including Control of the Airway**
      2. **Complete Trauma Evaluation**
      3. **Burn-specific Secondary Survey**
      4. **Fluid Resuscitation**
      5. **Maintenance of Torso Compliance and Extremity Perfusion**
      6. **Preparation for Burn Center Transfer of Selected Patients**
   C. **Overall Management Strategy**
   Patients with large burns typically present with a deep wound, associated with pain, impending sepsis, and potentially progressive multiorgan dysfunction. Immediate needs must be met, but a specific overall plan of care must also be generated. An organized plan of care can be viewed as having four phases (**Table 11-1**). The initial evaluation and resuscitation phase, from days 1 though 3, requires that an accurate fluid resuscitation be performed while the patient is thoroughly evaluated for other injuries and comorbid conditions. The second phase, initial wound exci-

Table 11-1.   Phases of burn care

Phase	Objectives	Time Period
1. Initial evaluation and resuscitation	Accurate fluid resuscitation and thorough evaluation	0–72 h
2. Initial wound excision and biologic closure	Exactly identify and remove all full-thickness wounds and achieve biologic closure	Days 1–7
3. Definitive wound closure	Replace temporary with definitive covers and close small complex wounds	Days 7–Week
4. Rehabilitation, reconstruction, and reintegration	Initially, to maintain range and reduce edema; subsequently, to strengthen and facilitate return to home, work, school	Day 1 through discharge

sion and biologic closure, is the maneuver that so profoundly changes the natural history of the disease. Typically, a series of staged operations are completed during the first few days after injury. The third phase, definitive wound closure, involves replacement of temporary wound covers with definitive covers, and closure and acute reconstruction of small but highly complex surface areas (e.g., the face and hand). The final stage of care is rehabilitation. Although rehabilitation begins early—even during resuscitation—it becomes involved and time-consuming toward the end of the acute hospital stay. Ideally, patients are ready to return home when they are discharged from the burn unit.

II.   Physiologic Implications of Burn Injury
A.   Predictable Physiologic Changes
Successfully resuscitated burn patients manifest a sequence of predictable physiologic changes (**Table 11-2**). Anticipation of these changes is possible.

1.   Early Ebb Phase and Later Hyperdynamic Phase
Cuthbertson first described the ebb and flow phases of injury. The ebb phase relates to a period of hours to a day after injury in which the patient is in a relative hypodynamic state that needs to be supported in the resuscitation period. The flow phase relates to the subsequent predictable development of high cardiac output, low reduced peripheral vascular tone, fever, and muscle catabolism that becomes particularly exaggerated in patients with large burns.

**Table 11-2.   Predictable physiologic
changes in burn patients**

Period	Physiologic Changes	Clinical Implications
Resuscitation Period (day 0 to 3)	Massive capillary leak	Closely monitor fluid resuscitation
Postresuscitation Period (day 3 until 95% wound definitive wound closure)	Hyperdynamic and catabolic state with high risk of infection	Remove and close wounds to avoid sepsis; nutritional support is essential
Recovery period (95% wound closure until 1 year after injury)	Continued catabolic state and risk of nonwound	Accurate nutritional support essential; anticipate septic events and treat complications

2.   Physiology of the Resuscitation Period

Unique to a patient suffering a serious burn is a massive, diffuse capillary leak, believed to be secondary to wound-released mediators, that results in the vascular extravasation of fluids, electrolytes, and even moderate-sized colloid molecules. Burn patients initially require massive fluid resuscitation. Formulas have been developed over the past 40 years that attempt to predict resuscitation volume requirements based on body weight or body surface area and burn size. Multiple other variables, however, affect resuscitation requirements, including *preexisting fluid deficits,* delay until resuscitation, inhalation injury, and the depth and vapor transmission characteristics of the wound itself. No two injuries are exactly alike and no formula has yet been developed that accurately predicts volume requirements in all patients. Inaccurate volume administration is associated with substantial morbidity. It, therefore, is essential that burn resuscitations be guided by hourly reevaluation of resuscitation endpoints, the formula serving only to help determine initial volume infusion rates and to roughly predict overall requirements.

3.   Postresuscitation Physiology

In those patients who are successfully resuscitated, volume requirements abruptly decline 18 to 24 hours after injury, as the diffuse capillary leak predictably abates. Subsequently, a diffuse inflammatory state evolves that is characterized by a hyperdynamic circulation, fever, and massively increased protein catabolism. Release of poorly characterized inflammatory mediators; the counter regulatory hormones cortisol, catecholamines, and glucagon; bacteria and their byproducts from the wound; and a compromised gastrointestinal barrier, pain, and infection are thought responsible for these changes.

B. Physiologic Support

The metabolic stress associated with a large burn is enormous. Support includes accurate fluid repletion, provision of an adequate quantity and quality of substrate, control of environmental temperature, prompt removal of nonviable tissue with physiologic wound closure, support of the gastrointestinal barrier, and proper management of pain and anxiety. A critical component is support of body temperature. Burn patients have enormous evaporative water and energy losses if they are maintained in the typical cool, dry air of a general hospital. Monitoring and support of body temperature is an important part of initial care. Burn units and operating rooms need to be engineered to maintain high ambient temperatures and humidity to avoid hypothermia.

III. Initial Evaluation

The initial management of a seriously burned patient is often completed within the trauma unit that first receives the patient and before transfer to a burn center. All of these patients should be approached as a potential polytrauma patient. The evaluation follows the primary and secondary survey format of the American College of Surgeons' Committee on Trauma's Advanced Trauma Life Support (ATLS) Course.

A. Primary Survey

The primary survey encompasses the first few seconds and minutes of the initial evaluation of the burn patient. Special points of emphasis for the burn patient include the following.

1. Airway Evaluation and Protection

The patency and security of the airway must be established, realizing that progressive mucosal edema can compromise airway patency over the first few hours after injury. This is especially true of young children, as airway resistance varies inversely with the fourth power of the airway radius. Endotracheal intubation should be performed if progressive airway edema is suspected. Do not wait until edema is symptomatic and intubation must be performed emergently. Facial and airway edema makes the burn patient's airway among the most challenging to intubate. Proper tube security is critical because inadvertent extubation in the patient with a burned, swollen face and airway is potentially lethal. A harness system using umbilical ties is recommended.

2. Vascular Access and Initial Fluid Support

Reliable and secure vascular access is essential. *In severely injured patients,* this usually requires central venous access, although the placement of central lines is most safely performed after immediate postburn hypovolemia has been corrected by volume administration.

3. Multiple Trauma Issues

All patients with multiple trauma must be approached as a polytrauma patient because other injuries are common. Initial evaluation of the trauma patient is outlined in Chapter 6, *Initial Evaluation and Resuscitation: Primary Survey and Immediate Resuscitation.*

4. Hypothermia

Severely burned patients have an inability to maintain their body temperature. Temperature should be monitored and hypothermia addressed.

B. Burn-specific Secondary Survey

In parallel with the trauma secondary survey, a number of burn-specific issues must be considered during the initial evaluation (**Table 11-3**).

1. History

The initial evaluation is the best time to elicit important points of medical history and mechanism of injury. These data should be actively sought from emergency personnel and family members because access to these individuals and their information often is transient. Important points include details of the injury mechanism, initial neurologic status, extrication time, and tetanus immune status.

2. Physical Examination

Burn and trauma patients require a comprehensive physical assessment at the time of their initial admission. Several aspects of this physical assessment are unique to burn patients.

a. Head, Eyes, Ears, Nose, and Throat. The head should be inspected for trauma. Pressure on the burned occiput should be avoided. The globes should be inspected before the development of massive adnexal edema, which can severely limit an adequate examination. Serious burns of the globe are generally apparent by a clouded appearance of the cornea. More subtle injuries are detectable after fluorescein staining. Adnexal burns are noted, but acute tarsorrhaphy is virtually never indicated. Ear burns are noted; pressure is avoided on the burned auricle and topical mafenide acetate is applied. *The tympanic membranes should be checked for perforation in the event of a blast injury.* Finally, signs of inhalation injury (e.g., carbonaceous debris and singed vibrissae) are noted on examination of the nose and throat. Devices used to secure the nasogastric and endotracheal tubes are adjusted to that they do not apply pressure on the nasal septum.

b. Neurologic. Assess the patient for central nervous system trauma. Imaging of the head and axial spine is indicated, depending on the mechanism of injury (see Chapters 14 and 15, *The Nervous System*). Pain and anxiety management, ideally, is begun during the initial evaluation. In paralyzed or obtunded patients, it is important to make sure there is no pressure on peripheral nerves, so that neuropathies are avoided. Finally, those burned in structural fires should be assessed

(*text continues on page 156*)

Table 11-3.   Important aspects of the burn-specific secondary survey

SYSTEM AND IMPORTANT CONSIDERATIONS

HISTORY
1. Important points include the mechanism of injury, closed space exposure, extrication time, delay in seeking attention, fluid given during transport, and prior illnesses and injuries.

HEENT
1. The globes should be examined and corneal epithelium stained with fluroscein before adnexal swelling makes examination difficult. Adnexal swelling provides excellent coverage and protection of the globe during the first days after injury. Tarsorrhaphy is virtually never indicated acutely.
2. Corneal epithelial loss can be overt, giving a clouded appearance to the cornea, but is more often subtle, requiring fluorescein staining for documentation. Topical ophthalmic antibiotics constitute optimal initial treatment.
3. Signs of airway involvement include perioral and intraoral burns or carbonaceous material and progressive hoarseness.
4. Hot liquid can be aspirated in conjunction with a facial scald injury and result in acute airway compromise requiring urgent intubation.
5. Endotracheal tube security is crucial and is best maintained with an umbilical tape harness, rather than adhesive tape, on the burned face.

NECK
1. The radiographic evaluation is driven by the mechanism of injury.
2. Rarely, in patients with very deep burns, neck escharotomies are needed to facilitate venous drainage of the head.

CARDIAC
1. The cardiac rhythm should be monitored for 24 to 72 hours in those with electrical injury.
2. Although elderly patients may develop transient atrial fibrillation if modestly over resuscitated, significant dysrhythmias are unusual if intravascular volume and oxygenation are adequately supported.
3. Those with a prior history of myocardial infarction can reinfarct with the hemodynamic stress associated with the injury and should be appropriately monitored.

PULMONARY
1. Ensure inflating pressures are less than 40 cm H_2O by performing chest escharotomies when needed.
2. Severe inhalation injury can lead to slough of endobronchial mucosa and thick bronchial secretions that can occlude the endotracheal tube; be prepared for sudden endotracheal tube occlusions.

VASCULAR
1. The perfusion of burned extremities should be vigilantly monitored by serial examinations. Indications for escharotomy include decreasing temperature, increasing consistency, slowed capillary refill, and diminished Doppler flow in the digital vessels. Do not wait until flow in named vessels is compromised to decompress the extremity.

continued

Table 11-3. *Continued*

SYSTEM AND IMPORTANT CONSIDERATIONS

2. Fasciotomy is indicated after electrical or deep thermal injury when distal flow is compromised on clinical examination. Compartment pressures can be helpful, but clinically worrisome extremities should be decompressed regardless of compartment pressure readings.

ABDOMEN
1. Nasogastric tubes should be in place and their function verified, particularly before air transport in unpressurized helicopters.
2. An inappropriate resuscitative volume requirement can be a sign of an occult intraabdominal injury.
3. Torso escharotomies may be required to facilitate ventilation in the presence of deep circumferential abdominal wall burns.
4. Immediate ulcer prophylaxis with histamine receptor blockers and antacids is indicated in all patients with serious burns.

GENITOURINARY
1. Bladder catheterization facilitates using urinary output as a resuscitation endpoint and is appropriate in all who require a fluid resuscitation.
2. It is important to ensure that the foreskin is reduced over the bladder catheter after insertion, as progressive swelling can result in paraphimosis

NEUROLOGIC
1. An early neurologic evaluation is important, as the patient's sensorium is often progressively compromised by medication or hemodynamic instability during the hours after injury. This may require computed tomography scanning in those with a mechanism of injury consistent with head trauma.
2. Patients who require neuromuscular blockade for transport should also receive adequate sedation and analgesia.

EXTREMITIES
1. Extremities at risk for ischemia, particularly those with circumferential thermal burns or those with electrical injury, should be promptly decompressed by escharotomy, fasciotomy, or both when clinical examination reveals increasing consistency, decreasing temperature, and diminished Doppler flow in digital vessels. Limbs at risk should be dressed so they can be frequently examined.
2. The need for escharotomy usually becomes evident during the early hours of resuscitation. Many escharotomies can be delayed until transport has been effected if transport time will not extend beyond 6 hours postinjury.
3. Burned extremities should be elevated and splinted in a position of function.

WOUND
1. Although wounds are often underestimated in depth and overestimated in size on initial examination, nevertheless, they should be evaluated for size, depth, and the presence of circumferential components.

Table 11-3. *Continued*

SYSTEM AND IMPORTANT CONSIDERATIONS

LABORATORY
1. Arterial blood gas analysis is important when airway compromise or inhalation injury is present.
2. A normal admission carboxyhemoglobin concentration does not eliminate the possibility of a significant exposure as the half-life of carboxyhemoglobin is 30 to 40 minutes in those effectively ventilated with 100% oxygen.
3. Baseline hemoglobin and electrolytes can be helpful later during resuscitation.
4. Urinalysis for occult blood should be sent for those with deep thermal or electrical injuries.

RADIOGRAPH
1. The radiographic evaluation is driven by the mechanism of injury and the need to document placement of supportive cannulae.

ELECTRIC
1. Monitor cardiac rhythm for 24 to 72 hours in high (>1000 V) or intermediate (>220 V) voltage exposures.
2. Low and intermediate voltage exposures can cause locally destructive injuries, but rarely result in systemic sequelae.
3. Carefully documented neurologic and ocular examinations are an important part of the initial assessment after high voltage exposures because delayed neurologic and ocular sequelae can occur.
4. Injured extremities should be serially evaluated for intracompartmental edema and promptly decompressed when it develops.
5. Bladder catheters should be placed in all patients suffering high voltage exposure to document the presence or absence or pigmenturia, which can be treated adequately with volume loading in most patients.

CHEMICAL
1. Irrigate wounds with tap water for at least 30 minutes. Irrigate the globe with isotonic crystalloid solution. Blepharospasm may require ocular anesthetic administration.
2. Exposures to hydrofluoric acid may be complicated by life-threatening hypocalcemia, particularly exposures to concentrated or anhydrous solutions. Such patients should have serum calcium closely monitored and supplemented. Subeschar injection of 10% calcium gluconate solution is appropriate after exposure to highly concentrated or anhydrous solutions.

TAR
1. Tar should be initially cooled with tap water irrigation and later removed with a lipophilic solvent.

(Adapted from Sheridan RL, Tompkins RG. Burns. In: Greenfield LJ, Mulholland MW, Oldham KT, et al., eds. *Surgery: scientific principles and practice.* Philadelphia: JB Lippincott, 1996;12:422–438, with permission.)

for carbon monoxide exposure by history, neurologic examination, and carboxyhemoglobin level because selected patients with significant exposures can benefit from hyperbaric oxygen treatment.

c.   Neck. The neck should be assessed for trauma, based on the mechanism of injury. This is particularly important in those suffering high voltage injuries. Extremely deep circumferential neck burns may require escharotomy to facilitate normal venous drainage of the head.

d.   Chest. The chest should be assessed for compliance, and deep eschars should be sectioned if they interfere with ventilation. Escharotomy is best done, bilaterally if needed, along the anterolateral chest wall. The presence of bilateral air movement should be verified.

e.   Cardiovascular. Most patients initially are hypovolemic and respond favorably to volume administration. Occasionally, patients with massive burns will have an element of primary myocardial dysfunction. These patients, identified with invasive monitoring, will benefit from the administration of a beta-adrenergic agonist (e.g., dobutamine).

f.   Genitourinary. In male patients, foreskin retracted over the glans should be reduced after catheterization of the bladder so that progressive edema does not result in acute paraphimosis. Occasionally, a deeply burned foreskin must be sectioned to permit bladder catheterization. Pregnancy tests should be routinely performed on all women burn patients of childbearing age.

g.   Musculoskeletal. Burned extremities must be assessed for other trauma and monitored for adequacy of perfusion. It can sometimes be difficult to identify fractures in this setting, so liberal use of radiography is appropriate. Fractured and burned extremities are initially stabilized with external splints. Progressive edema during resuscitation can result in the late development of profound limb ischemia, secondary to swelling within circumferential eschar or inelastic muscle compartments. Extremity perfusion should be monitored throughout the resuscitation period.

h.   Skin. First-degree burns are superficial and involve only the epidermis. The classic example is sunburn. These burns heal without scarring. Second-degree burns involved a portion of the dermis. Superficial second-degree burns are painful and sensate and blanch with pressure. They are usually associated with blisters. They generally heal within 3 weeks by generation of a new epidermis from the base of hair follicles and sweat glands, with minimal scarring. Deeper second-degree burns often have a nonblanching red stain that represents coagulated hemoglobin. Although these burns are sensate and can also heal, healing is prolonged and scar quality is often poor, resulting in functional and cosmetic defects. Skin grafting is often desirable. Third-degree burns are full thickness and involve the entire epidermis and dermis. They are insensate and often have a hard white, black, or brown appearance. Remaining hair shafts can be readily extracted from the eschar with no evident attachment, indicating that the base of the hair follicle is destroyed. Assessment of burn depth on admission is often misleading because injured cells can go on to die over the next several days, increasing the depth of the burn.

3. Initial Wound Evaluation and Management
Wounds are assessed for extent, using (a) a Lund-Browder or other burn diagram (**Fig. 11-1**), depth, (b) the practiced examiner's eye, and (3) the presence of circumferential components, which may require decompression to assure adequate perfusion.

4. Laboratory and Radiographs
Little laboratory evaluation is required beyond routine electrolyte and hematologic testing, except for carboxyhemoglobin and arterial blood gas determinations, in the proper clinical setting. Toxicology screens are often useful for many reasons, including identifying potential large fluid deficits associated with alcohol intake. Chest radiographs are appropriate to ensure proper placement of resuscitative cannulas and the absence of chest trauma. Inhalation injuries rarely cause early radiographic changes. The mechanism of injury will dictate the need for other radiographs.

5. Possibility of Abuse
All patients should be screened for abuse as the injury mechanism. Approximately 20% of burns in young children are reported to state authorities for investigation, but abuse occurs in all age groups. The evaluating team should consider this possibility and file any suspicious case with appropriate state agencies. Careful and complete documentation of the circumstances and physical characteristics of the injury *and the source of this information* are essential. Photographic documentation is ideal.

IV. Fluid Resuscitation
  A. Physiology of the Immediate Postburn Period
For perhaps the first hour after an extensive burn, patients experience little derangement in intravascular volume, which explains the common observation that, after even massive injuries, patients can be alert for the first hour after injury. As wound-released mediators are absorbed into the systemic circulation, and as stress- and pain-triggered hormonal release occurs, a diffuse loss of capillary integrity occurs that results in the extravasation of fluids, electrolytes, and even moderate-sized colloid molecules. For

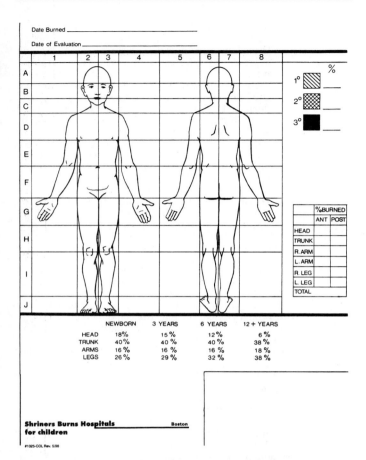

Figure 11-1.   A number of age-specific burn diagrams are available to facilitate accurate estimation of the extent of a burn, compensating for the varying anthropometrics among age groups.

reasons still unknown, this leak abates between 18 and 24 hours later in those successfully resuscitated. An increased leak can be seen in those whose resuscitations are delayed, thought to be caused by the systemic release of reactive oxygen species formed on reperfusion of marginally perfused tissues

B.   Resuscitation Formulas

Formulas have been developed over the past 40 years that attempt to predict resuscitation volume requirements. The multiple variables that have an impact on resuscitation requirements render all such formulas inherently inaccurate. No two injuries are exactly alike and no formula has yet been developed that accurately predicts volume requirements in all patients. Several formulas are widely used to determine initial infusion rates and to roughly guide resuscitation efforts. One such consensus formula is the modified Brooke, which is summarized in **Table 11-4.**

C. Monitoring

Inaccurate volume administration is associated with substantial morbidity. Resuscitation of burn patients must be guided by hourly reevaluation of resuscitation endpoints, which are summarized in **Table 11-5.** Oxygen delivery and consumption determinations have been advocated as guides to the adequacy of burn resuscitation, but no compelling data suggest such information provides clinically relevant guidance in this setting.

D. Recognition and Management of Resuscitation Problems

The infusion volume required by patients with large injuries can be enormous. It is essential to promptly recognize when resuscitation is not proceeding as it should, and what to do in such cases. At any point during a resuscitation, the total 24-hour volume can be predicted based on the known volume infused so far and the current rate of infusion. If this number exceeds 6 mL/kg/% burn/24 hours, it is likely that the resuscitation is not proceeding optimally. At this point,

Table 11-4. The modified Brooke formula

FIRST 24 HOURS

Adults and Children >10 kg

–Ringer's lactate solution: 2–4 mL/kg/%burn/24 h (first half in first 8 h)
–Colloid: none

Children <10 kg

–Ringer's lactate solution: 2–3 mL/kg/%burn/24 h (first half in first 8 h)
–Ringer's lactate solution with 5% dextrose: 4 mL/kg/h
–Colloid: none

SECOND 24 HOURS

All patients

–Crystalloid: To maintain urine output. If silver nitrate is used, sodium leeching will mandate continued isotonic crystalloid. If another topical is used, free water requirement is significant. Serum sodium should be monitored closely. Nutritional support should begin, ideally by the enteral route.
–Colloid: (5% albumin in Ringer's lactate solution):
0% to 30% burn: none
30% to 50% burn: 0.3 mL/kg/%burn/24 h
50% to 70% burn: 0.4 mL/kg/%burn/24 h
>70% burn: 0.5 mL/kg/%burn/24 h

(Adapted from Sheridan RL, Tompkins RG. Burns. In: Greenfield LJ, Mulholland MW, Oldham KT, et al., eds. *Surgery: scientific principles and practice.* Philadelphia: JB Lippincott, 1996;12:422–438, with permission.)

Table 11-5. Age-specific resuscitation endpoints

Endpoint	Target
Sensorium	Comfortable, arousable
Urine output	Infants: 1–2 mL/kg/h Children: 0.5–1 mL/kg/h All others: 0.5 mL/kg/h
Base deficit	<2
Systolic pressure	Infants: 60 to 70 mm Hg Children: 70 to 90 + (twice age in years) mm Hg Adolescents and adults: 90 to 120 mm Hg

(Adapted from Sheridan RL, Tompkins RG. Burns. In: Greenfield LJ, Mulholland MW, Oldham KT, et al., eds. *Surgery: scientific principles and practice.* Philadelphia: JB Lippincott, 1996;12:422–438, with permission.)

consider the use of low-dose dopamine, colloid administration, or the placement of a pulmonary artery catheter to gather additional information regarding the adequacy of ventricular filling and myocardial contractility. This is particularly important in older patients whose underlying cardiac disease is unmasked by the stress of burn resuscitation.

V. Subsequent Intensive Care

Some burn patients will go on to have some or all of their care within a trauma program. It is recommended that those patients whose injury severity meets American Burn Association Burn Center Transfer Criteria are subsequently transferred to American Burn Association or American College of Surgeons' verified burn centers for definitive care. Enhanced outcomes and reduced costs have been demonstrated when such patients are transferred to dedicated centers for comprehensive multidisciplinary care. It is useful for trauma programs to have established relationships with regional burn units. Important highlights of subsequent burn intensive care follow.

A. Neurologic Issues

Neurologic issues that must be considered include pain and anxiety management, the exposed globe, and peripheral neuropathies.

1. Pain and Anxiety Management

Uncontrolled pain and anxiety have adverse physiologic, as well as psychologic, sequelae. Both can contribute to the development of posttraumatic stress syndrome. Previously, inadequate pain management occurred because the extraordinary opiate doses required to address pain adequately in the seriously burned inspired fear of respiratory depression, addiction, and litigation.

The opiate tolerance that rapidly develops in patients with large open wounds can be remarkable. Despite this, addiction is rare; opiate requirements rapidly decrease after wound closure. In fact, the best way to manage pain in burn patients is with prompt biologic closure of the wounds.

Well-monitored administration of intravenous opiates and benzodiazepines is well tolerated by most patients with serious injuries and should be considered unless hemodynamic stability has not been achieved. This is particularly important in those patients who require periods of neuromuscular blockade. Smooth management of pain and anxiety is facilitated by an organized protocol that considers the unique needs of the ventilated acute, nonventilated acute, chronic, and reconstructive patient.

2. Ocular Exposure

Commonly, progressive contraction of the burned eyelids and periocular skin results in exposure of the globe. This predictably results in desiccation of the globe, which is followed by keratitis, ulceration, and globe-threatening infection. Frequent lubrication of the exposed globe with hourly application of ocular lubricants and surgically releasing the eyelid in those who do not rapidly respond help prevent these sequelae.

3. Peripheral Neuropathy

Peripheral neuropathies can develop rapidly in burn patients because of direct thermal damage to peripheral nerves or because of one of the many metabolic derangements that these patients can have. *Peripheral neuropathies can also occur as a result of electrical injury or carbon monoxide poisoning.* Some peripheral neuropathies can be avoided. Diligent monitoring of extremity perfusion avoids the morbidity of constricting eschar and missed compartment syndromes. Proper application of well-fitting splints avoids pressure-induced neuropathies. Careful positioning of deeply sedated or anesthetized patients avoids traction and pressure injuries.

B. Pulmonary Issues

1. Airway Security

The critical importance of secure control of the airway throughout the period of intubation cannot be overemphasized. Security of the endotracheal tube should be regularly verified and intensive care unit (ICU) personnel should be drilled and equipped to deal with sudden airway emergencies. The facial, neck, and oropharyngeal edema common in serious burns makes unplanned extubation an especially difficult problem.

2. Inhalation Injury

a. Diagnosis of Inhalation Injury. Inhalation injury is a clinical diagnosis based on a history of closed spaced exposure, *elevated carboxyhemoglobin level,* presence of singed nasal vibrissae, and carbonaceous sputum. Fiberoptic bronchoscopy facilitates diagnosis in equivocal cases and can help document laryngeal edema. Such information is useful when making decisions regarding preemptive intubation for evolving upper airway edema.

b.   Clinical Consequences and Management.
Five events with major clinical implications occur predictably in patients with inhalation injury.

(1)   Acute Upper Airway Obstruction.
Acute upper airway obstruction is anticipated and managed with endotracheal intubation.

(2)   Bronchospasm. Bronchospasm from aerosolized irritants is a common occurrence during the first 24 to 48 hours, particularly in young children. This is managed with inhaled beta$_2$ adrenergic agonists. Some young patients will require intravenous bronchodilators (e.g., terbutaline) or low-dose epinephrine infusions and, occasionally, steroids. Ventilatory strategies should be designed to minimize auto-positive end-expiratory pressure (PEEP).

(3)   Small Airway Obstruction. Small airway obstruction occurs as necrotic endobronchial debris sloughs and complicates clearance of secretions. Small endotracheal tubes can become suddenly occluded, and it is important to be prepared to evaluate and respond to a sudden deterioration of the patient ventilator unit (**Table 11-6**). Therapeutic bronchoscopy facilitates clearance of the airways.

(4)   Pulmonary Infection. Pulmonary infection develops in between 30% and 50% of patients with inhalation injury. Differentiating between pneumonia and tracheobronchitis (purulent infection of the denuded tracheobronchial tree) is often difficult, but generally of little clinical consequence. A patient with newly purulent sputum, fever, and impaired gas exchange should be treated; the antibiotic coverage is adjusted according to the results of sputum Gram stain and culture. Secretion clearance is a particularly important component of management, because inhalation injury to bronchial mucosa greatly impairs mucociliary clearance.

(5)   Respiratory Failure. Respiratory failure is common in those sustaining inhalation injury. It is managed as outlined in Chapter 7, *The Trauma Airway*. These patients do well with a pressure-limited ventilation strategy based on permissive hypercapnia. Patients who fail this approach should be considered for innovative methods of support (e.g., inhaled nitric oxide or high-frequency ventilation).

3.   Carbon Monoxide Exposure
a.   Physiology. Carbon monoxide is a common component of structural fires. It is readily absorbed, and avidly binds and inactivates heme-containing enzymes, particularly hemoglobin and the cytochromes. The formation of carboxyhemo-

Table 11-6. Addressing sudden deterioration of the patient–ventilator unit

In cases of a sudden deterioration of the patient–ventilator unit, you have to quickly act to see which of the four possibilities [(a)=mechanical problem; (b)=obstruction; (c)=displacement out (c1) or into mainstem (c2); (d)=pneumothorax] is present:

1. Disconnect patient from ventilator and ventilate with self-inflating bag (remember pop-off valve) and maximal FIO_2. This precautionary measure eliminates and treats possibility (a). If this is not the immediate solution . . .
2. Manually ventilate; if ventilation is not successful, you know that obstruction, possibility (b), is the problem. If the patient is "stable," suction the tube. If obstruction cannot be quickly cleared, extubate, mask ventilate, and reacquire the airway.
3. If the ventilations are successful, displacement either out of the trachea or into the mainstem or pneumothorax, possibility (c1), (c2), or (d) has occurred. Auscultate in the axillae. If there are R>>L sided sounds, probably (c2) has occurred. Accessing depth of tube insertion will help here. Back tube out cautiously and reassess. If you hear gurgling in the hypopharynx, displacement is probably out of the trachea (c1). Extubate, mask ventilate, and reacquire the airway.

   If you hear unilateral breath sounds, pneumothorax is a possibility (d). This can be difficult to differentiate from displacement into the mainstem, possibility (c2), at times, but is often accompanied by hemodynamic deterioration or hyperresonance (or a recent subclavian line insertion attempt). If you suspect pneumothorax (d), place a 14 g or 16 g catheter in the second interspace, midclavicular line, and later place a chest tube.
4. The final common pathway if things are not going right is extubation, mask ventilation, and reacquisition of the airway. *Remember:* oxygen buys you time. If you cannot reintubate (or if you cannot effectively mask ventilate), options include laryngeal mask airway, needle cricothyroidotomy, surgical cricothyroidotomy or tracheostomy, and percutaneous cricothyroidotomy.

globin results in an acute physiologic anemia, much like an isovolemic hemodilution. As a carboxyhemoglobin concentration of 50% is physiologically similar to a 50% isovolemic hemodilution, the routine occurrence of unconsciousness at this level of carboxyhemoglobin makes it clear that other mechanisms are involved in the pathophysiology of CO injury. It is likely that CO binding to the cytochrome system in the mitochondria, interfering with oxygen utilization, is more toxic than CO binding to hemoglobin. For unknown reasons, between 5% and 20% of patients with serious CO exposures have been reported to develop delayed neurologic sequelae.

b.   Clinical Issue. Carbon monoxide exposure is common in patients injured in structural fires.

Many are obtunded from a combination of CO, anoxia, and hypotension. Hyperbaric oxygen has been proposed as a means of improving the prognosis of those with serious CO exposures, but its use remains controversial. The question of whom to treat in the hyperbaric chamber commonly arises on a busy burn service.

c.   Management Options. These patients can be managed with 100% isobaric oxygen or with hyperbaric oxygen. If serious exposure has occurred, manifested by overt neurologic impairment or a high carboxyhemoglobin level, then hyperbaric oxygen (HBO) treatment is probably warranted if it can be administered safely. HBO treatment regimens vary, but an exposure to 3 atm for 90 minutes, with three 10-minute "air breaks" is typical. An air break refers to the breathing of pressurized room air, rather than pressurized oxygen, which decreases the incidence of seizures from oxygen toxicity. Because treatment is generally in a monoplace chamber, unstable patients are suboptimal candidates. Other relative contraindications are wheezing or air trapping, which increases the risk of pneumothorax; and high fever, which increases the risk of seizures. Before placement in the chamber, endotracheal tube balloons should be filled with saline to avoid balloon compression and associated air leaks. Upper body central venous cannulation should be avoided, if possible, to reduce the chance of a pneumothorax that can enlarge suddenly during decompression. Myringotomies are required in intubated patients.

d.   Cyanide Exposure. *Cyanide exposure* is often detectable in patients extricated from structural fires, but is rarely of the severity to justify the risk of treatment with amyl nitrate and sodium thiosulfate.

C.   Gastrointestinal Issues
1.   Ulcer Prophylaxis
Until the routine use of prophylactic therapies, burn patients had a virulent ulcer diathesis (Curling's ulcer) that was a common cause of death. Ulceration is believed to be secondary to periods of reduced splanchnic flow. Presently, it is advisable to treat most patients with serious burns with empiric histamine receptor blockers and antacids (see Chapter 26, *Abdominal Trauma*). Although it is unclear when to stop prophylactic therapy, most would agree that patients with closed wounds who are tolerating tube feedings are at low enough risk that this therapy can be stopped.

2.   Nutritional Support
Burn patients have predictable and protracted needs for supplemental protein and caloric support, which needs to be accurate because both underfeeding and overfeeding have adverse sequelae.

　　　a.   Route and Timing. Intragastric continuous tube feedings are ideal and usually successful. Tube feedings are begun at a low rate during resuscitation. Initially, a sump nasogastric tube is used so that gastric residuals can be used to help determine tolerance of the feedings. Parenteral nutrition is used if tube feedings are not tolerated. Highly catabolic burn patients poorly tolerate prolonged periods of fasting.

　　　b.   Targets. Nutritional targets in severely injured burned patients remain controversial. The many formulas propagated to predict these requirements vary widely in their predictions. The current consensus is that protein needs are about 2.5 g/kg/day, and caloric needs are between 1.5 and 1.7 times a calculated basal metabolic rate, or 1.3 to 1.5 times per measured resting energy expenditure.

　　　c.   Monitoring. Substrate support needs to be titrated to nutritional endpoints during a lengthy burn hospitalization if the complications of overfeeding or underfeeding are to be avoided. Regular physical examination, quality of wound healing, nitrogen balance, and indirect calorimetry are all useful in this regard. The combination of a highly catabolic state, the critical need to heal extensive wounds, and the length of time that support is required makes monitoring and adjustment of nutritional support particularly important in patients with extensive burns.

D. Infectious Disease Issues
　1.   Topical Wound Care
　　　The best way of avoiding wound sepsis is through prompt excision and successful closure of deep wounds. Topical agents are an adjunct in this regard, slowing the inevitable occurrence of wound sepsis in deep wounds and minimizing desiccation and colonization of healing wounds. Several agents are in wide general use, the most common itemized in **Table 11-7.**
　2.   Antibiotic Use
　　　Antibiotics are two-edged swords in this clinical setting. Burn physiology includes the routine occurrence of moderate fever, which is not necessarily a sign of infection. When unexpected fever occurs, a complete

Table 11-7.   Common topical agents

Silver sulfadiazine: Painless on application, fair to poor eschar penetration, no metabolic side effects, broad antibacterial spectrum

Mafenide acetate: Painful on application, excellent eschar penetration, carbonic anhydrase inhibitor, broad antibacterial spectrum

Silver nitrate (0.5%): Painless on application, poor eschar penetration, leeches electrolytes, broad spectrum (including fungi)

physical assessment is done; wounds are inspected for evidence of sepsis; directed laboratory studies and radiographs are taken; and cultures of blood, urine, and sputum are sent. If the patient appears unstable, empiric broad-spectrum coverage is reasonable, pending return of culture data. If no infectious focus is identified, then antibiotics are stopped. It is critically important that deteriorating burn patients be compulsively evaluated for occult foci of infection to allow prompt treatment before systemic sepsis develops.

3. Infection Control

Patients referred from other facilities often bring highly resistant bacterial species with them. Proper infection control practices are of particular importance to avoid cross contamination of vulnerable patients with these organisms. Universal precautions and compulsive handwashing are essential components of practice.

4. Recognition and Management of Burn Complications

Successful management requires that a predictable series of complications (**Table 11-8**), mostly infectious, are successfully treated as the wound is progressively closed. Compulsive attention to changes in clinical status facilitates early detection and successful intervention.

E. Rehabilitation

Rehabilitation efforts begin with resuscitation and proceed throughout critical illness.

1. Therapists

Physical and occupational therapists play important roles in the burn ICU. Initially, twice-daily passive ranging of all joints and static antideformity positioning is begun to prevent the development of contractures.

2. Perioperative Therapy

Physical and occupational therapists should be informed of the sequence of planned operations and the modifications of therapy plans that these imply. Therapists should be encouraged to range a patient's joints under anesthesia in conjunction with planned operations and to fabricate custom face molds and splints in the operating room, particularly in children who often poorly tolerate these activities when awake.

F. Intraoperative Support

Burn patients must have staged excision and closure of their wounds even if they are critically ill. Not to do so will render them even sicker. Close communication between the ICU and operating room teams is essential.

1. Environmental Considerations

Transport to and from the operating room must be carefully planned and properly attended. Operating rooms must be maintained hot and humid to minimize

(*text continues on page 169*)

**Table 11-8.   Systematic reassessment of
seriously Ill burn patients**

SYSTEMS AND COMPLICATIONS
NEUROLOGIC
1. Transient delirium, which occurs in up to 30% of patients, generally resolves with supportive therapy when the possibility of anoxia, metabolic disturbance, and structural lesions is eliminated by appropriate studies.
2. Seizures most commonly result from hyponatremia or abrupt benzodiazepine withdrawal.
3. Peripheral nerve injuries occur from direct thermal injury, compression from compartment syndrome or overlying inelastic eschar, major metabolic disturbances, or improper splinting techniques.
4. Delayed peripheral nerve and spinal cord deficits develop weeks or months after high voltage injury secondary to small vessel injury and demyelinization.

RENAL
1. Early acute renal failure follows inadequate perfusion during resuscitation or myoglobinuria.
2. Late renal failure complicates sepsis and multiorgan failure or the use of nephrotoxic agents.

ADRENAL
1. Acute adrenal insufficiency secondary to hemorrhage into the gland presents with hypotension, fever, hyponatremia, and hyperkalemia.

CARDIOVASCULAR
1. Endocarditis and suppurative thrombophlebitis are intravascular infections that typically present with fever and bacteremia without signs of local infection.
2. Hypertension occurs in up to 20% of children and is best managed with beta-adrenergic blockers.
3. Venous thromboembolic complications are so infrequent in patients with large burns that routine prophylaxis is not currently routine.
4. Iatrogenic catheter insertion complications are minimized by meticulous technique

PULMONARY
1. Carbon monoxide intoxication, which is best managed acutely with effective ventilation with pure oxygen, can be associated with delayed neurologic sequelae.
2. Pneumonia can occur with or without antecedent inhalation injury; it is treated with pulmonary toilet and antibiotics.
3. Respiratory failure can occur early postinjury secondary to inhalation of noxious chemicals or later in the course secondary to sepsis or pneumonia.

HEMATOLOGIC
1. Neutropenia and thrombocytopenia, as well as disseminated intravascular coagulation, are common indicators of impending sepsis and should prompt appropriate investigation.
2. Global immunologic deficits associated with burn injury contribute to a high rate of infectious complications.

continued

Table 11-8. *Continued*

SYSTEMS AND COMPLICATIONS

OTOLOGIC

1. Auricular chondritis secondary to bacterial invasion of cartilage results in rapid loss of viable tissue and is prevented by the routine use of topical mafenide acetate on all burned ears.

2. Sinusitis and otitis media can be caused by transnasal instrumentation and are treated by relocation of tubes, antibiotics, and judicious surgical drainage.

3. Complications of endotracheal intubation include nasal alar and septal necrosis, vocal cord erosions and ulcerations, tracheal stenosis, and tracheoesophageal and tracheoinnominate artery fistulae. The occurrence of such complications is minimized by compulsive attention to tube position, avoidance of oversized tubes, and attention to cuff pressures.

ENTERIC

1. Hepatic dysfunction, secondary to transient hepatic blood flow deficits and manifested as transaminase elevations, is extremely common during resuscitation from large burns; it resolves with volume restitution. Late hepatic failure, beginning with elevations of cholestatic chemistries and progressing through coagulopathy and frank failure, complicates sepsis and multiorgan failure.

2. Pancreatitis, beginning with amylase and lipase elevations and ileus and progressing through hemorrhagic pancreatitis, is generally coincident with splanchnic flow deficits early and sepsis-induced organ failures later in the hospital course.

3. Acalculous cholecystitis can present as sepsis without localized symptoms or signs. It is accompanied by rising cholestatic chemistries. A standard radiographic evaluation can be followed by bedside percutaneous cholecystostomy in unstable patients.

4. Gastroduodenal ulcerations, secondary to splanchnic flow deficits that degrade mucosal defenses, is extremely common and often life threatening if routine histamine receptor blockers and antacids are not administered.

5. Intestinal ischemia, which can progress to infarction, is secondary to inadequate resuscitation and splanchnic flow deficits.

OPHTHALMIC

1. Ectropia, from progressive contraction of burned ocular adnexae, results in exposure of the globe. This requires acute eyelid release. Tarsorrhaphy is rarely helpful, more often resulting in injury to the tarsal plate as contraction forces pull out tarsorrhapy sutures.

2. Corneal ulceration, which develops after initial epithelial injury or later exposure secondary to ectropion, can progress to full-thickness corneal destruction if secondary infection occurs. This is prevented by careful globe lubrication with topical antibiotics in the former case and acute lid release in the later.

3. Symblepharon, or scarring of the lid to the denuded conjunctiva following chemical burns or corneal epithelial defects complicating transcutaneous electric nerve stimulation, is prevented by daily examination and adhesion disruption with a fine glass rod.

Table 11-8.   *Continued*

SYSTEMS AND COMPLICATIONS
GENITOURINARY

1. Urinary tract infections, which can be minimized by maintaining indwelling bladder catheters only when absolutely required, are treated with appropriate antibiotics. Neither catheterization nor colonic diversion is necessarily required for management of perineal and genital burns.

2   Candida cystitis occurs in those patients treated with bladder catheters and broad spectrum antibiotics. Catheter change and amphotericin irrigation for 5 days is generally successful. If infections are recurrent, the upper urinary tracts should be screened ultrasonographically.

MUSCULOSKELETAL

1. Burned exposed bone is generally debrided with a dental drill until viable cortical bone is reached, which is then allowed to granulate and is autografted. Patients whose overall condition and wounds are appropriate are managed with local or distant flaps.

2. Fractured and burned extremities are best immobilized with external fixators, whereas overlying burns are grafted. Burn patients with coincident fractures in unburned extremities benefit from prompt internal fixation.

3. Heterotopic ossification, which develops weeks after injury, is seen most commonly around deeply burned major joints such as the triceps tendon; it presents with pain and decreased range of motion. Most patients respond to physical therapy, but some require excision of heterotopic bone to achieve full function.

SOFT TISSUE

1. Hypertrophic scar formation is a major cause of long-term functional and cosmetic deformities seen in burn patients. This poorly understood process is heralded by a secondary increase in neovascularity between 9 and 13 weeks after epithelialization. Management options include grafting of deep dermal and full-thickness wounds, compression garments, judicious steroid injections, topical silicone products, and scar release and resurfacing procedures.

(Adapted from Sheridan RL, Tompkins RG. Burns. In: Greenfield LJ, Mulholland MW, Oldham KT, et al., eds. *Surgery: scientific principles and practice.* Philadelphia: JB Lippincott, 1996;12:422–438, with permission.)

the occurrence of hypothermia in exposed burn patients. Intraoperative hypothermia is poorly tolerated, causes coagulopathies, and increases bleeding.

2.   Intraoperative Critical Care and Communication

Critical care must proceed during surgery. The surgical and anesthesia teams must be in constant communication. Each team must know what the other is doing to conduct the care properly. Avoid the use of succinylcholine in the burn patient.

VI.   Special Considerations
A.   Electrical Injury
Patients exposed to low and intermediate voltages can have severe local wounds, but rarely suffer systemic consequences. Exposure to high voltages commonly results in compartment syndromes, myocardial injury, fractures of the long bones and axial spine, and free pigment in the plasma that can cause renal failure if not promptly cleared. Those with high-voltage injuries should receive cardiac monitoring, radiographic clearance of the spine, and examination of the urine for myoglobin. Fluid resuscitation initially is based on burn size, but this generally does not correlate well with deep tissue injury, so resuscitation needs to be closely monitored and adjusted. Muscle compartments at risk should be closely monitored by serial physical examinations; they should be decompressed in the operating room when an evolving compartment syndrome is suspected. Wounds are débrided and closed with a combination of skin grafts and flaps.

B.   Tar Injury
Numerous thermoplastic road materials are the source of occupational injury. They are highly viscous and heated to between 300°F and 700°F. Wounds should be immediately cooled by tap water irrigation. Resuscitation is based on burn size and monitored. Wounds are dressed in a lipophilic solvent and then débrided, excised, and grafted. The underlying wounds are generally very deep.

C.   Cold Injury
Soft tissue necrosis from cold injury is often managed in the burn unit. Wound care is conservative until the extent of irreversible soft tissue necrosis is apparent, which often requires several weeks if not months. When definitely demarcated, surgical debridement, excision, and reconstruction or closure is carried out, if needed. Lesser injuries often heal without need for surgery. Cold-injured patients can manifest all the problems of systemic hypothermia when they present, and should be managed accordingly.

D.   Chemical Injury
Patients can be exposed to thousands of chemicals, which are often heated. It is important to consider the thermal, local chemical, and systemic chemical effects. Liberal consultation with poison control information centers for guidance regarding systemic effects is extremely useful. Most agents can be washed off with tap water. Alkaline substances can take longer to remove than the traditional 30 minutes. When the soapy feel that these alkalis typically impart to the gloved finger is gone or when litmus paper applied to the wound shows a neutral pH, irrigation can be stopped. Concentrated hydrofluoric acid exposure will cause dangerous hypocalcemia, and a subeschar injection of 10% calcium gluconate and emergent wound excision may be appropriate. Elemental metals should be covered with oil and white phosphorus should be covered in saline to prevent secondary ignition.

E. Toxic Epidermal Necrolysis

Toxic epidermal necrolysis is a diffuse process of unknown pathophysiology in which epidermal dermal bonding is acutely compromised. Patients commonly present with a drug exposure preceding the illness, and have both a cutaneous and visceral wound. This disease is similar in presentation to a total-body second-degree burn. With good wound care, most cutaneous wounds will heal without the need for surgery. Involvement of the aerodigestive tract mucosa can lead to sepsis and organ failures, particularly if septic complications are not promptly recognized and treated.

F. Purpura Fulminans

Purpura fulminans is a complication of meningococcal sepsis in which extensive soft tissue necrosis and often organ failures occur. It is believed to be secondary to a transient hypercoagulable state that occurs early in the primary septicemic event. These patients often present with sepsis-associated organ failures and extensive deep wounds. Both should be managed concurrently because the wounds are susceptible to infection if not promptly excised and closed.

G. Soft Tissue Infections

Patients with soft tissue infections share many characteristics of burn patients. Accurate classification of serious soft tissue infections is difficult, but all are approached in the same general fashion. These patients need to go directly to the operating room. Operative goals are exposure of the infection so that its anatomic extent can be accurately described and its microbiology determined by culture, Gram stain, and biopsy. Debridement under general anesthesia is repeated until infection is controlled, and the wounds are then closed or grafted. Broad-spectrum and then focused antibiotics are important adjuncts. Some patients, particularly those with clostridial infection, can benefit from adjunctive HBO; however, prompt surgery is the primary therapeutic modality.

H. The Burned Polytrauma Patient

Burn care priorities frequently conflict with orthopedic, neurosurgical, and other priorities. Thoughtful resolution of these differences is an important part of successful management (**Table 11-9**). These situations commonly require a great deal of judgment and liberal consultation.

I. Long-term Follow-up of the Burned Patient

Long-term follow-up of burn patients by the burn center in an outpatient setting is associated with improved quality of life. Issues commonly encountered following burn injury include the following.

J. Scarring and Contracture

Until improvement plateaus, joint contractures are addressed by physical and occupational therapy. Severe contractures should be treated with operative release. Hypertrophic scars with an erythematous heaped-up appearance can appear in a few months from the injury and peak 6 to 9 months following the injury. These are

**Table 11-9. Conflicting priorities of the
polytrauma burn patient**

Area of Conflict and Consensus Resolution

NEUROLOGIC

Patients with burns and head injuries must have cerebral edema
controlled during resuscitation; pressure monitors increase risk
of infection.

A very tightly controlled resuscitation with short-term placement
of indicated pressure monitors with antibiotic coverage is useful.

CHEST

Patients with blunt chest injuries and overlying burns may require
chest tubes through burned areas with risk of empyema and
difficulty closing the tract.

Use a long subcutaneous tunnel to minimize difficulty closing the
tract and remove tubes as soon as possible to decrease empyema
risk.

ABDOMEN

Blunt abdominal injuries can be hard to detect in cases of an overlying burn. A high incidence exists of wound dehiscence when
operating through a burned abdominal wall.

Liberal use of imaging to detect occult injuries and routine use of
retention sutures after laparotomy address this possibility.

ORTHOPEDIC

An overlying burn can compromise optimal management of a
fracture.

Most such extremities are best managed with prompt excision and
grafting of the wound with external fracture fixation.

best managed with pressure garments, silicone pads, and
steroid injections. They usually subside several years
after the injury.

K. Chronic Pain

Patients should be slowly weaned off narcotic pain medications during the rehabilitation phase. Radiographs of
painful joints should be obtained to rule out heterotopic
ossification. Light touch, minor temperature changes, or
a dependent extremity can set off scar pain, described as
intermittent, shooting, stabbing, pins and needles, or burning. Patients with scar pain often respond to gabapentin,
topical silicone, desensitization programs, and steroid
injections.

L. Itching

Itching, a common complaint following burns, is often
associated with hypertrophic scars. Systemic antihiista-
mine or topical doxepin cream produces relief and is useful for small areas..

M. Inpatient Records

Inpatient records should be reviewed to address any
follow-up issues required by the critical care course of
the patient.

N.   Substance Abuse and Psychiatric Issues
Substance abuse, psychiatric issues including posttraumatic stress disorder, and adjustment disorders should be documented and aggressively treated.
O.   Symptoms of Heat Exhaustion and Heat Stroke
Patients with extensive injuries should be alerted to signs and symptoms of heat exhaustion and heat stroke.
P.   Unprotected Exposure to the Sun
Unprotected exposure to the sun should be limited in the burned area.
Q.   Prevention
If appropriate, the mechanism of the accident should be examined and addressed with prevention in mind.
VII.   Conclusion
Seriously burned patients can do extremely well in the long term. Skillful resuscitation, initial evaluation, and long-term follow-up are essential if optimal outcomes are to be realized. Most initial burn care is provided within trauma programs, so it is important for these skills to be a part of the trauma unit armamentarium.

SELECTED READING

Sheridan RL. The acutely burned child: resuscitation through reintegration. Parts I and II. *Curr Probl Pediatr* 1998;28(4,5):105–167.

Sheridan RL, Baryza MJ, Pessina MA, et al. Acute hand burns in children: management and long-term outcome based on a 10-year experience with 698 injured hands. *Ann Surg* 1999;229(4):558–564.

Sheridan RL. Comprehensive treatment of burns. *Curr Probl Surg* 2001;38(9):657–756.

Sheridan RL, Hinson MM, Liang MM, et al. Long-term outcome of children surviving massive burns. *JAMA* 2000;283(1):69–73.

Sheridan RL, Remensnyder JP, Schnitzer JJ, et al. Current expectations for survival in pediatric burns. *Arch Pediatr Adolesc Med* 2000;154(3):245–249.

Sheridan RL, Zapol WM, Ritz RH, et al. Low-dose inhaled nitric oxide in acutely burned children with profound respiratory failure. *Surgery* 1999;126(5):856–862.

Trauma Anesthesia

Kristopher R. Davignon, MD,
and Keith Baker, MD PhD

I. Introduction

Anesthesia for the major acute trauma victim has progressed significantly over recent years.

II. Preparation

A level I trauma center must have operating rooms (OR) ready in advance to receive a critically ill patient on a moment's notice.

A. Operating Room Setup

Have the OR entirely ready to start a case.

1. The anesthesia machine should be checked for proper function and emergency equipment (AmbuBag, back-up oxygen tanks, manual blood pressure cuff, and stethoscope). The machine should be left on with 100% oxygen priming the circuit.

2. The operating table should be in the room and prepared for a patient (including arm boards).

3. The OR suite should be warmed well in advance. Warming the walls and equipment can reduce the radiant cooling of the patient. Warming the operating table can reduce conductive cooling.

B. Equipment and Medications

Equipment and supplies that need to be immediately available are shown in **Table 12-1**.

C. Communication

Clear and frequent communication between the OR, emergency room (ER), blood bank, and laboratory and radiology departments is essential. An efficient way should be in place for physicians, nurses and staff to communicate from the emergency department to the OR. If time allows, general information regarding the patient and his or her injuries should be relayed before patient transport. This can allow the OR staff to prepare special equipment to address potential problems (e.g., a difficult airway or lung isolation). Early relay of patient information also enables the OR staff to order blood products or any medications that may not have been anticipated by the general OR setup mentioned above. The blood bank, laboratory, and radiology departments must be aware of the acuity of the tests being ordered on a trauma patient and must be prepared to deliver results rapidly enough to use in a quickly changing situation.

III. Preinduction

A. Patient Arrival, Prioritization, and Task Assignment

When the patient arrives, the anesthesiologist must quickly prioritize the tasks that need to be carried out and

Table 12-1. Equipment and drugs available for trauma

In Room and Immediately Available
–Anesthesia machine with positive pressure ventilator
–Laryngoscope handles and blades (several sizes and types)
–Masks, endotracheal tubes, oral and nasal airways of different sizes
–Suction and suction devices (Yankauer)
–Electrocardiographic monitor
–Pulse oxymiter
–End-tidal CO_2 monitor
–Blood pressure cuff (several sizes)
–Intravascular pressure monitoring capabilities
–Oxygen analyzer
–Temperature monitor
–Sodium citrate
–Induction agents: pentothal, etomidate, ketamine
–Muscle relaxants: succinylcholine, nondepolarizing muscle relaxants
–Amnestics: benzodiazepine, scopolamine
–Inhalation agents
–Opiates
–Vasopressors/inotropes: ephedrine, phenylephrine, norepinephrine, dopamine, epinephrine, CaCl
–Atropine
–Lidocaine
–Defibrillator with internal and external paddles
–AmbuBag
–Rapid Infusion device with warmer
–Warming blankets
–Supplies for intravenous and intraarterial access
–9F introducer or equivalent large-bore venous access device
–Intravascular catheter (3 lumen)
–Intravenous infusion set with pressure bags or pumps

Available on Short Notice
–Misc. drugs: antiarrythmics, bronchodilators, diuretics, anti-histamines
–Difficult airway cart: fiberoptic bronchoscope, LMA or LMA fast track, topical anesthetics, jet ventilator, gum elastic bougie, Magill forceps
–Positive end-expiratory pressure (PEEP) valve
–Double lumen endotracheal tubes
–Pulmonary artery catheter

LMA, laryngeal mask airway.

delegate as necessary. The anesthesiologist's focus must be on taking care of the patient. Assume that you are the only one watching the patient's cardiovascular and respiratory status. Significant changes can occur in the short time that is taken to transport the patient from the ED to the OR and can go unrecognized in the commotion.

B. Directed Assessment

Clinical assessment must be rapid with special attention to the ABCs, level of consciousness, and ongoing resuscitative measures.

1.   Vital Signs
The term "vital signs" is self-explanatory. Be sure that the vital signs you see are recent. Quickly evaluate airway, breathing, and circulation (ABC).

2.   Primary and Secondary Survey Results
The team in the ED should have conducted a primary and secondary survey. Ask for a "list of injuries." This is a quick way to get a lot of information.

3.   History and Physical Examination— Allergies, Medications, Comorbid Medical Illnesses
The history and physical examination may have to be abbreviated because of lack of time. Key information should be sought first. Specifically, elicit any patient allergies and medications as well as major comorbid illnesses. Less critical information can be delineated during the case.

4.   Airway Evaluation
Is the patient intubated? If so, *confirm* bilateral breath sounds and end-tidal CO_2. Does the airway look difficult? Is there cervical spine injury? Take time to be sure there is no occult upper or lower airway injury by going over radiographs and speaking with the surgeons, if the clinical situation allows. If you anticipate any problems, be prepared (fiberoptic scope, laryngeal mask airway [LMA], surgical help available). **See Chapter 7,** *The Trauma Airway.*

5.   Assess Intravenous Access and Monitors in Situ
What type of intravenous (i.v.) access exists? What monitors exist? Confirm their placement. Are they sufficient for your anesthetic plan and the patient's injuries? See sections below.

6.   Laboratory Values
Review any laboratory findings available from the ER. Note what time they were drawn. If time is limited, at least try to note the hematocrit and coagulation studies, as they often have an impact on early resuscitative therapy.

7.   Assess Volume Status
Having a good sense of the patient's volume status will be important in treating the patient's hemodynamics. A hypovolemic patient should be resuscitated before induction, if possible.

    a.   Vital Signs. Vital signs are an easy way to get a sense of the patient's volume status. Hypotension and tachycardia are the hallmarks of hypovolemia. Normal vital signs, however, do *not* equal normovolemia. A young healthy trauma victim can have normal hemodynamics, despite significant volume loss.

    b.   History. Ask the ED staff what their estimates are for blood loss. Ask the staff what resuscitation has occurred in the interim from patient injury to present, including the patient's response.

    c. **Examination.** Note urine output, quantity, and color. Also note the jugular venous pulse. Examine the peripheral extremities for temperature and mottling and check for chest tube drainage and evidence of external bleeding.

    d. **Laboratory Studies.** With serial laboratory studies, often a trend can be noted. The hematocrit is most likely to help.

    e. **Radiology.** Ultrasound, computed tomography scan, or other radiographic studies may demonstrate fluid in the chest or abdomen. This may help assess blood loss or sequestration of fluid.

C. Anesthetic Plan Formation

   1. Regional Versus General Versus Combined Techniques

Much controversy exists among the anesthesia community to whether real differences in outcome variables exist between regional and general anesthetics. Risks and benefits are seen to each choice and an anesthetic plan must be individualized for each patient.

    a. **Regional**

      (1) Indications. Common indications for regional anesthesia include *rib fractures, pulmonary contusion, and peripheral procedures.* Regional anesthesia also has application for lower abdominal surgery, and can be used in combination with general anesthesia for upper abdominal and thoracic surgery.

      (2) Benefits. Regional anesthetics are valued for the lack of central nervous system (CNS) depression. They allow CNS monitoring by the awake patient and, thus, potentially eliminate the addition of more invasive neurologic monitors. Evidence suggests that deep venous thrombosis (DVT) risk is decreased postoperatively.

      (3) Contraindications (Relative and Absolute). Regional anesthetics are not appropriate in many situations associated with trauma. Coagulopathy, increased intracranial pressure (ICP), hypovolemia or shock from hemorrhage, and sepsis or bacteremia with intestinal perforation are just a few of the trauma situations in which regional anesthesia is not appropriate.

    b. **General**

      (1) Indications. A most common indication for general anesthesia in the trauma patient is "location of surgery not amenable to regional anesthesia." Others include the need for control of airway independent of surgical procedure (see Chapter 7, *The Trauma Airway*), massive transfusion requirement, the uncooperative patient, or need for mechanical ventilation.

(2) **Contraindications/Risks.** Few or no absolute contraindications are seen for general anesthesia in the truly emergent situation. Certain clinical situations, however, may merit the avoidance of a general anesthesia. For example, a small pneumothorax (that would not require a chest tube) may be preferably managed in a spontaneously breathing patient or a patient with pericardial effusion may benefit from the maintained, sympathetic outflow of being awake if the procedure would allow. As noted, a general anesthetic can require additional neurologic monitors (ICP in the setting of head injury).

2. Special Procedures and Flexibility

When formulating an anesthetic plan, the surgical procedure often has an impact on decisions and choices the anesthesiologist makes. Communicate with the surgical team and prepare for things such as *lung isolation, cardiopulmonary bypass or vascular cross clamping.* Often these require special equipment and drugs. Trauma anesthesia requires flexibility because of the ever-changing patient status. Constant communication with the surgical team is essential to good patient care.

D. Premedication

Premedication is very dependent on the patient's clinical situation and the anesthetic plan. Every trauma patient should be treated as having a full stomach. If the patient is awake and has maintained protective airway reflexes, a nonparticulate antacid (*Na citrate*) should be administered. *Metoclopramide* should be considered for gastric emptying, realizing that it can be contraindicated in certain abdominal injuries and the timing of its administration may not allow its effects to be clinically beneficial. Often H_1 and H_2 blockers are given to blunt histamine effects from drugs that will be administered or from rapid transfusion. H_2 blockers can also be beneficial in reducing both the risk of aspiration pneumonitis if given 60 minutes or more before induction and the incidence of gastric stress ulceration if prolonged intubation is anticipated. *Benzodiazepines* and *narcotics* are often administered in the preoperative phase, but careful attention must be paid to their effects on the respiratory and cardiovascular systems (especially when given in combination). **Antibiotics,** if indicated, should be administered as soon as possible.

E. Establish Necessary Intravenous Access

The trauma patient should have two large bore i.v. A single 8F or 9F catheter allows massive volume resuscitation and a second large i.v. will provide backup in case the primary i.v. fails and allows administration of drugs and platelets. This approach is preferable to the placement of several smaller i.v. (≤18 gauge), which may be required in large numbers to adequately resuscitate the trauma patient. Flow rates depend on many factors, including the pressure system, filters, temperature and type of fluids, as well as the caliber of the tubing, i.v. catheters and the vein. When using an "introducer" for volume access, recognize that the side arm can significantly limit flow. Turbulent flow caused by high flow rates and stopcocks increases resistance and diminishes the maximal flow rate of a given i.v. infusion set. PRBC with their increased viscosity also slow infusion rates by more than 50%. Pressure bags can increase infusion rates 200% to 300%. Many systems are currently marketed to deliver large volumes of warmed, de-aired fluid. The warming system should be capable of delivering up to 600 mL/min, which is limited primarily by warming capabilities.

In addition to having *enough* access, i.v. placement must be appropriate for the patient's injuries and positioning. Generally, i.v. access below the diaphragm may be ineffective for major abdominal trauma. Conversely, i.v. access above the diaphragm may be inappropriate for certain thoracic injuries.

F. Establish Necessary Monitors
Several monitors must be in place before induction; others can be placed after. This is a decision that must be based on the patient's clinical situation.

1. Electrocardiography
Five-lead electrocardiography (ECG) is essential. Generally, lead II is selected to monitor arrhythmias, whereas a lateral precordial lead is selected to monitor for ischemia. Traditionally, V_5 is selected, but recent evidence has shown V_4 to be superior for detection of ischemia (V_4 was 83% sensitive, V_3 or V_5 was 75% sensitive, and V_3 and V_4 in combination was most sensitive [97%]).

2. Oxygen Saturation
Oxygen saturation by pulse oximetry should be measured continuously. This can be difficult in the hypovolemic trauma victim with poor peripheral perfusion. Placement of the probe on the nose, ear, or even tongue has been described, all of which may improve the success of obtaining a trace.

3. End-Tidal CO₂
End-tidal CO_2 aids in detecting esophageal intubation, airway obstruction (particularly bronchospasm), pulmonary embolus (thrombus, air, or fat), and exsanguination.

4. Arterial Pressure
Intraarterial blood pressure monitoring is almost always indicated for major acute trauma. If noninvasive blood pressures are adequate, an automated cuff should be used to free the anesthetist for other manual tasks.

5. Central Venous Pressure
Central venous pressure (CVP) monitoring is rarely needed before induction. Its placement after induction can be helpful in monitoring fluid status and in administering fluids and drugs.

6.   Monitor Placement Considers Patient Injuries and Positioning

a.   Upper Extremity Versus Lower Extremity. Often a femoral arterial line is placed during trauma resuscitation because of its simplicity and ease of placement. In cases of major abdominal injury or the possibility of aortic compression or cross-clamping, this line will be inadequate for the operating room. Likewise, if injury to the upper extremity has occurred, a femoral or dorsalis pedis placement may be preferred.

b.   Right vs. Left. With any suspicion that the aorta may need to be cross-clamped proximal to the left subclavian artery, a right sided, upper-extremity arterial line is essential (radial, brachial or axillary). Some advocate placing bilateral arterial lines in such situations.

G.   Volume Resuscitation

It is essential to be sure the patient is appropriately resuscitated before induction. If further resuscitation is merited, warm fluid is used. Loss of sympathetic outflow after induction of anesthesia can lead to circulatory collapse in the hypovolemic trauma patient.

IV.   Induction

A.   Awake Versus Rapid Sequence Induction

Information on awake versus rapid sequence induction is found in Chapter 7, *The Trauma Airway*.

B.   Agents

The physiologic state of the patient will be the key determinant of induction agent. Each agent has profound physiologic effects on the cardiovascular system and intracranial pressure.

1.   Sodium Thiopental

A rapid acting drug, sodium thiopental (STP) is commonly used for induction of anesthesia. STP will produce some decrease in systemic vascular resistance as well as modest myocardial depression.

2.   Ketamine

Ketamine is generally thought to be hemodynamically stable because of its promotion of adrenergic outflow. It can increase intracranial pressure as well as intraocular pressure, which must be considered in the patient with closed head injury or injury to the globe. Although ketamine generally causes hypertension and tachycardia, it is a direct myocardial depressant. This effect can predominate in the trauma victim who has no further sympathetic reserve.

3.   Propofol

Profound reduction in systemic vascular resistance can cause hypotension with induction in the hypovolemic patient or a patient whose cardiovascular status is being maintained by excessive sympathetic tone.

4.   Etomidate

Etomidate has very little direct effect on the cardiovascular system. Etomidate's problems originate in its inhibition of steroidogenesis. Used as an infusion, it can be detrimental to the trauma patient. Etomidate is also known to cause significant postoperative nausea and vomiting.

5. Narcotics and Benzodiazepine
Narcotics and benzodiazepines have relatively mild direct effects on the cardiovascular system and, thus, can provide a relatively stable anesthetic induction. In the trauma patient, however, the abrupt loss of sympathetic tone associated with the anesthetized state can lead to hemodynamic collapse. In addition, the time to loss of lid reflex can be excessive. In the patient with a full stomach requiring a rapid sequence induction, this may not be the technique of choice.

6. Scopolamine
Anterograde amnesia and minimal cardiovascular effects make scopolamine a popular choice for sedating unstable trauma victims. Be aware that scopolamine will alter the pupillary examination because of its anticholinergic effects. It is not an anesthetic and, thus, patients may be awake and in pain. It reduces the likelihood that the patient will recall the event.

C. **Muscle Relaxants for Induction**
1. **Succinylcholine**
Succinylcholine is the gold standard for rapid sequence induction. With a rapid onset (60 to 90 seconds), succinylcholine offers profound muscle relaxation and excellent intubating conditions. It is not without detrimental effects, however.

a. **Hyperkalemia** after use of succinylcholine is well described. Succinylcholine should likely be avoided in patients with previous burn injury, major crush injury, previous upper motor neuron lesion, spinal cord injury, and muscular dystrophies. Its use in the setting of acute (<24 hours) burn, crush injury, or stroke is safe, however. Patients with renal failure must be carefully selected for the use of succinylcholine. Succinylcholine should be avoided in any patient with existing hyperkalemia.

b. Increases in **intracranial and intraocular pressure** have been demonstrated after the administration of succinylcholine. The clinical implications, however, seem to be minimal and succinylcholine is frequently used for rapid sequence induction in patients with intracranial pathology.

c. **Intragastric pressure** is increased with succinylcholine.

d. **Bradycardia and bradydysrhythmia** are seen, especially in children, after a dose of succinylcholine. This effect is rarely seen in adults after one dose of succinylcholine, but repeat doses can cause sinus arrest.

e. Succinylcholine has been shown to reduce increases in intragastric, intracranial, and intraocular pressure induced by succinylcholine. Precurarization can also lessen the incidence of bradydysrhythmia.

f. Succinylcholine does not cause fixed or dilated pupils.

2. Nondepolarizing Muscle Relaxants

Alternatives to succinylcholine are available for obtaining rapid control of the airway if contraindications exist.

a. Priming doses of nondepolarizing muscle relaxants (NDMR), given 1 to 2 minutes before the intubating dose, have been demonstrated to reduce the time to optimal intubating conditions. Subclinical blockade at the neuromuscular junction can be unpleasant and not without complication. Disadvantages include diminished airway reflexes and weakness of respiratory musculature, especially if the priming dose is incorrect or improperly timed.

b. High-dose vecuronium or cis-atracurium have been demonstrated to provide rapid paralysis. Vecuronium can provide intubating conditions in less than 2 minutes.

c. Rocuronium, with its rapid onset (90 to 100 seconds) and modest side effect profile, is an alternative to succinylcholine.

d. Rapacuronium, initially was thought to be a good alternative to succinylcholine. It had an onset of 60 to 90 seconds and a rapid redistribution (offset of single dose less than 20 minutes). Several reports of severe bronchospasm, however, have led to its removal from the US market.

e. New agents are currently being developed in the laboratory with continued hope for a new NDMR with profound and rapid onset and short duration of action to replace succinylcholine.

D. Surgical Help

Do not forget about surgical airway (see Chapter 7, *The Trauma Airway*).

V. Maintenance

A. Anesthetic agents

Several options exist to maintain the anesthetized state for surgery.

1. Volatile Agents

Volatile agents are the standard. Vascular dilatation and myocardial depression limit their use in large doses for major acute trauma.

2. Nitrous Oxide

Nitrous oxide is a very stable drug for the cardiovascular system. Its use, however, limits the inspired fraction of oxygen. In addition, because nitrous oxide expands air spaces, it should be avoided if suspicion exists for pneumothorax, pneumocephalus, or venous air embolism.

3. Ketamine

Ketamine infusions can provide a stable anesthetic. Postoperative analgesia is often profound. Because of its elevation on ICP, heart rate, and blood pressure, this is not an appropriate technique for every patient, especially those with head injury or those at risk for myocardial ischemia.

4. Narcotic/Benzodiazepine Infusion

Narcotic/benzodiazepine infusion is a technique commonly chosen for its hemodynamic stability. The relatively long duration of action of currently available benzodiazepines, however, limits its usefulness if an awake patient is desired at the end of the operative procedure.

5. Awareness

Awareness is a problem of real concern in major acute trauma. Because of the hemodynamic effects of many anesthetic agents and the often compromised cardiovascular status of the trauma patient, the patient can be under anesthetized. New devices, such as the bispectral index (BIS) monitor, can help with this problem, but no simple solution exists.

B. Muscle Relaxants for the Maintenance Phase

1. Pancuronium causes tachycardia and requires functioning kidneys for elimination. Prolonged duration of action can occur in the setting of renal dysfunction.

2. Vecuronium is without significant cardiovascular effects. Its metabolism is primarily hepatic. It can be administered by bolus dosing or as an infusion.

3. Curare causes significant amounts of histamine release, thereby inciting significant hypotension if given in large bolus doses. It is both metabolized by the liver and excreted unchanged by the kidney. Because of ganglionic blockade, mydriasis can result, compromising neurologic evaluation.

4. Atracurium causes histamine release. It also has a toxic metabolite, laudanosine, which results from its spontaneous degradation. Laudanosine can accumulate in cases of renal failure if atracurium is used for prolong periods as an infusion. Laudanosine has been shown to cause seizures in animal studies.

5. Mivacurium has an extremely short half-life because of extensive metabolism by plasma cholinesterase. As with curare and atracurium, it causes significant histamine release with bolus dosing.

6. Cis-atracurium, an isomer of atracurium, also undergoes spontaneous degradation and, thus, does not depend on organ-specific elimination. Cis-atracurium does not seem to have the histamine-releasing properties of atracurium. It is the closest thing available to a perfect muscle relaxant.

C. Establish Appropriate Monitoring in Addition to That Placed Before Induction (see III.f)

1. Foley Catheter

Urine output will give clues about volume status, renal function, urinary tract trauma, diabetes insipidus, and rhabdomyolysis.

2. Temperature

Core temperature can be measured in several places, including the rectum, bladder, tympanum, posterior nasopharynx, esophagus, and pulmonary artery. Measuring core temperature can be important diagnostically (i.e., sepsis) as well as therapeutically (i.e., adjustment of warming devises to avoid hypothermia).

3. Neuromuscular Monitoring

Many things alter the pharmacokinetics of muscle relaxants (i.e. temperature, magnesium levels, and liver and kidney function). Train-of -four monitoring is essential for appropriate dosing.

4. Arterial Line

An arterial line can be invaluable in trauma. Beat-to-beat data acquisition during critical periods (induction, rapid hemorrhage, clamping of great vessels) allows prompt institution of cardiovascular resuscitation. It can be helpful diagnostically (pulsus paradoxus with tamponade, cyclical change of pressure with positive pressure ventilation during hypovolemia). It also has great utility in facilitating frequent blood gas and laboratory determination.

5. Central Venous Pressure

Central venous access allows for delivery of drugs for rapid action and measurement of filling pressures, which can be helpful in assessing intravascular volume status, valvular injury, arrhythmias, and cardiac dysfunction (i.e., ischemia, tamponade, contusion, or even pneumothorax).

6. Pulmonary Artery Catheterization

Pulmonary artery catheterization (PAC) used to measure pressure is rarely needed during acute trauma in otherwise well patients. PAC can help the patient with right or left ventricular dysfunction, valvular heart disease, or acute respiratory distress syndrome (ARDS). This is often most true in the postoperative phases. PAC can be useful if the need for pacing exists. Placement of the introducer sheath before surgery begins allows a route for volume administration and, if the need arises, a PA catheter can be placed.

7. Transesophageal Echocardiography

Transesophageal echocardiography (TEE) can be helpful in certain types of trauma, particularly blunt chest trauma. TEE can assess intravascular volume, ventricular wall motion, valvular injury, pleural effusion, tamponade, pneumothorax, and proximal aortic injuries. It is prudent to keep in mind that TEE can be harmful if placed in the setting of esophageal injury.

D. Active Warming
The propensity for the trauma victim to become hypothermic is enormous. The mortality rate following trauma is directly proportional to the severity of hypothermia (preoperatively and intraoperatively). Intraoperative heat loss is particularly problematic in patients with spinal cord injuries, burns, and large superficial injuries.

    1. Forced Warm Air Blanket
    Upper versus lower. Coverage of the maximal body surface area is preferable, but if the possibility for aortic cross-clamp exists, lower body blankets should be avoided.

    2. Room Temperature. Turn it up!

    3. Fluid Warmers. Almost 135 kJ is required to warm 1 unit of blood to body temperature.

    4. Warm and humidified gases have little effect. Take care to prevent the temperature at the distal end of the endotracheal tube from exceeding 40°C.

E. Resuscitation
Ongoing resuscitation and the treatment of developing problems are two of the most important tasks of the anesthesiologist caring for the trauma victim. Optimization of intravascular volume, oxygen-carrying capacity, capacity for coagulation and thrombosis, alveolar gas exchange, and cardiac output are paramount. This includes administration of appropriate fluids, inotropic agents, vasopressors, and vasodilators as well as mechanical ventilation.

    1. Volume: Assessment and Repair
    Assessment of volume status has been touched on briefly as part of the preoperative assessment. The anesthesiologist must use all the information available, including physical examination, hemodynamic measurements, urine output, and laboratory data (**Table 12-2**). Laboratory data are of particular importance when determining what type of fluid to use during "repair." (e.g., hypovolemia with a hematocrit of 20% merits different treatment than hypovolemia with a hematocrit of 35%).

        a. Crystalloid. The trauma victim often needs large volumes of fluid for resuscitation. Therefore, crystalloid solution, generally lactated Ringer's (LR) solution, should be chosen (**Table 12-3**). LR is a balanced salt solution that allows large volumes of fluid to be administered without producing nonanion gap hyperchloremic metabolic acidosis, as can be seen with normal saline (NS).

        A few clinical scenarios are seen wherein NS is preferred over LR. In renal failure, the small amount of K^+ in LR may be problematic. In closed head injury where cerebral edema is a concern, the slightly higher osmolarity of NS may make it preferable over LR.

        b. Colloid. Much debate exists over the benefits of colloid solutions over crystalloid solutions for initial acute resuscitation. Existing data suggest

Table 12-2.   Assessment of hemodynamic variables

	Central Venous Pressure (CVP)	Pulmonary Capillary Wedge Pressure (PCWP)	Cardiac Output (CO)	Systemic Vascular Resistance (SVR)
Hypovolemic shock	↓	↓	↓	↑
Septic shock	↓	↓	↑ or ↓	↓
Neurogenic shock	↓	↓	↑ or ↓	↓
Cardiogenic shock	↑	↑	↓	↑
–Tamponade	CVP and PCWP equalize↓			↑
–Left ventricle failure	↓	↑	↓	↑
–Right ventricle failure	↑	↓ or ↑	↓	↑
–Acute Mitral Regurgitation (large V)	↑ or ↓	↑	↓	↑

that the mortality rate may actually be higher in patients resuscitated with colloid solutions over those resuscitated with crystalloid.

c.   Hydroxyethel starch, and albumin are commonly used plasma expanders in the absence of an indication for blood component therapy.

(1)   Hydroxyethel starch can be suspended in either NS (**Hespan,** Du Pont, Wilmington, DE) or LR solution (**Hextend,** Abbott, N. Chicago, Illinois). It has been shown that, in large volumes, Hespan will result in prolonged coagulation times. Because Hextend is suspended in a lactated salt solution, it prevents the formation of a hyperchloremic acidosis that results from Hespan, which is suspended in NS.

(2)   Albumin comes in 5% and 25% solutions. Albumin is derived from human plasma and is relatively expensive. It has not been shown to possess any advantage over more conventional fluids.

d.   Blood Products. Blood products (PRBC, fresh frozen plasma [FFP], cryoprecipitate, platelets) have well-established indications. Administration of blood products is not without potential risk and should not be used lightly **(see Table 12-3).** They are, however, the only solution to anemia, thrombocytopenia, and coagulopathy from factor deficiency (except factors VII and VIII, which are available as recombinant products). Generally, PRBC are transfused to maintain a hematocrit (HCT) >21% and often closer to 30%,

Table 12-3. Resuscitation solutions

	Na	Cl	K	Ca	Mg	Lactate	Dextrose	Osmol/L
Crystalloid								
–Lactated Ringer's	130	109	4	3	0	28	0	273
–D_5LR	130	109	4	3	0	28	50 g/L	525
–0.9% NaCl (NS)	154	154	0	0	0	0	0	308
–0.45% NaCl (1/2NS)	70	70	0	0	0	0	0	140
–D_5NS	140	140	0	0	0	0	50 g/L	532
–Plasmalyte	140	98	5	0	3	(acetate) 27	0	294
Colloid								
–Hextend (Hydroxyethylstarch (HES)—60 g/L) (COP (mm Hg) =)	143	124	3	5	0.9	28	0	
–Hespan (Hydroxyethylstarch (HES)—60 g/L) (COP (mm Hg) =)	154	154						
–5% Human Albumin (Albumin—50 g/L) (COP (mm Hg) =)	154	154						

NS, normal saline; COP, colloidal osmotic pressure.
All concentrations are in mmoles/L unless otherwise noted.

although few data exist to suggest an "optimal" HCT. One unit of PRBC has a volume of 250 to 400 mL and a hematocrit of 60% to 70%. Each unit of PRBC contains approximately 50 mL of plasma. Most blood is stored with citrate, which chelates calcium (to prevent coagulation). Thus, with massive transfusion, hypocalcemia can occur, which generally requires >1 unit of PRBC every 5 minutes. Hyperkalemia is also possible from massive transfusion because some potassium is extravasated from lysed red cells during storage (see Chapter 10, *Transfusion and Coagulation Issues in Trauma,* for more comprehensive information).

2. Vasopressor therapy is sometimes necessary, despite appropriate fluid administration; however, it is needed more often while fluid is being administered ("catch up"). The cause of hemodynamic instability must be considered any time vasopressor therapy is to be instituted.

a. Phenylepherine is a pure alpha-agonist. It provides some venoconstriction and much arteriolar constriction and, thus, improves venous return and notably increases afterload. It is an excellent pressor to combat mild vasodilation from loss of sympathetic tone caused either by regional or general anesthesia or neurologic injury. Reflex bradycardia mediated by the carotid sinus often occurs.

b. Norepinepherine has strong alpha- and modest beta-agonist properties. It is the drug of choice for sepsis because it provides both vasoconstriction and increases in myocardial contractility. Norepinephrine is superior to phenylephrine, particularly in the patient with poor left ventricular contractility or in whom such high doses of phenylephrine are associated with either reflex bradycardia or left ventricular failure from increased afterload.

c. Vasopressin has recently been used in sepsis to reduce requirements of other vasopressors. Very few data exist to demonstrate its effect on outcomes, but it is apparent that the addition of vasopressin reduces the doses of other vasopressors significantly, particularly in the face of an acidosis. Vasopressin (0.04 units/min) has been used successfully in sepsis. Higher doses (1 to 4 units/min) have been used to combat gastrointestinal bleeding. Vasopressin use is not without risk. Vasopressin is known to constrict splanchnic vessels and can cause intestinal ischemia. Because of its coronary vasoconstrictor effect, it can cause myocardial ischemia. This is rare in the low doses usually used for sepsis.

d. Epinepherine is a strong vasopressor. It has both alpha- and beta-agonist properties. Its beta agonist effect is somewhat stronger than that of norepinephrine. Epinephrine is the drug of choice for cardiac arrest and allergic reactions. It can also be used for severe hypotension, especially in the patient with a failing heart.

e. Calcium chloride provides brief improvements in blood pressure after bolus dosing of 2 to 5 mg/kg. This occurs even in the normocalcemic state. CaCl should be reserved for patients with ionized hypocalcemia. Calcium is a key player in myocardial and vascular smooth muscle contraction and it is via this pathway that CaCl has its effect. CaCl will increase both myocardial contractility and peripheral vascular tone.

3. Ionotropic Therapy

Although the need for vasopressors is much more common, occasionally inotropic therapy is indicated to support the trauma patient. Cardiac contusion often can cause ventricular dysfunction (particularly right ventricular failure), requiring myocardial support. Elderly patients with comorbid illness may also require an inotropic agent to maintain acceptable hemodynamics.

a. Dopamine is often a first line inotropic agent. It is a dose-specific agonist. At low doses, it primarily binds the dopamine receptor, providing splanchnic vasodilation. At slightly higher doses, it is primarily a beta-agonist, improving myocardial contractility (positive inotropic agent) as well as increasing sinoatrial conduction (positive chronotropic agent). At still higher doses, it becomes an alpha-agonist. *In vivo,* it is impossible to know at what dose what effect site will be occupied and, thus, titration of dopamine should be based on measured hemodynamic indices.

b. Dobutamine has strongest affinity for the $beta_1$ receptor. It provides both inotropic and chronotropic support. It increases cardiac index and stroke volume, but also increases heart rate and can lower systemic blood pressure (via peripheral $beta_2$ receptor binding).

c. Milrinone is a phosphodiesterase inhibitor. It increases cardiac output with perhaps less tachycardia than that associated with dopamine and dobutamine. Systemic hypotension is the major side effect of milrinone.

d. Intraaortic balloon pump (IABP) can be useful in severe, refractory left ventricular failure that is suspected to be reversible. The IABP reduces afterload and aids in ventricular ejection by inflating and deflating itself in the aorta in synchrony with the cardiac cycle.

F.   Ventilation Strategy

Ventilatory strategy is dependent on the physiologic status of the patient. Choosing a strategy merits consideration of all of the patient's injuries. The ventilatory decisions are then made based on a risk-to-benefit evaluation. Sometimes, separate injuries in the same patient cause conflict in ventilation strategy.

1. **Pulmonary Injury**

   Protective ventilation is used for pulmonary injury.

   a. **Low Peak Inspiratory Pressure (PIP) and Low Plateau Pressure (Pplat) to Avoid Barotrauma or Volutrauma.**

   b. **PEEP to Maintain Oxygenation**

   c. **Low FIO_2** to Avoid Oxygen Toxicity

   d. **Permissive Hypercapnia.** Recent evidence in intensive care unit (ICU) patients suggests it is not necessary to maintain a normal pH at the expense of high driving pressures to maintain minute ventilation. In fact, normal to low tidal volumes with mild acidosis is generally well tolerated.

   e. **ICU Ventilator.** An ICU ventilator may be required with severe lung injury. Many newer modes of ventilation do not exist on older anesthesia machine ventilators.

2. **Hypovolemia and Tamponade**

   Provide ventilation to maintain cardiovascular stability.

   a. **Low Tidal Volume (V$_T$)**

   b. **Low PEEP** is used to maintain ventricular filling in the face of already high "extracavitary" pressures.

3. **Closed Head Injury**

   Maintaining cerebral perfusion pressure in the brain-injured patient often can be assisted by an appropriate ventilation strategy.

   a. **Hyperventilation** with its associated alkalosis reduces ICP by vasoconstriction of cerebral vessels. This effect, however, is transient and autoregulation of cerebral blood flow shifts, ultimately making hyperventilation an ineffective long-term strategy. Hyperventilation is no longer recommended, except for acute management of high ICP.

   b. **PEEP alters ICP** via several mechanisms; however, the addition of PEEP to aid in oxygenation is usually well tolerated and can be accommodated by elevating the head of the bed 30 degrees.

G.   Laboratory Monitoring

When and what laboratory studies to obtain are truly dictated by clinical situation. Serum electrolytes, arterial blood gas, hemoglobin, and blood glucose are a bare minimum to have on admission. Coagulation parameters, platelet count, and calcium are also often helpful.

1. **Hemoglobin and Hematocrit** can help guide transfusion therapy as well as assess blood loss and intravascular volume.

2. Electrolytes

Serum **potassium,** which can change rapidly, has serious clinical implications. **Ionized calcium** can fall with rapid transfusion (especially if citrate clearance is impaired because of shock and poor tissue perfusion) and can have cardiovascular implications, clotting indications, and actions at the neuromuscular junction. **Hyperglycemia and hypoglycemia** often occur in head-injured patients and recent data suggest that tight control may improve outcomes in all critically ill patients.

3. Bleeding Parameters

Monitoring prothrombin time (PT), partial thromboplastin time (PTT), platelet count, and fibrinogen can be helpful in guiding transfusion of clotting factors.

H. Constant Vigilance for New and Undiagnosed Problems

Maintain constant vigilance for new and undiagnosed problems. Any new clinical findings should be discussed with the surgical team to ensure appropriate surgical interventions.

1. Internal or External Hemorrhage

2. Airway Injuries

3. Thoracic Injuries

    a. Pneumothorax is a common cause of hypoxia and hypotension. Undiagnosed pneumothorax is common in the trauma patient and should be anticipated. Increasing airway pressures often herald pneumothorax. Therapy is surgical thoracostomy.

    b. Diaphragmatic Injuries

    c. Pulmonary contusion resulting in significant impairment in oxygenation or ventilation can result from blunt chest trauma. Therapy is supportive.

    d. Aspiration can occur at any time. Often, it is not witnessed and clinical effects can be delayed. Pneumonitis occurs frequently and can be difficult to treat. Induction and emergence are times when the trauma patient is particularly susceptible to aspiration.

4. Cardiac Injuries

    a. Myocardial contusion with ventricular dysfunction.

        (1) Dysrhythmia

        (2) Complete Heart Block

    b. Aortic dissection must be considered in the differential diagnosis of hypotension after blunt thoracic trauma. TEE would provide fast and sensitive diagnosis.

    c. Tamponade from fluid or blood must be considered any time hypotension occurs.

    d. Septal Perforation

5. Abdominal Injuries

    a. Liver or spleen lacerations can result in significant hemorrhage that can go unnoticed.

Delayed hemorrhage from liver and spleen injuries can be a cause of hypovolemia, hypotension, and anemia intraoperatively or in the postoperative period.

b.   Retroperitoneal hemorrhage can hide large volumes of blood even during laparotomy and should be a part of the differential diagnosis of continued transfusion or volume requirement.

c.   Intraabdominal Hypertension

(1)   Bladder pressure can be helpful in monitoring increased abdominal pressures.

(2)   TEE may be the most effective way to evaluate volume status with elevated filling pressures produced by intraabdominal hypertension.

(3)   Impaired respiratory mechanics with increased airway pressures and decreased functional residual capacity can arise.

d.   Sepsis From Viscous Perforation

6.   Neurologic Injury

a.   Cushing reflex can herald an **increasing ICP** from hemorrhage, edema, or expanding hematoma.

b.   Spinal cord injury has the potential to cause hypotension (neurogenic shock).

7.   Urinary tract injuries may be noted by hematuria. These injuries can be from trauma or iatrogenic during laparotomy for intraabdominal trauma.

8.   Rhabdomyolysis is diagnosed by checking serum creatinine kinase. This is a common cause of acute renal failure after trauma, particularly crush injury, or any time there is prolonged ischemia to an extremity.

9.   Orthopedic Injuries

a.   Pelvic fracture with pelvic bleeding can cause hypovolemia and anemia.

b.   Long bone fracture can give rise to fat emboli syndrome.

c.   Peripheral compartment syndromes may require fasciotomy to prevent vascular compromise.

VI.   Emergence from Anesthesia

Emergence from anesthesia requires decisions regarding extubation and disposition. All aspects of the patient's clinical status must be considered.

A.   Postoperative disposition must be determined. Does the patient's cardiovascular or respiratory status require ICU level care?

B.   Postoperative Extubation

Criteria for extubation must be met.

1.   Hypothermia

A temperature of at least 36°C should be established before emergence and extubation.

2.   Hemodynamic stability must be maintained without significant intervention.

3. Cervical spine injury can deter extubation if intubation was difficult or if the patient has been placed in a halo brace. Ligamentous injury, however, can often not be ruled out in the patient with other "distracting" injuries and forces the team to treat the patient as though the neck may be "unstable."

4. Pulmonary dysfunction or insufficiency would preclude extubation. Acute lung injury and ARDS are frequent sequelae of trauma. Intraabdominal hypertension with impaired respiratory mechanics can help the anesthetist to decide to keep the patient intubated.

5. Difficult airway management from facial or laryngeal edema secondary to large volume resuscitation or facial injuries or a wired jaw from facial fractures all must be considered when deciding about extubation. Extubation should not be taken lightly in such patients!

C. Postoperative Pain Management Plan

A postoperative plan for pain management should be in place before emergence from anesthesia. Epidural analgesia for thoracic or upper abdominal injuries can help promote extubation. Regional analgesia can sometimes be used for peripheral procedures. Intravenous narcotics, especially administered in a patient-controlled fashion, provide excellent analgesia and patient satisfaction.

VII. Traps, Decision Dilemmas, and Conclusions

A. Airtrapping and Cardiac Arrest

During vigorous resuscitation, significant amounts of auto-PEEP can develop, which can lead to cardiac arrest. Allowing complete deflation between breaths will alleviate the problem.

B. Differential Diagnosis of Common Life-threatening Problems

1. Hypotension

Hypovolemia (absolute or relative) from epidural, anesthetic, surgical manipulation of venous return; arrhythmia, myocardial ischemia, pericardial tamponade, acute valvular disease, pulmonary embolus (any source: fat, air, clot), tension pneumothorax, sepsis or systemic inflammatory response syndrome (SIRS), neurogenic shock, anaphylaxis, intraabdominal compartment syndrome, auto-PEEP, hypoxia.

2. Hypertension

From Cushing reflex, inappropriate vasopressor administration, "light" anesthesia, vascular cross-clamp, sympathetic outflow secondary to volatile anesthetic (particularly desflurane).

3. Tachycardia

From arrhythmia, "light" anesthesia, hypoxia, hypercarbia, anemia, hypovolemia, side effect of inotropic agent or reflex from vasodilator, anaphylaxis, pulmonary embolus, cardiac contusion, tamponade, tension pneumothorax.

4. Bradycardia
From Cushing reflex, arrhythmia, narcotic effect, reflex from vasopressor, carotid artery manipulation, profound hypovolemia, myocardial ischemia.
5. Hypoxia and Hypoxemia
From improper endotracheal tube (ETT) placement (esophageal, right mainstem), ETT plug, bronchial plug, unintended delivery of low FIO_2 from machine, atelectasis, pulmonary edema (cardiogenic or otherwise), bronchospasm, pulmonary embolus, carbon monoxide poisoning, methemoglobinemia, cyanide poisoning, intrapulmonary vascular malformations and shunt, comorbid pulmonary pathology (pulmonary fibrosis, chronic obstructive pulmonary disease [COPD], sarcoidosis).

SELECTED READING

Capan LM, Miller SM, Turndorf H, eds. *Trauma: anesthesia and intensive Care.* Philadelphia: JB Lippincott, 1991.

Dutton RP. Shock and trauma anesthesia. *Anesthiol Clin North Am* 1999;17:83–96.

Grande CM, Stene JK, Berhard WN, eds. Overview of trauma anesthesia and critical care. *Crit Care Clin* 1990;6(1):1–219.

McCunn M, Karlin A. Nonblood fluid resuscitation. *Anesthesiol Clin North Am* 1999;17(1):107–124.

Landers DF, Dullye KK. Vascular access and fluid resuscitation in trauma: issues of blood and blood products. *Anesthesiol Clin North Am* 1999;17(1):125–140.

Longnecker DE, Tinker JH, Morgan GE, eds. *Principles and practice of anesthesiology,* 2nd ed. St. Louis: Mosby, 1998:2138–2164.

13

Prevention Strategies: Thromboembolic Complications, Alcohol Withdrawal, Infection and Gastrointestinal Bleeding

Ruben Peralta, MD, Alexander Iribarne, MS,
Oscar J. Manrique, MD,
and Robert L. Sheridan, MD

I. Thromboembolic Complications

A. Epidemiology

Pulmonary embolism (PE) and deep venous thrombosis (DVT) are part of a well-known spectrum of venous thromboembolic diseases (VTE). As described by Virchow more than a century ago, three major risk factors or components of VTE are seen: vascular wall injury, stasis, and hypercoagulability. In the United States, 250,000 patients are affected by VTE, and more than 200,000 complications and fatalities occur secondary to PE each year. The incidence of VTE in trauma patients varies, depending on the screening methods used, and can reach as high as 54% in patients with head injuries, 62% associated with spinal injuries, and 69% in patients with pelvic fractures. According to earlier reports, the incidence of venous thrombosis in trauma patients may be as high as 35%, with thrombus formation generally felt to occur soon after injury in both the injured and the uninjured extremity. VTE is one of the most frequent causes of hospitalization in adults. The highest incidence of VTE appears to be within 24 hours of an operation, and most occur within 2 weeks of surgery. Early identification and treatment, however, can decrease the frequency of complications.

B. Diagnosis and Risk Factors

Most of the clinical findings are uncertain and inadequately specific or sensitive for diagnosis of VTE. Signs and symptoms for PE range from mild anxiety with hyperventilation and tachycardia to profound dyspnea, cyanosis, hypotension, and cardiac arrest. The most common symptoms are dyspnea (75%), chest pain with or without pleuritic component (60%), and cough (30%). The most common signs are tachypnea, followed by rales and tachycardia. Localized tenderness along the deep veins, unilateral thigh or calf swelling more than 3 cms, and Homans' sign (slight pain at the back of the knee or calf when the ankle is slowly and gently dorsiflexed, with the knee bent) are the most frequent findings for DVT, but they are unreliable.

As many as two thirds of the patients with DVT have no symptoms or physical findings to suggest its occurrence.

Many tests are included for the screening and diagnosis of DVT and PE. Depending on the circumstances and conditions of the patient, other modalities such as contrast venography, hand-held venous Doppler, impedance plethysmography, phleborheography, and radiolabeled fibrinogen scanning can be used. Currently, the gold standard method for DVT diagnosis is venography, but it is time consuming and invasive. Duplex imaging, with it good sensitivity and specificity because it combines the flow analysis and the ultrasound image, make it the most used diagnostic modality. Characteristics of acute thrombosis include incompressibility of the interrogated vein, enlargement of the vein, and the lack of significant venous collaterals. Noted in chronic thrombosis are echogenic thrombi, a nonenlarged vein, and prominent collaterals. Depending on the localization of the thrombi, in general above the knee, PE can represent a greater risk because of the large volume of thrombus that can occlude the pulmonary circulation.

For PE, other studies such as ventilation or perfusion lung scanning, helical computed tomography (CT) of the chest, pulmonary angiography and echocardiography, could be performed. Pulmonary angiogram still is the gold standard.

Age is a major risk factor for VTE. Incidence increases at the age of 40, and rises more rapidly after the age of 55. Other major risk factors for this condition include immobilization, previous DVT or PE, malignancy, obesity, prolonged operation, fractures, major trauma, varicose veins, recent myocardial infarction, congestive heart failure, stroke, pregnancy, and head and spinal cord injury. Depending on the number of these risk factors, patients can be considered at low, moderate, high, and very high risk for developing DVT.

C. Treatment and Complications

For treatment and prophylaxis, the patients can be approached in two ways: mechanically and pharmacologically. Definitive randomized, controlled clinical studies on prophylactic measures in patients with multiple trauma do not exist, because of many reasons, including the heterogeneity of the trauma patient population. Mechanical approaches are aimed at reducing stasis or preventing propagation of preexisting thrombus. The second approach is drug therapy to alter part of the extrinsic clotting cascade.

1. Mechanical Treatment

Elastic compression is the cornerstone for controlling postthrombotic edema and the long-term morbidity of the postthrombotic syndrome. Few, if any, complications can be attributed to the use of these devices. Simple leg elevation reduces venous stasis but does not reliably reduce the incidence of DVT.

The most effective mechanical method is the intermittent pneumatic compression of the leg. Each
cycle generates a pressure between of 35 and 40 mm
Hg for a few seconds per minute. These pneumatic
garments have to be used at least 1 to 2 hours per
day, three or more times a day for effective control of
swelling.

No type I data support the use of vena cava filters
to prevent PE. Studies show that 10% of injured
patients who had a prophylactic vena cava filter
demonstrated vena cava thrombosis, and 50% of
these patients had long-term lower extremity edema.
The effectiveness of a vena cava filter in preventing
PE in patients with known proximal DVT has been
well established in the literature. The placement of
vena cava filters in trauma patients at high risk with
no documented DVT, especially in those patients who
have relative contraindications to anticoagulation,
has been variably adopted in trauma programs.
Severe closed head injury with a Glasgow Coma
Scale (GCS) score <8, spinal cord injury with paraplegia or quadriplegia, complex pelvic fracture with
associated long-bone fractures, and multiple long-
bone fractures, put patients at particular risk for PE
and are relative indications for filter placement, particularly if anticoagulation is contraindicated. Various effective devices are currently available. A
removable vena cava filter has been developed and is
currently used in an investigational protocol in our
institution. Placement of vena cava filters, however,
can result in complications such as DVT at insertion
site, migration, perforations of the inferior vena cava
and other major vessels and major hemorrhage; and
local trauma to the skin, vessels, and nerves at insertion site.

2. Pharmacologic Treatment

Anticoagulation continues to be the mainstay of
treatment for acute VTE. Currently, low molecular
weight heparin (LMWH) is considered to be the
most effective form of prophylaxis against VTE in
patients with multiple trauma, and it should be initiated as soon as possible if no contraindication
exists. Two large, prospective studies have documented the effectiveness of the LMWH enoxaparin
in preventing posttraumatic DVT. Both studies
showed benefits, but the difference in incidence of
DVT in these two studies demonstrates the difficulty in reaching any consensus in the management
of DVT prophylaxis. LMWH is normally administered subcutaneously (s.q.). Each dose is different,
depending on the weight of the patient (1 mg/kg s.q.
ever 12 h for DVT). LMWH does not require monitoring for therapeutic effects, and does not prolong
the activated partial thromboplastin time (aPTT) or

prothrombin time (PT) at prophylactic levels. When compared to unfractionated heparin LMWH for VTE confers a much lower risk of major bleeding complication (absolute risk reduction approximately 2 per 100 patients treated; relative risk reduction of 58% to 68%).

Treatment of established thrombus with low-dose, unfractionated heparin (LDUH) can be initiated with an 8000 to 10,000 IU bolus intravenously followed by 2000 IU/h. Effectiveness of LDUH therapy should be monitored with the aPTT or PT. An aPTT ratio of 1.5 to 2.5 times control levels (90 to 100 seconds) every 6 hours should be monitored and maintained. This level of anticoagulation is required for only 4 to 5 days, at which time the heparin can be discontinued because warfarin has reached its therapeutic levels. In patients whose baseline aPTT is prolonged (e.g., lupus-type inhibitor), the PT is preferred over the aPTT for monitoring heparin therapy.

Oral anticoagulation with warfarin and other vitamin K antagonists, inhibit vitamin K-dependent clotting factors II, VII, IX, X; and carboxylation of proteins C and S, reducing the incidence of recurrence of thrombosis in patients with VTE in more than 30% of patients treated. When practical, warfarin should be started within the first 72 hours of heparin therapy, with a dose of 10 mg the first day followed by 5 mg every day thereafter. The goal is to maintain an international normalized ratio (INR) of 2.0 to 3.0. Treatment duration should be evaluated, depending on the conditions, indications, and characteristics of each patient.

Regular platelet counts are recommended after the fourth day for patients receiving LDUH because of the approximately 5% incidence of heparin-induced thrombocytopenia (HIT), also known as the "white clot syndrome."

An immune mediated syndrome, HIT is caused by a heparin-specific immunoglobulin G (IgG) antibodies that bind to the membrane of the platelet, stimulating platelet activation and aggregation. It also can be induced by LMWH; however, this is more rare. It usually occurs 5 to 10 days after first exposure with heparin, but can be sooner with repeat exposure. The diagnosis should be suspected in a patient who develops thrombosis on heparin or when platelet count falls to <100,000 or a decline by 50% from baseline counts during heparin therapy. Management consists of discontinuation of all heparin, including heparin line flushes. Adjunctive treatments may include lepirudin; a direct thrombin inhibitor, argatroban; a selective thrombin inhibitor; or fondaparinux, a new synthetic antithrombotic agent that specifically inhibits factor Xa.

Although rarely used in a patient with multiple trauma, because of the risk of severe bleeding, dissolution of thrombus by pharmacologic means can eliminate deep venous obstruction and maintain valvular function. Recombinant tissue plasminogen activator (rt-PA) is the preferred plasminogen activator for treating patients with VTE, both systemically and via catheter-directed techniques. Administering smaller doses of rt-PA in higher volumes over a prolonged period has demonstrated good efficacy with significantly reduced bleeding complications.

Operative venous thrombectomy techniques have improved significantly during the past 20 years. Some studies indicate significantly better patency and fewer postthrombotic symptoms in patients having thrombectomy.

A clear DVT prevention protocol should be part of every trauma program. Our current program is summarized in **Table 13-1.**

II. Alcohol Withdrawal
A. Introduction
Alcoholism and its associated complications continue to be a tremendous problem in trauma. Alcohol withdrawal is defined as the development of a predictable constellation of signs and symptoms following the abrupt discontinuation of, or rapid decrease in, alcohol intake. Alcohol consumption is a major factor in the cause of both intentional and unintentional trauma. More than 50% of fatal car accidents are alcohol related. It has been estimated that societal costs attributed to alcohol abuse were $116.7 billion in 1986 and included more than 69,000 deaths. In a recent study, it has been demonstrated that among blunt trauma patients in vehicular accidents, approximately two thirds had abused alcohol. Also, only 55.2% of the trauma centers that participated in the study routinely obtained blood alcohol levels for patients on admission and less than one third used alcoholism counselors.

B. Diagnosis and Risk Factors
Obtaining blood alcohol levels (BAL) is an important first-line goal in working up a possibly intoxicated trauma patient. The most common system for measuring and reporting BAL is calculated using the weight of alcohol (milligrams) and the volume of blood (deciliter). This yields a blood alcohol concentration that can be expressed as a percentage (i.e., 0.10% alcohol by volume) or as a proportion (i.e., 100 mg/dL). This system is the one prescribed by almost every state, and is sometimes referred to as the "weight by volume" (w/v) method. A few states prescribe a "weight by weight" (w/w) method (milligrams of alcohol in milligrams of blood). BAL depends on:

1. Blood volume (which will increase with weight)
2. The amount of alcohol consumed over time (the higher the drinking rate, the higher the BAL)

Table 13-1. MGH trauma service: suggestions for DVT prophylaxis in trauma patients

No uniform agreement exists about what constitutes ideal practice in DVT prophylaxis in trauma and burns, and because of this there is no single best practice. Consequently, substantial practice variation exists nationally. What follows is a four-step process to determine DVT prophylaxis and monitoring practices in trauma. This is based on a review of available literature, published guidelines, and institutional experience.

STEP ONE: Determine risk level (high or low)

Patients at HIGH risk have one or more of the following characteristics:
–Pelvic fractures
–Lower extremity crush injury or long bone fractures
–Multiple trauma or extensive burns with anticipated protracted bed rest
–Prior history of DVT
–Morbid obesity
–Spinal cord injury

All other patients can generally be considered at LOW risk.

STEP TWO: Determine if anticoagulation might be best avoided

Anticoagulation is often best avoided if any of the following are present:
–Solid organ injury being managed nonoperatively
–Brain or spinal cord injury without written clearance from neurosurgery
–Rib fractures (epidural may be needed)
–Laparotomy within 24 h
–Ongoing bleeding from pelvic or long bone fractures
–Incomplete evaluation of the multiple trauma patient

STEP THREE: Prescribe treatment

Three patient categories based on risk level and desire to avoid anticoagulation.
–HIGH RISK/AVOID ANTICOAGULATION: sequential compression with leg or foot pumps
–HIGH RISK/ANTICOAGULATION LIKELY SAFE: subcutaneous LMWH at prophylactic dose may add sequential compression with leg or foot pumps
–LOW RISK: elastic stockings, encourage ambulation and exercise

STEP FOUR: Prescribe monitoring

Monitoring suggestions are different for each of the three patient categories based on risk level and desire to avoid anticoagulation.
–HIGH RISK/AVOID ANTICOAGULATION: regular clinical examination and ultrasound screening every Monday and Thursday
–HIGH RISK/ANTICOAGULATION LIKELY SAFE: regular clinical examination
–LOW RISK: regular clinical examination

NOTE: IVC FILTERS are indicated in occasional patients
–DVT found clinically or on LENI's and anticoagulation contraindicated
–Pulmonary embolus despite anticoagulation
–Patient at extremely high risk (determined case by case) especially if anticoagulation contraindicated

MGH, Massachusetts General Hospital; DVT, deep venous thrombosis; LENIS, lower extremity non-invasive study; IVC, inferior vena cava.

Clinically, levels of BAL correlate as follows:

- **0.02:** Mellow feeling; slight body warmth; less inhibited
- **0.05:** Noticeable relaxation; less alert; less self-focused; coordination impairment begins
- **0.08:** Drunk driving limit; definite impairment in coordination and judgment
- **0.10:** Noisy; possible embarrassing behavior; mood swings; reduction in reaction time
- **0.15:** Impaired balance and movement; clearly drunk
- **0.30:** May lose consciousness
- **0.40:** Most lose consciousness; some die
- **0.50:** Breathing stops; many die

Once patients have been treated for their immediate trauma, the emergency room or critical care staff is often faced with the clinical manifestations of alcohol withdrawal. These can be subtle and frequently missed. In the central nervous system, ethanol (in concentrations high enough to intoxicate humans) interferes with neuronal cell activation and enhances neuronal cell inhibition. During withdrawal, a person's central nervous system experiences a reversal of this effect: excitatory processes are enhanced and inhibitory processes are reduced. Clinically, such symptoms are organized, as *alcohol withdrawal syndrome,* which is a cluster of symptoms observed in persons who stop drinking alcohol following continuous and heavy consumption. Early symptoms usually begin within 5 to 10 hours after the last alcoholic drink and typically peak at 24 to 48 hours. Symptoms can include tremulousness, seizures, hallucinations, tachycardia, hypertension, tachypnea, fever, diaphoresis, nausea and vomiting, anxiety, depressed mood, irritability, nightmares, and insomnia. Alcohol-withdrawal seizures commonly occur 6 to 48 hours after the last drink, peaking at 24 hours. Later symptoms typically beginning between 48 and 96 hours after the last drink include delirium tremens (DTs), which involves profound confusion, disorientation, altered level of consciousness, hallucinations, agitation, delusions, sleep disturbances, and severe autonomic nervous system overactivity. The peak intensity of DTs is at 4 to 5 days and visual hallucinations are especially common; the patient may often report seeing insects or small animals.

C. Treatment and Complications

In caring for the trauma victim who is alcohol intoxicated, the first goal of the physician is clearly to stabilize vital signs or any other life-threatening injuries. Once stabilized, the issue of alcohol intoxication can be addressed. First, determine if the BAC corresponds to the physical examination and the person's apparent degree of intoxication. For example, the lower the BAC, the less likely that prominent symptoms (e.g., lethargy) can be explained by alcohol, which may require a search for other causes. Next, ask if any evidence of serious neurologic injury exists, if such has not already been completely ruled out in the initial trauma evaluation. Deeply lethargic or comatose patients should have CT scans in the event that a neurovascular lesion may present as a symptom of alcohol intoxication. Finally, assess any medical conditions that can mimic those of alcohol intoxication (e.g., hypoglycemia, seizure disorders, illicit drugs). Furthermore, look for evidence of chronic alcohol abuse (e.g., spider angiomas, hepatomegaly, jaundice). No specific treatment can reverse the effects of alcohol intoxication. Intravenous fluids and B complex vitamins can be administered for dehydration as a precaution against vitamin deficiency. In cases of stupor or coma, the patient should be intubated to support respirations and protect the lungs from aspiration.

Often in the recovery phase or the hours shortly after admission the physician will have to manage the symptoms of alcohol withdrawal syndrome. Usually, the agent chosen is a benzodiazepine or a barbiturate with a longer biologic half-life than alcohol. Residual symptoms can be managed with adjunctive medications (e.g., antiemetic for nausea). An appropriate benzodiazepine for the treatment of alcohol should be selected, based on the patient's age and hepatic function. The effectiveness of phenobarbital has been reported to be superior to that of diazepam for DTs. Promethazine or hydroxyzine can be administered for the treatment of nervousness or nausea. Finally, for delirious, hallucinating, and combative patients, haloperidol is the agent of choice, in combination with the above withdrawal agents. The ability of haloperidol to lower seizure threshold is controlled by concomitant administration of an anticonvulsant.

D. Injury Prevention

Although definitive treatment of alcohol withdrawal must be the primary goal in treating the patient suffering from alcohol withdrawal syndrome, prevention is the ideal way to reduce the burden of injury associated with alcohol intoxication. Patients with symptoms of alcohol withdrawal should be informed about the dangers, both in terms of their personal health and public safety, of chronic alcohol abuse. Furthermore, such patients should be provided with easy access to alcohol abuse support groups (e.g., Alcoholics Anonymous) and, if severe enough, alcohol detoxification centers. Our trauma service, use a multidisciplinary approach for the management of alcoholic patients (**Tables 13-2, 13-3**).

III. Infection

A. Introduction

Surgical site infections (SSI) are currently the third most common nosocomial infection encountered in hospitals in

(*text continues on page 205*)

Table 13-2. Complications of Alcohol Abuse

INJURY MECHANISM
- motor vehicle accidents
- falls
- burns
- assaults

NEUROLOGIC
- alcohol withdrawal, seizures
- Wernicke encephalopathy (ataxia, confusion, ophthalmoplegia)
- alcoholic peripheral neuropathy
- cerebellar degeneration

PSYCHIATRIC
- abuse of other substances
- Korsakoff syndrome (amnesia and confabulation)
- dementia
- depression
- hepatic encephalopathy
- personality disorders
- agressive or combative behaviors

SOCIAL
- chronic and acute legal problems
- financial instability
- homelessness
- estrangement from family
- isoloation
- gambling
- abusive behaviors
- suicide

DERMATOLOGIC
- spider angiomas
- palmar erythema
- acne rosacia

CARDIOPULMONARY
- alcoholic crdiomyopathy
- aspiration pneumonia
- chronic tobacco related lung disease

HEMATOLOGIC
- alcoholic bone marrow suppression
- anemia
- thrombocytopenia
- hepatic dysfunction with coagulapathy

GASTROINTESTINAL
- alcholic cirrohis
- hepatitis
- pancreatitis
- gastirc and esophagael varicies
- varicael bleeding
- ascites
- spontaneous bacterial peritonitis
- coagulapathy

NUTRITIONAL
- chroninc malnutrition
- thaimine deficiency
- folate deficienc
- electrolyte abnormalities (especially magnesium, potassium, calcium, phosporous)
- alcoholic ketoacidosis

Table 13-3: Important Considerations in
Alcohol Withdrawal Management

ASSESSMENT
COSIDERATIONS

assess injury mechanism for relation to intoxication

assess patients for chronic alcohol abuse

assess for other substance abuse

assess blood alcohol concentration if measured

consider use of structured assessment scales (CAGE, AUDIT)

consider laboratory screen for hepatic function and coagulation

assess risk of withdrawal (chronic abusers)

PROPHYLAXIS
CONSIDERATIONS

consider use of prophylactic benzodiazepines for chronic abusers

consider administion of thaimine

consider administion folate

consider DVT prophylaxis

NURSING
CONSIDERATIONS

consider more frequent monitoring of vital signs

be alert for inappropriate agitation and confusion

be alert for autonomic hyperactivity (inappropriate elevation of pulse, temperature, excessive sweating)

consider aspiration precautions

consider fall precautions

be prepared to follow restraint policy if needed

TREATMENT
CONSIDERATIONS

some patients will develop life-threatenting autonomic dysregulation and agitation despite prophylactic use of benzodiazepines

consider transfer to intensive care unit if needed

CASE MANAGMENT
CONSIDERATIONS

discuss problem frankly with patient

consider addiction services consultation

consider psychiatry consultation

consider homelessness consultation

consider discussions with family if appropriate legally (see chapter 46)

consider discussion with primary care provider if appropriate legally (see chapter 46) the United States. The diagnosis of surgical wound infection is usually made between postoperative days 4 and 8, but can occur at any time within 30 days of the operation. The most common symptoms and signs include fever, purulent drainage, local signs of inflammation, and isolation of organisms from the wound.

B. Risk Factors

In 1964, the National Research Council (NRC) proposed the idea of using wound classification to predict risk for surgical site infection. This classification has four categories:

1. Class I: Clean
2. Class II: Clean-Contaminated
3. Class III: Contaminated
4. Class IV: Dirty

The expected wound infection in each one of these classifications is 1.5%, 7.5%, 15% and 40%, respectively. Statistics, however, indicate that the traditional wound classification system does not stratify the total risk of infection very well. In 1970, the Efficacy of Nosocomial Infection Control (SENIC) project, simplified the index of factors for predicting the risk for surgical site infection. The four factors (surgical procedure on the abdomen, surgical procedure more than 2 hours, a contaminated or dirty infected surgical site, and having three or more distinct discharge diagnoses, excluding a wound infection) have a value of one point each. The more points (risk factors) the patient, has the higher the risk for infection. Patients with a risk index of 0 were considered at low risk, with an overall infection rate of 1%. Patients with one risk factor were considered at medium risk, with an overall infection rate of 3.6%. Finally, patients with 2, 3, or 4 risk factors have an overall infection rate of 8.9%, 17.2%, and 27% respectively. In 1991, however, the National Nosocomial Infection Surveillance classification system was proposed based on the SENIC project. This new classification uses three criteria: wound class, The American Society of Anesthesiologists score (ASA >3), and the length of the procedure (>75th percentile for similar procedures). Each group represents one point, scoring high risk of infection for patients with 3 points. Clean wounds can be further stratified as class 0, 1, or 2, for which the infection rate is 1%, 2.3%, and 5.4% respectively. Currently, the Centers for Disease Control and Prevention (CDC) recommends prophylactic antibiotics for operations associated with a high risk of infection or for those in whom the occurrence of an infection can produce severe consequences.

Other important risk factors can be categorized as patient-related factors such as diabetes mellitus, age above 50 years or younger than 1 year, malnutrition, and cigarette smoking. Other risk factors are classified as perioperative factors (e.g., prophylaxis, hair removal, technical proficiency, and foreign material in the surgical site).

C. Pitfalls in Antibiotic Prophylaxis

The inability to distinguish between contamination, infection, and inflammation is one of the most common pitfalls in the current clinical practice, leading to continued use of antibiotics for unnecessarily long periods of time. Other reasons for the inappropriate use of antimicrobial prophylaxis is administration of antibiotics in the absence of infection, poor choice of drug, wrong dosage, excessive duration, and misguide prophylaxis. In many studies, excessive duration seems to be the most common mistake. Long duration of antibiotic prophylaxis increases hospital costs, raises bacterial resistance, alters the normal bowel flora, and produces adverse reactions (e.g., direct toxicity and impairment of the immune system). In addition, the unnecessary extension of prophylactic treatments can lead to allergic reactions and superinfection.

Current guidelines for use of prophylactic antibiotics are based on the traditional wound classification system, which suggests that all categories of wounds, except clean wounds, be given prophylactic antibiotics. Patients with clean wounds receive prophylactic antibiotics only in cases wherein an implantable device (e.g., vascular prostheses) is used or presence of other foreign materials. The surgical wound class and the site of the surgery largely determine the choice of antibiotics. One of the most important issues for antibiotic prophylaxis is to maintain effective antibiotic levels throughout the procedure. The agent of choice should provide adequate coverage against the flora residing in the surgical field. In addition, using broad-spectrum antibiotics for prophylaxis is discouraged because it serves only to increase the rate of bacterial resistance.

In patients who develop sudden organ failure secondary to overwhelming infection, a limited role may be seen for the use of activated protein C infusion.

IV. Gastrointestinal Bleeding

A. Epidemiology

Gastrointestinal (GI) bleeding from stress ulcers still remains a major problem for the patient in the intensive care unit (ICU). More than 300,000 new cases of stress ulcers are diagnosed each year in the United States, and approximately 4 million people receive some form of ulcer treatment.

Numerous clinical entities are associated with stress ulcers. Head injury, burns, shock, and sepsis are some of the most common diseases associated with stress ulceration. However, no common causative mechanism explains why these lesions develop. Depending on a patient's baseline condition, stress ulcers have some variants. In 1823, Swan described Curling ulcers that are associated with burns. This condition was subsequently named after T. B. Curling who reported some cases in 1842. Curling ulcers are distributed along the entire GI tract. These ulcers are typically small, rarely exceeding 2.5 cm in diameter, and bleeding is usually mild. The other variant is Cushing ulcers, which are associated with head trauma, and are a common problem for the neurosurgical ICU patient. These ulcers are distributed more commonly in the stomach and duodenum.

B. Pathophysiology

Stress ulcers are numerous small lesions occurring in the superficial gastric mucosa. The major clinical consequence is bleeding, which potentially compromises the already ill patient. The pathogenesis of these ulcers is incompletely understood, but probably involves compromise of the mucosal defense mechanism. In addition, mucosal ischemia, acid secretion, and infection with *Helicobacter pylori* appear to play a major role in the development of these lesions. Together, these factors lead to an imbalance in the endocrine system, mucosal defense, and gastric acid secretion.

C. Diagnoses and Differential Diagnosis

Critically ill patients may have no symptoms of gastroduodenal ulceration. In most circumstances, endoscopy is the preferred method of diagnosis. Painless bleeding is the most common presentation in the critically ill.

D. Prophylaxis and Treatment

The American Society of Hospital Pharmacists (ASHP) published the current therapeutic guidelines for stress ulcer prophylaxis. These guidelines provide an extensive analysis of the available clinical trials and meta-analyses from the last couple of years.

Measures of the efficacy of prophylaxis was based on three points:

1. Episodes of clinically important GI bleeding defined as gastroduodenal bleeding associated with clinically important complications (e.g., hemodynamic compromise and the need for blood transfusions or surgery).
2. Mortality caused by clinically significant bleeding
3. Adverse effects of prophylaxis agents, including the risk of nosocomial pneumonia.

Conclusions of ASHP are that stress ulcer prophylaxis should be administered to patients who will remain on a ventilator for more than 48 hours or any ICU patient with a coagulopathy. In addition, prophylaxis was recommended for patients with a history of GI ulceration or bleeding within 1 year before hospital admission and in patients with at least two of the following risk factors: sepsis, ICU stay of more than 1 week, occult bleeding lasting 6 days or more, and use of high-dose corticosteroids (>250 mg/day of hydrocortisone or the equivalent).

Prophylaxis is also recommended for ICU patients with a GCS of ≤10 or thermal injuries to >35% of their body surface area (BSA), and with partial hepatectomy, multiple trauma, transplantation, hepatic failure, and spinal cord injuries. The major complication of prophylaxis is pneumonia, but clinical data still need to demonstrate this as a significant event. Monitoring is recommended for all patients receiving prophylaxis treatment, with a focus on bleeding and drug effects. H_2 blockers, antagonist, sucralfate, and proton pump inhibitors all constitute reasonable prophylaxis.

SELECTED READING

Anda RF, Williamson DF, Remington PL. Alcohol and fatal injuries among US adults. Findings from the NHANES I Epidemiologic Follow-up Study. *JAMA* 1988;260(17):2529–2532.

Comerota AJ. Deep venous thrombosis. In: Cameron JL, ed. *Current surgical therapy,* 7th ed. Vol. 1. St. Louis: Mosby, 2001:999–1007.

Frank T, Padberg J. Prevention of venous thromboembolism in the surgical patient. In: Cameron JL, ed. *Current surgical therapy,* 7th ed. Vol. 1. St. Louis: Mosby, 2001:1023–1027.

Geerts WH, et al. A prospective study of venous thromboembolism after major trauma. *N Engl J Med* 1994;331(24):1601–1606.

Hatton J, et al. A step-wise protocol for stress ulcer prophylaxis in the neurosurgical intensive care unit. *Surg Neurol* 1996;46(5):493–499.

Kamerow DB, Pincus HA, MacDonal DI. Alcohol abuse, other drug abuse, and metabolic disorders in medical practice. Prevalence, costs, recognition, and treatment. *JAMA* 1986;255: 20054–20057.

Knight R, et al. Prophylactic antibiotics are not indicated in clean general surgery cases. *Am J Surg* 2001;182(6):682–686.

Knudson MM, et al. Use of low molecular weight heparin in preventing thromboembolism in trauma patients. *J Trauma* 1996;41(3): 446–459.

Lee Green MM. *Guidelines for clinical care: venous thromboembolism (VTE).* Ann Arbor: University of Michigan Health System, 2001.

Livingston EH. Stomach and duodenum. In: Norton JA, et al., eds. *Surgery: basic science and clinical evidence.* Vol. 1. New York: Springer, 2001:489–515.

Mulholland MW. Duodenal ulcer. In: Greenfield LJ, ed. *Surgery: scientific principles and practice,* 3rd ed. Vol. 1. Philadelphia: Lippincott Williams & Wilkins, 2001:750–766.

Muscarella, P., Steinberg SM. Postoperative wound infection. In: Cameron JL, ed. *Current surgical therapy,* 7th ed. Vol. 1. St. Louis: Mosby, 2001: 1277–1282.

Nathan S, et al. Severe gastrointestinal bleeding resulting in total gastrectomy in a patient with major burns. *Burns* 1999;25(6):531–536.

Pillai TA, Jalewa AK, Chadha IA. Antibiotic prophylaxis—Hobson's choice in burns management. *Burns* 1998;24(8):760–762.

Rodriguez JL, et al., Early placement of prophylactic vena caval filters in injured patients at high risk for pulmonary embolism. *J Trauma* 1996;40(5):797–802; discussion 802–804.

Shepard AD, Shin LH. Pulmonary thromboembolism. In: Cameron JL, ed. *Current surgical therapy,* 7th ed. Vol. 1. St. Louis: Mosby, 2001; 1014–1018.

Soderstrom CA, Cowley RA. A national alcohol and trauma center survey. Missed opportunities, failures of responsibility. *Arch Surg* 1987;122(9):1067–1071.

Solomkin JS. Perioperative antimicrobial prophylaxis. In: Baker RJ, Fisher JE, eds., *Mastery of surgery,* 4th ed. Philadelphia: Lippincott Williams & Wilkins, 2001;146–154.

Villaveces A, Cummings P, et al. Association of alcohol-related laws with deaths due to motor vehicle and motorcycle crashes in the United States, 1980–1997. 2003. *Am J Epidemiol* 2003;157(2): 131–140.

Wakefield LJG.a.T.W. Venous and lymphatic systems. In: Lazar MWM, Greenfield J, Oldham KT, et al., eds. *Surgery: scientific principles and practice,* 3rd ed. 2nd ed. Philadelphia: Lippincott William & Wilkins 2001;1873–1888.

Wittmann MSaD. Let us shorten antibiotic prophylaxis and therapy in surgery. *Am J Surg* 1996;172(6a):26s–32s.

III

Evaluation and Management of Specific Injuries

Nervous System 1: Head Injury

Yogish D. Kamath, MD,
and Lawrence F. Borges, MD

I. Epidemiology

Trauma is estimated to cause of approximately 150,000 deaths per year in United States. One third of these deaths result from severe head injury. About one million visits to hospital emergency rooms (ER) occur as a result of head trauma and approximately 230,000 in-patient admissions result from to traumatic brain injury (TBI). Efficient implementation of trauma systems and TBI management protocols will improve outcome and minimize disability.

II. Mechanisms

A. Blunt and Penetrating Trauma

Blunt trauma usually occurs from motor vehicle accidents, falls, assault, and industrial accidents. Gunshot or missile wounds and stab wounds result in penetrating trauma.

B. Primary Brain Injury

Primary brain injury occurs at impact and is irreversible.

C. Secondary or Delayed Brain Injury

Secondary brain injury occurs as a result of several factors, including development of intracranial hematomas, contusions, cerebral edema, anoxia and other metabolic abnormalities, hydrocephalus, infections, pneumocephalus, seizures, and so forth. Secondary injury is often preventable and, in many cases, reversible. In gunshot or missile wounds, the extent of injury may not be limited to the missile tract because of an associated blast effect or pressure wave from dissipation of energy from high velocity missile deceleration.

III. Classification

Head injury is classified as *open* or *closed,* based on whether a breach of scalp with or without underlying skull fracture or exposure of brain tissue has occurred. A more useful classification is based on a Glasgow Coma Scale (GCS) score (see Chapter 8, *Secondary Survey of the Trauma Patient*).

1. **Mild:** GCS of 14 to 15; loss of consciousness, if present, is brief (<5 minutes)
2. **Moderate** GCS of 9 to 13
3. **Severe:** GCS of ≤8, which, by definition, is coma

IV. Initial Evaluation of the Head-Injured Patient

Initial evaluation must be integrated with the primary and secondary patient surveys conducted in the ER. Airway, breathing, and circulation (ABC) management takes precedence.

A. History

Detailed history must be obtained expeditiously from emergency medical services (EMS), bystanders, and the patient to assess the following:

1. **Mechanism of Injury**

The mechanism of injury includes information on the speed at which the motor vehicle accident (MVA) occurred, vehicular damage, restraints, ejection from vehicle, assault weapon, type of missile or firearm, alcohol or substance use, and so on. A high index of suspicion should be maintained for associated injuries to craniocervical junction or upper cervical spine (C-spine), when a significant mechanism exists for severe head injury.

2. **On-Scene Neurologic Examination**

Information from emergency personnel must be obtained, when available. Loss of consciousness, changes in neurologic examination while en route to the ER, history of nausea or vomiting, side of the pupil to dilate first, and so on must be elicited.

3. **Time Course of Events**

Determine the possibility of multisystem trauma and so on.

4. **Neurologic Symptoms**

Consider any neurologic symptoms described by patient (headache, changes in vision, speech, hearing, motor strength or sensation, pain in neck or spine).

5. **Alcohol or Substance Use**

B. **Examination**

1. **Vital Signs**

A combination of hypertension, bradycardia, and respiratory irregularity (Cushing reflex) indicates increased intracranial tension causing transtentorial herniation. Hypotension is unlikely to result from head injury, except in following circumstances: neonates or infants who can lose significant proportion of total blood volume in an intracranial hemorrhage and adults with significant loss of blood from scalp injuries or associated spinal cord injury with neurogenic shock. Hypothermia needs to be treated because it will worsen coagulopathy and alter neurologic status.

2. **Dilated Pupil**

Unilateral or bilateral, a dilated pupil is a surgical emergency. Expeditious cranial imaging takes precedence over a detailed secondary survey. Treatable causes of cerebral herniation from increased intracranial tension must be diagnosed and treated emergently. Emergency cranial burr hole exploration may be necessary if hemodynamic compromise precludes adequate cranial imaging.

3. **Level of Consciousness or Cognition (Glasgow Coma Scale)**

Serial neurologic examinations are necessary to diagnose delayed deterioration from causes of secondary brain injury.

4. **Inspection**

Note lacerations or defects in scalp, periorbital ecchymoses (raccoon eyes), and retroauricular ecchymoses (Battle's sign) indicative of anterior cranial skull base and petrous temporal fractures, respectively; open skull fractures; and craniocervical or facial deformities indicative of injuries to craniofacial skeleton. Bleeding in the ear canals or cerebrospinal fluid (CSF) otorhinorrhea can also indicate skull fractures and increased risk of ascending infection. Probing of scalp defects to assess whether an associated cranial defect exists is to be avoided, because this can further the injury and increase the risk of infection. Skull fractures or defects by missiles are best assessed by diagnostic imaging (computed tomography [CT] scan or skull radiographs).

5. Cranial Nerves

Assess for traumatic cranial neuropathies or brainstem injury. Assessment of olfaction has little utility in examination of the unconscious and semiconscious patient. Loss of olfaction, when detected in the setting of concussion, can indicate the severity of the shear forces.

6. Pupils

Assess size, shape, and reaction to light on each side. Presence of an afferent pupillary defect may be detected by swinging flashlight test (i.e., Marcus Gunn pupil: slower and smaller direct light reflex with intact consensual reflex). When present, this can be indicative of a compressive traumatic optic neuropathy.

7. Vision

Visual acuity can be tested with a pocket vision screener card or finger counting or by perception of motion or light as is applicable. Visual fields can be assessed bedside by confrontation.

Funduscopic examination may show papilledema, retinal hemorrhages, retinal detachment, or evidence of injury to the globe. Pharmacologic mydriasis must be avoided, however, until a reliable method has been established to monitor the neurologic status of the patient (reliable clinical examination or intracranial pressure monitoring devices).

8. Ocular Movements

Ocular movements can be assessed in a conscious cooperative patient. Doll's eye maneuvers must be avoided in the setting of trauma because of the possibility of worsening an associated C-spine injury. Rigid cervical collars should be in place until C-spine trauma is excluded reliably.

9. Facial Motor and Sensory Function

Presence of facial bone fractures can limit the examination. Facial nerve injury must be identified early because surgical decompression may be required. Corneal reflex can be used in assessing trigeminal and facial nerve function in an unconscious patient.

10. Hearing and Equilibrium

Inspect external auditory canals and tympanic membranes before assessing hearing. Conductive hearing loss can indicate ossicular disruption, which may need surgical correction. Other causes of vertigo or dizziness may need to be ruled out before attributing posttraumatic dizziness to concomitant vestibular concussion.

Lower cranial nerve (9–12) dysfunction is uncommon in trauma; however, in cases of posttraumatic dysarthria, it should be ruled out. When present, lower cranial nerve dysfunction increases the risk of aspiration.

11. Limbs

Full motor, sensory, and reflex examination must be done in all four extremities. Any flaccidity or rigidity, weakness, or sensory impairment should lead to consideration of associated spinal cord injury. Specific patterns of posturing (decerebrate, decorticate, or triple flexion-withdrawal reflex) or spinal shock need to be recognized.

12. Spine

Patient can be logrolled carefully to inspect and gently palpate the whole spine for any evidence of deformity or tenderness. A rectal examination can be done at this time to assess rectal tone, voluntary sphincter contraction, anal wink, and bulbocavernosus reflex. A rectal examination must be done in all unconscious patients and all conscious patients in whom a suspicion of spinal cord injury exists. Assess gait, when practical.

V.   Treatment Plan for Head-Injured Patient After Initial Assessment

Accurate assessment of risk of intracranial injury and subsequent triaging for discharge to home, admission for observation, or transfer to another facility equipped to manage the patient must be made after initial assessment; then supplemented, if necessary, with diagnostic studies.

Patients with **mild** head injury, no loss of consciousness or evidence of intoxication, and minimal symptoms (e.g., mild headache or dizziness) can be discharged home with standard head-injury instructions, provided they are observed by reliable family members and have access to appropriate emergency medical care in a timely fashion. Worsening headache should prompt reevaluation and admission. Admission and further work-up are required for patients with (a) any other neurologic symptoms; (b) moderate and severe head injury; (c) findings on head CT scans; (d) substance abuse; (e) suspicious circumstances of injury; (f) lack of access to appropriate care in a timely fashion; and (g) lack of proper supervision in the immediate period after trauma.

VI.   Diagnostic Studies

A.   Skull Radiograph

Skull x-ray studies are of limited value in modern management of head trauma. Because CT scans offer accurate and comprehensive diagnostic information, no place is seen for routine skull x-ray studies in the management of head trauma. They can be used to locate a radio-opaque foreign body, when such are missed on CT scans.

B.   Head Computed Tomography Scan

Nonenhanced CT scan of the head has become the standard for diagnostic assessment of head trauma. It provides information on intracranial hemorrhage, cerebral edema, skull fractures, pneumocephalus, hydrocephalus, and infarction (of 6 to 24 hours). Contrast-enhanced CT scans can be appropriate when cerebral vascular integrity needs to be assessed with CT angiograms, as in penetrating head injury or basal skull fractures involving vascular structures, or to assess other incidental lesions. Single pass, whole-body contrast CT scans are currently being evaluated as quick diagnostic tools in trauma.

C. Magnetic Resonance Imaging of Brain

Magnetic resonance imaging (MRI) of the brain is not usually necessary in acute head trauma. It is helpful in prognostication by detecting diffuse axonal injury (DAI), brainstem injury, preexisting neurologic disorders, and so forth, when done after the acute phase of trauma.

D. Cerebral Angiogram

In tertiary trauma centers, CT angiogram of the brain has essentially supplanted invasive cerebral angiograms. It can be useful in penetrating head injury, when CT scan is unavailable.

E. Nuclear Cerebral Perfusion Studies

Nuclear cerebral perfusion studies can be appropriate to assess presence or absence of cerebral perfusion, when apnea test is deemed inappropriate for brain-death evaluation in severe head injury (e.g., high cervical spine injury).

VII. In-Hospital Management of Head-Injured Patients

All patients admitted need serial neurologic examinations. Patients with *mild* head injury with benign findings on head CT (no potentially expansive lesions) can be admitted to the floor with frequent neurologic monitoring, preferably every 2 hours. *All others* need admission to the ICU with hourly neurologic examinations. Follow-up CT scans of the head can be performed if neurologic examination does not show improvement or deteriorates.

A. Head Elevation

Intracranial pressure (ICP) can be reduced by 30 to 45 degrees of head elevation.

B. Bedrest

C. Avoid Hypothermia

Acetaminophen and a cooling blanket helps in avoiding hypothermia.

D. Maintain Normovolemia

Administer isotonic fluids (NS + 20 mEq KCl/L) at maintenance rates to maintain normovolemia and avoid secondary injury.

E. Nothing by Mouth

The patient should have nothing by mouth until alert and able to protect the airway from aspiration.

F. Orotracheal Intubation and Assisted Ventilation

In severe head injury and in situations with risk of airway compromise (e.g., facial fractures, and severe intoxication), orotracheal intubation and assisted ventilation can be used.

G. Avoid Jugular Venous Compression

Avoid jugular venous compression from tracheal tapes, head rotation, or tight cervical collars.

H.   Serial Monitoring

Electrolytes, blood gasses, osmolality, serum levels of antiepileptic drugs, and coagulation parameters must be monitored serially.

I.   Maintain Normotension

Cerebral perfusion pressure (CPP) of 70 mm Hg and above (in patients with an ICP monitor) or, alternatively, a mean arterial pressure (MAP) of 90 mm Hg and above are to be maintained to optimize cerebral perfusion. Autoregulation of cerebral blood flow, which can be impaired in head injury, can contribute to secondary head injury from hypotension and hypovolemia. (CPP = MAP – ICP).

J.   Continuous Intracranial Pressure Monitoring

Continuous ICP monitoring is required for patients with severe head injury or those with moderate head injury who are having emergent non-neurologic surgical procedures requiring anesthesia.

K.   Steroids

Steroids have not been proven beneficial for patients with head injury.

L.   Antiemetics and Mild Analgesics

M.   Antiepileptic Treatment

Antiepileptic treatment has not been shown to prevent the development of *late* posttraumatic seizures. It is, however, of significant benefit in preventing *early* posttraumatic seizures (in the first 1 to 2 weeks). *Immediate* posttraumatic seizures can be treated with benzodiazepines.

N.   Intravenous Mannitol

Intravenous mannitol can be used to control ICP. Mechanism of action is deemed to be multifactorial, including osmotic diuresis, antioxidant effect, and free-radical scavenger action. Mannitol can be used as a temporizing measure in patients en route to the operating room (OR) for either mass lesions or deteriorating neurologic examination. When given for ICP control, a bolus of 0.25 to 1 g/kg, with maintenance of 0.25 to 0.5 g/kg every 6 to 8 hours, is recommended. Monitoring of serum sodium and osmolality are essential to avoid adverse effects of hypernatremia and hyperosmolarity.

O.   Diuretics

Diuretics can be used in addition to mannitol.

P.   Hypertonic Saline

Boluses of hypertonic saline at various concentrations (2% to 23%) have been used in refractory intracranial hypertension in adult and in pediatric patients with head injury.

Q.   Short-Acting Sedatives and Paralytics

Short-acting sedatives and paralytics can be used as adjuncts in the medical management of refractory intracranial hypertension.

R.   Hyperventilation

Hyperventilation is to be avoided because it can lead to cerebral ischemia from persistent vasoconstriction. When done as a temporizing measure, PCO_2 must be kept at approximately 30 to 35 mm Hg.

S. Induced Coma
See further below for details.

VIII. Intracranial Pressure Monitoring

    A. Indications

        1. In Severe Head Injury (GCS of ≤8)

        2. In patients who cannot be monitored by clinical neurologic examinations (e.g., emergent surgery for other systemic injuries, pharmacologic paralysis, severe intoxication)

        3. In patients whose condition deteriorates and who do not demonstrate a focal, surgically treatable lesion on head CT

        4. In induced coma for treatment of head injury

    B. Types

Different types of ICP monitors have been described, including subdural, intraparenchymal, and intraventricular. Intraparenchymal fiberoptic and intraventricular locations are most commonly used. Where possible, intraventricular catheters are preferable because they allow therapeutic drainage of CSF in addition to ICP monitoring. If the ventricles are very narrow from cerebral edema or mass lesions, however, intraparenchymal fiberoptic bolts are an easier alternative.

    C. Risks and Complications

        1. Infection

        2. Malposition

        3. Hemorrhage

IX. Decompressive Surgery in Severe Refractory Intracranial Hypertension

Decompressive hemicraniectomy or bifrontal craniectomy, contusion debridement, and temporal and frontal lobectomies have been proposed as treatment of refractory intracranial hypertension. Although the outcome improvement in head injury has not been conclusively established, studies indicate that decompressive surgery is beneficial in younger patients with good initial GCS score, who present early after trauma and subsequently deteriorate.

X. Pentobarbital Therapy

In refractory intracranial hypertension, induced coma may be used. Although the reduction in ICP from barbiturates has been conclusively established with induced coma, improvement in outcome has been controversial. Such therapy works mainly by reducing cerebral metabolic activity, thereby reducing cerebral metabolic oxygen requirement. Commonly practiced regimens aim at maintaining a serum level (3 to 5 mg% for pentobarbital) or obtaining *burst suppression* on electroencephalogram (EEG) (true barbiturate coma). An intravenous (i.v.) bolus or boluses (5 to 10 mg/kg), followed by a maintenance drip (1 mg/kg/h) can be used. Monitoring of cardiac function with Swan-Ganz catheters (because of cardiac depressant action of pentobarbital), serum drug levels, electroencephalogram (EEG) and brainstem auditory evoked response (BAER) have been advocated to guide therapy.

XI. Diffuse Axonal Injury

Diffuse axonal injury (DAI) is shear injury to axons from sudden deceleration, acceleration, or rotational forces, in a diffuse distribution, especially involving deeper structures. This should be considered in patients with severe neurologic deficits with normal CT or in patients where the neurologic deficits are out of proportion to those expected from lesions on head CT. Hemorrhagic foci in deep white matter, corpus callosum, or brainstem are suggestive of DAI. MRI of the brain may demonstrate the lesions; however, it is useful only for prognostication. Microscopic examination reveals axonal retraction balls, microglial stars, and white matter tract degeneration.

XII. **Skull Fractures**

A. **Classification**

1. **Open or Closed**

Open or closed skull fractures are based on presence or absence of overlying scalp laceration

2. **Calvarial, Basal Skull, Sinus, and Maxillofacial Fractures**

3. **Depressed or Not Depressed**

B. **Indications for Surgery**

1. **Significant Depression**

Significant depression, more than calvarial thickness, except when over venous sinuses (surgery entails risk of massive bleeding or air embolism). In the absence of focal deficits, cosmesis is the only reason for elevation of fractures with lesser degree of depression.

2. **Compressive Fractures**

Focal deficits corresponding to brain subjacent to the fracture, compressive optic or facial neuropathy

3. **Persistent Cerebrospinal Fluid Leak**

Most traumatic CSF leaks heal spontaneously, however.

4. **Open Fractures**

Open fractures with dural or brain exposure.

C. **Antibiotic Therapy in Basal Skull Fractures**

Although no conclusive evidence exists, empiric broad-spectrum antibiotic treatment is generally used for 1 to 2 weeks, especially in pediatric patients, for basal skull fractures, or fractures overlying air-sinuses or external auditory canal.

D. **Frontal Sinus Fractures**

1. **Anterior Wall**

Nondisplaced fractures are treated conservatively. Significant cosmetic deformity may warrant surgery.

2. **Posterior Wall**

Displaced posterior wall fractures need surgery, commonly obliteration of frontal sinus with removal of mucosa, fat graft packing, and vascularized pericranial graft overlay, to reduce the risk of intracranial infection and delayed CSF rhinorrhea. Surgery for minimally displaced or nondisplaced fractures of posterior wall is controversial.

3. **Fractures in the Region of Frontonasal Duct**

Some ear, nose, and throat surgeons recommend endoscopic reconstruction or stenting of the frontonasal duct.

E. **Pediatric Skull Fractures**
   1. **"Pond" Fractures (Ping-Pong Ball Fractures)**
   Circular depression fractures of incompletely ossified membranous calvarial bone are seen in children, commonly under 2 to 3 years of age. The bone buckles, however, does not break, which is akin to greenstick fractures of long bones in children. Most correct spontaneously.
   2. **Growing Fractures**
   Linear or stellate pediatric calvarial fractures occasionally fail to heal, when associated with a dural tear and interposition arachnoid membrane between the bone edges. These can enlarge over time. Common in children under 3 years of age, these are treated surgically with closure of dural tear. All pediatric calvarial fractures, therefore, need to be followed for at least 3 months to detect occurrence of these fractures.
   3. **Sutural Diastasis**
   Sutural diastasis should be treated expectantly when overlying venous sinuses.

XIII. **Extraaxial Lesions**
   A. **Acute Epidural Hematoma**
      1. **Source:** Mostly Arterial (85%), Venous (15%).
      2. **Classic Presentation**
      Initial loss of consciousness (from concussion), a lucid interval of few hours, followed by signs of deterioration (decreased sensorium, ipsilateral mydriasis, contralateral hemiparesis). Ipsilateral hemiparesis can occur from compression of contralateral peduncle against tentorium (**Kernohan's notch or phenomenon**) and is a false localizing sign.
      3. **Classic Findings on CT**
      Classic finding on CT is a biconvex hyperdense lesion. Hyperacute epidural hematoma (EDH) may be isodense (**Fig. 14-1**).
      4. **Treatment is Surgical**
      Craniotomy for hematoma evacuation, bleeding source coagulation, and obliteration of the epidural space by dural tenting and tack-up sutures.
   B. **Acute Subdural Hematoma**
      1. **Causative**
      Injury in acute subdural hematoma (SDH) is much more severe than in EDH.
      2. **Underlying Brain Injury**
      Underlying brain injury is common, making prognosis worse than EDH.
      3. **Computed Tomography**
      A crescentic, hyperdense lesion is seen on CT.
      4. **Treatment**
      Treatment depends on clinical presentation, lesion size, and presence of mass effect. In general, lesions >1 cm in thickness are evacuated via craniotomy. Keep in mind the possible need for decompressive

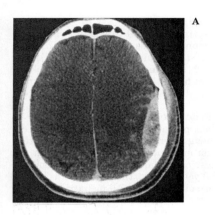

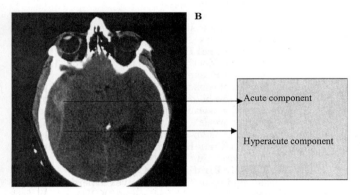

Acute component

Hyperacute component

Figure 14-1.   (A) Acute epidural hematoma. (B) Epidural hematoma with hyperacute and acute components.

        hemicraniectomy while preparing for surgery, because of possibility of underlying brain injury.

        5.   Prognosis

        The prognosis in cases of SDH is poorer than in EDH, and is secondary to associated brain injury.

XIV.   Late Complications of Head Injury
- **A.   Communicating Hydrocephalus**
- **B.   Late Posttraumatic Seizures**
- **C.   Endocrine Dysfunction**
- **D.   Central Nervous System Infections**
- **E.   Dementia or Encephalopathy**
- **F.   Traumatic Aneurysms**

XV.   Penetrating Trauma

General management of penetrating trauma is similar to blunt trauma. Cerebral angiography may be needed, if concern exists for possible vascular injury from the missile or weapon.

A. **Gunshot Wounds to the Head**
  1. **Injury**
  Injury is twofold, from the bullet itself and from the blast wave, shock wave, or cavitation effect.
  2. **Prognosis**
  Prognosis is poor if the initial examination results are poor or if the bullet crosses the midline or involves the basal structures or brainstem.
  3. **Surgery**
  In patients presenting with reasonable neurologic status, the surgical procedure is aimed at wound debridement and removal of large accessible fragments.
B. **Stab Wounds**
  Embedded weapons should be removed in the OR, preferably with craniotomy around the entry site to allow emergency access to neurovascular structures.

SELECTED READING

Greenberg MS. *Handbook of neurosurgery,* 5th ed. New York: Thieme, 2000.

Horn P, Munch E, Vajkoczy P, et al. Hypertonic saline solution for control of elevated intracranial pressure in patients with exhausted response to mannitol and barbiturates. *Neurol Res* 1999;21(8): 758–764.

Joint project of Brain Trauma Foundation, American Association of Neurological Surgeons. Management and prognosis of severe traumatic brain injury—joint section on neurotrauma and critical care, 2000.

Khanna S, Davis D, Peterson B, et al. Use of hypertonic saline in the treatment of severe refractory posttraumatic intracranial hypertension in pediatric traumatic brain injury. *Crit Care Med* 2000; 28(4):1144–1151.

Munch E, Horn P, Schurer L, et al. Management of severe traumatic brain injury by decompressive craniectomy. *Neurosurgery* 2000; 47(2):315–322.

Polin RS, Shaffrey ME, Bogaev CA, et al. Decompressive bifrontal craniectomy in the treatment of severe refractory posttraumatic cerebral edema. *Neurosurgery* 1997;41(1):84–92.

Qureshi AI, Suarez JI, Castro A, et al. Use of hypertonic saline/acetate infusion in treatment of cerebral edema in patients with head trauma: experience at a single center. *J Trauma* 1999;47(4):659–665.

Taylor A, Butt W, Rosenfeld J, et al. A randomized trial of very early decompressive craniectomy in children with traumatic brain injury and sustained intracranial hypertension. *Childs Nerv Syst* 2001; 17(3):154–162.

Nervous System 2: Spinal Cord and Peripheral Nerve Injuries

Yogish D. Kamath, MD,
and Lawrence F. Borges, MD

I. Spinal Cord Injury

A. Epidemiology

Approximately 11,000 new cases of traumatic spinal cord injury occur in the United States every year. Of these cases, 52% involve tetraplegia and 46% paraplegia. Initial treatment expenses range from $160,000 to half million dollars per patient, depending on level of injury. Lifetime costs range from half to 2.1 million dollars, depending on age at the time of injury.

B. Initial Evaluation

In a trauma setting, presume spinal cord injury until it is ruled out by clinical examination and imaging studies, as necessary. An expeditious, complete neurologic examination must be performed as part of the initial evaluation. Rectal examination must be performed as part of the initial evaluation and must include testing for voluntary contraction and sensation, in addition to reflexes.

If pharmacologic interventions, unconsciousness, or hemodynamic instability from other systemic injuries precludes a complete examination, spinal cord injury must be presumed until ruled out and steroids must be started empirically (except in pediatric age group).

Sacral sparing: preservation of perianal sensation, voluntary anal sphincter control, or voluntary toe flexion indicates incomplete spinal cord injury. Anal reflex is thought to be the first reflex to return after spinal shock from acute spinal cord injury. Presence of anal or bulbocavernous reflexes alone does not qualify an injury as incomplete as these reflexes are thought to have shorter polysynaptic reflex loops in spinal cord than other superficial reflexes.

Absence of spinal column injuries does not rule out spinal cord injury. Spinal cord injury without any radiographic abnormality (SCIWORA) is common in children, mostly because of the ligamentous laxity of the pediatric spine.

Examiner should be aware of discrepancy in vertebral column levels and spinal cord levels because of differential growth rates of spine and spinal cord with associated ascent of spinal cord.

C. Points to be Clarify in Examination

1. Level of Injury

Controversy exists to the definition of level of spinal cord injury. A simple, practical definition is used by American Spinal Injury Association (ASIA) scoring system for spinal cord injury. Most caudal level of normal function is considered as the level of spinal cord injury.

2. Complete or Incomplete Lesion
As per the ASIA scoring system, complete lesion is defined as lack of all motor or sensory function below the level of injury, including sacral 4–5 segments.

D. ASIA Classification for Spinal Cord Injury (with Dermatomal Chart) with Scoring System
The ASIA classification for spinal cord injury is the scoring system (**Fig. 15-1**) recommended for use in all spinal cord injury patients.

E. Spinal Shock
Transient loss of all neurologic function can occur below the level of spinal cord injury, resulting in atonia and areflexia for periods lasting a few hours to 1 to 2 weeks. Resolution may reveal one of two patterns: (a) either recovery of voluntary motor and sensory function or (b) emergence of spastic paralysis as a result of upper motor neuron injury. This should not be mistaken for *neurogenic shock* resulting in hypotension from loss of sympathetic function secondary to spinal cord injury.

F. Indications for Steroid Treatment
Based on the time between injury and presentation in the emergency room, intravenous methylprednisolone is administered as follows:

1. Bolus Dose: 30 mg/kg given over 15 minutes, followed by 45-minute pause.
2. Maintenance: 5.4 mg/kg/h for 23 hours for those who presented within 3 hours of injury; for 48 hours for those who presented after 3 hours but before 8 hours from the time of injury. In the 48-hour group, higher sepsis and pneumonia rates were noted.

Safety or benefits of use of steroids in pregnant women or children with spinal cord injury are not well established. Cauda equina syndrome, gunshot wounds, patients with life-threatening morbidity, pregnant women, narcotic addiction, children aged less than 13 years, and those on maintenance steroids before injury were excluded from the study. Steroid usage in gunshot injuries to spinal cord has not been conclusively shown to be beneficial and can increase the risk of sepsis.

G. Radiographic Evaluation
1. Magnetic resonance imaging (MRI) has largely supplanted most other diagnostic studies. In some centers, diffusion MRI techniques are available, enabling differentiation between edematous and infarcted tissue.
2. Computed tomography (CT) scan with myelogram can be used when MRI is not available.

H. Indications for Emergent Surgery
Although this issue remains controversial, in general, emergent decompressive surgery, combined with stabilization, is carried out for incomplete injury with persistent or progressive spinal cord compression as demonstrated by

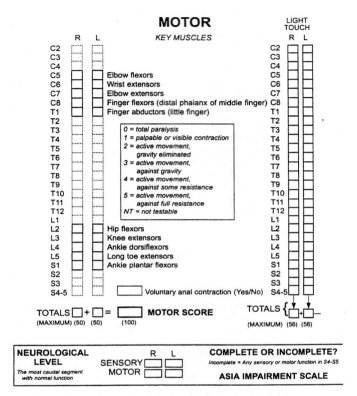

Figure 15-1. American Spinal Injury Association (ASIA) classification for spinal cord injury (with dermatomal chart) and scoring. (This form may be copied freely but should not be altered without permission from the American Spinal Injury Association.)

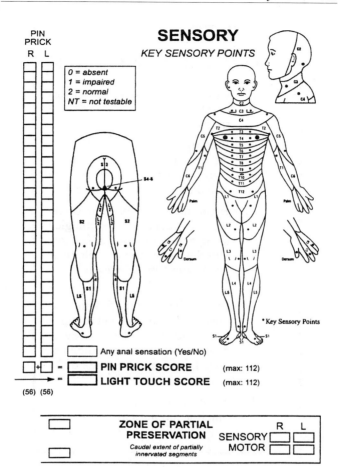

PIN PRICK

R L

0 = absent
1 = impaired
2 = normal
NT = not testable

SENSORY

KEY SENSORY POINTS

Any anal sensation (Yes/No)

☐ + ☐ = ☐ **PIN PRICK SCORE** (max: 112)

→ = ☐ **LIGHT TOUCH SCORE** (max: 112)

(56) (56)

* Key Sensory Points

☐	**ZONE OF PARTIAL PRESERVATION**		R	L
	Caudal extent of partially innervated segments	SENSORY	☐	☐
☐		MOTOR	☐	☐

ASIA IMPAIRMENT SCALE

☐ **A = Complete:** No motor or sensory function is preserved in the sacral segments S4-S5.

☐ **B = Incomplete:** Sensory but not motor function is preserved below the neurological level and includes the sacral segments S4-S5.

☐ **C = Incomplete:** Motor function is preserved below the neurological level, and more than half of key muscles below the neurological level have a muscle grade less than 3.

☐ **D = Incomplete:** Motor function is preserved below the neurological level, and at least half of key muscles below the neurological level have a muscle grade of 3 or more.

☐ **E = Normal:** motor and sensory function are normal

CLINICAL SYNDROMES

☐ Central Cord
☐ Brown-Sequard
☐ Anterior Cord
☐ Conus Medullaris
☐ Cauda Equina

Figure 15-1.   *(Continued).*

clinical and radiologic studies. Early surgery for complete spinal cord lesions, although traditionally not recommended, still remains controversial. Early decompressive surgery for complete lesions is recommended by some neurosurgeons. If such early surgery is undertaken, hypotension must be avoided during induction and maintenance of anesthesia.

I. Incomplete Spinal Cord Injuries

1. Central Cord Syndrome

a. Most common incomplete injury

b. Classic presentation is that of greater motor deficit in upper extremities than in lower, in a background of varying degrees of myelopathy.

c. Results from edema or ischemia of central vascular watershed region of cervical cord where long tract fiber tracts are somatotopically arranged such that cervical fibers are medial and are more susceptible to edema or injury.

d. Causes include hyperextension in a stenotic canal from degenerative disease; less commonly disc herniation or bony trauma.

e. MRI does not always show cord edema or ischemia. Central cord syndrome is a clinical diagnosis.

f. Recent studies indicate early decompression is beneficial in cases caused by trauma from disc herniation or fracture. Early surgery is safe but does not show significant benefit in cases caused by stenosis from spondylosis.

2. Anterior Cord Syndrome

a. **Occurs from infarction in territory of anterior spinal artery.**

b. Corticospinal and spinothalamic tracts in anterior and lateral columns of spinal cord are involved, whereas posterior columns are spared. Clinical picture, therefore, is one of dense bilateral paralysis and loss of pain and temperature sensation with preservation of fine touch, vibration, position sense, and deep pressure sensation—all below the lesion.

c. MRI helps differentiate surgically correctable causes (fracture fragment or disc herniation) from spontaneous thrombosis.

d. Despite surgical treatment, surgical results are poor.

3. Posterior Cord Syndrome

a. Results from contusion of posterior columns

b. Minimal long tract findings, sensory more than motor

c. Rarely, surgical treatment, unless laminar fracture and hematoma with cord compression are noted.

4. Brown Séquard Syndrome

a. Classic form, which is rare, is most commonly caused by penetrating trauma.

   b.   Underlying pathology is hemisection of the cord, thereby interrupting all tracts on the affected half of the cord.

   c.   Clinically, is seen ipsilateral hemiparesis and posterior column function (tactile discrimination, vibration, position sense, deep pressure) loss with contralateral pain and temperature (spinothalamic) sensory loss.

   d.   Although surgery for penetrating trauma does not the reverse the injury, unilateral nature of injury entails a good prognosis.

   e.   Surgical exploration is often needed for penetrating trauma to repair the dura and stop cerebrospinal fluid (CSF) leak.

J.   Postoperative Care and Rehabilitation

Important considerations are briefly mentioned below.

   1.   Deep Venous Thrombosis
   2.   Spasticity
   3.   Constipation and Bladder Dysfunction
   4.   Dysautonomia (Autonomic Dysreflexia, Shoulder-Hand Syndrome)
   5.   Syringomyelia
   6.   Pressure Ulcers
   7.   Osteoporosis
   8.   Heterotopic Calcification
   9.   Depression

K.   ASIA Spinal Injury Worksheet

See the ASIA spinal injury worksheet (pdf document) (**Fig. 15-1**), available from: http://www.asia-spinalinjury.org/publications/2001_Classif_worksheet.pdf

II.   Peripheral Nerve Injury

   A.   Anatomy of Peripheral Nerve

   Peripheral nerves, shown in (**Figure 15-2**), consist of the following:

   1.   Epineurium
   Outer collagen and elastic layer covering the whole nerve made of several nerve fascicles

   2.   Perineurium
   Collagenous covering of each fascicle within a nerve

   3.   Endoneurium
   Collagenous covering of each myelinated nerve fiber or groups of unmyelinated nerve within a fascicle

   4.   Interfascicular Epineurium
   Connective tissue between the fascicles

   5.   Mesoneurium
   Connective tissue interface between epineurium and surrounding structures

   B.   Causes of Peripheral Nerve Injury
   1.   Penetrating Trauma
   2.   Stretch or Traction
   3.   Contusion or Blunt Trauma
   4.   Gunshot Wounds
   5.   Thermal
   6.   Radiation

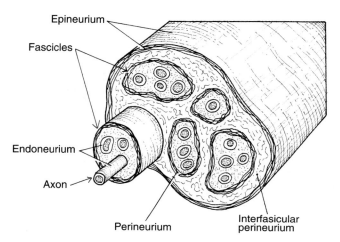

Figure 15-2. Anatomy of peripheral nerve.

C. Changes in the Nerves After Injury

The changes in the nerves vary widely, depending on severity of injury.

1. Neuronal changes include neuronal swelling and chromatolysis of Nissl's granules starting as early as 4 days and peaking in 20 days from injury.

2. Axonal changes were classified by Seddon and Sunderland.

Seddon's classification is as follows.

a. Neuropraxia. This is the mildest form of injury with pathology limited to a biochemical lesion. Commonly caused by mild compression or contusion to nerve. Axonal transport is impaired; however, most of microscopic anatomy is preserved. No Wallerian degeneration is seen and recovery is certain.

b. Axonotmesis. Involves loss of continuity of axons and its myelin, but the connective tissue framework is preserved. Commonly caused by crush or stretch injury. Distal Wallerian and proximal retrograde degeneration occurs. Electromyography (EMG) shows denervation injury as early as 10 days. Regeneration is facilitated by preservation of connective tissue framework and Schwann cells.

c. Neurotmesis. Involves loss of continuity of axons and connective tissue framework as well; commonly caused by severe crush or traction or laceration. EMG shows denervation changes similar to axonotmesis. Distal Wallerian and proximal retrograde degeneration occurs. Regeneration is complicated by neuroma formation and scarring and is often incomplete. This category was classified further in Sunderland's classification (grade 4 involving axonotmesis and injury to endoneurium, grade 4 involving grade 5 being complete transsection).

With the exception of mild compressions and complete transsections, most lesions have components of both axonotmesis and neurotmesis. Partially transected nerves show a clear zone of neurotmesis and an adjoining zone of axonotmesis.

D. Evaluation

In addition to a comprehensive neurologic examination, a tailored, detailed examination of extremities for each nerve may be necessary.

1. All cases of lacerations, penetrating injuries, and bone fractures must be examined by senior medical personnel to rule out associated peripheral nerve injury, because it may be possible to perform a primary anastomose to clean cut nerve ends at the same time for best chances of recovery.

2. All cases of head injury or unconscious patient must be examined for peripheral nerve dysfunction.

3. Look for findings that may indicate associated nerve injury (e.g., Horner's syndrome accompanying avulsion of C8-T1 roots).

E. Diagnostic Studies

In the acute stage, little use is seen for diagnostic studies.

1. **Electromyography and Nerve Conduction Studies**

Earliest EMG changes are noticeable in 2 weeks. EMG and nerve conduction studies (NCS) are used to determine baseline extent of injury, extent of degeneration, and spontaneous regeneration and to aid in deciding time of surgery.

2. **Computed Tomography Scan**

The CT scan provides little information about nerve injury.

3. **Myelography**

Myelography can show pseudomeningocele, indicating avulsion of spinal nerve roots.

4. **Magnetic Resonance Neurography**

Magnetic resonance neurography is a developing diagnostic modality and has potential to be useful in both acute stage and afterward.

F. Treatment

1. **Timing of Surgery**

In acute stage, preferably only primary end-to-end repair of clean-cut injuries is preferred. With loss of nerve segments in injury, the proximal and distal ends can be tagged with nonabsorbable sutures for easier identification in future surgeries.

2. **Timing of Delayed Surgery**

Sufficient time must be allowed for completion of Wallerian and retrograde degeneration and for spontaneous regeneration. Follow-up during this period is based on clinical examination (Tinel's sign: tapping on the regenerating proximal end may produce sharp pain or tingling sensation), EEG/NCS and imaging (e.g., myelography, MR neurography). These changes can take from 2 months to as long as 2 years in cases of longer nerves with longer segments of degeneration. Keep in mind the nature of the pathologic lesion (neuroma or scar) and the possibility of irreversible disuse atrophy while waiting for spontaneous regeneration in deciding the timing of surgery.

3. **Common Operations**
   a. **External Neurolysis**
   b. **Scar or Neuroma Excision**
   c. **End-to-End Suture**
   d. **Nerve Grafting**
   e. **Split Repair**
   f. **Neurotization or Nerve Hitching**
   g. **Tendon Transfers.** Where nerve repair is not possible or has failed.

G. **Common Traumatic Nerve Injuries**
   1. **Radial Nerve**
      a. **Injury at Upper Arm Level**
         (1) Deltoid and latissimus dorsi are not affected
         (2) Very proximal nerve lesions can involve triceps paralysis
         (3) Brachioradialis, elbow extension, forearm supination, wrist extension (wristdrop), and finger extension (fingerdrop) are impaired, with a variable sensory loss over dorsum of hand over little, ring, or middle fingers.
      b. **Injury at Mid Arm Level in Radial Groove**
         (1) Commonly associated with humeral shaft fractures.
         (2) Triceps is spared.
         (3) Other motor and sensory deficits are similar to those seen in injury at upper arm level.
      c. **Injury at Elbow Level**
         (1) Commonly caused by penetrating wounds
         (2) Triceps and brachioradialis are spared. Involvement of the rest of the muscles supplied by radial nerve causes loss of supination of forearm, wristdrop, fingerdrop, and sensory loss over radial nerve distribution as described above.
      d. **Injury at Forearm Level.** Posterior interosseous nerve injury
         (1) At the elbow, the radial nerve divides into the PIN and superficial sensory branch, after giving branches in the elbow to brachialis, brachioradialis, and the ECRL.
         (2) Can be caused by penetrating trauma or associated forearm bone fractures

(3) Wristdrop is minimal or absent because of preservation of ECRL. Fingerdrop (loss of finger extension) is the major feature with no sensory loss.

2. Median Nerve

a. Injury at Arm Level

(1) Penetrating injury is the common cause of injury at this level.

(2) Motor and sensory loss in the entire distribution of the nerve

(3) Muscles involved are forearm pronators (pronator teres and quadratus), Long flexors of distal thumb (*flexor pollicis longus*), Long finger flexors (*flexor digitorum superficialis,* and lateral half of *flexor digitorum profundus* supplying index and middle fingers), lumbricals of index and middle fingers, muscles of thenar eminence (flexor, adductor, opponens pollicis), and *palmaris longus.*

(4) "Simian hand" or "ape thumb" deformity results from loss of thenar muscle function.

(5) Pilate hand, pope hand, or pointing index finger results from loss of finger flexor function, complete in index and partial in middle fingers.

b. Injury at Forearm Level—Anterior Interosseous Syndrome

(1) Penetrating injury or contusive injury can cause this syndrome.

(2) Anterior interosseous branch of median nerve is involved with selective motor loss of *flexor digitorum profundus* and *flexor pollicis longus,* with no sensory loss.

c. Injury at Wrist Level

(1) Injury at wrist level is commonly part of a complex injury to nerves, tendon, vessels, and so forth.

(2) Thenar muscles and index and middle finger lumbricals are denervated.

(3) Sensory loss is mostly over the distal palm and over thumb, index, and middle fingers, as median nerve gives a thenar sensory branch just proximal to wrist supplying sensation over proximal thenar eminence.

3. Ulnar Nerve

a. Injury at Wrist

(1) **Guyon's Canal.** An area volar to *flexor carpi retinaculum* in palm traversed by ulnar nerve, where it is subject to compression or injury, because of superficial location.

(2) **Motor Deficits.** Includes loss of most intrinsic hand muscles, especially the hypothenar muscles, interossei, *musculi lumbricals* to little and ring finger, and *adductor pollicis.*

(3) Ulnar Claw Hand (Main en Griffe).
Unopposed finger extension at metacarpophalangeal joints (because of loss of *musculi lumbricals*) and flexion at interphalangeal joints
from preserved long forearm flexors.

(4) Froment's Sign. Flexion of distal phalanx of the thumb on attempted adduction of
thumb to index finger (as in holding a card
between index and thumb). Loss of *adductor
pollicis* function is substituted by *flexor pollicis longus.*

(5) Sensory Loss. Is usually limited to volar
aspect of little and ring finger (medial half) and
over proximal medial palm

b. Injury Proximal to Wrist. In addition to
the above-mentioned injuries, injury proximal to
the wrist can involve *flexor carpi ulnaris* (loss of
wrist flexion), *flexor profundus* for ring and little
finger, and sensory loss over dorsal surface of little finger and medial half of ring finger.

4. Sciatic Nerve and its Branches

a. Injury to Deep Peroneal Nerve. Footdrop
(*tibialis anterior, extensor hallucis longus, extensor digitorum*) with loss of sensation over first
web space.

b. Injury to Superficial Peroneal Nerve. Loss
of *peroneus longus* and *brevis* (foot eversion), and
loss of sensation over lateral surface of distal leg
and dorsum of foot.

c. Injury to Common Peroneal Nerve. A combination of superficial and deep peroneal nerve
deficits.

d. Injury to Tibial Nerve. Prominent features
are loss of *tibialis posterior, gastrocnemius* and
soleus function with loss of plantar flexion of foot
and weakness of foot inversion; flexors of toes are
also lost. Sensory loss involves posterior distal
leg, sole of foot, and lateral border of foot.

**e. Injury Below Sciatic Notch and Above
the Take-off of Common Peroneal Nerve.**
Includes features of both common peroneal nerve
and tibial nerve injury; in addition, hamstrings
can be involved, causing knee flexion weakness.

H. Brachial Plexus Injuries (Fig. 15-3)

1. Common Causes

a. Penetrating injuries—stab and gunshot
wounds

b. Traction injuries

c. Laceration from rib fractures

d. Compression from hematomas

2. Clinical Features

a. Examination must include inspection and
evaluation of muscular function of shoulder, neck,
and upper back, in addition to routine neurologic
examination of upper extremities.

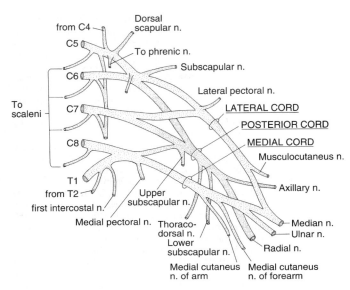

Figure 15-3.   Brachial plexus injuries.

    b.   Look for shoulder girdle asymmetry, drooping shoulder, shoulder girdle muscle atrophy, winging of scapula, or rhomboid atrophy.
    c.   Evaluate latissimus dorsi and rhomboids.
    d.   Evaluate diaphragmatic function.
    e.   Look for evidence of Horner's syndrome, indicating interruption of sympathetic outflow.

3.   Indicators of Preganglionic Versus Postganglionic Injury
    a.   Results of surgical treatment of preganglionic injuries remain poor.
    b.   Presence of rhomboid paralysis (dorsal scapular nerve), serratus anterior paralysis (long thoracic nerve), Horner's syndrome (T1), and denervation of paraspinal musculature with preservation of sensory nerve action potentials indicate preganglionic injury with poor prognosis.
    c.   Replantation of avulsed ventral spinal roots to spinal cord or repair by coaptation of other nerves to the injured nerve have modest success in functional recovery.

4.   Erb's Palsy (Erb-Duchenne Palsy)
    a.   Caused by injury to upper brachial plexus (C5-C6) roots.
    b.   Mechanism is usually abrupt and forceful distraction of shoulder, from cervical spine or neck, as in motorcycle injury or childbirth.

    c. Muscles paralyzed are deltoid, supraspinatus, infraspinatus, biceps, rhomboids, brachioradialis, and supinator.

    d. Characteristic position of paralyzed arm: arm hangs at side, internally rotated and extended at elbow (Porter's tip position or bellhop's tip position)

5. Klumpke's Palsy

    a. Lower brachial plexus root avulsion (C8-T1)

    b. Mechanism is forceful abduction of arm as in attempting to prevent a fall by an outstretched arm.

    c. Muscles paralyzed are intrinsic muscles of hand, with preserved long forearm flexors leading to clawing. Horner's syndrome may also be seen (T1).

    d. Characteristic **claw hand** deformity (similar to ulnar claw hand described above)

6. Diagnostic Imaging

    a. Chest x-ray study may show first rib fractures

    b. CT scan is mostly useful in detecting associated injuries that can indicate brachial plexus involvement

    c. Myelography may show pseudomeningocele, indicating root avulsion

    d. Magnetic Resonance Neurography

    e. Angiography to evaluate associated vascular injury.

7. Management of Brachial Plexus Injuries

    a. In Acute Stage. In clean, sharp injuries, initial exploration with tension-free end-to-end anastomosis is recommended within 72 hours, as early exploration makes anatomic identification easy in the absence of scarring and reduces the need for grafting.

    b. Lacerations from Blunt Mechanisms. Ends of nerves are tacked down in the acute stage and are best explored in a delayed fashion, when extent of injury to stumps is evident, retraction are complete, and stumps can be trimmed and grafted.

    c. Gunshot Wounds. Exploration in the acute stage is not recommended because injuries are axonotmetic or neurotmetic in nature and are best explored in a delayed fashion.

    d. Stretch Injuries are explored in a delayed fashion.

SELECTED READING

Bracken MB, Shepard JJ, Collins WF Jr, et al. A randomized controlled trial of methylprednisolone or naloxone in the treatment of acute spinal cord injury. The results of the National Acute Spinal Cord Injury. *N Engl J Med* 1990;322:1459–1461.

Bracken MB, Shepard JJ, Collins WF Jr, et al. Methylprednisolone or naloxone in the treatment of acute spinal cord injury: one year follow-up results of the National Acute Spinal Cord Injury Study. *J Neurosurg* 1992;77:324.

Bracken MB, Shepard MJ, Holford TR, et al. Administration of methyl-prednisolone for 24 or 48 hours OR tirilazad mesylate for 48 hours in the treatment of acute spinal cord injury. *JAMA* 1997;277: 1597–1604.

Bracken MB. Steroids in acute spinal cord injury (Cochrane review). *Cochrane Database Syst Rev* 2002;(3):CD 001046.

Carlstedt T, Anand P, Hallin R, et al. Spinal nerve root repair and reimplantation of avulsed ventral roots into the spinal cord after brachial plexus injury. *J Neurosurg* 2000;93(2 Suppl.):237–247.

Greenberg MS. *Handbook of neurosurgery,* 5th ed. New York: Thieme, 2000.

Guest J, Eleraky MA, Apostolides PJ, et al. Traumatic central cord syndrome: results of surgical management. *J Neurosurg* 2002; 97 (1 Suppl.);25–32.

Heary RF, Vacarro AR, Mesa JJ, et al. Steroids and gunshot wounds to the spine. *Neurosurgery* 1997;41(3);576–583.

Kline DG, Hudson AR. *Nerve injuries: operative results of major nerve injuries, entrapments, and tumors.* Philadelphia: WB Saunders, 1995.

Malessy MJ, Thomeer RT. Evaluation of intercostal to musculocuta-neous nerve transfer in reconstructive brachial plexus surgery. *J Neurosurg* 1998;88(2):266–271.

National spinal cord injury information network. *Facts and figures at a glance.* Available at http://www.spinalcord.uab.edu; accessed May 2001.

Williams PL, Bannister LH. *Gray's anatomy: the anatomical basis of medicine & surgery,* 38th ed. New York: Harcourt Health Sciences Group, 1995.

16

Evaluation and Acute Management of Maxillofacial Trauma

Jeffrey A. Hammoudeh DDS, MD,
Leonard B. Kaban, DMD, MD,
and Thomas B. Dodson, DMD, MPH

I. Introduction

The evaluation and acute management of maxillofacial injuries are important skills for trauma surgeons. Although commonly not life threatening, maxillofacial injuries involve areas of complex, visible anatomy and resultant deformities can be functionally and psychologically debilitating. As such, the goal is to restore the form and function of the maxillofacial unit. Once the airway is stabilized and hemorrhage is controlled, evaluation of maxillofacial injuries becomes part of the advanced trauma life support (ATLS) secondary survey. This chapter provides an overview of the initial assessment and acute management of common maxillofacial injuries. It is assumed that the patient is otherwise stable and ready for definitive assessment of these skeletal and soft tissue injuries.

II. Epidemiology of Maxillofacial Injuries

Most maxillofacial injuries are caused by blunt trauma in the setting of interpersonal violence or motor vehicle accidents (MVA). Stricter laws and enforcement of regulations on alcohol consumption while driving, as well as increased compliance with the use of seat belts, safer automobiles, airbags, and better informed drivers have all contributed to a decrease in the total number of maxillofacial injuries secondary to MVA.

III. Applied Anatomy

Anatomic details important for initial evaluation and management of the patient with a maxillofacial injury are highlighted below.

A. Neuroanatomy

Patients with maxillofacial injuries commonly have concomitant central nervous system (CNS) and peripheral nerve injuries. Relevant CNS and ophthalmologic anatomy are reviewed in other chapters. Cranial nerves at risk in maxillofacial trauma include olfactory (I), optic (II), oculomotor (III), trochlear (IV), trigeminal (V, three divisions), abducens (VI), facial (VII, all branches), and hypoglossal (XII). Peripheral nerves at risk for injury that provide innervation to the maxillofacial region include the cervical plexus (C_2 and C_3) and the greater auricular nerve.

    1. A careful, well-documented postinjury, pretreatment examination of the 1st to 7th (facial) and 12th (hypoglossal) cranial nerves is important to establish baseline nerve function. Patients can have sensory deficits, including hypoesthesia, paresthesia or anesthesia and motor deficits resulting in facial paresis or limitation of extraocular movements. The oculomotor (III), trochlear (IV), and abducens (VI) nerves innervate the extraocular muscles and injuries or entrapment can result in extraocular muscle dysfunction and diplopia. The olfactory (I) and optic (II) nerves may be injured in midface with resultant loss of smell or visual acuity.

2.   The ophthalmic (V_1), maxillary (V_2), and mandibular (V_3) divisions of the trigeminal nerve have intrabony components at risk for injury. When a patient presents with altered sensation, the surgeon, therefore, must rule out facial skeletal injury. The ophthalmic branch (V_1) provides general sensation to the dorsum of the nose, upper eyelid, frontal sinus, and forehead. Using a cotton tip applicator twisted to form a point, light touch and brush stroke direction can be rapidly assessed. Altered sensation in this region suggests direct injury to the nerves, an underlying fracture of the supraorbital rim, or fractures involving the roof of the orbit or the superior orbital fissure.

The maxillary branch (V_2) terminates as the pterygopalatine, infraorbital, and zygomatic nerves. Light touch should be assessed in the region of the infraorbital nerve (i.e., alar base of the nose, upper lip, anterior maxilla, and anterior maxillary dentition). Paresthesia suggests a midface fracture involving the orbital floor, inferior orbital rim, or the maxilla.

The major branches of V_3 include the buccal, auriculotemporal, lingual, and inferior alveolar nerves (IAN). The IAN passes through a bony canal in the mandible and innervates the mandibular teeth, associated intraoral soft tissues, and gingiva before exiting the mental foramen to supply sensation to the chin and lower lip. This nerve is commonly injured in mandibular fractures.

3.   The facial nerve (VII) provides motor innervation to the muscles of facial expression, as well as the occipital, auricular, platysma, and stylohyoid muscles. Facial lacerations can result in injury to this nerve producing ipsilateral paralysis of the muscles of facial expression. The facial nerve also provides special sensory fibers for taste to the anterior two thirds of the tongue. These fibers (chorda tympani) travel with the lingual nerve. The facial nerve fibers carry preganglionic visceral efferent fibers to the lacrimal and salivary glands.

The facial nerve (VII) trunk exits the skull via the stylomastoid foramen in close proximity to the mandibular condyles. It travels forward and enters the superficial lobe of the parotid gland and separates into temporal, zygomatic, buccal, marginal mandibular, and cervical branches.

The facial nerve is at risk from penetrating injuries and it is critical to document its function during the initial facial skeletal evaluation. A vertical line is dropped from the lateral canthus of the eye. Facial nerve injury can be classified as high or low risk in relation to this landmark. High-risk injuries are located proximal (or lateral) to the vertical line and require further investigation and surgical repair as indicated. Injuries distal (or medial) to the line usually involve much smaller, minor terminal branches. In such cases, surgical repair may be unnecessary and is technically impractical. Most of these injuries recover without treatment.

B. Salivary Glands

The three major salivary glands are the parotid, submandibular, and sublingual. The facial nerve branches travel through the parotid gland. Parotid salivary secretions travel via Stensen's duct, which wraps around the masseter and perforates the buccinator muscle to enter the oral cavity at the level of the second maxillary molar. Any laceration that is parallel to a line from the commissure of the lip to the tragus of the ear is at high risk for duct laceration or nerve injury. The paired submandibular gland secretions enter the oral cavity via Wharton's duct. Duct injuries can occur with trauma involving the floor of the mouth.

C. Skeletal Anatomy

The maxillofacial skeleton consists of three anatomic regions: (a) upper face (frontal bone); (b) midface (orbit, nasal bones and cartilages, nasal septum, ethmoid, zygomatic bones, and maxilla with its associated dentition), and (c) lower face (mandible with its associated dentition).

1. Frontal Bone

The frontal bone, which protects the brain, contains the frontal sinus. It forms the orbital roof and articulates with the maxilla, zygoma, nasal bones, ethmoid, temporal, sphenoid, and parietal bones. The frontal sinus has anterior and posterior tables and is lined by sinus mucosa. Drainage occurs via the frontonasal duct into the nose below the superior turbinate. When fractures involve the frontal sinus, it is important to determine if the injury involves the anterior or posterior walls or both. The potential for a dural tear or laceration, with associated cerebral spinal fluid (CSF) leakage, is associated with posterior table fractures.

2. Maxilla

The maxilla, which contains the maxillary sinuses and dentition, has four processes: frontal, alveolar, palatine, and zygomatic. These processes articulate with adjacent bones at suture lines that serve as potential sites of bony separation. In adults, the maxilla is fused in the midline at the palatine suture, but fractures can result in separation of the maxilla into two segments at this location.

3.   Zygoma

The zygoma (cheekbone), a paired structure support-ing the upper cheek, is an important esthetic compo-nent of the face. Although injuries to this area are not life threatening, early diagnosis and management are important to provide a satisfactory esthetic correction. Late treatment results are commonly disappointing. The zygoma articulates with the frontal, temporal, sphenoid, and maxillary bones. Fractures of the zygomaticomaxillary complex (ZMC) are also known as "tripod fractures." This term should be avoided, as it is anatomically incorrect. The zygoma has four articulations, not three (i.e., the frontozygomatic, zygomaticomaxillary, zygomaticotemporal, and zygo-maticosphenoid sutures).

4.   Nose

With its associated structures, the nose is an impor-tant esthetic element of the face that is commonly injured. The abundant blood supply is from branches of the internal and external carotid arteries. The exter-nal carotid artery contributes to the maxillary and facial arteries. The internal carotid artery branches (i.e., anterior and posterior ethmoidal arteries) are sometimes the source of prolonged nasal bleeding.

5.   Mandible

Prominently positioned, the mandible is the second most frequently fractured facial bone—after nasal fractures. It has a U-shaped body with paired vertical rami, condyles, and coronoid processes. All these com-ponents of the lower jaw are at risk for fracture. The mandible contains the inferior alveolar nerve, man-dibular dentition, and it articulates with the temporal bone at the temporomandibular joint (TMJ). Mandibu-lar fractures disrupt the usual relationships between the muscles of mastication and the dentition. Neuro-sensory function can also be affected. These fractures usually result in the following:

    a.   Alterations in the occlusion (e.g., "my bite has changed")

    b.   Pain with function (jaw motion or chewing)

    c.   Inferior alveolar nerve paresthesia

    d.   Deviation of the jaw on opening

    e.   Mandibular hypomobility secondary to me-chanical obstruction or trismus (muscle spasm)

IV.   Evaluation and Management of Acute Maxillofacial Injuries

A.   History

If the patient is alert or if witnesses are available, ask about and document the timing and mechanism of injury. A good history can guide in the identification of all the primary and associated injuries. For example, a patient who sustains a chin laceration after a fall may also have a fracture of the symphysis of the mandible. Additionally, retain a high index of suspicion for fractures of one or both mandibular condyles (*contrecoup* injury) and injuries to

the cervical spine (flexion or extension). Presence of paresthesia, malocclusion, and visual disturbances by history
suggests underlying maxillofacial skeletal fractures.

B. Physical Examination

Inspection and palpation can identify most maxillofacial
injuries. Inspect the scalp and facial soft tissues for lacerations, foreign bodies, asymmetry, and open fractures.
Periorbital ecchymosis (i.e., "raccoon eyes") suggests midface fractures and mastoid ecchymosis (i.e., "Battle's
sign") suggests a basilar skull fracture. In the alert patient,
evaluate facial expressions to assess integrity of the 7th
cranial nerve (i.e., ask the patient to raise the eyebrows,
squeeze the eyes shut, smile, and pucker the lips). Ocular
examination needs to be completed in detail as outlined in
Chapter 17, *Ocular and Adnexal Trauma.* At a minimum,
check the pupils for reactivity, gaze, and size and correlate with the clinical neurologic examination. Assess visual
acuity and extraocular muscle function and document
the presence of diplopia. Examine the nose for deviation,
bleeding, rhinorrhea, or any evidence of septal hematoma.
To complete the nasal examination, use a nasal speculum
and a good light. Evaluate the ear for evidence of soft tissue injury to the auricle or ear canal or otorrhea. Using an
otoscope, evaluate the ear for evidence of hemotympanum
or tympanic membrane perforation. With good light, examine the oral cavity to identify soft tissue injuries, occlusal
abnormalities and injured or missing teeth, and assess
mandibular range of motion (normal range < 35 to 55 mm).
Loose teeth pose a risk for aspiration and missing teeth
should be accounted for to rule out aspiration. Ecchymosis in the maxillary buccal vestibule suggests midface
fracture, whereas ecchymoses in the floor of the mouth or
mandibular buccal vestibule suggests fractures of the lingual or buccal cortices of the mandible, respectively.

After inspection, palpate the facial soft tissues, feeling for
bony steps, embedded foreign bodies (e.g. glass, teeth, and
road debris), and mobility of the maxilla or mandible. Complete the cranial nerve examination with an emphasis on
the branches of the 5th cranial nerve. Paresthesia involving the trigeminal nerve suggests an underlying maxillofacial fracture of the orbit, midface, or mandible. Use a cotton
tip applicator or fingertip to assess rapidly for the presence
of light touch sensation and brush stroke direction. Ocular
and facial nerve injuries are critical injuries to be identified
in a rapid fashion.

C. Imaging

Imaging confirms the diagnosis and provides details necessary for treatment planning. For injuries involving the
upper or midface, fine cut (1 to 2 mm) computed tomography (CT) in the axial plane, with reformatted images in the
sagittal and coronal planes, is indicated. Three-dimensional
reformations of the axial CT scan also can facilitate diagnosis and treatment planning. For mandible fractures,
panoramic radiographs or a mandible series (i.e., anterior-
posterior, lateral, oblique, and Towne views are generally

adequate). After consulting with the maxillofacial surgery service, other specialized imaging may be indicated.

V. Evaluation and Acute Management of Maxillofacial Skeletal Injuries

A. Midface Injuries

1. Nasal fracture

Nasal fractures are the most common maxillofacial skeletal injuries. The patient reports a blunt injury to the nasal region and complains of pain, swelling, difficulty breathing through the nares, and bleeding. Physical findings include edema, epistaxis, and septal deviation. The examination should include inspection of the septum, with a nasal speculum and a good light source, to assess septal deviation and to rule out a septal hematoma. Septal hematomas should be promptly drained, when identified, to avoid nasal obstruction and to minimize the risk of septal perforation or necrosis. Palpation of the nose often reveals crepitus, mobility, and a palpable nasal bone step. These findings can be obscured if significant swelling is present. The diagnosis is made clinically and confirmed radiographically with a CT scan.

Most nasal fractures can be managed by observation or closed reduction under local anesthesia. When manipulating the fracture, it is imperative to obtain profound anesthesia and vasoconstriction. Lidocaine (1% to 2%) with epinephrine (1:200,000 is adequate), supplemented with 4% topical cocaine for mucosal hemostasis, is commonly used. Closed reduction is facilitated by the use of an Ash forceps or Goldman displacer.

Nasal packing with iodoform, oxidized cellulose, absorbable gelatin, or petrolatum-impregnated gauze can be used to stabilize the septum or control hemorrhage. The packing is inserted with a bayonet and compressed as far posteriorly as possible (**Fig. 16-1**). After packing the nose to support the septum, an external nasal split can be applied. Precut aluminum splints are simple to use. Water-activated splints (e.g., Aquaplast [Rolyan AbilityOne, Germantown, WI]) convert a soft, pliable sheet into a firm, custom-formed nasal split. The splint should not be applied directly to the skin. Half-inch adhesive tape strips should be placed horizontally over the nose to serve as a foundation on which the external nasal splint is applied.

Posterior nasal packing is indicated in the setting of severe septal mobility or continuous, uncontrolled bleeding. A posterior nasal pack compresses the nasopharyngeal region, thereby stopping hemorrhage by pressure. Several accepted methods can be used to place a posterior nasal pack. Use of a Foley catheter is effective, rapid, and simple. After appropriate local anesthesia is delivered, a Foley catheter is inserted into the nares and advanced until in the oropharynx. The balloon is inflated with approximately 10 mL of

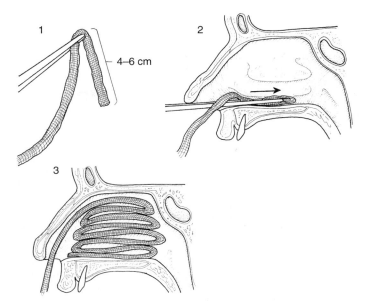

Figure 16-1. **Anterior nasal packing to support the septum after fracture reduction. It can also be used to control epistaxis.**

sterile saline (**Fig. 16-2**). Vaseline-impregnated gauze is packed into the nose on either side of the septum. If bleeding persists, consider placing another Foley catheter in the contralateral nares to provide more compression in the posterior oral pharynx, or use a dual cuffed catheter. After hemostasis is achieved, the catheter is secured into position and left in place for 3 days. The balloon is then deflated and the catheter removed if the bleeding does not recur. When posterior nasal packs are placed, the patient should be placed on

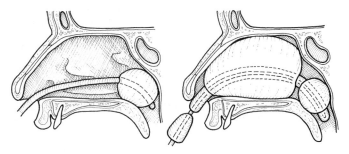

Figure 16-2. **A Foley catheter being used to control posterior nasal epistaxis.**

antibiotics and admitted for observation. Maxillofacial surgery consultation should be obtained.

Intractable epistaxis is uncommon but can be life threatening. Direct approaches to control hemorrhage in this region include ligation of the ethmoidal, internal maxillary, or external carotid arteries or embolization by interventional radiology.

2.   Zygomaticomaxillary Complex Fractures

Zygomaticomaxillary complex (ZMC) fractures are the second most common midface fractures after nasal fractures. Most patients describe a blunt force to the side of the face as the cause of injury. They may complain of double vision, pain, swelling, limitation of mandibular opening (trismus), and altered sensation in the distribution of the infraorbital nerve (second division of the trigeminal nerve). Inspection may reveal periorbital ecchymosis and edema, subconjunctival hemorrhage, flattening of the malar eminence, depression of the zygomatic arch, downward displacement of the lateral canthus (antimongoloid slant), trismus, and ecchymosis in the buccal vestibule. A bony step, which can be painful, is palpable at the frontozygomatic suture or at the infraorbital rim. Swelling, however, can mask the findings on palpation. A detailed ocular examination is indicated for all patients sustaining orbital trauma.

The diagnosis is confirmed by axial and coronal CT scans. Three-dimensional reconstruction and direct sagittal views of the orbit are also helpful. In the absence of CT technology, consider obtaining Waters and submental vertex plain film views.

The ZMC fractures are usually treated electively after the swelling subsides (3 to 5 days). Permitting resolution of facial edema facilitates the dissection and assessment of the esthetic deformity. Indications for repair are cosmetic (flattening of the malar eminence, facial asymmetry) and functional (i.e., enophthalmos, extraocular muscle dysfunction, trismus secondary to impingement of the fractured segments on the temporalis muscle, or a neurosensory deficit involving the infraorbital nerve). Surgical management ranges from observation, closed reduction (Gillies approach), or open reduction, with or without internal fixation, depending on the degree of displacement and stability of the fracture after reduction.

Isolated zygomatic arch fractures are common. Typical presentations include flattening or a palpable depression over the arch and trismus caused by impingement of the arch on the temporalis muscle or coronoid process of the mandible. Indications for operative intervention include trismus or evident depression of the arch producing asymmetry. Arch fractures, which can be reduced in the outpatient setting with local anesthesia and sedation, rarely require internal fixation.

3. Maxilla

Maxilla fractures, which are uncommon, result from a significant blunt force to the midface. Maxillary fractures are frequently associated with multisystem injuries.

a. Le Fort Classification. Maxillary fractures occur in predictable patterns and are classified as Le Fort I, II, and III fractures (**Fig. 16-3**). The Le Fort I level or Guérin fracture is horizontal and extends from the anterior nasal spine posteriorly to the lateral pterygoid plates above the level of the apices of the teeth. The Le Fort II level (pyramidal fracture) extends from nasofrontal suture inferiorly and laterally to the zygomaticomaxillary suture, then posteriorly to the lateral pterygoid plates. Le Fort III level (craniofacial dysjunction) fractures are manifest by disruption at the nasofrontal and frontomaxillary sutures extending to orbital wall and traveling posteriorly to a high level at the pterygoid plates. Anatomically, the Le Fort III fracture includes the ZMC and maxilla as its primary anatomic components. It is rare to encounter pure, isolated forms of the Le Fort fractures in the setting of high speed or high impact trauma. Most patients have some combination of fractures (e.g., Le Fort III on one side and Le Fort I or II on the contralateral side).

b. Findings. The alert patient complains of malocclusion, pain, swelling, and infraorbital paresthesia. Inspection reveals periorbital and facial edema, subconjunctival hemorrhage, epistaxis, and commonly CSF rhinorrhea. The experienced clinician may also note facial disproportion with abnormal lengthening of the midface, although this may be a subtle finding. Palpation reveals a mobile midface, infraorbital and occasionally supraorbital hypoesthesia, palpable steps at the nasofrontal and zygomaticofrontal, and zygomaticotemporal (arch) sutures.

Evaluate midface mobility by placing the thumb on the lingual surface of the anterior teeth and the index finger on labial surfaces, stabilize the head with the other hand, and attempt to move the maxilla in an anterior-posterior direction. To ascertain the maxillary fracture level, while manipulating the maxilla with one hand, place the other hand sequentially over the anterior nasal spine (Le Fort I), the frontonasal junction (Le Fort II and III), and the zygomaticofrontal sutures (Le Fort III) and assess for the presence of mobility.

As with other midface injuries, axial CT imaging with reformatted coronal, sagittal, and three-dimensional views are ideal to confirm the diagnosis and plan treatment.

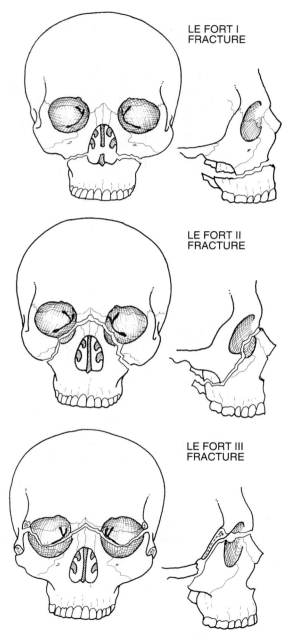

LE FORT I
FRACTURE

LE FORT II
FRACTURE

LE FORT III
FRACTURE

Figure 16-3.   Le Fort fracture patterns.

c. **Management.** In most circumstances, the management of maxillary fractures can be accomplished after the patient has been stabilized and the swelling has subsided. Because the teeth and intraoral soft tissues are often involved, it is best to treat the injuries as soon as possible to avoid complications (e.g., infection). Consultation with the ophthalmology service is mandatory to evaluate ocular injury as with other midface fractures.

Operative management of the fractures is indicated to restore form and function. In the setting of a minimally displaced fracture in an edentulous patient, however, soft diet and observation may be all that is required. The standard of care for displaced or mobile midface fractures is open reduction and rigid internal fixation, which permits the earliest possible return of function.

4. Nasoorbitoethmoid Complex Injuries

Nasoorbitoethmoid (NOE) complex fractures, which result from direct injury to the central midface, are challenging injuries to manage. The injury includes fractures of the nasal, orbital, and ethmoid bones, and injury to associated structures (i.e., medial canthus, lacrimal apparatus). Typical physical findings on inspection include periorbital edema and ecchymosis, subconjunctival hemorrhage, epistaxis, widening and flattening of the nasal dorsum, and telecanthus. The normal intercanthic distance is 32 to 35 mm. Disruption of the attached medial canthal ligament results in traumatic telecanthus. If left untreated, a significant cosmetic deformity will result.

Palpation of the face can elicit pain, steps at the infraorbital rims or nasal bones, and crepitus, commonly secondary to subcutaneous emphysema or comminuted fractures. The diagnosis of a NOE fracture is by clinical examination and confirmed by thin CT scan slices of the region. As with other midface fractures, treatment is delayed until the patient is stable and some resolution of the acute facial edema has occurred.

Consultation should be obtained and definitive management rendered by a maxillofacial trauma surgeon. NOE fractures can have associated CSF rhinorrhea that should be followed closely, although most CSF leaks resolve spontaneously or after fracture treatment. A *persistent* CSF leak requires neurosurgical consultation.

B. Mandibular and Dentoalveolar Fractures

Although nasal fractures are the most common facial fractures, mandibular injuries are the second most common fractures overall and the most common requiring hospitalization. Most mandibular fractures are caused by interpersonal violence or MVA. The anatomic distribution is as follows: body 28%, condyle 25%, angle 25%, symphysis 17%, ramus 4%, and coronoid 1%. Fractures involving the teeth are considered compound or open fractures. As with other fractures, describe the location, type, and degree of displacement when communicating with consultants.

1. History

The alert patient commonly complains of pain, swelling, altered sensation in the lip on the affected side (i.e., "numb lip") and a malocclusion (i.e., "my bite does not feel right"). When possible, obtain details regarding the mechanism of injury and where the injury impact was located because predictable patterns of fracture need to be considered. For example, a chin laceration suggests an injury directly to the anterior mandible and *contrecoup* injury to the condyles. Whereas fractures of the symphysis are uncommon, condylar or subcondylar fractures are commonly associated with trauma to the anterior mandible. A blow producing a body or angle fracture is commonly associated with a *contrecoup* injury of the condylar or subcondylar region on the opposite side.

2. Physical Examination

Findings on inspection include swelling, intraoral and extraoral ecchymoses and lacerations, trismus, fractured or displaced teeth, and a malocclusion. Bimanual palpation helps confirm the fracture location and degree of mobility. Neurosensory function of the IAN using light touch and brush stroke direction should be assessed. Fractures involving the angle or body, which are associated with injury to the inferior alveolar nerve as it passes through its bony canal, result in paresthesia of the lip.

3. Imaging

In contrast to imaging of midface fractures, plain films (i.e., mandible series or panoramic radiographs) are generally adequate or frequently preferable to CT imaging for mandibular fractures. Three-dimensional, reformatted CT images can be helpful to visualize the fracture, but are usually not necessary. In the multisystem trauma cases, however, CT scans may be the only images available.

4. Management

Acute management of mandible fractures includes pain control, initiating antibiotic therapy for open fractures, and preliminary immobilization of the fractures. Narcotic analgesics, topical ice therapy, and a non-chewable diet (i.e., blenderized or pureed) all contribute to pain control. Virtually all mandible fractures in tooth-bearing regions are considered compound fractures contaminated with oral flora. To decrease the risk for infection, broad-spectrum antibiotics should be started immediately (e.g., penicillin (2 million units intravenously [i.v.] every 4 hours), clindamycin (600 mg i.v. every 6 hours), or cefazolin (1 g i.v. every 8 hours). The use of a Barton head dressing can provide some temporary immobilization of the fracture. Ask the patient to bite the teeth together and then apply the Barton dressing.

A maxillofacial surgeon should render definitive management of the fractures. Options range from observation to closed reduction and maxillomandibular fixation to open reduction and rigid internal fixation permitting immediate return to function.

5. Dentoalveolar Fractures

Fractures of the teeth and alveolus, although common, are often not seen in the emergency department. Frequently, the patient's dentist manages these injuries on an outpatient basis. Patients complain of loose teeth, bleeding from the gingiva, pain, and a malocclusion. Inspection reveals an injury to the dentition resulting in chipped, fractured, displaced, or avulsed teeth and, possibly, an associated alveolar bone fracture. Palpation reveals mobility of the alveolar segment and associated dentition. Imaging recommendations include a panoramic radiograph and dental films. Obtain a dental or oral surgical consultation for definitive management of dentoalveolar injuries. If a tooth is avulsed, attempt to replace it into the socket and contact a dentist or oral surgeon for definitive management. Antibiotic coverage is indicated (e.g., oral penicillin [500 mg four times/day] or oral clindamycin [300 mg four times/day]) and the patient should be urged to follow up with the dental or oral surgical service for definitive management. Also consider prescribing an antibacterial mouth rinse such as 0.12% chlorhexidine (30 mL; swish for 30 seconds and spit, twice a day for 7 days).

C. Skull Fractures Associated with Maxillofacial Injuries

1. Frontal Sinus Fractures

Frontal sinus fractures result from blunt trauma over the region of the frontal sinuses. In the absence of a depression in the frontal bone, it is difficult to appreciate a frontal sinus fracture by physical examination. Inspection may reveal an associated laceration, edema, or an evident depression over the frontal sinus. Palpation may reveal crepitus, a step, or hypoesthesia. Associated injuries can include damage to the sinus lining, nasofrontal duct, or brain. Imaging recommendations include CT scanning in at least the axial plane, with appropriate reformatting. The maxillofacial or neurosurgical consultant provides definitive management if the inner table of the skull and the dura are involved.

Although the management of frontal sinus fractures is controversial, some general comments can be made. In most circumstances, imaging defines the extent of the frontal sinus injury and guides subsequent clinical decision-making. No treatment is indicated for an isolated, nondisplaced or minimally displaced anterior table fracture. Reduction and rigid plate fixation are commonly recommended for a displaced anterior table fracture. Esthetically, a depression on the forehead is undesirable. Functionally, the displaced anterior table can obstruct the frontonasal duct. Additionally, it is hypothesized that damage to the sinus lining or obstruction of the duct can predispose the patient to frontal sinus infections that can extend locally into the brain or produce septicemia. Nondisplaced fractures of the posterior table without an associated CFS leak need no operative intervention. Displaced posterior table fractures are commonly explored in concert with the neurosurgical service.

2.   Temporal Bone

Temporal bone fractures are usually identified when a craniofacial CT is done to assess other midface and skull injuries. It is important to recognize this fracture because important associated structures, including the facial nerve and auditory ossicles, are often damaged. If a temporal bone fracture is present, it is important to get a temporal bone CT scan in the coronal, sagittal, and axial cuts, with reconstruction. This helps to assess the extent and displacement of the skull base fracture. Skull base compression or fracture can present with facial nerve palsy. Otolaryngology consultation should be obtained to help evaluate and manage these injuries.

3.   Skull Base Fractures

Skull base fractures are associated with severe midface fractures as a result of the magnitude and direction of the force of injury. Most patients are unable to give a history and the physical examination is difficult. Clues to the presence of this fracture are mastoid ecchymoses ("Battle's sign") and periorbital ecchymoses ("raccoon eyes"). Seen may be evidence of a CSF leak (otorrhea or rhinorrhea) or of neurovascular insult manifested by central or peripheral neurologic deficits. A neurosurgical consult is indicated.

VI.   Evaluation and Acute Management of Maxillofacial Soft Tissue Injuries

A.   Principles of Evaluation and Management

To the inexperienced observer, a patient with facial lacerations often has the appearance of having exsanguinating hemorrhage because a small blood volume and clot, sometimes mixed with saliva, can accumulate on the face, making blood loss appear greater than it actually is. During the secondary survey, quickly identify the extent of the soft tissue injury, explore the wound, and identify active bleeders, if possible. Acute management is geared toward controlling bleeding by application of pressure and packing the exposed wound with gauze dressing. Do not blindly clamp bleeding areas because the risk to vital structures (e.g., the facial nerve or parotid duct) is great. A Barton dressing can be used to stabilize the bleeding until imaging studies are complete and the patient is anesthetized to repair the lacerations.

Meticulously clean and examine the wound to (a) determine its extent, (b) assess for evidence of fractures, and (c) identify and remove any foreign material embedded in the wound. Then, it is possible to identify the anatomy and reposition and repair the involved structures. Verify the tetanus immunization status of the patient. If the wound is contaminated, extensive, or necrotic, a dose of a broad-spectrum antibiotic (e.g. cefazolin (1 g i.v. every 8 hours) is given. Once the wound is cleaned, hemostasis achieved, and the wound dressed, definitive management can be delayed until the patient is hemodynamically stable, if necessary.

B. Management Recommendation for Specific Soft Tissue Injuries

1. Abrasions

Copiously irrigate the wound and apply a thin layer of topical antibiotic ointment.

2. Simple Lacerations

Adequate pain control is critical to the successful management of lacerations. In most circumstances, 1% to 2% lidocaine with 1:200,000 epinephrine provides excellent local anesthesia and vasoconstriction. Attempt to infiltrate the local anesthetic solution some distance from the wound or give a nerve block to prevent distortion of the laceration margins. Copiously irrigate the wound with saline, prepare with antiseptic solution, and drape the wound for sterile closure. With adequate lighting, explore the wound and remove any foreign material. Judiciously excise only necrotic tissue. If a layered closure is indicated, close the deep layers with a 3-0 to 5-0 resorbable suture (e.g., chromic gut), reapproximate the dermal layer with 4-0 to 5-0 resorbable suture (e.g., polyglactin or poliglecaprone), and close the skin with 5-0 or 6-0 interrupted monofilament suture (e.g., nylon). Apply a light dressing using a topical antibiotic ointment. Facial skin sutures should be removed by day 5 in adults and day 3 in children. Systemic antibiotics are usually not indicated.

3. Complex Lacerations

In most cases, lacerations are considered complex if a risk exists of injury to vital structures, the wounds are extensive, or tissue is avulsed. To manage complex lacerations, follow the basic principles outlined above and pay close attention to reapproximating the deep layers; identifying and retracting or repairing vital structures (i.e., nerves); and identifying superficial landmarks and placing tagging sutures to facilitate the accurate reapproximation of the wound edges. In most cases, even in the setting of apparently avulsed tissue, facial lacerations can be closed primarily. Complex lacerations may require some undermining of adjacent tissue to get a tension-free closure. Dress the wound with a topical antibiotic. Systemic antibiotics are commonly indicated. A broad-spectrum antibiotic with coverage of skin flora (e.g., first generation oral cephalosporin [cephalexin] 500 mg four times/day for 7 days) is adequate.

4. Avulsions

After copious irrigation, attempt primary closure by careful undermining of the associated area. If closure of the wound edges by suturing is not possible, achieve coverage with a thin split-thickness skin graft that can serve as temporary or permanent closure. Alternatively, dress the wound with petrolatum type gauze at the base, then an absorbant layer and a transparent, adhesive layer. Definitive closure, if necessary, can be carried out later.

5. Scalp Lacerations

The soft tissue covering the cranium is composed of five layers: skin, connective tissue, aponeuroses (galea), loose connective tissue, and periosteum (SCALP). The same principles of repair of simple lacerations apply to repair of scalp wounds. The scalp is highly vascularized and it is important to obtain hemostasis quickly by repairing the galea aponeurosis. The closure should be in three layers, first approximating the galea aponeurosis with 3-0 or 4-0 resorbable suture, completing the dermal closure, and finally reapproximating the skin with 4-0 monofilament, nonresorbable suture or staples.

6. Eyelid Lacerations

This topic is covered in detail in Chapter 17, *Ocular and Adnexal Trauma.*

7. Parotid Duct Injuries

The parotid duct, which is approximately 7 cm long and 2 to 4 mm in diameter, crosses the masseter muscle and then pierces the buccinator muscle to empty into the oral cavity. The duct runs parallel and near the buccal branch of the facial nerve. Parotid duct injury, therefore, should be suspected in any patient with a buccal branch paresis after facial laceration. Consultation should be requested from the maxillofacial trauma service.

Retrograde injection of methylene blue via Stensen's duct facilitates locating parotid duct lacerations and confirms the integrity (or lack thereof) of the duct. If a repair of the duct is indicated, it should be completed in the operating room under magnification.

8. Facial Nerve Injuries

Facial nerve injuries can occur as a result of either penetrating or blunt trauma to the region of the parotid gland. After completing the primary and secondary surveys, in the hemodynamically stable patient, the timely identification of facial nerve function and treatment of facial nerve injuries is important. Ideally, the injury should be repaired within 72 hours. The goal of nerve repair is to achieve primary junction of the proximal and distal segments without tension.

The repair should be completed in the operating room using magnification.

9.   Intraoral Lacerations

Oral lacerations are challenging because they are bloody, bathed in saliva, obscured by the teeth and other soft tissues, and difficult to visualize. In most circumstances, applying the principles of repair of simple lacerations in the setting of adequate lighting and suction will result in a satisfactory outcome. A short course of antibiotics may be indicated (i.e., oral penicillin V potassium [500 mg po four times/day for 5 days] or oral clindamycin [300 mg three times/day for 5 days]) to decrease the risk of posttraumatic wound infection.

The tongue is well vascularized and lacerations can result in extensive hemorrhage, edema, and hematoma formation, with resultant airway compromise. Ventral and dorsal surfaces of the tongue can be lacerated by the teeth during jaw closure. In the setting of a dorsal laceration of the tongue, inspect the ventral surface and repair it, as needed. Hospital admission for observation may be indicated if concern regarding the airway exists. Systemic corticosteroids (i.e., dexamethasone) can be used to decrease swelling and help maintain a patent airway. Taper dose, as indicated clinically, for significant edema; give 10 mg i.v. on the initial trauma day, then taper to 8 mg i.v. on posttrauma day 1; 6 mg i.v. on posttrauma day 2; 4 mg i.v. on posttrauma day 3; 2 mg i.v. posttrauma day 4; then discontinue. Another alternative is to give the first and or second dose i.v., then switch to oral dexamethasone for posttrauma days 3 and 4 at the same dosage.

10.   Facial Lacerations Communicating with the Oral Cavity

A common situation encountered in the emergency department is a lip laceration that involves the vermillion border. After obtaining adequate local anesthesia and copiously irrigating the wound, place a 5-0 monofilament nonresorbable suture at the skin-vermilion border to reapproximate this cosmetically significant landmark. Repair the intraoral lacerations, in layers if indicated, using a 3-0 resorbable suture (i.e., chromic gut). After the intraoral laceration is closed and the vermilion landmark is satisfactory, direct attention to closing the extraoral laceration, as described above. Topical antibiotic ointment is applied to the extraoral wound. Consider using 0.12% chlorhexidine oral mouth rinse (30 mL; swish and spit for 5 days) and an oral broad-spectrum antibiotic (cephalexin [500 mg po four time/day for 5 days] or oral clindamycin [300 mg three times/day for 5 days]) to decrease the risk for posttraumatic wound infection.)

C.   Location of the Repair
Lacerations can be effectively closed in the emergency department or in the operating room. Factors to consider in choosing the operative setting include the following:
1. Time needed to repair the wound
2. Age of the patient
3. Cooperation or stability of the patient
4. Need for excellent lighting or possible use of the microscope to facilitate the exploration or repair of vital structures (e.g., facial nerve or parotid duct)
5. Need for additional resources (e.g., surgical assistant, suction, excellent instrumentation)

D.   Maxillofacial Gunshot Injuries
Edema secondary to maxillofacial gunshot wounds has the potential to progress rapidly and to involve the retropharyngeal space, especially when the tongue, floor of the mouth, and mandible are involved. Volume resuscitation is carried out and if the patient has significant injuries necessitating an emergent operation, exploration should be carried out in the operating room. Maxillofacial gunshot injuries can involve zones 2 and 3 in the neck, with an associated increased risk for vascular injury. The zones of the neck are described in other chapters as is the diagnoses and management of the vascular injuries to the zones.

In most cases CT imaging, especially with three-dimensional reformatting, should demonstrate the skeletal injuries. If the injuries are isolated to the mandible, panoramic radiographs are often useful to supplement the CT scan. Depending on the anatomic region injured, appropriate consultations can be requested from neurosurgery, ophthalmology, and maxillofacial surgery.

Copiously irrigate the wound with pulsatile lavage and inspect each wound carefully to identify and remove missiles and missile fragments, teeth and parts of teeth, shattered bone, or other foreign bodies. Carefully and judiciously débride nonviable tissue. Other considerations include reduction and stabilization of skeletal injuries, evaluation and repair of damaged vital structures (i.e. facial nerve and salivary ducts), and primary closure, if possible, of the soft tissues. Antibiotic coverage for *Staphylococcus aureus* and oral flora is indicated (cefazolin [1 g i.v. every 6 hours] or clindamycin [600 mg i.v. every 8 hours]).

VII.   Conclusion
In the patient with multiple trauma, communication between the general trauma surgeon and consultants is critical. Even in the patient with multiple systems injuries, the maxillofacial surgery service should be consulted as soon as the patient is stabilized and the injuries recognized. Early diagnosis and management of maxillofacial injuries minimizes the need for additional trips to the operating room and exposures to general anesthetics. If the patient is hemodynamically stable, it is possible to repair facial fractures at the same time as general or orthopedic injuries are being addressed. For the hemodynamically or neurologically unstable patient, the maxilla or mandible can be reduced and stabilized at bedside using a variety of techniques. Temporary immobilization minimizes

infection and facilitates bone healing. For planning purposes, when definitively treating the facial injures, it is common for the maxillofacial consult to request that oroendotracheal tube be converted to a nasoendotracheal tube or the service will plan for a tracheostomy. Many previous texts have discouraged nasoendotracheal intubation in the setting of midface injuries because of the risk of cranial intubation. This is a myth to be discarded. Given competent clinicians working with current anesthesia techniques, the risk of cranial intubation is nil. In the hemodynamically stable patient, cleared for treatment by the trauma service, definitive treatment of the maxillofacial injuries should be rendered in an expeditious manner to enhance the posttraumatic clinical outcomes and minimize the length of hospitalization.

SELECTED READING

Barber DH, et al. Mandibular fractures. In: Fonseca JR, Walker RV, eds. *Oral and maxillofacial trauma,* 2nd ed. Vol. 1. Philadelphia: WB Saunders, 1997.

Dean SJ. Maxillary, Midfacial, and Mandibular Injuries. In: Nwariaku F, Thal E, eds. *Parkland trauma handbook,* 2nd ed. London: Mosby International Ltd., 1999.

Dean SJ. Soft tissue injuries to the face. In: Nwariaku, Thal, eds. *Parkland trauma handbook* 2nd ed. London: Mosby International Ltd., 1999.

Ellis E. Fractures of the zygomatic complex and arch. In: Fonseca, Walker, eds. *Oral and maxillofacial trauma,* 2nd ed. Vol. 1. Philadelphia: WB Saunders, 1997.

Haung RH, Morgan JP. Management of human and animal bites. In: Fonseca, Walker, eds. *Oral and maxillofacial trauma,* 2nd ed. Vol. 2. Philadelphia: WB Saunders, 1997.

Lenhart ED, Dolezal FR. Fractures of the nose. In: Weinnzweig J, ed. *Plastic surgery secretes,* 1st ed. Philadelphia: Hanley & Belfus, Inc., 1999.

Lew D, Sinn PD. Diagnosis and treatment of midface fractures. In: Fonseca, Walker, eds. *Oral and maxillofacial trauma,* 2nd ed. Vol. 2. Philadelphia: WB Saunders, 1997.

Manson PM. Facial injuries. In: Cameron JL. *Current surgical therapy,* 6th ed. St. Louis:, Mosby, 1998:990–999.

Osborne ET, Bays AR. Pathophysiology and management of gunshot wounds to the face. In: Fonseca, Walker. *Oral and maxillofacial trauma,* 2nd. Vol. 2. Philadelphia: WB Saunders, 1997.

Polley WJ, Flagg SJ, Cohen M. Fractures of the mandible. In: Weinzweig J, ed. *Plastic surgery secretes,* 1st ed. Philadelphia: Hanley & Belfus Inc., 1999.

Powers PM, Beck WB, Fonseca JR. Management of soft tissue injuries. In: Fonseca, Walker. *Oral and maxillofacial trauma,* 2nd ed. Vol. 2. Philadelphia: WB Saunders, 1997.

Weinzweig J, Bartlett PS. Fractures of the orbit. In: Weinzweig J, ed. *Plastic surgery secretes,* 1st ed. Philadelphia: Hanley & Belfus Inc., 1999.

17

Ocular and Adnexal Trauma

Nicoletta Fynn-Thompson, MD,
and Lynnette Watkins, MD

I. Introduction

The incidence of ocular and adnexal (lids, orbit and lacrimal system) injury in the trauma setting is large; and should not be overlooked. Up to 90% of patients with facial fractures have some degree of ocular trauma, from subconjunctival hemorrhage to open globe injury. The economic impact of ocular and adnexal injuries is significant. This impact was studied at the Massachusetts Eye and Ear Infirmary (MEEI) in 1988, and the total annual cost of all eye injuries seen at MEEI was calculated at $5 million. Indirect costs (e.g., loss of workdays, time lost from school, training, housework) are also significant. This study estimated the time of paid labor lost in the patient population seen at MEEI annually was 60 work years. Most of these injuries, particularly those occurring in the workplace and during recreational activities, are preventable.

II. Epidemiology

Approximately 25% of all serious eye injuries are work related. The National Institute of Occupational Safety and Health estimated that 900,000 occupational eye injuries occurred in 1982. Of work-related injuries, 60% occur in mens aged 20 to 29 years. Approximately 100,000 of these injuries are sports related. Sports-related and recreational injuries are common and severe, most of which occur in playing basketball, baseball, and racket sports. Nonpowder firearms (e.g., air guns and BB guns) have a high rate of penetrating ocular trauma and lead to more severe eye injuries with a worse visual prognosis. Ocular injury secondary to assault is a growing problem, especially in urban centers. Injury to the eye after a motor vehicle collision, usually involving the anterior segment, is frequently seen.

III. Initial Evaluation.

A. Essential Equipment for Evaluation

The patient with ocular trauma should be evaluated in a fully equipped eye room with a slit lamp, which may not be possible. A portable eye equipment bag should, therefore, be available. The bag should contain a near reading card, eye occluder, pinhole, penlight with cobalt blue filter, eyelid retractors or lid speculum, fluorescein strips, eye pads, gauze pads, metal eye shield (Fox shield), tape, sterile normal saline, Jewelers forceps, no. 15 blade, clamp, Westcott scissors, intraocular pressure (IOP) measuring device (Tono-Pen or Schiøtz tonometer), portable slit lamp, and direct ophthalmoscope. Medications should include an ocular anesthetic (e.g., 0.5% proparacaine) and dilating and cycloplegic drops (e.g., 2.5% phenylephrine and 1% tropicamide, respectively).

B. Key Questions for Evaluation

The first step in the evaluation of a patient with ocular trauma is obtaining an accurate history from the patient, family, or witnesses. Mechanism of injury, events preceding the injury, and other details (e.g., ocular history and previous ophthalmic surgery [e.g., cataract, refractive, or retinal surgery]) should be determined. Use of contact lens, spectacles, and protective eyewear at the time of the incident should also be noted. Medical history, with special emphasis on bleeding disorders, anticoagulation use, and tetanus immunization status, must also be determined. If the patient presents with a chemical injury, copious irrigation should be instituted before obtaining a history (if no obvious evidence of open globe injury is present).

C. Basic Eye Evaluation

    1. Visual Acuity

Visual acuity should be recorded using a near card (with reading or bifocal glasses at 14 inches) or Snellen distance chart (at 20 feet). Each eye should be tested separately, with a pinhole occluder. If the visual acuity is not obtainable with either method, assess the patient to whether he or she can see counting fingers, hand motions, or light perception. If the patient has no light perception, the test should be repeated by several other observers. It is important to have this measurement confirmed by an ophthalmologist, because a poor visual acuity portends a poor prognosis and has a significant impact on future management of the patient.

    2. External Examination

A thorough understanding of the normal anatomy of the eye and adnexal structures is helpful in all stages of the basic eye examination (**Figs. 17-1, 17-2, 17-3**). The first step in this evaluation should include a thorough external examination. Abnormal position of the globe relative to bony structures should be recorded. Enophthalmos (sinking in of the globe) can indicate orbital or sinus fractures. Proptosis of the globe (protrusion of the eye relative to the face) can indicate retrobulbar hemorrhage or edema, subperiosteal hemorrhage, or orbital emphysema (air in the orbit). Associated injuries to the face, head, and neck should also be inspected. The orbital bones should be palpated to assess for *stepoff* or asymmetry indicating a potential fracture. Patients may also complain of numbness or hypesthesia of the face and upper teeth. The presence of foreign bodies should be noted. Periorbital and lid ecchymosis should be noted. Tense, edematous lids with decreased vision are signs of an orbital compartment syndrome, which requires urgent lateral canthotomy and cantholysis. Eyelid and brow lacerations and puncture wounds should be inspected. The presence of orbital fat in a lid laceration should be recorded, because of possible levator aponeurosis involvement. Lacerations of the lid margin and medial lacerations should be inspected for

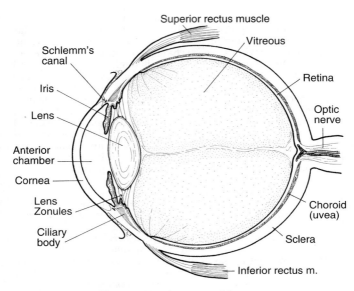

Figure 17-1. Anatomy of the eye.

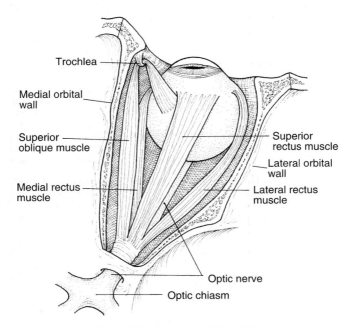

Figure 17-2. Anatomy of the orbit.

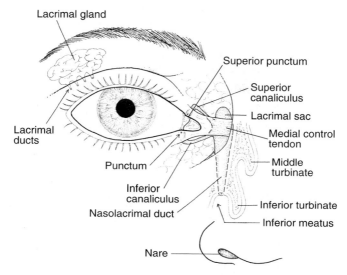

Figure 17-3. Anatomy of the lacrimal drainage system.

lacrimal drainage system involvement. The depth and extent of injury should be determined by gentle probing with a cotton-tipped swab. The presence of abnormal lid position or ptosis should also be documented.

3. Pupil Examination

The pupils should be checked for reactivity, presence of an afferent pupillary defect, and symmetry. An afferent pupillary defect is present if the abnormal pupil dilates instead of constricts when a bright light stimulus is swung in front of the abnormal eye. An eccentric or peaked pupil suggests ocular injury, particularly an open globe injury.

4. Extraocular Motility

Extraocular motility should also be tested. Limitation of extraocular motility can be secondary to traumatic cranial neuropathies or muscle restriction secondary to entrapment of orbital tissue or extraocular muscle in an orbital fracture.

5. Visual Fields

Visual field defects can be obtained on confrontational visual field testing. Central, paracentral, and arcuate defects can be caused by optic nerve lesions. Retinal lesions cause peripheral defects. Bitemporal defects can be seen in optic chiasmal trauma. Other types of visual field defects (e.g., hemifield and quadrant defects) can be caused by trauma of the cortex and other areas along the visual pathway.

6.   Anterior Segment Examination

In an ideal situation, every patient should have an examination with slit-lamp biomicroscopy. If this is not possible, a careful penlight examination should be performed. Until an open globe injury has been ruled out, no pressure should be placed on the globe. Retractors (e.g., a Desmarres retractor, lid speculum, or bent paper clip) should be used. The conjunctiva should be assessed for chemosis (swelling), hemorrhage, laceration, or the presence of a foreign body. If a foreign body is present, it is important to rule out perforation of the globe. The lids should be everted for inspection. The cornea should also be assessed for the presence of abrasions, lacerations, or embedded foreign bodies using fluorescein stain. The anterior chamber (the space between the cornea and the iris) is best viewed with a slit lamp to look for shallowing, which would indicate either leakage or misdirection of aqueous humor. Traumatic iritis or hyphema (blood in the anterior chamber) can also be visualized. If only a penlight examination is possible, layered hyphema can be seen with gross inspection of the anterior chamber. The iris should be inspected for defects or perforation and pupil shape, which can indicate traumatic mydriasis and the presence of peaking, which can indicate a penetrating globe injury. The lens should be evaluated for dislocation or cataract formation. With a low suspicion for open globe injury, IOP should be measured. Low IOP can be seen in traumatic iritis or occult open globe injury. High IOP can be seen with chemical injuries and hyphemas. A high IOP does not rule out an open globe injury.

7.   Posterior Segment Examination

The vitreous and retina should be examined with a direct ophthalmoscope to rule out vitreous or retinal hemorrhage, posterior vitreous detachment, retinal tears or detachment, or intraocular foreign body. The optic nerve should be viewed to assess for abnormalities, including hemorrhages, edema, or avulsion. An ophthalmologist should follow up this posterior segment examination with careful indirect ophthalmoscopy to evaluate the retinal periphery.

IV.   Diagnostic Imaging

Diagnostic imaging is an important tool in assessing the anatomy of both the injured eye and adnexa and its surrounding normal structures. Plain x-ray films, computed tomography (CT), ultrasound, and magnetic resonance imaging (MRI) are all available and useful modalities in the setting of acute trauma. Clinical judgment, however, must be used in deciding the imaging of choice. All of these modalities have advantages and disadvantages.

A.   Plain X-ray Films

Plain x-ray films are a fast, cost-effective imaging modality that can identify foreign material (e.g., metal) in the eye and orbit. This imaging modality can also demonstrate many types of orbital and skull fractures. Plain films, however, are less effective in localization of foreign bodies (particularly if they are intraocular or extraocular) and identification of radiolucent foreign bodies (e.g., glass, plastic, wood).

B. Computed Tomography

Computed tomography scan has become the diagnostic imaging of choice in the setting of ocular trauma. This diagnostic modality provides excellent bone and soft tissue contrast. It provides excellent detection and localization of fractures, as well as radiopaque and most radiolucent foreign bodies. It also demonstrates associated soft tissue injury, particularly in the setting of fractures, where radiographic evidence of incarceration of orbital tissues can be seen. The sinuses and brain can also be seen simultaneously, allowing assessment of concurrent sinus and intracranial injuries. Helical CT scanning provides a quick, detailed image and allows for three-dimensional reconstruction. Carotid-cavernous sinus fistulas and arteriovenous malformations can be seen with contrast-enhanced CT. Disadvantages of CT include artifact formation with metallic foreign material and bone artifact at the skull base, which limits visualization. Also, CT imaging can miss wooden foreign bodies.

C. Magnetic Resonance Imaging

Magnetic resonance imaging is a diagnostic imaging modality that is important primarily with trauma patients with suspected neurologic or neuro-opthalmic injury. MRI demonstrates superior visualization of the posterior cranial fossa, optic nerve, and intracranial pathology. It also better demonstrates wooden foreign bodies. MRI should not be used as a first-line imaging modality in the acute setting of trauma. MRI should be used only when the presence of a metallic foreign body is ruled out. Movement of a metallic foreign body can occur during imaging, which can lead to further intraocular, intraorbital, or intracranial injury. MRI does not provide good visualization of bone detail and, thus, is not helpful in the setting of fractures. MRI is also expensive and requires longer scanning times, which can be a problem in the trauma setting.

D. Ocular Ultrasound

Ocular ultrasound is useful in the setting of ocular trauma to assess the posterior segment (retinal detachments, vitreous hemorrhage) when visualization is limited by anterior segment pathology (e.g., hyphema, traumatic cataract, corneal edema). This imaging should be used only after an open globe injury has been ruled out. Other associated injuries can preclude use of this modality.

V. Indications for Ophthalmologic Consultation

Following is a brief list of situations that mandate **immediate** referral to an ophthalmologist.

- Vision loss presenting after traumatic injury
- Obvious open globe injury
- Intraocular or intraorbital foreign body
- Chemical eye injuries (particularly alkaline injuries)
- Lid lacerations that involve the lid margin (particularly

avulsion injuries), have prolapsed orbital fat, or in a medial location (potentially involving the lacrimal drainage system)
- Orbital compartment syndrome secondary to hemorrhage, edema, or emphysema (air in the orbit)
- Patient presents with flashes and floaters (worrisome for a retinal tear or detachment)

If an open globe injury is suspected, the injured eye should be covered with a metal shield. The head of the bed should be elevated. The patient should have nothing to eat (NPO), and given a tetanus booster (if indicated). Intravenous (i.v.) access should be established, broad-spectrum i.v. antibiotics should be instituted. Vancomycin and ceftazidime are drugs of choice at MEEI, because of their broad antimicrobial coverage, including *Bacillus cereus*. Antiemetics are important to avoid vomiting, which could increase IOP and potentially facilitate expulsion of intraocular contents. Diagnostic tests should be performed before transfer and copies of radiographs and scans sent to the referring ophthalmologist.

Intraorbital foreign bodies that are protruding should be gently covered with a Styrofoam cup or loose bandage. The object should not be removed. Lid lacerations should be gently covered with sterile saline gauze.

VI. Anterior Segment
   A. Conjunctival Injuries
      1. Subconjunctival Hemorrhage
      Subconjunctival hemorrhage is the appearance of a blood underneath the conjunctiva in a diffuse or focal pattern. Patients normally do not complain of pain. These areas are often bright red or reddish-purple. This will initially spread and gradually absorb over several weeks. If subconjunctival hemorrhage is associated conjunctival emphysema (air beneath the conjunctiva), an associated orbital fracture should be ruled out. With extensive bullous or elevated subconjunctival hemorrhage present (particularly if it is 360 degrees around the cornea), an open globe injury must be ruled out. The patient must be taken to the operating room by an ophthalmologist for exploration under general anesthesia.

      2. Conjunctival Foreign Bodies
      Foreign bodies embedded in the conjunctiva frequently occur after occupational accidents. Patients complain of foreign body sensation, pain, tearing, and redness. The foreign bodies may be metallic or organic materials. In the setting of grinding, sawing, or hammering (especially without protective eyewear), it is mandatory to rule out penetrating trauma by careful examination of the entire globe. Imaging techniques can be valuable for further testing, especially in the setting of high-velocity injuries. It is important to evert the lids to determine if foreign bodies are present underneath the lid, which can then cause concurrent linear corneal abrasions. Conjunctival foreign bodies are removed by copious irrigation, and sweeping the conjunctiva with a cotton-tipped swab or removal with fine forceps. Topical anesthetic should be instilled before removal and

broad-spectrum antibiotic ointment (e.g., bacitracin or bacitracin/polymyxin) should be instilled after removal. Follow-up with an ophthalmologist should be within 1 week. If removal of the foreign body is incomplete, an ophthalmologist should be consulted to complete this procedure to prevent infection.

3. Conjunctival Lacerations

Conjunctival lacerations are common with the presence of foreign bodies. They are best viewed with fluorescein staining. Usually, associated subconjunctival hemorrhage occurs. It is important to inspect the extent of the injury and the possibility of scleral involvement, with the aid of a topical anesthetic. A dilated funduscopic examination should also be performed. Small, conjunctival lacerations do not need to be surgically repaired. Larger lacerations (>1 cm) should be closed with an absorbable suture. Broad-spectrum antibiotic ointment should always be prescribed, with subsequent evaluation in 1 week. A protective shield should be worn by the patient to prevent further injury at bedtime.

B. Scleral Injuries

1. Foreign Bodies

Scleral foreign bodies are present in cases of a concurrent full-thickness conjunctival laceration with a foreign body present in the sclera. If the foreign matter is not fully embedded into the sclera, it can be removed with topical anesthetic and a cotton-tipped swab or fine forceps. If the depth of the foreign body cannot be determined, however, removal should be deferred and exploration done in the controlled setting of the operating room. If the foreign body is successfully removed, then prophylactic broad-spectrum antibiotic ointment should be prescribed, and a metal shield placed over the affected eye.

2. Ruptures and Lacerations

Scleral ruptures and lacerations are partial or full-thickness defects of the eye wall. Full thickness scleral ruptures or lacerations are, by definition, open globe injuries. Scleral ruptures are *secondary to blunt injury*. Scleral lacerations are *secondary to penetrating injury*. Lacerations can be classified as penetrating (entry wound only) or perforating (entry and exit wounds present). The conjunctiva is often (although not always) lacerated. Only surgical exploration can completely assess the extent of a scleral injury, because rupture sites often occur at the limbus, around the optic nerve (peripapillary region), posterior to muscle insertions, and at previous surgical incision sites. A Seidel test with sterile application of 2% fluorescein to the affected eye is helpful in the evaluation of a scleral laceration. Dilution of the 2% fluorescein by the aqueous humor can be seen as a yellow area with a cobalt blue light or a yellow-green area on an orange background with white light. If a partial-thickness laceration is present, topical antibiotic ointment or drops and a protective shield should be placed onto the affected eye. The depth of the laceration determines surgical intervention. A full-thickness scleral laceration is an open globe injury and requires prompt surgical attention by an ophthalmologist. Full-thickness scleral lacerations often have prolapse of brown tissue (uvea). In cases of obvious scleral laceration, it is best to avoid instillation of drops and shield the eye. Imaging (CT or plain films) is recommended to rule out an intraocular foreign body.

C. **Corneal Injuries**

1. **Abrasions**

Corneal abrasions are defects of the corneal epithelium that can be caused by various mechanisms (e.g., foreign body, scratch, finger poke). The foreign body can be contaminated; therefore, risk of secondary infection is always a possibility. The patient may complain of blurred vision, pain, foreign body sensation, photophobia (pain exacerbated by light), and tearing. Fluorescein staining of deepithelialized cornea confirms the diagnosis. Examination of the conjunctiva and eyelid eversion is important to rule out the presence of a foreign body. Treatment consists of a broad-spectrum antibiotic ointment (bacitracin/polymyxin) and a cycloplegic eyedrop for relief of pain secondary to ciliary muscle spasm. Patching of the eye is not recommended if the abrasion is contact lens related or secondary to an organic foreign material (e.g., tree branch, fingernail) because of increased risk of subsequent infection. In the absence of these situations, the injured eye can be patched for larger abrasions (>3 mm) for comfort after instilling antibiotic ointment. The patient must be seen the following day and the patch removed. Patients with corneal abrasions secondary to a shearing injury are at increased risk of recurrent erosion syndrome. Recurrent erosion occurs because of damage to the epithelial and basement membrane complexes, leading to areas of irregular epithelium and epithelial defects that present symptomatically with pain and photophobia. Treatment consists of pressure patching, antibiotic ointment, gentle corneal epithelial debridement, and placement of a bandage contact lens. Incisional and laser surgical methods are used for severe cases.

2. **Foreign Bodies**

Corneal foreign bodies occur predominantly from occupational injuries. Often, protective eyewear is not worn. The patient complains of blurred vision, pain, foreign body sensation, photophobia, and tearing. The foreign body may be seen with the use of fluorescein staining. If it is a metallic substance, a rust ring may be evident. It is important to determine the depth of corneal involvement with embedded foreign bodies. The depth of the anterior chamber should also be assessed to rule out corneal perforation. Because the foreign material can be contaminated, subsequent infection is possible, especially with organic material.

On examination, concurrent foreign bodies of the conjunctiva and sclera should also be ruled out. A dilated funduscopic examination should be performed to rule out the possibility of an intraocular foreign body. Treatment is extraction of the foreign body. The eye should be anesthetized with topical anesthetic. First, copious irrigation should be attempted to dislodge the foreign material. If this is unsuccessful, removal with a 27- or 30-gauge needle or high-speed burr can be attempted under magnification with a slit lamp. Foreign bodies that are deeply embedded or incompletely removed should be evaluated by an ophthalmologist for further management. If corneal perforation is suspected, a Seidel test (**see Section IV.A.2.**) can be performed to rule out aqueous leakage. In this setting, surgical exploration is required for closure of the entry site once the presence or absence of an intraocular foreign body is determined. Dilated fundus examination and diagnostic imaging are essential to evaluate intraocular foreign body. If the corneal foreign body is superficial and easily removed, the patient should be treated with antibiotic ointment and followed closely. If a concurrent corneal infection is present, the foreign body and injured corneal area can be cultured to aid in appropriate therapy.

3. Chemical Eye Injuries

Chemical eye injuries are potentially devastating injuries that can lead to permanent visual loss. Early, aggressive management with copious irrigation is imperative. Alkaline injuries are more devastating than acid injuries because of their ability to penetrate the eye. Alkaline injuries cause fat saponification, which results in damage of the entire depth of the cornea, as well as other anterior segment structures. Acid injury forms precipitates on the corneal surface, which limits penetration of the chemical and, thus, corneal and anterior segment damage. A lid speculum can be used to keep the eye open. Any retained particles or debris should be removed. Check the pH by placing litmus paper into the fornices. Irrigation should be continued until the pH is neutral. An urgent ophthalmology consult should be requested. For minor injuries with only minimal epithelial defects and preservation of corneal clarity, treatment with antibiotic (erythromycin) or antibiotic steroid ointment (tobramycin/dexamethasone or sulfacetamide/prednisolonee) is recommended. Topical steroids, cycloplegic agents, citrate, ascorbic acid, and IOP lowering agents are just some of the medications used to treat the patient with a chemical eye injury. Patients with opaque corneas, limbal ischemia, and limbal necrosis have a poorer visual prognosis.

4. Thermal Burn

Corneal thermal burn injuries are frequently seen in burn patients with facial involvement. Usually, associated lid burns with lid scarring and cicatricial changes are seen. Corneal injuries from thermal burn present with opaque corneas with irregular epithelial edges and epithelial defects. Exposure keratopathy secondary to lagophthalmos (incomplete closure of the lids) can exacerbate the underlying thermal injury. Treatment includes frequent lubrication with topical antibiotic or antibiotic steroid ointment to the cornea and conjunctiva, and artificial tears. Temporary closure of the eyelids (suture tarsorrhaphy) may be necessary to treat severe keratopathy. Skin dressings for burns should be followed by a burn specialist. An ophthalmology consult is required.

5.   Ruptures and Lacerations

Corneal lacerations can be classified as penetrating (entry wound only) or perforating (both entry and exit wounds) injuries. Corneal injuries can be partial thickness or full thickness, which can be determined with Seidel testing (**see Section VI.A.2.**). Full thickness corneal and corneo-scleral lacerations are, by definition, open globe injuries. Symptoms of corneal laceration include pain, photophobia, decreased vision, and foreign body sensation. Signs include red eye, corneal edema, and epithelial and stromal defect. Associated findings include a shallow anterior chamber, abnormal or irregular pupil, hyphema, and cataract. Vitreous (clear gelatinous material) can also be seen in severe cases of corneal laceration and in corneoscleral lacerations (lacerations involving both the cornea and sclera). Partial-thickness lacerations can be observed closely with treatment consisting of broad-spectrum antibiotic drops or ointment, and cycloplegic agents. Pressure patching or bandage contact lens can also be placed. If the laceration is deep, it may require surgical closure. If the Seidel test (**see Section VI.A.2.**) is positive, the laceration is full thickness and requires urgent surgical intervention for closure of the globe. Orbital radiographs or CT scanning should be performed to evaluate for an intraocular foreign body. In cases of open globe injury, an immediate ophthalmology consult should be obtained. The injured eye should be protected with a Fox shield. The patient should be given i.v. antibiotics, tetanus booster, and kept NPO in preparation for surgery.

D.   Iris, Ciliary Body, and Anterior Chamber Injuries

1.   Iris Sphincter Tears

Iris sphincter tears are small radial tears commonly seen following blunt trauma to the anterior segment. These tears are often seen in association with hyphema. Patients complain of glare, monocular diplopia (double vision), and photophobia. Gross examination shows a dilated, often irregular pupil. Slit-lamp examination shows irregularities of the iris sphincter. Treatment for iris sphincter tears includes surgical reconstruction of the pupil (pupilloplasty). Patients who decline to have surgery can be fit with a tinted contact lens to decrease glare symptoms and improve cosmesis.

2. Iridodialysis

Iridodialysis is traumatic separation of the iris root from the ciliary body after blunt trauma. It is often associated with hyphema. Anterior segment examination shows a disinserted iris root and polycoria (multiple pupils). The patient may complain of monocular diplopia. Treatment is surgical (pupilloplasty) or a cosmetic contact lens, when indicated.

3. Cyclodialysis

Cyclodialysis is caused by a traumatic cleft between the ciliary body and its insertion into the scleral spur. Diagnosis is made only after evaluation of the anterior chamber angle with gonioscopic lens examination (gonioscopy). Cyclodialysis can cause hypotony (abnormally low IOP). Acute "spikes" of IOP elevation can occur when the cleft intermittently closes. Treatment consists of surgical or laser closure of the cyclodialysis cleft and management of abnormal IOP.

4. Angle Recession

Angle recession occurs when a tear between the longitudinal and circular muscles of the ciliary body occurs after blunt trauma to the anterior segment. This diagnosis is made with gonioscopy. Patients with this entity have a higher lifetime risk of developing glaucoma in the affected eye, particularly if more than two thirds of the angle is involved. Treatment consists of topical intraocular medications, laser, and surgery to control elevated IOP.

5. Hyphema

Hyphema is caused by the disruption of the vessels in the iris and ciliary body following blunt trauma. Penlight or slit-lamp examination reveals circulating red

Table 17-1. Differential diagnosis of the red eye in the trauma patient

Subconjunctival hemorrhage
Conjunctival laceration
Conjunctival foreign body
Corneal foreign body
Corneal abrasion
Chemical eye injury
Thermal corneal injury
Traumatic iritis
Traumatic cataract (with lens capsule disruption)
Traumatic glaucoma (direct injury, lens particle-induced glaucoma)
Open globe injury
Hyphema
Posttraumatic endophthalmitis (after intraocular foreign body or open globe injury)
Carotid-cavernous sinus fistula (may be delayed in onset)

blood cells in the anterior chamber (microhyphema) or the presence of a layered clot or hemorrhage in the inferior anterior chamber visible on gross inspection (hyphema). IOP should be checked, as it can be elevated by blockage of the trabecular meshwork with red blood cells.

The primary goal of treatment is to reduce the probability of rebleeding and prevent episodes of increased IOP. Studies show that episodes of rebleeding frequently occur 2 to 5 days after injury with clot lysis. Daily evaluation of these patients by an ophthalmologist is essential to monitor and treat potential complications. Rebleeding can cause prolonged increases in IOP, leading to optic nerve damage and vision loss. Rebleeding also causes corneal blood staining, which is staining of the corneal endothelium with hemosiderin and erythrocyte breakdown products. Treatment includes topical steroid medication to decrease inflammation. Cycloplegics are often prescribed to ease inflammation and ciliary muscle spasm and to facilitate fundus examination. Bedrest is enforced with elevation of the head of the bed at 30 degrees. Aspirin use is contraindicated. Aminocaproic acid, an antifibrinolytic agent that is thought to decrease the rate of clot lysis, is used for severe cases with high risk of rebleeding. Surgical lavage of the anterior chamber can also be done to remove the hemorrhage. Close follow-up by an ophthalmologist is imperative to monitor for glaucoma, rebleeding, and corneal blood staining. Hyphema and angle recession with subsequent development of glaucoma may occur months after the injury.

6. Traumatic Iritis

Traumatic iritis is a transient problem caused by mild iris injury. Iris pigment is liberated and seen floating in the anterior chamber, depositing on the lens, corneal endothelium, and trabecular meshwork. It can be associated with elevated or decreased IOP. Treatment includes the use of a cycloplegic agent for comfort and to prevent posterior synechiae and topical steroids to decrease the inflammation.

E. Glaucoma Associated with Ocular Trauma

1. Immediate Causes of Traumatic Glaucoma

Immediate causes of increased IOP include presence of inflammatory cells or red blood cells (hyphema) in the anterior chamber. These cells can obstruct drainage at the trabecular meshwork. Another cause for immediate rise in IOP is severe trabecular meshwork disruption from direct impact or in the setting of chemical injury. Acute rises in IOP after trauma can result from lens particle glaucoma (phacolytic glaucoma). This occurs because of disruption of the lens capsule that allows lens particles to be released into the anterior chamber, obstruct the trabecular meshwork, and cause an inflammatory reaction. Treatment consists of topical medication to lower IOP and inflammation,

**Table 17-2.   Differential diagnosis
of vision loss in the trauma patient**

Hyphema
Open globe injury
Corneal abrasion
Chemical eye injury
Thermal corneal injury
Traumatic iritis
Traumatic glaucoma
Traumatic cataract
Traumatic optic neuropathy
Vitreous hemorrhage
Retinal detachment
Posttraumatic endophthalmitis (possibly associated with intra-
    ocular foreign body or subsequent to open globe injury)
Cortical blindness
Orbital hemorrhage
Orbital compartment syndrome
Carotid-cavernous sinus fistula

then surgical removal of lens particles. IOP can acutely rise with lens subluxation or dislocation causing pupillary block (bowing of the iris forward causing closure of the anterior chamber angle and trabecular meshwork) and alteration of the anterior segment anatomy and drainage pathway. An ophthalmology consult should be obtained for IOP management.

2.   Delayed Causes of Traumatic Glaucoma
Angle recession or direct trabecular meshwork damage with resultant scarring can cause delayed glaucoma after trauma. Studies have shown that the patient has a 10% chance of developing chronic glaucoma when the angle is recessed >180 degrees (assessed via gonioscopy). Treatment is with topical or oral IOP-lowering agents. A second cause of delayed increased IOP is ghost cell glaucoma. With blunt trauma, there is disruption of the anterior hyaloid face. Blood and hemosiderin collect in the vitreous and anterior chamber. Approximately 1 to 3 weeks after trauma, as blood clears the anterior chamber, the cells in the vitreous become tan colored (khaki-colored) and less pliable. These cells migrate into the anterior chamber, causing blockage of the trabecular meshwork. Treatment is with topical or oral IOP-lowering agents. Anterior chamber lavage of these cells can be done to treat a persistently elevated pressure. An ophthalmology consult should be obtained for further management.

F.   Lenticular Injuries

1.   Lens Subluxation and Dislocation
Lens subluxation (partial dislocation) and dislocation can result from blunt or penetrating trauma. Sudden

anterior or posterior compression of the globe can cause partial or complete disruption of the zonular or lens support fibers. Initial visual symptoms may not occur until several days after the injury. The patient may complain of fluctuating vision (from marked astigmatism or functional aphakia), monocular diplopia, or glare. Lens dislocation can be subtle and only apparent on dilated examination. Findings from careful examination of the anterior chamber depth and presence of lens instability (phacodonesis) or iris instability (iridodonesis) can be variable. Vitreous herniation through ruptured zonules into the anterior chamber may be seen. If the anterior or posterior lens capsule is disrupted, removal is more urgent and can be required because of movement of the lens into the anterior chamber or pupillary block. Dislocation of the lens anteriorly can also cause acute corneal edema and corneal decompensation. Posterior dislocation of the lens into the vitreous can cause inflammation (vitritis) and macular edema, with resultant vision loss. These patients should be referred to an ophthalmologist for medical management of astigmatism and myopia or surgical removal of the lens.

2. Traumatic Cataracts
Traumatic cataracts can develop after blunt or penetrating trauma. A contusion cataract is the development of a lens opacification secondary to nonpenetrating, blunt ocular trauma. If the lens capsule remains intact, the cataract can develop months from the time of injury. Observation is recommended, and removal only necessary for glare or decreased vision secondary to lens opacities. The presence of lens particles will cause severe inflammation, hastening the removal of the cataract. All patients should be referred to an ophthalmologist for management.

3. Lenticular Injuries from Secondary Mechanism
    a. Glassblower's cataract, which occurs secondary to thermal and infrared radiation, is seen in glassblowers. The lens capsule peels away in sheets or scrolls. Treatment includes observation (if mild) or cataract extraction (if severe). Safety goggles can prevent this condition.
    b. Electrical cataract are seen after electrocution to the head and face. These cataracts, which occur because of protein coagulation of the lens, present as stellate opacities of the cortex. Glare, photophobia, and vision loss are complaints. These cataracts can regress, mature, or progress. Treatment is based on degree of visual disability and includes observation or cataract extraction.

G. Intraocular Foreign Bodies Located in the Anterior Segment
Intraocular foreign bodies can cause potentially devastating injuries because of the traumatic injury from the for-

eign body and the potential risk of intraocular infection (posttraumatic endophthalmitis). These types of injuries occur in patients performing high-velocity activity (hammering, sawing, grinding) often without safely eye protection. The foreign bodies are usually metallic, organic, plastic, or glass. Other concurrent injuries include corneal, corneoscleral, or scleral lacerations; traumatic cataract; iris injury; iritis; and hyphema. The foreign body may or may not be visible. These patients should have radiographic imaging (CT or plain films). Treatment of these injuries requires closure of the laceration or entry wound and surgical removal of the foreign body through a separate corneal or beveled scleral incision by an ophthalmologist in the controlled setting of the operating room. Preoperative patient management is similar to that for patients with an open globe injury (i.v. antibiotics, tetanus booster, nothing by mouth status, eye shield) (**see Section VII.C**).

VII. **Posterior Segment**
   A. **Vitreal Injuries**
      1. **Posterior Vitreous Detachment**
      Posterior vitreous detachment results from trauma to the globe causing the vitreous to disinsert from its attachments at the vitreous base, peripapillary region (the optic nerve area), and the macula. The patients commonly complain of floaters (mobile black or dark spots located within their visual field), which occasionally form a ring (Weiss ring). Flashes of light can also occur from pulling and irritation of the retinal tissue during the vitreous detachment. The visual acuity should be documented and a dilated fundus examination performed. An ophthalmologist should be consulted to examine the patient using indirect ophthalmoscopy and perform scleral depression to assess the extent of the vitreous detachment, vitreous hemorrhage, retinal dialysis, retinal tears, or retinal detachment. Hemorrhage in the vitreous associated with a vitreous detachment is worrisome, because in 70% of cases an associated retinal tear or detachment is seen (Note: 15% of patients who present with a retinal tear or detachment have no evidence of vitreous hemorrhage). All patients with flashes and floaters should be referred to the ophthalmologist the day of presentation for examination.

      2. **Traumatic Vitreous Hemorrhage**
      Traumatic vitreous hemorrhage can occur from either blunt or penetrating ocular trauma. It results from breaks in the retinal blood vessels, retinal breaks, injury to the uveal tract, and scleral rupture or laceration. The patient may complain of decreased vision and the presence of floaters. Dense vitreous hemorrhages may only allow a red reflex to be seen without retinal details on dilated examination. If vitreous hemorrhage is suspected, an ophthalmologist should be consulted to perform a dilated fundus examination to assess for the presence of red blood cells in

the vitreous cavity. The presence of retinal breaks, retinal detachments, retinal dialysis, and scleral laceration (open globe injury) should be investigated. The patient presenting with vitreous hemorrhage and bullous subconjunctival hemorrhage must be considered to have an open globe injury until proven otherwise. Ocular ultrasound can be used to detect retinal pathology once an open globe injury is excluded.

B. Retinal and Choroidal Injuries

1. Commotio Retinae (Berlin's Edema)

Commotio retinae (Berlin's edema) is caused by blunt injury resulting in retinal shearing of the photoreceptor layer, with subsequent retinal whitening opposite the site of direct impact on the anterior portion of the globe. The patient may complain of decreased vision if the retinal whitening is located within the macula. The discoloration may be confined to the macula or involve more extensive areas in the peripheral retina. On funduscopic examination, the outer retina develops a cloudy, grayish-white opacification. Prognosis is often good. Vision loss can occur if the macula is involved. An ophthalmologist should be consulted to perform a dilated fundus examination and rule out the presence of associated intraretinal and subretinal hemorrhages, choroidal rupture, macular and retinal detachment, or macular hole. Treatment is observation.

2. Retinal Hemorrhages

Retinal hemorrhages are classified by their location: preretinal, intraretinal, and subretinal. Preretinal hemorrhages are located between the retina and the vitreous and are boat shaped. These types of hemorrhages are seen in shaken-baby syndrome (child abuse), posterior vitreous detachments, and retinal tears. Intraretinal hemorrhages are flame or dot-shaped and appear in various types of ocular injury. Subretinal hemorrhage occurs beneath the retina and retinal vessels and is dark in appearance. It is also associated with various types of trauma, particularly choroidal ruptures.

3. Purtscher's Retinopathy

Purtscher's retinopathy is caused by multiple embolic events to the retinal vasculature causing retinal ischemia and hemorrhages. It has been associated with severe head, chest, and long-bone trauma that causes either fat (in long-bone fractures) or air (in compressive chest injuries) embolization. Less traumatic causes include acute pancreatitis and amniotic fluid embolism. The patient may complain of decreased vision (more commonly bilateral) and visual scotomas. An ophthalmology consult should be obtained. Dilated fundus examination reveals retinal whitening (caused by ischemia) associated with multiple intraretinal hemorrhages (within the superior and inferior arcades), large cotton-wool spots, and optic disc edema. Treatment is observation.

4.   Retinal Tears and Detachments
Several types of retinal breaks occur in the setting of trauma. They include retinal tears, giant retinal tears, retinal dialysis, and rhegmatogenous retinal detachments. Traumatic retinal dialysis, tears, or detachments from trauma most commonly result from vitreoretinal traction secondary to transmission of blunt forces to the vitreous gel. Patients may complain of decreased vision, floaters, flashes, or a "shade" covering their vision. Slit-lamp examination may reveal the presence of pigmented cells or red blood cells in the anterior vitreous space, indicating a vitreous hemorrhage from rupture of a retinal vessel. A dilated examination must be performed by an ophthalmologist with scleral depression to determine the location, quantity, and extent of retinal damage, as well as to identify retinal tears. A retina specialist should manage these problems surgically.

5.   Macular Holes
Macular holes secondary to trauma are caused by vitreous traction, retinal necrosis (secondary to macular edema or cyst formation), and subfoveal hemorrhages. The fovea (center of the macula) is susceptible to traumatic injury because it is very thin. Macular holes can be associated with posterior vitreous detachment. In the presence of a full-thickness macular hole, the patient complains of decreased vision, a central scotoma or blind spot, and metamorphopsia (distortion of images). Ophthalmic consultation is necessary to perform a dilated fundus examination to determine the depth of the hole (lamellar versus full thickness).

6.   Direct Choroidal Rupture
Direct choroidal rupture (separation of the vascular layer beneath the retina) occurs at the site of contusive impact following trauma, usually anterior and parallel to the ora serrata. Indirect choroidal ruptures are caused by the antero-posterior compression of the trauma. These ruptures are curvilinear and occur in the peripapillary and macular region. The patient may complain of decreased vision. Initial examination reveals subretinal and choroidal hemorrhage, and intraretinal, preretinal, and vitreous hemorrhage. These hemorrhages can obscure the rupture site, which becomes evident during serial examinations.

7.   Choroidal Effusion and Suprachoroidal Hemorrhage
Choroidal effusion presents as a smooth, dome-shaped elevation of the retina and choroids. It is often seen in the setting of severe blunt trauma and open globe injury. Suprachoroidal hemorrhage results from bleeding of the short posterior ciliary artery and, possibly, the long posterior ciliary arteries as a result of significant trauma. The patient complains of ocular pain and significant decreased

vision. Examination reveals loss of the red reflex, a firm globe, and anterior displacement of the lens. Expulsion of intraocular contents can occur in this setting. Immediate ophthalmology consult is needed for further management.

C.   Intraocular Foreign Bodies of the Posterior Segment

Intraocular foreign bodies of the posterior segment lodge in the retina. Often, a concurrent corneal, corneoscleral, or scleral laceration is seen. Most foreign bodies are metallic and magnetic. Other types of foreign bodies include glass, plastic, and organic foreign bodies (e.g., wood). Slit lamp and dilated fundus examination performed by an ophthalmologist are required to investigate the diagnosis and determine the location of the injury. The view, however, can be obscured by hemorrhage, cataract, and inflammation. Radiographic imaging is important in this situation. Plain films and CT imaging are useful in determining that an intraocular foreign body is present. CT is superior because of the greater soft tissue/bone contrast and availability of thin slices to localize small metallic foreign bodies. CT is less precise in the detection of wood, plastic, and glass. MRI is contraindicated because of the risk of movement of the foreign body by the magnet, causing further intraocular injury. Timing of foreign body removal depends on its type and location. Organic material must be removed early, to decrease the chance of bacterial or fungal endophthalmitis (infection of the posterior segment). Foreign bodies with high copper content (>85%), which can cause intraocular inflammation, also should be removed without delay. Inert materials (e.g., glass, plastic) can be removed later, because of the lower incidence of inflammation. A retinal specialist should remove these foreign bodies through a scleral incision (sclerotomy), with the use of an ophthalmic magnet if the foreign body is metallic and magnetic. Systemic i.v. antibiotics are required for these patients because of the risk of posttraumatic endophthalmitis (**see Section VI.G**).

VIII.   Neuro-ophthalmic Injuries (All suspected neuro-opthalmic injuries should be evaluated by an opthalmologist)

A.   Pupillary Abnormalities

1.   Traumatic Mydriasis

Traumatic mydriasis (dilation of the pupil) occurs from direct trauma to the iris or in association with intracranial pathology. Patients experience blurred vision and photophobia as a result. Hyphema and other iris pathology may also be present. Examination in the dark may also reveal poor dilation or pupil nonreactivity. Symptomatic cases can warrant surgical management. Mydriasis after traumatic injury can also be secondary to compression of the third cranial nerve. The patient may have an epidural hemorrhage, cerebral hemorrhage, or cerebral edema, which can cause uncal herniation. Uncal herniation can cause compression of the ipsilateral third cranial nerve by forcing it against the posterior clinoid.

2. Traumatic Miosis

Traumatic miosis (constriction of the pupil) is associated with Horner's syndrome. If no other findings are noted, the injury may be to the sympathetic plexus within the neck and a carotid artery dissection must be ruled out. If other cranial nerves (e.g., cranial nerve VI) are involved, the cause may be traumatic injury of the cavernous sinus. The triad of ocular findings seen in Horner's syndrome includes ptosis, miosis, and anhidrosis (loss of sweating mechanism on ipsilateral side of the face). If Horner's syndrome is suspected, MRI or magnetic resonance angiography (MRA) should be obtained immediately to assess for a carotid-cavernous fistula, traumatic intracavernous carotid aneurysm, or dissection of the extracranial portion of the internal carotid artery. Transfermoral angiography may also be necessary in the evaluation of these entities.

B. Optic Nerve and Visual Pathway Injuries

1. Traumatic Optic Neuropathy

Traumatic optic neuropathy can result from either a direct or an indirect cause. *Direct optic nerve trauma* results when an object has penetrated the orbit or intracanalicular space and directly injured the optic nerve. *Indirect optic neuropathy* develops in the setting of closed head trauma. CT scan of the orbits should be obtained with 1.5-mm axial and coronal cuts and special attention to the optic canal. The presence of a foreign body, optic canal fracture, optic nerve hemorrhage, or optic nerve avulsion should be ruled out. Treatment of this disorder is controversial. Some recommend high-dose i.v. corticosteroids. Optic canal decompression has been recommended in some studies if a foreign body, bone fragment, or hematoma is present and impinging on the optic nerve.

2. Chiasmal Syndrome

Chiasmal syndrome can develop from closed or penetrating trauma. The exact mechanism of chiasmal injury in closed head trauma has not been thoroughly explained; however, tears and axonal disruption secondary to fractures or contusions have been postulated to cause some damage.

3. Trauma to the Optic Radiations

Trauma to the optic radiations of the visual pathway can occur in the temporal or parietal lobes, as a result of penetrating or closed head trauma. These cases are usually associated with other neurologic deficits. Damage to the optic radiations produces homonymous hemianopic or quadrantanopic defects. Cortical blindness results from penetrating or closed head trauma.

C. Traumatic Ocular Motor Nerve Palsies

1. Oculomotor Nerve (Cranial Nerve III) Injury

Oculomotor nerve palsy is secondary to either direct injury or indirect injury as a result of transtentorial herniation, skull fracture, or aneurysm of the posterior communicating artery. Injuries that cause a third nerve palsy are usually severe. *The patient who presents with a third nerve palsy after minor trauma should be evaluated for a vascular lesion or tumor.* The most common site of injury is in the subarachnoid space near the posterior clinoid space. Symptoms that present include binocular diplopia, which is oblique and variable depending on the position of gaze, and ptosis of the upper lid. The pupil can be dilated and unreactive, with loss of accommodation. Patients often have associated neurologic findings. CT and MRI imaging should be obtained to rule an associated skull fracture or aneurysm.

2.   Trochlear Nerve (Cranial Nerve IV) Injury
Most causes of trochlear nerve injury are contusion or avulsion of the nerve from the posterior aspect of the midbrain. Symptoms include binocular vertical or torsional (oblique) diplopia, which increases with downgaze and in the contralateral direction of gaze to the affected superior oblique muscle.

3.   Abducens Nerve (Cranial Nerve VI) Injury
Abducens nerve injury is the most common ocular nerve to be affected by trauma. It results from severe closed head injury. Acceleration deceleration forces are exerted on the nerve. Symptoms include binocular horizontal diplopia worse at distance and in the direction of the action of the paretic muscle. Symptoms can resolve and not require surgery, therefore the palsy should be observed for 6 months or more before considering corrective muscle surgery.

IX.   Adnexal Trauma (Orbit, Eyelid, and Lacrimal System Injury)

A.   Orbital Trauma
Orbital trauma can occur as a result of blunt or penetrating injury. The patient with orbital trauma can present with mild or severe injury. Evaluation of the globe to assess for ocular injury is important. CT is the imaging of choice to determine the type of fractures, locate intraorbital foreign bodies, and identify the secondary complications of trauma (e.g., hemorrhage, orbital emphysema).

1.   Orbital Contusion
Orbital contusion presents as periocular ecchymosis and edema, which is usually secondary to blunt trauma.

2.   Orbital Hemorrhage
Orbital hemorrhage is a collection of blood in the intraconal, extraconal, or subperiosteal space in the orbit that accumulates secondary to trauma. This condition presents as pain, decreased vision, afferent pupillary defect, motility limitation, tense orbit, proptosis, and increased IOP. Decreased vision can occur from compression of the optic nerve by the intraorbital contents. Urgent lateral canthotomy and cantholysis must be performed to release the eyelids and relieve pressure

in the orbit. Orbital CT imaging should be performed to assess the size and location of the hemorrhage.

3.   Intraorbital Foreign Body

Intraorbital foreign body must be suspected in the trauma patient presenting with significant edema, ecchymosis, proptosis, eyelid and conjunctival laceration, and motility limitation. Orbital CT is important to evaluate the type and location of the orbital foreign body. MRI is *contraindicated* in this situation because of the risk of further injury with the movement of the foreign body caused by the magnet. Small, inert foreign material (e.g., lead, steel, aluminum, glass, plastic, stone) are tolerated well and may not need immediate removal. Materials with high copper content are not well tolerated and should be removed promptly.

4.   Orbital Fractures

a.   Orbital Floor Fractures. Fractures of the orbital floor or "blowout floor fractures" are the most common orbital fractures. These fractures occur in the posterior medial portion of the orbital floor. Prolapse of orbital fat and muscle into the maxillary sinus can occur, causing motility limitation and pain (entrapment). Muscle entrapment should be repaired to decrease risk of muscle ischemia and permanent muscle damage and intractable diplopia. Other complications of floor fractures include globe ptosis, enophthalmos, diplopia, and hypesthesia of the lower face, cheek, and upper teeth. Proptosis of the affected area can occur if a retrobulbar hemorrhage is also present.

b.   Medial Orbital Wall Fractures. Fractures of the medial orbital wall can occur in isolation, or in association with orbital floor and nasoorbital ethmoid fractures. The medial wall consists of the lamina papyracea, a thin plate of bone that is easily broken with blunt crush injuries to the face. Patients can present with motility limitation (most severe on lateral gaze), globe retraction, enophthalmos, lid and orbital emphysema, telecanthus (widening of the area between the medial canthi), epistaxis, cerebrospinal fluid rhinorrhea, ecchymosis and edema.

c.   Lateral Wall and Zygomatico-Complex (ZMC) Fractures. Patients with lateral wall and zygomatico complex fractures complain of diplopia, numbness of the cheek (hypesthesia), and trismus (pain on chewing). On examination, patients have flattening of the cheek, globe displacement, lateral canthal dystopia (downward displacement of the lateral canthal tendon), enophthalmos, prominent superior sulcus, and lower lid retraction. These fractures can also have concomitant intraocular injury and vision loss. Orbital hemorrhage, edema, and emphysema can also occur. Treatment includes repair of the fractures with miniplate fixation or wiring, through an external approach or lateral canthotomy and inferior fornix approach.

d.   Orbital Roof Fractures. Orbital roof fractures, which are rare in adults, are secondary to severe crush injuries from falls, motor vehicle accidents, and blows to the head and face with heavy materials. Because of the lack of frontal sinus pneumatization, roof fractures are more commonly seen in children. Treatment of roof fractures should be done in conjunction with a neurosurgeon or otolaryngologist in cases with intracranial or sinus injury. Anterosuperior orbitotomy via a transcranial or coronal flap approach with subspecialty collaboration is used.

e.   Le Fort Fractures. Three types of Le Fort fractures are seen. Only Le Fort II and III fractures involve the orbit. Le Fort I fractures are low, transverse maxillary fractures. Le Fort II fractures involve the medial portion of the orbital floor, and nasal and lacrimal bones. Le Fort III fractures (i.e., craniofacial dysjunction) include the lateral wall, medial wall, and the orbital floor.

f.   Orbital Apex Fractures. The optic canal can be fractured in cases of orbital apex fractures, causing traumatic optic neuropathy and vision loss. Traumatic optic neuropathy can also occur in the absence of orbital apex or canal fracture.

g.   Nasoorbital Ethmoid Fractures. Nasoorbital ethmoid fractures, which are secondary to midface crush injuries, are associated with Le Fort fractures, floor fractures, and medial wall fractures. These injuries are associated with a high rate of vision loss and lacrimal system injury. Patients with these fractures also present with cerebrospinal fluid leaks 42% of the time. Treatment includes restoration of the lacrimal drainage system (see below) and repair of the fractures and medial canthal dehiscences through a coronal or external Lynch incision.

5.   Carotid-Cavernous Sinus Fistula
A high-flow fistula can occur between the cavernous sinus and the internal or exernal carotid arteries (or their arterial branches). Patients present with conjunctival injection and "corkscrew vessels," conjunctival edema, pulsatile proptosis, motility limitation, increased IOP, and an orbital bruit. Symptoms include pain and hearing a "swishing noise." Orbital imaging with CT and MRI show dilation of the superior ophthalmic vein, proptosis, and enlargement of the cavernous sinus. Angiography is required to identify and locate the fistula site. Vision loss occurs from corneal exposure caused by severe proptosis or optic neuropathy from severe orbital congestion and increased IOP. Treatment consists of embolization with coils or beads.

B. Eyelid Trauma

   1. Contusions

   Eyelid contusions are secondary to blunt injury, and present with ecchymosis and lid edema. These injuries are often associated with ocular injuries of varying degrees of severity.

   2. Avulsions

   Eyelid avulsions are tearing or shearing injuries. Avulsions of the eyelids occur most often medially, at the weakest portion of the eyelid. These avulsions can be partial or complete injuries.

   3. Eyelid Lacerations

   Eyelid lacerations are classified by (1) their anatomic location and (2) whether they involve the eyelid margin (**Fig. 17-4**). Foreign material must be removed (particularly, vegetative material) to avoid infection, dermal tattooing, and hypertrophic scarring. Most of these lacerations can usually be repaired in a minor procedure room or emergency room setting.

C. Lacrimal System Trauma

Trauma to the lacrimal drainage system occurs at one of three sites: the canaliculi, the lacrimal sac, and the nasolacrimal duct.

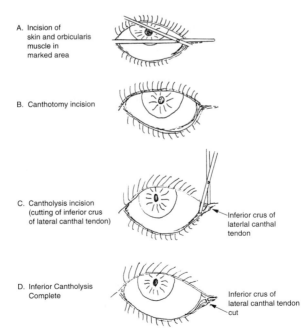

A. Incision of skin and orbicularis muscle in marked area

B. Canthotomy incision

C. Cantholysis incision (cutting of inferior crus of lateral canthal tendon) — Inferior crus of laterial canthal tendon

D. Inferior Cantholysis Complete — Inferior crus of lateral canthal tendon cut

Figure 17-4.   Lateral canthotomy and cantholysis.

1. Canalicular Laceration

Early repair of canalicular lacerations is essential to normal lacrimal function.

2. Lacrimal Sac Trauma

Tears and trauma of the lacrimal sac are seen in association with lacerations of the medial canthal angle and nasoorbital ethmoid fractures. Patients complain of tearing and pain. Treatment includes silicone intubation alone or dacryocystorhinostomy (creation of an anastomosis between the lacrimal sac and nasal cavity using a bony osteotomy) by an oculoplastic surgeon.

3. Nasolacrimal Duct Obstruction

Nasolacrimal duct obstruction is seen in nasoorbital ethmoid fractures or fractures associated with midfacial trauma. The nasolacrimal canals are damaged in midfacial fractures, with subsequent nasolacrimal duct obstruction. Silicone intubation of the nasolacrimal duct or dacryocystorhinostomy can relieve this disorder with varying degrees of success.

X. Pediatric Ocular Trauma

A. Epidemiology

Ocular trauma is the leading cause of noncongenital, unilateral blindness in American children. Children comprise a disproportionate number of those affected by ocular trauma, with approximately 29% of ocular trauma occurring in children under 10 years of age.

B. Special Considerations in Evaluation and Management of the Pediatric Patient

1. Obtaining a History and Performing the Physical Examination

Obtaining a history in a pediatric trauma case can be challenging. Some incidents can be poorly supervised or a result of child abuse, making an accurate account of events difficult to obtain, and the child may be unconscious. It is important to determine from a detailed history the mechanism of injury, timing of injury, witnesses to the event, and presence of supervision. Medical history is also important. Previous ocular surgeries, ocular trauma, and other ocular disorders should be elucidated. A history of amblyopia or "lazy eye" is important because this information helps to establish baseline visual acuity.

2. Risk of Amblyopia

Amblyopia is defined as decreased visual acuity not entirely explained by an organic lesion. The risk of amblyopia in the injured eye is present in any child younger than 9 to 10 years of age. There are many causes of amblyopia secondary to ocular and adnexal trauma. These include refractive disorders from corneal astigmatism after laceration repair, aphakia after cataract extraction, sensory deprivation from cataract, hyphema, vitreous hemorrhage, retinal injury, or traumatic ptosis. Diplopia from strabismus secondary to extraocular muscle palsy or muscle entrapment can force the child to suppress the visual image of the deviated eye and cause loss of vision and amblyopia. Thus, timely repair of corneal lacerations and retinal detachments, removal of traumatic cataracts, and treatment of ptosis and hyphema is important. Once this is completed, prevention of amblyopia should begin. This involves occlusion therapy with a patch or atropine penalization (pharmacologic blurring) of the eye with better visual acuity. Any child with an ocular or adnexal injury should be under the care of an ophthalmologist to monitor and treat amblyopia, in addition to restoring the integrity of the globe to prevent infection.

XI. Rehabilitation

Visual rehabilitation after ocular trauma is extremely important. Once the globe integrity has been restored and the eye has had ample time to heal, maximizing visual recovery is crucial. Patients with corneoscleral lacerations have significant corneal scarring and astigmatism. These patients can benefit from refraction, contact lens fitting, or corneal transplantation. Patients who are aphakic (without a lens) after lens extraction for traumatic cataract will benefit from a contact lens or secondary intraocular lens implant. Patients with residual diplopia from extraocular muscle injury or paresis should be seen for prism evaluation or surgical correction. It is essential that patients with subnormal vision caused by ocular trauma in one eye be prescribed polycarbonate (protective) eyewear with safety frames to be worn at all times. This protects the uninjured eye and prevents further injury to the traumatized eye.

Patients with severe open globe injuries and uveal disruption and prolapse are at risk for sympathetic ophthalmia, a rare disease in which inflammation of the normal (sympathizing) eye develops secondary to trauma of the injured (inciting) eye. Eyes with severe injury and complete loss of vision function are often surgically removed (enucleation) to prevent sympathetic ophthalmia.

SELECTED READING

Albert DA, Jakobiec FA, eds. *Principles and practice of ophthalmology.* Philadelphia: WB Saunders, 2000:5180.

Bosniak S, ed. *Principles and practice of ophthalmic plastic and reconstructive surgery.* Vol. 2. Philadelphia: WB Saunders, 1996:1085.

Friedman NJ, Pineda R, Kaiser PK. *The Massachusetts Eye and Ear Infirmary illustrated manual of ophthalmology.* Philadelphia: WB Saunders, 1998.

National Society to Prevent Blindness. *Vision problems in the US.* New York, 1980.

Negrel AD, Thylefors B. The global impact of eye injuries. Ophthalmic Epidemiol 1997;5(3):143–169.

Schein OD, Hibberd PL, Shingleton BJ, et al. The spectrum and burden of ocular injury. *Ophthalmology* 1988;95:300–305.

Shingleton BJ, Hersh PS, Kenyon KR. *Eye trauma.* Boston: Mosby Year Book, 1991.

Shingleton BJ, Mead MD. *The New England Eye Center handbook of eye emergencies.* Thorofare, NJ: Slack Inc., 1998.

The Wills Eye manual: office and emergency room diagnosis and treatment of eye disease, 3rd ed. Philadelphia: Lippincott Williams & Wilkins, 1999.

18

Neck Injuries

Ruben Peralta, MD, and Oscar J. Manrique, MD

I. Epidemiology and Mechanisms

In the neck, important anatomic structures are localized in a small area, unprotected by bone or muscular covering, making them vulnerable to anterior and lateral penetrating and blunt trauma. In general, 5% to 10% of all traumatic injuries involve the neck. In the late 1800s, mortality rates were reported to be 60% for cervical vascular injuries. During World War II, common carotid artery injuries were associated with a mortality rate as high as 47%. During the Vietnam War, mortality rates were reduced to 15%. Gradual improvement in evacuation, prehospital care, operative techniques, and postoperative management contributed to the continued decline in surgical mortality from cervical vascular injuries.

Penetrating injuries are most common and most severe, with fatality rates ranging from 1% to 2% for stab wounds, 5% to 12% for gunshots wounds, and up to 50% for rifle or shotgun blasts. The course of a stab wound is more limited and direct than that of a gunshot wound; however, seemingly innocuous cuts and lacerations have the potential to cause major damage. The path of a gunshot is totally unpredictable. Missiles have the ability to bounce, tumble, ricochet, shatter, and embolize. As the missile compresses the surrounding tissue on entry, a temporary cavity is produced. The higher the energy imparted to the tissue, the more extensive is the inapparent compressive damage.

Significant blunt neck trauma is less common, but can be particularly difficult to manage because it often involves the airway. Motor vehicle crashes account for most neck injuries, which are usually caused by acceleration deceleration forces. High-speed collisions and high-velocity missile wounds account for the most devastating problems.

II. Important Surgical Anatomy

The neck is divided into a number of anatomic triangles and zones (**Figs. 18-1 and 18-2**). The sternocleidomastoid (SCM) muscle divides the neck into the anterior and posterior triangles. The anterior triangle of the neck, bounded by the SCM, the midline, and the mandible, contains most of the major vascular and visceral structures, and carrying a high likelihood of vascular, airway, or esophageal injury in penetrating trauma. The posterior triangle, which is bounded by the SCM, the trapezius, and the clavicle, has relatively few important structures except inferiorly just above the clavicle. The neck has also been divided into three anatomic zones (**Fig. 18-2**).

A. Zone I

Zone I, which represents the base of the neck, extends from the clavicles to the cricoid cartilage. This area includes the proximal carotid, subclavian, and vertebral arteries; the upper lung; esophagus; trachea; and cervical nervous

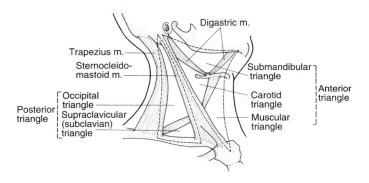

Figure 18-1. Neck triangles.

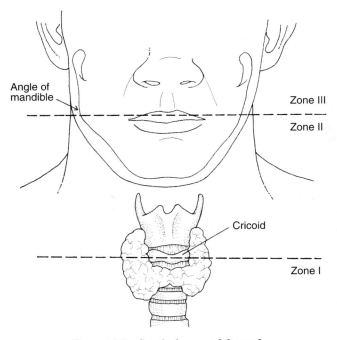

Figure 18-2. Surgical zones of the neck.

system (brachial plexus and spinal cord). Injuries at this zone carry the highest mortality rate because of the risk of major vascular and intrathoracic injuries.

B. Zone II

Zone II, the mid and largest area of the neck, extends from the cricoid cartilage to the angle of the mandible. The structures of this zone include the carotid and vertebral arteries, jugular vein, larynx, esophagus, trachea, vagus, and recurrent laryngeal nerve, as well as the spinal cord. The pharynx, distal carotid, and vertebral arteries; parotid gland; and cranial nerves can be injured in this area. This is the most frequent site of penetrating neck trauma, but carries a lower mortality rate than either zone I or III injuries because injury is usually apparent and exposure of vital structures is more readily accomplished.

C. Zone III

Zone III includes the area from the angle of the mandible to the base of the skull. The pharynx, parotid gland, distal carotid, vertebral arteries, and cranial nerves can be injured in this area. Vascular injuries high in this zone involving the upper portions of the internal carotid or vertebral arteries can be difficult to expose and manage.

III. Initial Evaluation

The major concern in any case of neck injury, whether blunt or penetrating, is the establishment and maintenance of an adequate airway. As with all trauma patients, systematic evaluation should be follow as indicated in the Advanced Trauma Life Support (ATLS) protocols (see Chapter 6, *Initial Evaluation and Resuscitation*). If a patient has any difficulty with oxygenation, ventilation, or depressed sensorium, endotracheal intubation should be performed. Ventilation assessment is also important because tracheal and esophageal injury can lead to a tension pneumothorax, requiring urgent decompression. Supplemental oxygen should always be administered, and adequate lighting and suction are essential. Clearance of the bony spine is discussed elsewhere (see Chapter 33, *Orthopedic Trauma 1*).

The history and physical examination are the most essential points in arriving at an early and accurate diagnosis of neck injury. The neurologic examination is key and should include the upper extremities, especially in cases with penetrating trauma to the lower neck. If the patient has sustained blunt or penetrating trauma or a cervical fracture is suspected, immobilize the neck in a neutral position until injury or lesion has been ruled out. The physical examination should be complete and focused on the structures in the neck that may be injured. An algorithm for clearance of the bony cervical spine is illustrated in **Table 18-1.**

Always suspect airway injury by the presence of abnormal ventilatory exchange, subcutaneous emphysema, bubbling of air from the wound, crepitus, hemoptysis, difficulty with phonation, and stridor. Laryngeal trauma is usually manifested by a fracture of the thyroid cartilage, subluxation of the arytenoid cartilages, dislocation of the cricothyroid joint, or subcutaneous emphysema. Patients with laryngeal trauma complain of tenderness, voice change, and, possibly, shortness of breath. Laryngeal intubation is contraindicated in suspected or proved laryngeal fractures because of the possibility of making a partial obstruction a complete one.

Table 18-1. Simplified cervical spine clearance protocol in patients with multiple trauma

This protocol only applies to patients with no signs or symptoms of possible spinal cord injury.

Both bones and ligaments must be cleared, but not necessarily at the same time. Often, the ligaments can be cleared by a negative clinical examination (**NCE**) when the patient has become sober or has recovered sufficiently from a concussion.

TO CLEAR THE BONES
Patient is awake, alert, sober, and without significant distracting injury: NCE[a]

All others:
  —Spiral computed tomography scan with out of collar lateral[b]
  OR
  —Adequate five-view cervical spine series[b]

TO CLEAR THE LIGAMENTS
Patient is awake, alert, sober, and without significant distracting injury:
  —NCE[a]
  OR
  —Active flexion-extension views (typically, if there is pain or distracting injury in those whose bones have been cleared)

All others:
–**If clinical suspicion is high:** passive flexion-extension views under fluoroscopic control by attending surgeon, orthopedist, or radiologist[b]
–**If clinical suspicion is low:** neck magnetic resonance imaging[b]

[a] A NCE can be performed only if the patient is sober, awake, alert, and without significant distracting injuries. It requires that the alert patient deny significant neck pain; physical examination reveal, no significant tenderness of the cervical spine; and the patient is able to move the neck through a full voluntary range of motion without significant pain.
[b] NO radiology study of the cervical spine is considered normal until there is an interpretation signed by an attending radiologist. Until such is available, the cervical spine is considered NOT clear and immobilization should be continued.

Evaluate potential vascular injuries bilaterally by carefully assessing pulses, bruits, the size and progression of hematomas, and evidence of neurologic deficits suggestive of strokes. Nerve injuries can be manifested by sensory deficits, Horner's syndrome, drooping of the mouth, or deviation of the tongue. Assess brachial plexus injuries, which can be detected by motor and sensory examination of the upper extremities. Penetrating wounds should not be probed, cannulated, or locally explored. Opening a wound tract can dislodge a clot, allowing uncontrollable bleeding. Although nasogastric tubes are often used in trauma patients, an exception should be made in the patient with a potential vascular injury of the neck. Because of the risk of dislodging a clot through gagging, retching, and vomiting, it is best to defer insertion until just before the induction of anesthesia in the operating room. The use of a nasogastric tube is important, because it can help identify an injury high in the digestive tract if blood is aspirated. It will also provide a pathway through which the gastric contents can be evacuated, reducing the chance of aspiration in the perianesthetic period.

Unstable patients with clear indications for surgery (e.g., shock, expanding hematomas, uncontrollable bleeding) must be taken directly to the operating room. If the patient is stable and diagnosis is in question, or additional information is required to better plan the operative procedure, a thorough secondary survey should be done. A secondary survey can include computed tomography (CT) angiography, arteriography, endoscopy, contrast studies, and magnetic resonance imaging (MRI) (**Fig. 18-3**).

IV.   Noninvasive Diagnostic Methods

Once the patient has been stabilized, the next step will be to operate promptly, perform diagnostic tests, or simply observe. No disagreement exists about the need for immediate surgery on patients who are hemodynamically unstable or who have had severe hemorrhage or expanding hematoma. Patients who are hemodynamically stable can have further diagnostic evaluation of the cardiovascular, respiratory, and digestive systems. Magnectic resonance imaging (MRI) is used to identify ligamentous injuries (Table 18-1).

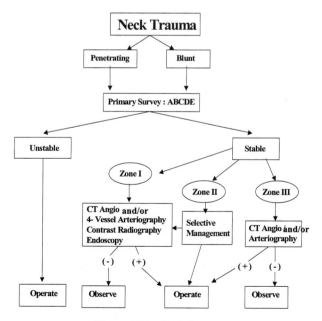

Figure 18-3.   Neck trauma.

A. **Radiography**
   1. **Neck**
   Lateral radiographs of the neck are indicated in all patients who have had penetrating injuries to the neck or severe blunt trauma above the shoulders. Anteroposterior and lateral films may reveal subcutaneous emphysema, airway compression, damage to laryngeal structures, tracheal deviation, cervical spine injury, and increased thickness of the anterior paravertebral tissues secondary to bleeding or edema. Normally, the distance between the posterior margin of the upper airway and the anterior margin of the vertebral bodies in front of C-3 and C-4 is usually no more than 4 to 5 mm, and less than 5 to 10 mm in front of C-5, C-6, and C-7. Interstitial emphysema along the facial planes of the neck or mediastinum following blunt trauma is almost diagnostic of tear in the aerodigestive tract. Position of missile fragments can also be noted and documented.
   2. **Chest**
   Radiographs of the chest may reveal subcutaneous emphysema, tracheal deviation, pneumothorax, hemothorax, fractured ribs, flail segments, pneumo or hemopericardium, or widening of the mediastinum. Traditional teaching is that, fractures of the first two ribs are highly associated with tracheobronchial, myocardial or vascular injury. In addition, chest radiography is particularly important with zone I injuries because of associated thoracic injuries in at least 27% of the patients.
B. **Endoscopy**
Pharyngoesophageal injuries, which can be difficult to diagnose, occur in up to 7% of penetrating injuries of the neck. Surgery is recommended for all patients for whom the course or extent of the penetrating wound suggests pharyngoesophageal damage. Endoscopy is the best method for evaluating the airway in the neck. Bronchoscopy and laryngoscopy, when done together, are highly accurate for detecting upper airway injuries; however when they are done individually, an occasional false negative result occurs. The combination of a barium swallow and rigid endoscopy, which should rule out most significant esophageal injuries, is recommended for any penetrating injury that is thought to be in proximity to the esophagus.
C. **Contrast Studies**
Extravasation of swallowed contrast material is diagnostic of a pharyngeal leak. A negative contrast swallow, however, is not reliable, particularly in the neck and especially when done with water soluble contrast. Therefore, a barium swallow, using anteroposterior and lateral views with cineradiography is recommended. Barium can cause increased inflammation and infection if it were to enter the mediastinum, but water soluble contrast can cause severe pneumonitis if it is aspirated.

D. Computed Tomography Scan

Proper CT scanning requires a cooperative or sedated patient and should not be attempted with an insecure airway injury or unstable vital signs. One of the advantages of CT scans is the ability to demonstrate most bony or soft-tissue injuries and to delineate fascial planes in detail. The extent of soft-tissue injury and hematoma formation can also be documented with CT. In addition, clinically subtle injuries to laryngeal cartilages can usually be demonstrated on CT.

Computed tomography scans are also useful for patients with neurologic deficits, whose condition can only be demonstrated by this technique. Such injuries can include occult cervical spine fractures, epidural hematomas, or a partially transected spinal cord. CT angiography can often demonstrate cervical vascular injuries that are not clinicaly obvious.

E. Catheter Angiography

Arteriography for cervical trauma is extremely reliable. In the absence of obvious arterial injury, precisely performed arteriography is an effective way to evaluate arterial integrity. Documentation of vessel patency can be important to intraoperative decisions about repair or reconstruction in patients with neurologic deficits. Arteriography is generally recommended for patients with injuries in either zone I or III. Less agreement is seen about the need for angiography with zone II injuries, as operative access to this area is relatively easy to obtain. Angiography will reliably rule out an injury, allowing those who advocate nonoperative management to observe the patient with confidence. In addition, angiography can demonstrate unsuspected vertebral artery injuries that might otherwise go undetected at the time of operation.

This technique is also recommended in selected patients with blunt trauma. Blunt injuries to the carotid vessels are relatively uncommon, but can cause thrombosis and delayed neurologic deficits, resulting in mortality rates of up to 40%. The acquisition of multiple views, composed of at least an anteroposterior and lateral view, plus oblique views, and the use of subtraction techniques and image magnification are all helpful in identifying subtle injuries. With the increasing technology of new generation CT scanners, it appears that the CT angiography protocol will help in making a precise diagnosis, will be an excellent screening tool in the near future, and will make others test unnecessary.

V. Indications for Surgery

Neck exploration should be performed in the operating room under general anesthesia. Clear indications for surgery include unstable patient, uncontrollable bleeding, expanding hematomas, and stridor, regardless of the zone of injury (I, II, III).

Of patients with penetrating neck trauma (depending on the mechanism), 25% to 50% present with obvious signs of injury requiring prompt operation. An additional 10% to 20% of patients without clinical signs of injury are discovered to have significant vascular, esophageal, or airway injury after further diagnostic testing. Some controversy exists with regard to the evaluation of stable patients with penetrating zone II injuries. While some advocate diagnostic neck exploration, others advise non-operative diagnostic methods to reduce the negative exploration rate.

VI. Techniques of Neck Exploration

The first priority of neck exploration is always to ensure airway patency. The patient should be placed in supine position, with the neck in extension and head rotated away from the side to be explored. If any doubt of cervical spine injury exists, however, the neck should be maintained in a neutral position. Preparation and draping should extend from the chin to the umbilicus and should include all the anterior and lateral neck and chest so that a median sternotomy or anterolateral thoracotomy can be performed, if necessary. No limited explorations or probing of neck injuries should be conducted in the emergency department.

A. Unilateral Neck

Unilateral neck explorations are usually best done through an incision along the anterior border of the SCM muscle. This incision provides ready access to the trachea, thyroid gland, larynx, and carotid artery. Care must be taken to avoid damaging the sympathetic chain, which lies posterior to the carotid sheath on the prevertebral muscles.

B. Midneck

For patients whose preoperative evaluation suggests bilateral neck injuries or damage of the larynx and trachea, a low "collar" incision 1 to 2 cm above the heads of the clavicles should be performed. When injuries are limited just to the larynx, a horizontal incision placed over the mid-portion of the thyroid cartilage can be done.

C. Lower Neck

The right subclavian artery, both subclavian veins, and distal two thirds of the left subclavian artery can usually be exposed through a supraclavicular incision. If the origin of the innominate, left common carotid, or right subclavian arteries need to be exposed, a median sternotomy incision with supraclavicular extension should be performed. Control of the proximal third of the left subclavian artery is achieved through a left aneolateral thoracotomy in the third intercoastal space. As previously described, distal control of the left subclavian artery requires a supraclavicular incision. For definitive repair of left subclavian injuries a trapdoor incision may be required in some cases. (see Chapter 22, Vascular Trauma 1: Great Vessels and Neck).

D. Upper Neck

Structures near the base of the skull can be accessed by dividing the SCM muscle near its insertion into the mastoid process or dislocating the temporomandibular joint by pulling the mandible forward. Avoid injury of the hypoglossal nerve and the spinal accessory nerve.

VII. Vascular Injuries

A. Presentation

Blood vessels are the most commonly injured structures in the neck. Arterial injury accounts for approximately 12% to 13% of all penetrating neck injuries, whereas the incidence of venous injury is approximately 18%. The mortality rate for vascular injury in the neck is approximately 15%, making this often a life-threatening condition.

B. Diagnosis

Careful inspection, palpation, and auscultation of the neck, face, upper extremities, and chest should be performed. Vascular injury can be obvious, as evidenced by active hemorrhage, either from the neck wound or the presence of oral or pharyngeal penetration from the mouth. Other suggestive signs include an expanding hematoma, a bruit indicating an arteriovenous fistula, or absence of carotid, superficial temporal, facial, or upper extremity pulses. In addition, carotid or vertebral artery injuries can present with hemiplegia, hemiparesis, aphasia, monocular blindness, and decreased level of consciousness. A clear or milky drainage from a wound on the left side of the neck indicates a thoracic duct injury.

C. Management

The initial management of any patient with neck injury depends on how stable is the patient, current conditions, and compromised zones. Management can be divided into two categories: mandatory operation versus selective observation. If the patient is hemodynamically unstable, surgical exploration is indicated. After controlling the airway, the next priorities are control of bleeding and treatment of shock. External bleeding is best controlled by precise digital pressure.

Intraoral bleeding is more difficult to control but gauze packing can facilitate hemostasis. Intravenous lines should be placed in the contralateral upper extremity. In zone I, penetrating wounds are likely to injure the large vessels in the thoracic outlet. Preoperative arteriography is recommended in all patients with zone I penetration if they are hemodynamically stable and do not have evidence of active hemorrhage. Arteriography is recommended because zone I injuries are commonly clinically occult and because extensive surgical exposure, including thoracotomy, may be required for their control and repair. Similarly, arteriography is recommended for penetrating injuries in zone III.

In addition, surgical exposure of the internal carotid and vertebral vessels at the base of the skull can be difficult and precise definition of the anatomy and extent of the injury by arteriography can alter the operative approach. Arteriography will also identify thrombosis of the distal intracranial vessels and help assess the adequacy of crossover circulation in the circle of Willis. The role of angiography in identifying injuries in zone II is more controversial. Surgical access and exposure for symptomatic vascular injuries is relatively easy, and the morbidity from surgical exploration of zone II is very low. The indications for neck exploration in stable patients with zone II penetrating injuries is evolving.

The morbidity and mortality for patients having repair of the carotid artery are significantly lower than those who have ligation (15% to 50%) unless there is an established neurologic defect. If a patient is unstable or has another life-threatening condition, ligation is indicated. Distal bleeding control of the carotid artery can be achieved by placing a Fogarty catheter distally and inflating the balloon. The patient should also receive systemic heparinization, if not contraindicated, and, if the repair requires more than 10 to 15 minutes. Intrapetrous injury, clot, or dissection of the internal carotid artery can be managed with embolization. Vertebral artery injury, which is uncommon, is often not discovered except by angiography. The hemodynamically stable patient can be managed by surgical ligation, radiologic embolization, or observation. In venous injuries, ligation is acceptable if the contralateral vein is not injured. Always attempt to prevent embolism in these injuries.

VIII. Cervical Esophageal Injuries

    A. Presentation

Esophageal and pharyngeal injuries are the third most common type of injury in penetrating neck trauma. Because of the intimate anatomic relationship of the esophagus to major vascular structures in the mediastinum, many patients with esophageal injuries die at the scene of the traumatic event. Penetrating wounds of the esophagus are infrequent. Once a decision is made to explore for esophageal injury, a meticulous, exploration is mandated.

    B. Diagnosis

Esophageal injury is often difficult to diagnose. Initially, symptoms are subtle or absent, and the diagnosis is often overlooked, even in the presence of major injuries to adjacent structures, until complications resulting from salivary contamination have occurred. A factor that challenges the early diagnosis is the low index of suspicion, which too often delays diagnosis and increases the likelihood of complications and death. In addition, making the diagnosis is relatively difficult, particularly when the esophageal laceration is associated with additional major injuries. Subcutaneous emphysema in the neck, mediastinal emphysema seen on chest x-ray film, or blood recovered from a nasogastric tube following a transthoracic penetrating injury are some of the findings that seriously raise the possibility of esophageal perforation. Contrast esophagography is indicated to confirm the diagnosis, and to localize the site of perforation.

    C. Management

Patients with penetrating neck trauma who present with minimal clinical findings should be evaluated initially with contrast studies. A high index of suspicion for esophageal injuries must be maintain because they can be missed by physical examination, radiologically and endoscopically. If either of the diagositc evaluation tools is positive, then neck exploration is recommended. if the results of esophagography are equivocal, then esophagoscopy should be performed. If contrast studies (CT Angio/arteriography, esophagography and endoscopy are negative, then the patient can be observed safely.

    Otherwise, after identification of all wounds, devitalized tissue is débrided and minor injuries are closed in one or two layers. Larger esophageal wounds require débridement and mobilization of the esophagus to allow for wound closure without tension. Air insufflation of the esophagus through a proximal nasogastric tube can help to localize the esophageal wound that is not readily apparent on exploration. All esophageal injuries are drained. Soft, Silastic suction drains are preferred. If there is extensive tissue loss to prelude primary repair, a cervical esophagostomy should be performed as a temporizing measure. Definitive complex reconstruction of the esophagus should be done at a later time.

IX. **Laryngotracheal Injuries**
   A. **Presentation**
   Approximately 10% to 20% of patients with penetrating wounds of the neck sustain injuries to the laryngotracheal complex. Blunt laryngeal trauma typically results from an anterior impact that drives the larynx posteriorly against the rigid cervical spine. In general, blunt and penetrating laryngotracheal injuries can usually be suspected based on a combination of location of the neck wound, history, physical examination, and plain films of the neck.
   B. **Diagnosis**
   Laryngotracheal injuries are frequently occult and often initially overlooked as attention is directed to injuries of the head, face, and thorax. Delayed recognition of blunt laryngeal trauma is the single greatest contributor to mortality. Hoarseness is the most common symptom, followed by shortness of breath, inability to tolerate supine position, pain, dysphagia, and aphonia. Tenderness is the most common clinical sign identified, followed by subcutaneous emphysema, neck contusion, tracheal deviation, and hemoptysis. Unlike blunt laryngeal trauma, penetrating injuries to the trachea and larynx are usually readily apparent and obvious in their clinical presentation. Subcutaneous emphysema, pain, hoarseness, and respiratory distress are all hallmarks of tracheal injury. These symptoms and signs, however, do not correlate with the severity of the injury and they are not accurate indicators of the need for surgical repair. The definitive diagnosis of laryngeal injury depends on adequate visualization of the larynx and trachea. For this reason, diagnostic studies such as flexible and rigid laryngoscopy, bronchoscopy, and computed tomography should be performed.
   C. **Management**
   As with any trauma victim, the first priority for those with laryngotracheal injuries is to secure an adequate airway. Operative repair is not usually required for patients with simple laryngeal edema, hematomas without mucosal disruption, small lacerations of the endolarynx not involving the anterior commissure or the free margin of the vocal cord, and small lacerations of the of the supraglottic larynx. Indications of primary open repair of the larynx include all penetrating tracheal or laryngeal wounds, vocal cord disruption, mucosal tears with exposed cartilage, thyroid separation, thyroid or cricoid cartilage fractures, and hypopharyngeal perforations. The basic points of

operative care are débridement of devitalized cartilage, reduction of cartilaginous fractures, mucosal coverage of exposed cartilage, and closure of tracheal defects. Simple tracheal lacerations can be repaired in a single layer with absorbable suture. Complex tracheal injuries require tracheostomy. In extensive injuries, delayed reconstruction with cartilage graft and flaps may be necessary. Prompt diagnosis and treatment results in a lower rate of infection, decreased formation of granulation tissue, and reduced scarring and stenosis.

X. Postoperative Care

In the immediate postoperative period, patients with injuries to the neck must be observed for hemodynamic stability. Three key assessments include (1) patency of the airway, (2) evidence of controlled bleeding, and (3) maintenance of neurologic function. It is important to assess the adequacy of the airway before extubation. Patients must also be continually evaluated for delayed chest problems (e.g., pneumothorax, hemothorax, emphysema, mediastinitis). Drains are left in place long enough to serve the purpose for which they were inserted. The use of antibiotics is less well defined. In the absence of aerodigestive injuries, little indication is seen for their use.

SELECTED READING

Bee TK, and Fabian TC. Penetrating neck trauma. In: Cameron JL, ed. Current surgical therapy. St. Louis: Mosby 2001:1170–1174.

Borgstrom D. and Weigelt J. Neck: aerodigestive tract. In: Ivatury RR, Cayten CG, eds. *The textbook of penetrating trauma*. Baltimore: Williams & Wilkins, 1996:479–487.

Diebel RF. Injuries of the neck. In: Wilson RF, Walt AJ, eds. *Management of trauma. Pitfalls and practice*. Baltimore: Williams & Wilkins, 1996:270–282.

Gracias VH, Reilly PM, Philpott J, et al. Computed tomography in the evaluation of penetrating trauma. *Arch Surg* 2001;136:1231–1235.

Ivatury RR. Esophagus. In: Ivatury RR, Cayten CG, eds. *The textbook of penetrating trauma*. Baltimore: Williams & Wilkins, 1996:555–563.

Jacobson LE and Gomez GA. Neck. In: Ivatury RR, Cayten CG, eds. *The textbook of penetrating trauma*. Baltimore: Williams & Wilkins, 1996:258–270.

Jurkovich GJ. Definitive care phase: neck injuries. In: Lazar MWM, Greenfield J, Oldham JK, et al., eds. *Surgery. Scientific principles and practice*. Baltimore: Lippincott Williams & Wilkins, 2001:311–319.

Lucas CE and Ledgerwood AM. Neck: vessels. In: Ivatury RR, Cayten CG, eds. *The textbook of penetrating trauma*. Baltimore: Williams & Wilkins, 1996:488–496.

Peralta R, Hurford WE. Airway trauma. *Int Anesthisiol Clin* 2000;38(3):111–127.

Schenarts PJ, Diaz J, Kaiser C, et al. Prospective comparison of admission computed tomographic scan and plain films of the upper cervical spine in trauma patients with altered mental status. *J Trauma* 2001;51(4):663–669.

Thal ER. Injury of the neck. In: Feliciano DV, et al., eds. *Trauma*. Norwalk: Appleton and Lange, 1996:329–343.

19

Chest Trauma 1: Chest Wall, Pleural Space, and Lung Parenchyma

Christopher R. Morse, MD,
and James S. Allan, MD

I. Introduction: Background and Epidemiology

Estimates are that one quarter of all traumatic deaths occur secondary to thoracic injuries and ensuing complications from them. Blunt trauma to the chest (principally from motor vehicle collisions) accounts for 70% to 80% of all thoracic trauma, and one third of all patients hospitalized after a motor vehicle collision have evidence of thoracic trauma. Penetrating injuries (primarily from gunshot and stab wounds) account for the remaining 20% to 30% of traumatic thoracic injuries.

The most frequent cause of immediate death from a thoracic trauma is an injury to the heart or thoracic aorta. Rapid treatment of other serious intrathoracic processes that can cause respiratory and hemodynamic compromise (e.g., pneumothorax, hemothorax, pericardial tamponade), however, can be lifesaving.

II. Mechanisms of Injury in Thoracic Trauma

Thoracic trauma has been classically described as either "blunt" or "penetrating," and certain mechanisms of trauma are highly associated with particular patterns of traumatic injury. An awareness of the clinical significance of a certain mechanism of injury, when considered in conjunction with specific anatomic findings on physical examination, allows better assessment and prioritization of a patient's medical needs.

A. Blunt Chest Wall Trauma

Blunt chest trauma typically occurs as a consequence of experiencing a rapid acceleration-deceleration force or as a result of extrinsic thoracic compression (crush injuries). These mechanisms of injury are most commonly seen in motor vehicle collisions, but also can be seen in association with falls, assaults, and other circumstances where an external force is applied to the chest wall. Simple rib fractures (without significant pulmonary contusion) constitute most blunt thoracic injuries. More complex injuries, including pneumothorax, hemothorax, flail chest, pulmonary contusion, and pulmonary laceration, can also be encountered.

Acceleration-deceleration injuries, such as those sustained in a motor vehicle collision, should raise suspicion for shear injuries to the bronchi and thoracic aorta. Blunt force injuries tend to damage those structures immediately adjacent to the point of impact. Typical patterns of blunt-force injury include:

1. Rib fracture or flail segment with an associated pulmonary contusion

2. Rib fracture or flail segment with an associated pneumothorax and/or hemothorax
3. Sternal fracture with underlying cardiac contusion (steering wheel impact)

In addition, age is an important consideration in the evaluation of blunt chest wall trauma. The increased flexibility of a child's chest wall places children at considerable risk for injury to the thoracic viscera, even in the relative absence of obvious chest wall trauma. Conversely, elderly patients are significantly more susceptible to extensive chest wall trauma (and secondary visceral injury) from mechanisms of injury that involve relatively weaker impact forces.

B.   Penetrating Chest Wall Trauma

Penetrating thoracic trauma has its highest incidence in young adulthood and is seldom seen in children and the elderly. Most penetrating injuries to the chest wall occur as a result of gunshot or stab wounds, and patients who survive the initial injury often present with hemodynamic and respiratory compromise from pneumothorax, hemothorax, or pericardial tamponade. Gunshot injures can be caused by high-velocity projectiles (typical of rifle injuries) or low-velocity projectiles (typical of handgun injuries). Injuries that occur from low-velocity projectiles tend to be confined to the projectile's actual path of penetration. Most civilian handgun injuries fall into this category. High-velocity projectiles, however, induce significant collateral damage in an injury zone that radiates perpendicular to the projectile's path of penetration. The severity of a shotgun injury is highly dependent on the patient's distance from the shotgun discharge. In general, penetrating chest trauma most frequently results in pneumothorax, but a plethora of injuries can be found, depending on the path and force of the penetrating object.

With penetrating wounds are seen predictable patterns of injury, depending on the specific area of the chest involved. Wounds to the upper chest raise the potential for injury to the following structures: trachea, great vessels, esophagus, thoracic duct, lung parenchyma, and bronchi. Penetrating wounds to the middle third of the chest raise the potential for injury to the following structures: heart, aorta, lung parenchyma, and bronchi. Because of the dome-shaped configuration of the diaphragm and respiratory movement, injuries from penetrating wounds to the lower third of the chest can be variable. They often involve both intrathoracic and intraabdominal structures, including the heart, descending aorta, lung parenchyma and bronchi, diaphragm, abdominal viscera (including the esophagus, diaphragm, spleen, liver, stomach, colon, and pancreas), and abdominal vasculature (including the aorta and its branches, inferior vena cava, and portal vein).

III.   General Evaluation and Management of the Thoracic Trauma Patient

    A.   Initial Evaluation and Management

        1.   Airway

        The initial evaluation and management of any trauma patient follows a proscribed sequence of priorities.

First, it is essential to establish a patient airway. If a patient is conscious and alert, airway management may simply entail careful observation. However, the patient with a questionable or compromised airway generally requires intubation (with attention to cervical spine immobilization). Occasionally, surgical cricothyrotomy may be necessary when intubation is not otherwise possible.

In considering the thoracic trauma patient, keep in mind that semielective endotracheal intubation can often exacerbate a patient's condition for several reasons. First, the conversion of a spontaneously breathing patient to one who is being ventilated with positive pressure greatly increases the risk of developing a tension pneumothorax or an air embolism. Second, positive-pressure ventilation also impairs venous return, which may already be compromised in the hypovolemic trauma patient. Third, semi-elective intubation usually requires the administration of pharmacologic sedation, which can blunt a patient's life-sustaining sympathetic response at a most inopportune time. When possible, nonemergent intubation (and the administration of any sedation) should be performed in the operating room after the patient has been prepped and draped (while conscious).

2. Breathing

Following airway management, attention is directed to ensuring adequate ventilation and oxygenation. It is important to recognize that ventilation and oxygenation are two related, but separate, processes. To this end, it is crucial that a trauma victim is able to exchange a sufficient minute volume to clear carbon dioxide to prevent (or compensate for) the development of an acidosis of any cause. It is also important that oxygenation is optimized by the administration of high levels of supplemental oxygen.

At this point, those intrathoracic injuries that could be contributing to respiratory embarrassment must also be addressed. This may require the following:

1. Needle or tube decompression of a tension pneumothorax
2. Nasogastric or orogastric decompression of a distended stomach, especially in the presence of a diaphragmatic injury
3. Semiocclusive coverage of an open pneumothorax in the spontaneously breathing patient (sucking chest wound)

3. Circulation

Following management of the airway and respiration, attention should be directed toward insuring that a patient has adequate perfusion. Adequate perfusion is defined simply as the circulation of a sufficient volume of blood, at a sufficient pressure, with a sufficient oxygen carrying capacity to meet the metabolic needs of the end-organs (most importantly, the brain, heart, kidneys, and liver).

The first step to insuring adequate perfusion is to establish immediate control of all sources of external bleeding. This can usually be accomplished by direct external pressure. Next, intravascular volume must be rapidly restored by the intravenous administration of isotonic crystalloid followed by blood products when the estimated blood loss is significant. It is important neither to over-dilute the patient with crystalloid nor to over-transfuse with blood products. A hematocrit of 25% is adequate for most trauma patients without other significant underlying diseases.

If the patient's clinical condition continues to deteriorate despite the administration of several liters of intravascular fluid or if the patient has an ongoing volume requirement, it is likely that the patient is bleeding internally. Sources of internal bleeding in the thoracic trauma patient include:

1. Intercostal arterial bleeding
2. Great vessel injury
3. Parenchymal and hilar lung injuries
4. Penetrating cardiac injuries or cardiac rupture

Attention must then be directed to the immediate identification of the source of this bleeding and correcting it surgically. If a hemothorax is suspected on the basis of either the mechanism of injury or on physical examination, the rapid insertion of a chest tube can be both diagnostic and therapeutic. It is not necessary to wait for radiographic evidence of pneumothorax or hemothorax before performing tube thoracostomy.

At this point, other causes of circulatory collapse that can be quickly corrected must be identified. They can include:

1. Tension pneumothorax requiring needle or tube decompression
2. Pericardial tamponade necessitating emergency surgical decompression (see Chapter 21, *Chest Trauma 3*).

Finally, consider other less common causes of shock in the thoracic trauma patient such as:

1. Cardiac contusion
2. Air emboli
3. Loss of vascular tone caused by spinal cord injury

B. Secondary Survey
   1. History
In addition to the common elements of a medical history (previous medical history, medications, allergies), particular attention should be paid to the circumstances surrounding the traumatic event. For example, in a motor vehicle collision, be aware of the presence of adverse prognosticators such as the following:

1. High-speed collision
2. Unrestrained occupant
3. Person ejected from the vehicle
4. Prolonged extrication time
5. Death or a major injury at the scene

As another example, in gunshot injures, try to determine factors such as the type and caliber of the weapon used and the distance from which it was fired.

It is also important to be aware of any medications that could impair the patient's ability to survive a traumatic injury. In particular, identify the patient who is taking beta-blockers or anticoagulants.

2. Physical Examination

The physical examination of the trauma patient has been reviewed extensively in Chapters 6 and 8. In the patient with suspected chest trauma, it is important to inspect and palpate the chest and back, looking for signs of penetrating or blunt trauma. Particular attention should be paid to observing any chest wall asymmetry, paradoxic respiratory motion, soft tissue injury, point tenderness, and subcutaneous emphysema. Notice the position of the trachea as well. Inspect neck veins because distended neck veins can suggest a tension pneumothorax or cardiac tamponade. (Note that the absence of neck vein distension does not rule out these entities, particularly if the patient is hypovolemic.) Auscultation of breath and heart sounds is also an important modality in the early identification of intrathoracic injuries.

3. Diagnostic Modalities

Of all the diagnostic modalities that can be used in the evaluation of chest trauma, the anteroposterior (AP) chest radiograph is of paramount importance. Most major intrathoracic injuries can be identified on a plain chest radiograph. Some potential findings on the chest film include pneumothorax, hemothorax, pneumomediastinum, mediastinal widening, bony chest wall injuries, and diaphragmatic rupture. Foreign bodies in the soft tissues or chest cavity can also be identified, and it is usually helpful to localize all penetrating wounds with radiopaque markers before radiography. Prior placement of an orogastric or nasogastric tube is also helpful, particularly when diaphragmatic rupture is suspected. If the patient's condition does not warrant a chest computed tomography (CT) scan or emergent operative intervention, an upright posteroanterior (PA) and lateral chest radiograph should be obtained because these radiographs have a greater sensitivity to intrathoracic injuries.

For stable patients, the contrast-enhanced CT of the chest is also an essential component in the evaluation of chest trauma. The chest CT scan is particularly helpful when the mediastinal contour is abnormal on the initial chest radiograph. The chest CT scan also provides detailed anatomic information about chest wall and intrathoracic injuries and has recently supplanted other modalities (i.e., angiography) in the assessment of great vessel injuries. Keep in mind that hemodynamically unstable trauma patients generally should not be sent to the CT scanner. This group of patients usually requires immediate operative exploration and stabilization.

Other common diagnostic tests useful in the evaluation of chest trauma include the electrocardiogram, arterial blood gas analysis, contrast arteriography or aortography, surface and transesophageal echocardiography, bronchoscopy, and thoracoscopy.

IV. Treatment of Specific Traumatic Conditions of the Chest Wall, Pleural Space, and Lung Parenchyma

A. Rib Fractures

Rib fractures, which are the most common thoracic injury, are reported in 35% to 40% of all trauma patients. With the increased use of CT scanning in the evaluation of chest trauma, a greater number of subtle rib fractures are being found that are not readily apparent on the chest radiograph. Ribs four through ten are those most often fractured, and these fractures tend to occur near the angle of the rib because of external compression of the rib cage. Fractures that occur posteriorly usually imply direct blunt force trauma to the affected region, and are often associated with greater underlying injuries (e.g., pulmonary contusion). This is particularly true of fractures of the first and second ribs, given the high-energy transfer necessary to injure these well-protected ribs. Recognize that first and second rib fractures carry a 64% rate of association with other major intrathoracic injury. Because of the particular risk of associated aortic injury in these patients, many authors recommend routine angiography or CT in this subpopulation and also in patients with scapula fractures. Additionally, closed head injuries and significant abdominal injuries are more common in the setting of high rib and scapula fractures (35% and 33%, respectively). Fracture of ribs ten through twelve should raise suspicion for abdominal visceral injury. In both of these scenarios (fracture of the first and second rib or fracture of ribs ten through twelve), a hemodynamically stable patient should have a CT scan of the chest, abdomen, or both, given the high association of aortic and abdominal injuries respectively.

Focal pleuritic chest wall pain and point tenderness on physical examination are the most common findings in patients with rib fractures. In the absence of other associated injuries, the management of rib fractures focuses on pain control to avoid splinting and hypoventilation, which can ultimately result in posttraumatic pneumonia. One or two rib fractures can be managed with oral pain medications on an outpatient basis. Three or more fractures, however, can mandate more intensive pain control. Epidural anesthesia has been shown to result in lower morbidity and mortality rates than parenteral narcotics with multiple rib fractures. Another alternative pain control method is an intercostal nerve block. Intercostal nerve blocks need repeat administration, however, and a risk of pneumothorax is seen with the administration of these nerve blocks. Intrapleural catheter anesthesia has also been used in the treatment of rib fractures. Again, a risk is seen of pneumothorax, and intrapleural catheter anesthesia has been shown to be less effective than epidural anesthesia. Transcutaneous electric nerve stimulation has been described for chronic pain from rib fractures, but it has no role in the acute setting. Early mobilization and aggressive chest physiotherapy (either by manual percussion or by high-frequency chest wall oscillation) and pulmonary toilet are also important in the management of rib fractures. If the patient is unable to clear secretions, bronchoscopy may be indicated. There is no indication for operative fixation for simple rib fractures. Taping, casting, and binding also have been shown to increase the incidence of posttraumatic pneumonias and, therefore, should be avoided.

Outcome data for rib fractures are related to the number of ribs injured, the patient's age, and the patient's underlying pulmonary status. Reported mortality from isolated fib fractures in the elderly is as high as 10% to 20% because of the decreased ability to clear secretions leading to the development of atelectasis and subsequent pneumonia. The mortality from rib fractures in children is also a surprisingly high (5%). This mortality principally results from other associated intrathoracic injuries, as the energy transfer required to fracture ribs in children is much higher because of their flexible thoracic cages.

B. Flail Chest

By definition, a flail chest is the fracturing of at least three consecutive ribs in two locations each. The flail chest can also involve the disruption of the costochondral junction(s). The key defining feature of a flail chest is the finding of a segment of chest wall that has become destabilized and, thus, is able to move paradoxically with respiration. Flail chest occurs in an estimated 5% of thoracic trauma. The presence of a flail chest should increase the suspicion for major intrathoracic injury. It occurs more commonly in the elderly and only occurs in 1% of children after significant thoracic trauma because of the flexibility of the chest wall. The diagnosis is most often made during the initial physical examination, but a flail segment can also be identified on chest radiograph or CT scan.

The paradoxical chest wall motion in flail chest leads to a reduction in vital capacity and ineffective ventilation, thus increasing the work of breathing. Initially, it was thought that the respiratory embarrassment caused by a flail chest resulted principally from ineffective air movement. It is now known, however, that underlying pulmonary contusions and splinting secondary to pain are the dominant causes of respiratory failure with a flail chest.

With this recognition, management of the patient with flail chest focuses on effective pain control and aggressive pulmonary toilet, as described above for simple rib fractures. Several operative interventions for stabilization of the flail chest have been described; however, chest wall fixation is usually performed only when a thoracotomy is done for other indications and the flail segment is large.

If the flail chest is associated with a large pulmonary contusion (see below), it may be necessary to intubate the patient to provide ventilatory assistance and to optimize oxygen delivery. Keep in mind that intubation is done for respiratory insufficiency, not just simply to "splint" the chest wall. The patient can be extubated when pain control is achieved, pulmonary mechanics are adequate, and oxygenation is acceptable.

The overall outcome of patients who sustain a flail chest injury has improved with the institution of selective intubation and mechanical ventilation. Mortality rates have declined from approximately 35% in the 1990s to approximately 15% in the early 1990s. The remaining mortality is thought to be secondary to underlying pulmonary contusions and other associated injuries. Further, some evidence indicates that flail chest can have long-term consequences. Impaired pulmonary function has been documented with abnormal spirometry in patients who have dyspnea and persistent pain following injury.

C. Sternal Fractures

Sternal fractures are an uncommon injury present in only 4% of patients involved in motor vehicle collisions. The incidence is highest in elderly patients and usually results from sternal impact against a steering wheel. Sternal fractures are typically transverse fractures located in the upper half of the sternum. They are frequently associated with other significant thoracic injuries, including cardiac contusion. On physical examination, swelling, deformity, and point tenderness may be noted. The patient may have an overlying hematoma or ecchymosis. Occasionally, the imprint of a steering wheel can be identified (the "steering wheel sign.") In the radiologic evaluation of a potential sternal fracture, a lateral chest film is necessary, as the fracture is rarely visible on the AP film. Management of sternal fractures includes achieving adequate pain control and pulmonary toilet. In addition, cardiac contusion must be ruled out or treated (see Chapter 21, *Chest Trauma 3*). Severely displaced sternal fractures with disruption of the sternocostal junctions may require operative reduction and fixation. Posterior dislocation or fracture-dislocation of the sternoclavicular joints can also result in both tracheal and superior vena caval compromise by means of extrinsic compression. If necessary, a closed reduction of this injury can be accomplished by extending the shoulders and elevating the clavicular heads with the aid of a pointed clamp (e.g., a surgical towel clip).

D. Pulmonary Contusion

Pulmonary contusion is the result of hemorrhage into the alveolar and interstitial space without gross parenchymal disruption. Pulmonary contusions should be suspected in any patient with significant blunt chest wall trauma. Contusions are usually apparent on the initial CT scan of the chest, but may not always be seen on the initial chest radiograph. In the first few hours to days following the injury, however, a significant amount of focal edema can develop in the region of a pulmonary contusion, leading to a worsening clinical and radiographic picture.

From both a clinical and radiographic viewpoint, it is occasionally difficult to differentiate pulmonary contusion from aspiration pneumonitis or pneumonia, which is also common in trauma patients. Several important differences, however, help make this distinction. First, pulmonary contusions are present immediately following the trauma, whereas an infiltrate from aspiration can take hours to days to appear on radiographs. Second, infiltrates from aspiration are usually confined to specific pulmonary segments, whereas pulmonary contusions are found immediately adjacent to an area of chest wall trauma. Finally, the patient with aspiration can have increased tracheal secretions on suctioning or on bronchoscopy.

Most pulmonary contusions are small and contribute little to overall morbidity. Larger pulmonary contusions, however, lead to decreased lung compliance and the development of V/Q mismatching, resulting in hypoxemia and increased work of breathing. Occasionally, large pulmonary contusions can lead to the acute respiratory distress syndrome (ARDS) and the need for mechanical ventilation. Progression to ARDS is associated with a poor prognosis. Respiratory failure is more common in patients with a large contusion, increasing age, underlying pulmonary disease, and inadequate pain control.

Management of pulmonary contusions includes general supportive care and judicious fluid administration aimed at maintaining euvolemia and avoiding fluid overload. No clear benefit has been demonstrated by the empiric use of steroids or antibiotics in the treatment of pulmonary contusions. Mortality rates vary according to age, associated injuries, and underlying pulmonary disease.

E.   Pulmonary Lacerations

Lacerations of the lung parenchyma can occur from either penetrating or blunt thoracic trauma, and usually result in some degree of pneumothorax or hemothorax. Initial management is typically accomplished with the insertion of a chest tube, which alone may be sufficient therapy for smaller lacerations. More severe lacerations often result in significant intrapleural hemorrhage, large air leaks, or both. Ongoing bleeding, massive air leaks, and the failure of the lung to reexpand following tube thoracostomy indicate the need for operative repair, which can usually be accomplished by staple or suture closure of the laceration. Bronchoscopy should also be performed to evaluate the bronchi for more significant injuries and to evacuate blood and secretions from the airways. Proximal injuries to the major bronchi require more complex repair techniques (see Chapter 20, *Chest Trauma 2*).

F.   Pneumothorax

Posttraumatic pneumothorax typically occurs when air escapes from a lacerated or punctured lung into the pleural space. Pneumothorax also can occur when a major airway or hollow viscus (esophagus) is disrupted within the chest. In all of these scenarios, the air trapped in the pleural space may or may not be under pressure. If the air in the pleural space is under pressure, the patient is said to have a *tension pneumothorax*. Otherwise, the patient is deemed to have a *simple pneumothorax*. Both of these pneumothoraces are said to be "closed."

Air can also enter the pleural space through a traumatic injury to the chest wall. This type of pneumothorax is termed an *open pneumothorax*. If the patient is attempting to breathe spontaneously with an open pneumothorax, air will enter and exit the wound with respiration, giving rise to the term "sucking chest wound." Tension can develop in this scenario as well, if the chest wound acts as a one-way valve only admitting air into the pleural space.

Patients with pneumothoraces will present with varying degrees of respiratory compromise and pleuritic chest pain. Definitive diagnosis can be made through auscultation or chest radiography. All pneumothoraces cause the lung to collapse away from the chest wall, preventing the proper expansion of the lung that should occur with a spontaneous inspiratory effort. The elevated intrathoracic pressure associated with a tension pneumothorax has the added effect of impeding venous return to the heart. This can result in hemodynamic compromise and eventual cardiac arrest.

A small, simple pneumothorax may first be noted on the chest radiograph because subtly decreased breath sounds can be difficult to appreciate during a trauma resuscitation. These pneumothoraces are best treated with tube thoracostomy, particularly if positive pressure ventilation is contemplated for another reason. It is also permissible to observe very small pneumothoraces with serial chest radiographs, if the patient has no other significant injuries and exhibits no signs of respiratory or hemodynamic compromise.

In contrast, a tension pneumothorax is a clinical emergency that should be readily apparent. It should be immediately suspected in any trauma patient who presents in shock or cardiovascular collapse. A tension pneumothorax should also be suspected in any previously stable patient who develops cardiopulmonary collapse following the initiation of positive pressure ventilation. On physical examination will be found diminished breath sounds and hyperresonance over the affected hemithorax, and, perhaps, jugular venous distension (if the patient is otherwise euvolemic). The trachea may be deviated away from the affected hemithorax. Tension pneumothoraces should be treated before confirmatory radiography. Immediate needle decompression is indicated and can be achieved by inserting a large-bore needle or catheter into the pleural space through the second intercostal space at the midclavicular line (see below). This should be immediately followed by chest tube placement (see below).

An open pneumothorax can cause significant respiratory embarrassment to the spontaneously breathing patient. Management in the field involves placing an impermeable dressing over the wound and securing it on three sides. This restores the integrity of the chest wall, but allows a means of egress for any air that would otherwise accumulate in the pleural space under tension. In the trauma room, a chest tube should be placed with an impermeable dressing over the wound. Operative intervention is necessary with débridement of devitalized tissue and closure of chest wall. If the defect is too large to be closed primarily, a myocutaneous flap can be rotated to provide coverage. The use of Marlex or other synthetics should be avoided in the trauma setting, given the high rates of infection secondary to wound contamination.

Failure of a lung to reexpand following tube thoracostomy should lead to suspecting either a tracheobronchial injury or a large or deep pulmonary laceration. Further evaluation is indicated, and operative treatment may be necessary (see Chapter 20, *Chest Trauma 2*).

G.   Subcutaneous Emphysema

The presence of subcutaneous emphysema in a trauma patient suggests that the patient has sustained an injury to the airway or the lung parenchyma, and efforts need to be made to rule out the presence of an injury that would require further intervention. These efforts typically include chest radiography and CT scan. Bronchoscopy or endoscopy might also be necessary to rule out an injury to the trachea, bronchi, or esophagus (see Chapter 20, *Chest Trauma 2*). Often, a pneumothorax is found in association with subcutaneous emphysema, although it may not be readily apparent on the initial AP chest radiograph. If a pneumothorax is identified, a chest tube should usually be inserted, especially if the subcutaneous emphysema is progressive, and certainly if positive pressure ventilation is in progress or anticipated. If a pneumothorax is not seen (on plain radiography and CT scanning), the patient needs to be carefully observed. If positive pressure ventilation is anticipated or in use, bilateral tube thoracostomies are recommended in the absence of lateralizing findings.

H.   Hemothorax

Hemothorax refers to the accumulation of blood within the pleural space. Common sources for intrathoracic bleeding include injuries to the intercostal vessels, pulmonary parenchyma, major pulmonary vasculature, and the heart and great vessels. Large hemothoraces are usually apparent on plain radiography, but smaller hemothoraces may be missed on the initial trauma radiograph, because these are often done with the patient supine. A chest CT (assuming that the patient is hemodynamically stable) should reliably identify most hemothoraces. In the hemodynamically unstable patient with chest trauma, it is entirely appropriate to place chest tubes empirically to assess for intrapleural bleeding.

Initial treatment for all hemothoraces is the placement of a large (≥28F) chest tube. Reexpansion of the lung often tamponades bleeding that arises from minor injuries to the lung parenchyma. If the chest tube adequately drains the hemothorax and if the bleeding is stopped, no other therapy may be needed. Exploratory thoracotomy is generally recommended, however, if the initial chest tube drainage is more than 1500 mL or the chest tube drainage continues at a rate of more than 200 mL/h for 2 to 4 hours.

Bleeding intercostal arteries are best controlled with proximal ligation. If the intercostal artery is transected at the intervertebral foramen, a laminectomy may be indicated to achieve proximal control and to ensure that blood does not accumulate under pressure in the spinal canal. Usually, pulmonary lacerations associated with significant bleeding can be managed by local wedge resection or suture repair. Formal lobectomy is rarely necessary and the mortality rate from pneumonectomy in the trauma patient is exceedingly high and should be considered only in dire situations. The management of great vessel injuries is discussed in Chapter 21, *Chest Trauma 3.*

Finally, an inadequately drained hemothorax should be evacuated because the potential exists for the formation of a fibrothorax with permanent limitation of lung function. Also, traumatic hemothoraces carry an increased risk of empyema. If bleeding has stopped, however, such drainage can be accomplished several days following the acute injury using minimally invasive techniques (video thoracoscopy).

I.   Diaphragmatic Injuries

Traumatic diaphragmatic injuries can occur from either blunt or penetrating trauma. Blunt rupture of the diaphragm occurs as the result of the development of a pressure differential across the diaphragm, typically from sudden compressive abdominal forces. The blunt diaphragmatic rupture occurs most commonly on the left side and generally presents as a clinically apparent herniation of abdominal contents into pleural space. Initial management should include the placement of a nasogastric or orogastric tube to decompress the intrathoracic viscera. Acute surgical repair is indicated and should be performed via laparotomy, given the high likelihood of associated intraabdominal injuries. In the event of associated intrathoracic injuries, the laparotomy can be extended into a thoracoabdominal incision, or a separate anterolateral thoracotomy can be performed.

Penetrating injuries to the diaphragm are usually considerably smaller and are often found incidentally at the time of exploration for other injuries. Small diaphragmatic lacerations can be difficult to detect radiographically, and visceral herniation is often not present initially. Over time, however, small diaphragmatic injuries will enlarge and delayed herniation can occur. These chronic diaphragmatic defects frequently develop adhesions to the pulmonary parenchyma and chest wall and, thus, are best repaired via thoracotomy, as opposed to laparotomy.

J.   Traumatic Asphyxia

Traumatic asphyxia is a rare constellation of findings that occurs when the thorax is subject to a severe compressive force. Such a force results in a transient, but extreme, elevation in superior vena caval pressure. As a result, patients develop plethora and petechiae of their upper torso, neck, face, and head. Subconjunctival hemorrhage also occurs, reddening the sclerae. In severe cases, cerebral edema can be present. Care for patients with these findings is supportive and directed toward the identification and treatment of the underlying thoracic crush injuries.

K. Traumatic Chylothorax

The presence of a chylous collection in the chest following trauma or the drainage of chyle through an indwelling chest tube suggests an injury at some level to the thoracic duct. Such an injury may not be immediately apparent because of the characteristic milky drainage being obscured by blood. Also, the typical milky appearance of chyle only occurs in patients who have some form of enteric nutrition that includes a fat source. Thus, if the patient is not allowed anything by mouth, a chyle leak may not be immediately apparent. Occasionally, these leaks will close spontaneously with drainage, parenteral nutrition, and bowel rest. It is generally more expeditious, however, simply to ligate the thoracic duct at the diaphragm through either a small right thoracotomy or using by a minimally invasive approach.

V. Cardiac Arrest or Impending Cardiovascular Collapse in the Trauma Patient

Special considerations are necessary for the trauma patient who presents to the emergency room in posttraumatic cardiac arrest or who presents on the verge of cardiovascular collapse with profound hemodynamic and respiratory instability. The first and most important consideration is *not* to perform time-consuming diagnostic tests. In this dire situation, use clinical judgment and act empirically because time is of the essence. The second consideration needs to be the establishment of adequate ventilation and oxygenation through a secure airway. The third consideration is the rapid reestablishment of perfusion by restoring cardiac function and intravascular volume. Finally, also realize that blunt trauma victims who present in cardiac arrest have essentially a 100% mortality rate, and that attempts at resuscitation may not be indicated, particularly in the mass casualty setting. Penetrating trauma victims who present similarly, however, can have survival rates exceeding 50%, thus resuscitative measures are generally indicated for them. This survival difference is because many penetrating traumatic injuries are focal problems that can be rapidly addressed.

Four clinical scenarios are the ones most likely to result in a favorable outcome for the trauma patient who presents in extremis. Nonetheless, it is not inappropriate to initiate resuscitative measures, including emergency thoracotomy and cardiac resuscitation on any trauma patient who has some probability of functional recovery. These rapidly treatable injuries are discussed below.

A. Tension Pneumothorax

Tension pneumothorax is best treated with needle decompression (see below) or rapid tube thoracostomy (if the operator is facile with this skill and equipment is immediately available).

B. Massive Hemothorax

Mass hemothorax is best controlled with emergency anterolateral thoracotomy (left or right), with manual occlusion of bleeding point and prompt restoration of intravascular volume using blood products.

C. Cardiac Tamponade

Cardiac tamponade is best addressed via an emergency left anterolateral thoracotomy with pericardial decompression (see Chapter 21, *Chest Trauma 3*), manual occlusion of the bleeding point, and prompt restoration of intravascular volume using blood products.

D. Infradiaphragmatic Hemorrhage

Infradiaphragmatic hemorrhage is best addressed via an emergency left anterolateral thoracotomy, followed by low thoracic aortic cross-clamping, and immediate exploratory laparotomy with ongoing volume resuscitation.

VI. Considerations in the Operative Management of Thoracic Trauma

A. Maintenance of Body Temperature

The proper management of any trauma patient requires that the patient's body temperature be maintained. Hypothermia is known to induce coagulopathy and also to lower the ventricular fibrillatory threshold. Furthermore, hypothermia is extremely difficult to correct once it has occurred. The simplest way to keep a trauma patient warm is to keep the ambient room temperature warm. If this simple technique is used, there is no need to waste time with the application and use of a wide variety of warming devices that have been heavily marketed for this purpose. It, therefore, is recommended that the temperature of the operating room and any resuscitative fluids be maintained above 85°F. In situations involving massive volume transfusion, warming of resuscitative fluids is indicated.

B. Surgical Preparation

In general, all trauma patients should be positioned supine. This position affords the greatest flexibility in terms of addressing both known and unexpected injuries. Also, it places the patient in the most accessible position for a variety of resuscitative procedures, including the establishment of intravenous and intraarterial access, as well as cardiopulmonary resuscitation.

The surgical skin preparation should be performed with warm povidone-iodine solution. This solution has the advantage of having a dark color, which facilitates rapid skin coverage, and does not induce evaporative heat losses as do alcohol-based solutions. The patient with truncal trauma should be prepared from the mandible to the knees, and the preparation should be carried down to the table. The groins, neck, and axillae should always be included into the surgical field to facilitate vascular access (including cardiopulmonary and veno-veno bypass), if needed.

As mentioned above, critically ill patients with thoracic injuries should generally be prepared awake, before they are sedated and intubated.

VII. Thoracic Procedures and Incisions

A. Chest Tube Placement (Tube Thoracostomy)

Chest tube placement, which is the most common procedure in thoracic trauma, is often alone sufficient to successfully manage chest trauma in patients who present to the emergency room alive. The most common site for insertion in the trauma patient is the fifth or sixth intercostal space at the midaxillary line. After copious instillation of local anesthesia, a 1- to 2-cm incision is made in the skin. A Kelly clamp or hemostat is used to tunnel over the rib and enter the pleural space. Insert the index finger into the pleural space before tube placement to ensure that the thoracic cavity has been entered, the chest is free of adhesions, and the intraabdominal organs have not herniated through the diaphragm. At a minimum, a 28F chest tube should be inserted posteriorly and superiorly in the chest cavity. The tube should be secured to the chest wall and connected to a collection system. A chest radiograph should be done to confirm chest tube placement. The administration of systemic pain medication or sedatives for the insertion of a chest tube is discouraged and is generally unnecessary, if the operator is proficient in the administration of local anesthetics.

Once a chest tube is placed, it is important to note the amount of acute and ongoing blood loss from the pleural space. It is also important to characterize the extent of the air leak and to determine whether the lung has reexpanded.

B.   Needle Decompression of the Tension Pneumothorax

The rapid decompression of a tension pneumothorax can be easily accomplished by inserting a large-bore needle or catheter (14 gauge) into the pleural space. This is best accomplished by inserting the needle or catheter over the top of the second rib in the midclavicular line. By inserting the needle along the superior aspect of the rib, the operator avoids injury to the intercostal vessels that course along the underside of each rib. Successful entry into a tension pneumothorax will be heralded by the escape of air under pressure through the needle or catheter. This procedure should always be followed by a tube thoracostomy, as soon as the appropriate equipment and personnel are available. Note that this procedure is likely to cause a pneumothorax in the event that it is mistakenly performed on a patient without a pneumothorax. Again, chest tube insertion would probably be indicated.

C.   Anterolateral Thoracotomy

The right or left anterolateral thoracotomy (**Fig. 19-1**) is usually performed in the fifth intercostal space. It is an excellent incision to emergently access most intrathoracic structures. The left anterolateral thoracotomy is the most common emergency resuscitative incision. Through this

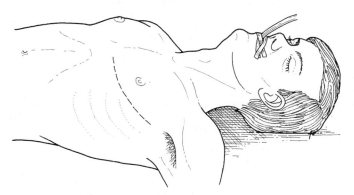

Figure 19-1.   Anterolateral thoracotomy.

approach, the pericardium can be opened, the heart can be accessed, the pulmonary hila can be secured, and the descending thoracic aorta can be cross-clamped. The antero-lateral thoracotomy is also the easiest way with which to gain rapid proximal control of the left subclavian artery. This incision is performed on a supine patient, allowing easy access to the neck, axillae, abdomen, and groin for contemporaneous operative procedures. Access to posterior mediastinal structures is the principal limitation of this exposure.

D. Bilateral Thoracosternotomy (Clamshell Incision)

The bilateral thoracosternotomy is a trans-sternal extension of bilateral anterior thoracotomies (**Fig. 19-2**). It

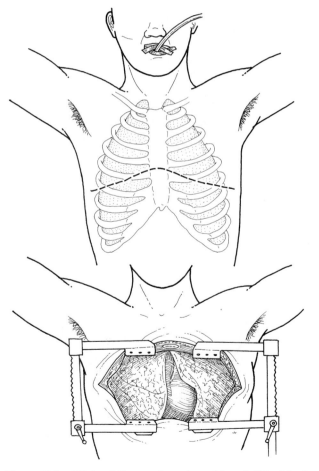

Figure 19-2. Bilateral thoracosternotomy (clamshell incision).

provides outstanding exposure to both pleural spaces and the mediastinum and can be accomplished relatively quickly. The transverse sternotomy can be made using a sternal saw, a Lebsche knife, a Gigli saw, or even a heavy scissors or bone cutter, if other instruments are not available. This incision also allows easy access to other vital areas for contemporaneous operative procedures. As with unilateral anterolateral thoracotomies, access to posterior mediastinal structures is the principal limitation of this exposure.

E.   Posterolateral Thoracotomy

The traditional posterolateral thoracotomy (**Fig. 19-3**) is an acceptable approach for *isolated* trauma to the intrathoracic segments of the trachea and esophagus, trauma to the hila and major bronchi, and injuries to the descending thoracic aorta. The principal drawback of the posterolateral thoracotomy is the lack of easy access to the contralateral thorax and, to a lesser extent, the mediastinum. For the most part, the patient's lateral position also obviates contemporaneous surgery on other vital areas, and complicates resuscitative efforts.

F.   Trap-Door Thoracotomy

The trap-door thoracotomy (**Fig. 19-4**) is essentially a combination of an upper median sternotomy with a supra-

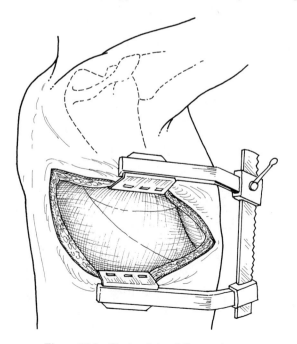

Figure 19-3.   Posterolateral thoracotomy.

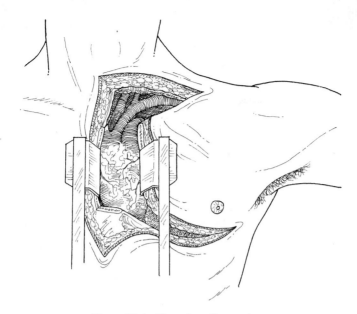

Figure 19-4.   Trap-door thoracotomy.

clavicular extension and an anterolateral thoracotomy. At times, the clavicle is also resected for increased exposure. This incision is generally performed on the left chest to obtain exposure for proximal subclavian injuries.

G. Median Sternotomy

The median sternotomy is an extremely convenient approach for the management of anterior penetrating injuries to the heart, proximal injuries to the right subclavian vessels, and proximal injuries to the carotid and jugular vessels. This incision, however, provides limited access to the pleural spaces and the posterior mediastinum. A bilateral thoracosternotomy may be more useful in situations where both cardiac and pleural access are desired.

SELECTED READING

Baue AE, et al. *Glenn's thoracic and cardiovascular surgery.* Stamford, CT: Appleton and Lange, 1995.

Mattox KL, et al. Thoracic trauma. *Surg Clin North Am* 1989;69:1.

Richardson DJ, et al. Complex thoracic injuries. *Surg Clin North Am* 1996;76(4):725–748. 1996.

Shields TW, et al. *General thoracic surgery.* Philadelphia: Lippincott Williams & Wilkins, 2000.

Chest Trauma 2: Tracheobronchial and Esophageal Injuries

Francis Fynn-Thompson, MD,
and James S. Allan, MD

I. Tracheobronchial Injuries

A. Introduction and Epidemiology

Although rare, tracheobronchial injuries are among the most dangerous and challenging of all traumatic injuries. Until recently, these injuries were generally considered to be universally fatal. Even today, it is estimated that nearly 80% of patients with blunt tracheobronchial injuries never survive to reach the hospital. For those victims who are fortunate enough to present for emergency care, a high index of clinical suspicion is required to make the appropriate diagnosis in a timely fashion. Successful patient outcome requires prompt recognition and expeditious management of difficult airway injuries that require careful operative planning.

B. Surgical Anatomy

To a large extent, the anatomy of the tracheobronchial tree dictates the nature and location of tracheobronchial injuries. The trachea is a tubular structure 10 to 13 cm in length that originates from the glottis and extends distally to its bifurcation at the carina. With the head and neck in a neutral position, approximately half of the trachea can be found in the neck, whereas the other half lies within the thorax. Remember, however, that the trachea is mobile and its anatomic position can be greatly modified by extension or flexion of the head and neck. The anterior two thirds of the trachea is composed of 18 to 20 C-shaped cartilaginous arches interconnected by thin membranous interspaces. The posterior wall of the trachea is entirely membranous and lies in close apposition to the esophagus. The trachea's semirigid architecture allows it to remain flexible, while providing sufficient rigidity to prevent its collapse in response to the excursions in intrathoracic and intraluminal pressure that occur during respiration. Nonetheless, the relatively weak membranous portions of the trachea are susceptible to rupture when sufficient pressures or forces are applied.

The cervical trachea, the most anterior structure in the neck, is poorly protected from injury. It is frequently the site of both blunt and penetrating injury. In contrast, the intrathoracic trachea is fairly well protected and well supported by surrounding structures and, thus, is injured less frequently. At about the level of T3-T4, the trachea bifurcates into the main bronchi. As the main bronchi branch laterally away from the trachea, the airways become significantly more mobile and less well protected. This creates transition points near the origins of the main bronchi that are very susceptible to shear injuries resulting from acceleration-deceleration forces. The susceptibility of the bronchi to injury is also intensified by the fact that the cartilaginous support of the tracheobronchial tree lessens as a person moves more peripherally.

The anatomic distribution of tracheobronchial injuries is given in **Figure 20-1.**

C. Mechanisms of Injury

As with other organ systems, it is convenient to classify the mechanisms of tracheobronchial trauma as either blunt or penetrating. It is also important to remember that both blunt and penetrating injuries to the cervical trachea are associated with concomitant esophageal and cervical spine trauma.

1. Penetrating Tracheobronchial Injuries

Stab wounds and gunshot wounds account for most of the penetrating injuries to the tracheobronchial tree. In the civilian setting, such injuries are typically limited to trauma caused by the direct path of a bullet or knife. In the military setting where high-velocity gunshot wounds are more likely encountered, tracheobronchial injuries can also occur secondary to cavitating forces that radiate laterally from the path of a high-speed projectile. Gunshot wounds can be found anywhere along the tracheobronchial tree, whereas knife wounds occur almost exclusively in the cervical trachea. Penetrating intrathoracic tracheobronchial injuries are commonly found in association with a *transmediastinal* bullet wound, which is also often associated with injuries to the heart and great vessels, contributing significantly to mortality. Iatro-

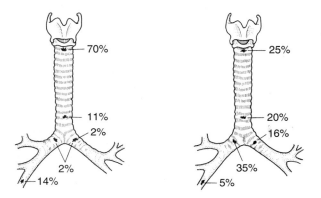

Figure 20-1. Anatomic distribution of tracheobronchial injuries.
(From Huh J, Milliken JC, Chen JC. Management of tracheobronchial injuries following blunt and penetrating trauma. *Am J Surg* 1997;63(10):896–899, with permission.)

genic injuries to the tracheobronchial tree also have been reported consequent to bronchoscopic interventions, traumatic intubations, and overinflation of endotracheal tube cuffs.

2. Blunt Tracheobronchial Injuries

Blunt traumatic injuries, most commonly resulting from motor vehicle collisions, often occur from the application of a sudden deceleration force to the thorax. As mentioned, this force can cause a shear injury that typically occurs at the level of the proximal bronchi. Acute chest compression, especially in the setting of a closed glottis, can also dramatically increase intratracheal and intrabronchial pressures, leading to ruptures that typically occur at the junction of the membranous and cartilaginous portions of the airway wall. Because of its anterior position, the cervical trachea is also subject to blunt-force injury. The typical mechanism involves a direct blow to the cervical trachea when the neck is hyperextended, crushing the trachea against the vertebral bodies (the so-called "clothesline" injury). Blunt-force injuries to the larynx, which can also occur through similar mechanisms, are discussed in Chapter 18, *Neck Injuries*.

D. Clinical Presentation

The clinical presentation of tracheobronchial trauma can be variable and is most often dictated by the location and severity of the specific injury.

Cervical tracheal trauma is usually readily apparent, and typically involves some obvious soft-tissue injury to the anterior or lateral neck. Subcutaneous emphysema in the neck is often present with varying degrees of airway compromise, ranging from hoarseness to complete airway obstruction. Respiratory compromise is typically more apparent during inspiration, when negative pressure within the extrathoracic airway favors tracheal collapse.

The initial presentation of intrathoracic tracheobronchial trauma depends on whether the airway disruption communicates with the pleural space or is confined by the tissues of the mediastinum and the visceral pleura. Injuries contained within the mediastinum and the visceral pleural envelope often present with pneumomediastinum, but also can be clinically silent. In fact, up to 10% of tracheobronchial injuries have no clinical or radiographic abnormalities whatsoever—a fact that can be explained by the strength of the peritracheal and peribronchial adventitial tissues in maintaining airway integrity, at least temporarily. In contrast, injuries that freely communicate with the pleural space often cause ipsilateral or bilateral pneumothoraces that do not resolve with standard chest tube drainage. A persistent air leak after routine tube thoracostomy is highly suggestive of a tracheobronchial disruption. Keep in mind that a relatively stable, contained tracheobronchial injury can suddenly become a surgical emergency (because of tension pneumothorax) when a patient is converted to positive-pressure ventilation.

In addition to the findings mentioned, a complete proximal bronchial disruption can give rise to a characteristic radiographic finding known as the "fallen lung sign." The fallen lung sign is best appreciated on an upright chest radiograph, which will show a collapsed, atelectatic lung balled-up in the lower medial pleural space. The fallen lung sign represents the lung dangling on its vasculature after losing the rigid support of the main bronchus.

E.   Diagnosis and Initial Management

A high index of suspicion for a tracheobronchial injury must be maintained when evaluating any patient with thoracic trauma. The presence of pneumothorax, pneumomediastinum, or subcutaneous emphysema (on chest radiograph, chest computed tomography [CT], or physical examination) should further raise the concern for tracheobronchial injury. The persistence of a pneumothorax in association with a large ongoing air leak following tube thoracostomy is pathognomonic for a bronchial disruption or a deep parenchymal lung injury, both of which will require operative repair.

If a tracheobronchial injury is suspected, every effort should be made to transport the patient immediately to the operating room. The patient should not be sedated or converted to positive-pressure ventilation if breathing spontaneously and with adequate minute ventilation and oxygenation. Occasionally, the administration of a helium-oxygen gas mixture (heliox) to the nonhypoxic patient with a compromised airway can be beneficial and buy a few minutes of valuable time. It is inappropriate to perform manipulative diagnostic examinations of a potentially compromised airway outside of the operating room environment or in the absence of a properly trained surgeon.

In the setting of potential tracheobronchial trauma, consider completing the overall trauma evaluation using modalities that can be performed in the operating room. These can include plain radiographs, portable ultrasound, diagnostic peritoneal lavage, intracranial pressure monitoring, and empiric surgical exploration. It is not appropriate to send a patient with a potentially compromised airway to the radiology department for an extended series of CT scans and plain radiographs.

Bronchoscopy is the most reliable tool for assessing the integrity of the tracheobronchial tree. Both flexible and rigid bronchoscopy should be available, because these modalities are complementary in the diagnosis and initial management of these injuries. Flexible bronchoscopy allows for visualization of the larynx, cervical trachea, and the major lobar bronchi without the need for general anesthesia. It also allows for the controlled insertion of an endotracheal tube, particularly when cervical stabilization is necessary. The rigid bronchoscope, on the other hand, provides superior visualization of the proximal airway, and allows blood and debris to be expeditiously cleared from the airway. The rigid bronchoscope is also an invaluable tool for establishing an airway in the setting of glottic, laryngeal, and high tracheal injuries.

Finally, recognize that proximal bronchial injuries are often associated with injuries to the hilar vasculature, which can lead to massive intrathoracic bleeding and hemoptysis. In the event of such a major hilar injury, emergency anterolateral thoracotomy and hilar clamping can be lifesaving (**Fig. 20-2**).

F.   Definitive Care

1.   Tracheal Injuries

Once the diagnosis of a tracheal injury is established, the first priority should be airway management, which must be individualized for each patient. Aggressive manipulation and instrumentation of the airway can have disastrous consequences in these patients. In the setting of a tracheal disruption, endotracheal intuba-

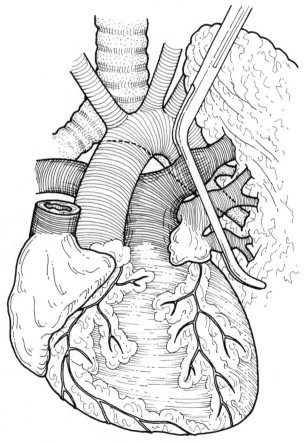

Figure 20-2.   Hilar clamping to control massive hilar injury.

tion can lead to the creation of a false passage, which can further disrupt the trachea and permanently obliterate the true lumen. For this reason, pursue other means of establishing an airway. In many instances, an awake fiberoptic intubation (done in a fully equipped operating room) will be possible, after the pharynx and trachea are topically anesthetized. If the airway is compromised at the glottic or high tracheal level, consider performing a tracheostomy under local anesthesia to secure a distal airway. Most distal tracheal disruptions are best managed with rigid bronchoscopy facilitated by the use of short-acting anesthetic agents. Again, keep in mind that the conversion to positive-pressure ventilation can result in the sudden appearance or worsening of pneumothorax, pneumomediastinum, and subcutaneous emphysema. In cases of a complete transection of the cervical trachea, the distal end will typically retract into the mediastinum. The distal end of the transected trachea can usually be secured and directly intubated by a rapid exploration of the traumatic wound.

Most tracheal injuries can be approached and repaired through a low collar incision, followed by the elevation of subplatysmal flaps. Lateral retraction of the strap muscles affords exposure to the trachea. Care should be taken to preserve the lateral attachments of the trachea, which carry the trachea's segmental blood supply. The recurrent laryngeal nerves should also be preserved. This is best accomplished by performing all dissection directly on the surface of the trachea, thereby lateralizing all peritracheal structures. Additional dissection for the sole purpose of identifying the recurrent nerves is generally not necessary or desirable. Occasionally, it is necessary to add a partial or complete median sternotomy to reach the distal trachea and the top of the carina. This is accomplished by dissecting between the superior vena cava and the aorta and opening the superior aspect of the posterior pericardium. Isolated injuries to the distal intrathoracic trachea and carina can also be approached via a right thoracotomy.

Simple lacerations and limited disruptions can be repaired using interrupted absorbable sutures and should be buttressed with viable tissue (e.g., a pedicled strap muscle flap or an intercostal muscle flap). Circumferential disruptions can also be repaired directly. In the circumstance where adjacent tracheal and esophageal injuries are concomitantly repaired, it is important to interpose some viable tissue (e.g., strap muscle) between the two suture lines to prevent fistulization.

2. Bronchial Injuries

The initial management of the patient with a proximal bronchial injury is often facilitated by the bronchoscopically guided placement of a double-lumen endotracheal tube into the uninjured bronchus. Because of the potential for exacerbation of a bronchial injury, unguided intubations should be avoided. Proper lung isolation minimizes the air leak through the injured bronchus and also prevents the soiling of the injured lung with secretions and blood.

Bronchial injuries are best approached via a posterolateral thoracotomy. The bronchial injury should be exposed with a limited dissection at the site of the injury, taking care to preserve the adjacent peribronchial tissue that supplies blood to the bronchus. The adjacent pulmonary arterial vessels are mobilized sufficiently to allow direct suture repair of the ruptured bronchus. Again, extensive dissection should be avoided. Repairs or reanastomosis can be accomplished using simple absorbable sutures. The bronchial repair should then be buttressed with healthy vascularized tissue (e.g., pericardial fat flap or a pedicled intercostal muscle flap). If an intercostal muscle flap is to be used circumferentially, it should be stripped of periosteum to prevent delayed reossification of the flap.

Keep in mind that massive injuries to the hilum, particularly in cases of extensive tissue destruction, devascularization, or associated major vascular injury, can be treated with urgent lobectomy or pneumonectomy. The decision to resect is a risk-to-benefit analysis that must weigh the likelihood of successful repair against the long- and short-term morbidity of a large pulmonary resection.

3. Nonoperative Management of Tracheobronchial Injuries

Occasionally, very minor injuries (e.g., a small laceration to the membranous wall of the trachea or bronchus) detected on bronchoscopy can be managed nonoperatively. This course of management is advisable only for spontaneously breathing patients who have no evidence of air leak or sepsis. Antibiotic therapy is mandatory and the patient must be watched carefully for complications (e.g., pneumothorax and abscess formation). Careful clinical observation and serial evaluation with CT are advisable if nonoperative therapy is chosen. This approach must be immediately abandoned if any complications arise.

II. Esophageal Trauma

A. Introduction and Epidemiology

Esophageal injuries are rare and account for less than 1% of all patients with traumatic injuries admitted to the hospital. Traumatic perforation of the esophagus, especially of the intrathoracic esophagus, can be one of the most rapidly lethal injuries of the gastrointestinal tract unless properly and expeditiously managed. Approximately 60% of esophageal perforations occur in the thorax, whereas cervical and intraabdominal perforations account for 25% and 15% of all perforations, respectively.

B. Surgical Anatomy

The esophagus is a narrow, muscular tube that extends approximately 25 cm from the cricopharyngeus muscle to the cardia of the stomach. The arterial supply of the esophagus is composed of branches from the inferior thyroid arteries, the aorta, the bronchial arteries, the intercostal arteries, phrenic vessels, and the left gastric artery. Two layers of muscle surround the esophageal mucosa and submucosa: an inner circular layer and an outer longitudinal layer. The esophagus has no serosal covering, which contributes to the difficulty of surgical repair. The paraesophageal tissues communicate freely with other structures of the mediastinum, thus contamination from an esophageal leak can rapidly lead to mediastinitis, sepsis, and mediastinal abscess formation. Also, the entire membranous portion of the trachea is in intimate contact with the proximal esophagus and, thus, simultaneous injury to both of these structures is common.

C. Mechanisms of Injury

Injuries to the esophagus can arise from either penetrating or nonpenetrating mechanisms. The management strategy is dictated by the extent and location of the injury and, to a lesser extent, the duration of the injury.

1. Penetrating Esophageal Injuries

With increasing utilization of diagnostic and therapeutic instrumentation of the esophagus, it is not surprising that most penetrating injuries of the esophagus are iatrogenic. In fact, it is currently estimated that between 50% and 60% of all esophageal perforations are iatrogenic. These iatrogenic injures can occur at any level of the esophagus, but commonly arise in areas with preexisting pathology. Such injuries can be very small, as in the case of a guidewire penetrating the esophageal wall during the course of therapeutic esophageal dilation. Conversely, overzealous passage of scopes, ultrasound probes, dilators, nasogastric tubes, or the misplacement of endotracheal tubes can cause large rents in the esophageal wall at a variety of levels.

Noniatrogenic penetrating wounds, which are relatively less common, are confined primarily to the cervical esophagus. Because of the central location of the esophagus and its small diameter in relation to the surrounding vital organs, noniatrogenic penetrating trauma to the intrathoracic esophagus is relatively uncommon. The notable exceptions are perforations caused by foreign body ingestions, caustic ingestions, and transmediastinal gunshot injuries.

2. Nonpenetrating Esophageal Injuries (Postemetic Esophageal Disruptions)

Rupture of the esophagus in the absence of penetrating trauma or neoplasm was first described in 1724 by the Dutch physician, Hermann Boerhaave: a syndrome of full-thickness esophageal rupture following forceful emesis. Boerhaave's syndrome accounts for about

15% of all esophageal perforations, and a slightly greater percentage if neoplastic causes of esophageal perforation are excluded. An analogous syndrome can result when blunt force abdominal trauma is sustained. The typical scenario involves the unrestrained driver who impacts the steering wheel with a full stomach. These postemetic disruptions typically occur at the level of the distal intrathoracic esophagus, and result in immediate mediastinal contamination. Most, but not all, of these disruptions will also communicate with the left pleural space. Left untreated, these postemetic esophageal disruptions are usually fatal within several days.

D. Clinical Presentation

Clinical signs and symptoms are present in 60% to 80% of patients with esophageal perforation and vary depending on the location, size, and duration of the injury. Cervical perforations often present with neck pain (especially with movement or palpation), dysphagia, odynophagia, and subcutaneous emphysema. Intrathoracic perforations can present with chest pain (usually subxiphoid), subcutaneous emphysema, and varying degrees of dysphagia or odynophagia. If the disruption is in communication with the pleural space, the patient will also have signs and symptoms characteristic of pneumothorax and phrenic irritation. Intraabdominal perforations manifest clinically as acute abdominal pain with signs and symptoms of peritonitis. Patients with an intrathoracic or intraabdominal perforation are also more likely to exhibit early signs of sepsis.

E. Diagnosis and Initial Management

1. Radiographic Evaluation

a. Plain Radiography and Computed Tomography. As with the clinical presentation, radiographic findings are dictated by three principal factors: the time elapsed since the injury, the site and severity of the perforation, and the integrity of the mediastinal pleura. Findings on plain radiographs or CT of the neck and chest can include pneumothorax, pneumomediastinum, pleural effusion, air dissecting in the retropharyngeal soft tissues, and cervical emphysema. Abdominal plain films can show free intraperitoneal air. Any of these findings should prompt a more definitive study with contrast esophagography, endoscopy, or both. Keep in mind that contrast esophagography and endoscopy are complementary, and that the use of both of these modalities increases diagnostic accuracy.

b. Contrast Esophagography. The contrast esophagogram is the gold standard of radiographic evaluation for esophageal injuries. The contrast esophagogram can confirm the diagnosis, demonstrate the size and location of the perforation, and show whether it communicates with the pleural space. Most radiologists initially choose water-soluble contrast (e.g., diatrizoate meglumine) because of being relatively inert to the mediastinum, if extravasated. If no gross perforation is identified with a water-soluble agent, barium is then used, which has the advantages of superior radiographic density and mucosal coating. Barium, however, can cause an intense mediastinal reaction if extravasated. If the patient's mental status is impaired or if the patient has an endotracheal tube in place, contrast can be introduced through a nasogastric or orogastric tube positioned near the area of interest. Keep in mind that pulmonary aspiration of contrast (particularly water-soluble agents) can cause a significant pneumonitis.

2. Endoscopy

Injuries to the esophagus can often be identified by esophagoscopy as well, and the combination of esophagoscopy with contrast studies improves diagnostic accuracy considerably. Esophagoscopy, however, does have some inherent limitations, particularly in diagnosing small injuries. Also, the high cervical region is difficult to visualize using flexible fiberoptic scopes. For this reason, a complete esophagoscopy should also include examination of the hypopharynx and cervical esophagus with both laryngoscope and rigid esophagoscope.

3. Initial Management

The initial management of the esophageal perforation is directed toward the stabilization of the patient in anticipation of urgent surgery. This can include volume resuscitation, ventilatory support, oxygen therapy, and the drainage of any pneumothorax or effusion with a tube thoracostomy. In addition, broad-spectrum intravenous antibiotic therapy should be instituted, including coverage for oral anaerobic organisms. Obviously, the patient should not be permitted to have any oral intake.

F. Definitive Care

1. Injuries to the Cervical Esophagus

The cervical esophagus begins at the cricopharyngeus muscle and extends down to the thoracic inlet. Virtually all injuries to the cervical esophagus should be explored through a collar-type incision or an incision along the anterior border of the sternocleidomastoid muscle. The main purpose of cervical exploration is to provide ample drainage in the region of the injury. In addition to directly draining the area of injury, is it usually prudent to place additional drains in the retropharyngeal space and the superior mediastinum. Closed suction drainage is convenient to manage, but Penrose-type drains are also acceptable.

It is often not possible to clearly identify a cervical esophageal injury, despite a thorough neck exploration,

particularly when the injury is small. With adequate
drainage, however, most cervical esophageal injures
heal well without the need for direct repair. If a cervical injury is identified, it should be closed primarily
and the repair should be buttressed with healthy tissue (e.g., a pedicled strap muscle flap). With an associated tracheal injury, it is mandatory to interpose
healthy tissue between the esophageal and tracheal
repair to prevent fistulization.

It is also customary to place a gastrostomy tube
(for gastric decompression) and a jejunostomy tube
(for enteral nutrition) at the time of neck exploration.
During the postoperative period, the patient should
be maintained on broad-spectrum antibiotics, which
can be adjusted according to culture results. Any
signs of persistent sepsis must be aggressively investigated with CT of the neck and chest to rule out the
presence of an undrained cervical or mediastinal
collection (abscess). A contrast esophagogram is typically performed on postoperative day 7. If the esophagus is intact, oral intake can be slowly advanced and
the cervical drains can be removed.

2.   Injuries to the Thoracic Esophagus
The level of the esophageal injury seen on endoscopy
dictates the operative approach to the thoracic esophagus. Injuries to the proximal and midthoracic esophagus are best approached through a right thoracotomy.
Disruptions of the distal intrathoracic esophagus are
best approached via a left thoracotomy. Several key
objectives need to be achieved in the proper management of a perforated intrathoracic esophagus. First,
mediastinal contamination (and pleural contamination, if present) must be addressed. This generally
requires a combination of débridement, irrigation,
and drainage (typically with multiple thoracostomy
tubes) of all contaminated tissues and spaces. Second,
one should endeavor to primarily repair the intrathoracic esophageal injury, even if the injury presents or
becomes apparent in a delayed fashion. Third, the
repair should be buttressed with healthy, vascularized tissue (e.g., a pedicled intercostal muscle flap or
an omental flap).

The esophageal repair itself can be performed in
either one or two layers; however, it is imperative
that the full extent of the mucosal disruption be identified by extending the rent in the overlying muscle
layers, if necessary. The underlying mucosal tear is
typically longer than the muscular disruption. Many
surgeons prefer to perform the esophageal repair with
a bougie or nasogastric tube in place to prevent inadvertent esophageal narrowing. After completion of
the repair, the buttressing tissue must be tightly
secured around the repair, so that it is able to contain
the esophageal leak that would result, if the primary
repair failed to heal. Again, it is crucial for the medi-

astinum and pleural space to be adequately debrided and drained.

Following the esophageal repair, it is again customary to place a gastrostomy tube (for gastric decompression) and a jejunostomy tube (for enteral nutrition). Some surgeons also like to leave a nasogastric tube across the repair, mainly to afford a redundant means of gastric decompression. Others like to place the tip of the nasogastric tube immediately above the repair to act as a sump tube to scavenge saliva. The use of a diverting cervical esophagostomy (spit-fistula) is generally not necessary.

As with all esophageal injuries, the patient should be maintained on broad-spectrum antibiotics, adjusted according to culture results, during the postoperative period. Any signs of persistent sepsis must be aggressively investigated with the use of CT and contrast esophagography to rule out any undrained mediastinal or pleural collections (abscesses) or a recurrent leak, respectively. A contrast esophagogram is typically performed on postoperative day 7. If the esophagus is intact, oral intake can be advanced slowly and the thoracostomy tubes can be removed.

On occasion, the nature of an intrathoracic esophageal injury or the medical condition of the patient will preclude a primary repair of the injury. In this situation, an esophageal T-tube can be placed through the injury to create a controlled esophageal-pleural-cutaneous fistula. In addition to the T-tube, it is imperative that the mediastinum and pleural space be adequately débrided and drained. In this situation, a gastrostomy tube and jejunostomy tube are also advisable. Some surgeons also choose to exclude the injured esophageal segment by creating a diverting esophagostomy and ligating or stapling the gastroesophageal junction, until the perforation heals. Finally, on a rare occasion, a severe injury to the esophagus can warrant esophageal resection, with either immediate or delayed reconstruction, depending on the medical condition of the patient, the degree of local sepsis, and the quality of the tissues to be used in the reconstruction.

3.   Injuries to the Intraabdominal Esophagus

The injured intraabdominal esophagus is generally approached via laparotomy. All intraperitoneal contamination must be evacuated and, again, the esophagus should be repaired primarily, as discussed above. Within the abdomen, the omentum is the most convenient buttressing tissue. Alternatively, the fundus of the stomach itself can be used to reinforce the repair. In the absence of extensive intraabdominal contamination or other injuries, it is not mandatory to leave behind intraperitoneal drains. Considerations regarding the use of antibiotics and the placement of nasogastric, gastrostomy, and jejunostomy tubes are identical to those discussed above for intrathoracic injuries. Again, any signs of persistent sepsis must be aggressively investigated with the use of CT and contrast esophagography to rule out the presence of undrained collections (abscesses) or a recurrent leak, respectively. If all goes well, a contrast esophagogram is typically performed on postoperative day 7. If the repair is intact, oral intake can be slowly advanced.

4. Nonoperative Management of Minor Esophageal Injuries

The decision to manage an esophageal injury in a nonoperative fashion is one that is fraught with potential risk. Although there are some circumstances where the nonoperative management of a minor esophageal injury can be considered, the nonoperative management of a cervical esophageal injury is seldom advisable. The risk associated with neck exploration to secure cervical drainage is very small compared with the relatively high risk of death associated with descending mediastinitis consequent to an undrained cervical esophageal perforation.

Nonoperative management of intrathoracic and intraabdominal injuries can be considered provided the following criteria are met. First and foremost, the patient should not be exhibiting any clinical signs of sepsis (e.g., fevers, chills, rigors, leukocytosis, thrombocytopenia, coagulopathy, hypotension, azotemia). Second, the injury should be small (e.g., a small perforation caused by an errant guidewire or biopsy instrument during an endoscopic procedure). Third, the associated esophageal leak should not communicate freely with the pleural space or the peritoneal cavity. Fourth, contrast should not be able to accumulate in the periesophageal tissues. If these criteria are met, attempts can be made to manage the esophageal injury with broad-spectrum antibiotic coverage, parenteral nutrition, and the complete restriction of oral intake.

Any patient managed nonoperatively requires close clinical observation. Serial contrast esophagography is necessary to ensure that the patient's injury is healing. Serial CT is essential to rule out the development of extraluminal collections or abscesses whose presence can be temporarily masked by the use of broad-spectrum antibiotics. Failure to heal, the development of a collection or abscess, or the presence of other signs and symptoms of local or systemic sepsis mandate immediate operative intervention.

SELECTED READING

Bacha EA, Mathisen DJ, Grillo HC. Airway trauma. In: Westaby S, Odell JA, eds. *Cardiothoracic trauma.* New York: Oxford University Press, 1999:265–279.

DeGroot KM. Penetrating trauma to the chest wall, lung, esophagus, trachea and thoracic duct. In: Westaby S, Odell JA, eds. *Cardiothoracic trauma*. New York: Oxford University Press, 1999:167–182.

Huh J, Milliken JC, Chen JC. Management of tracheobronchial injuries following blunt and penetrating trauma. *Am Surg* 1997; 63(10):896–899.

Mathisen DJ, Grillo H. Laryngotracheal trauma. *Ann Thorac Surg* 1987;43(3):254–262.

Meredith JW, Riley RD. Injury to the esophagus, trachea and bronchus. In: Mattox KL, Feliciano DV, Moore EE, eds. *Trauma*, 4th ed. New York: McGraw-Hill, 1999:507–521.

Pate JW. Tracheobronchial and esophageal injuries. *Surg Clin North Am* 1989;69(1):111–123.

Richardson JD, Miller FB, Carillo EH, et al. Complex thoracic injuries. *Surg Clin North Am* 1996;76(4):725–748.

Rossbach MM, Johnson SB, Gomez MA, et al. Management of major tracheobronchial injuries: a 28-year experience. *Ann Thorac Surg* 1998;65(1):182–186.

Wright CD, Grillo HC. Injury to the esophagus. In: Westaby S, Odell JA, eds. *Cardiothoracic trauma*. New York: Oxford University Press, 1999:252–264.

21

Chest Trauma 3: Blunt and Penetrating Injuries to the Heart and Central Vessels

David Tom Cooke, MD, and
Thomas MacGillivary, MD

I. Introduction

Trauma is the most common cause of fatality in individuals 15 to 40 years of age. Most of these injuries result from motor vehicle collisions. The heart is injured in 20% to 25% of all fatal traffic deaths, with an overall rate of cardiac injury in blunt chest trauma of 15%. In addition, the rate of penetrating wounds to the chest from assaults is increasing, with gunshot wounds to the chest becoming more common. This chapter discusses the features of cardiac and central vessel injury in trauma and recommends ways to manage these cases.

Cardiac injuries were thought to be uniformly fatal until the 19th century. In 1810, Larrey performed the first pericardial window in a patient with pericardial tamponade after a self-inflicted stab wound to the chest. He relieved a liter of fluid, and the patient recovered, but died 23 days later from mediastinitis. In 1829, Larrey reported the first case of recovery from pericardial tamponade, this time passing a catheter through the existing stab wound, relieving the tamponade. The first successful repair of a cardiac wound was by Rehn in 1896, when he sutured closed an injury to the right ventricle (RV). In 1897, Duval described the median sternotomy as an incision to expose the heart, and in 1906 Spanagaro introduced the left anterolateral thoracotomy, which is currently the incision of choice for emergent entry into the chest. The importance of the rapid recognition and treatment of cardiac injuries was emphasized by experiences learned in World War I and World War II.

II. Initial Evaluation

In the initial evaluation of a patient with thoracic trauma, adhere to the protocols of the American College of Surgeons' Advanced Trauma Life Support guidelines. The "airway, breathing, and circulation (ABC) approach to of trauma treatment should be followed, including intubation if indicated, and large bore intravenous access above and below the diaphragm. Blunt injury to the heart should be suspected in any patient with blunt chest wall trauma. Also, any penetrating injury to the chest that lies within the "precordial box" (**Fig. 21-1**) should be suspected of having injured the heart until such is proved otherwise. The *box* is the area between the midclavicular lines laterally, inferior to the clavicles and superior to the costal margins.

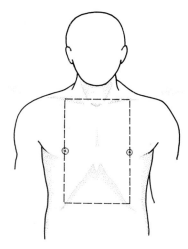

Figure 21-1. Precordial box.

III. Diagnostic Methods

A. Physical Examination

The physical examination uncovers the basics of the initial survey. Breath sounds are auscultated at the midaxillary line, and pneumothorax or hemothorax should be suspected in the absence of breath sounds. Muffled heart sounds should be worrisome for pericardial tamponade or injury. The presence of murmurs should alert the examiner to possible valvular or septal injury. Full neck veins can suggest tamponade.

B. Chest Radiographic Study

A chest radiography study is useful in identifying associated evidence of cardiac injury, which includes multiple fractured ribs, fracture of the sternum, pneumothorax, and hemothorax. The presence of congestive heart failure on chest x-ray film can suggest cardiac contusion.

C. Echocardiography

Two-dimensional transthoracic echocardiography (TTE), by a skilled surgeon, emergency medical physician, or cardiologist, is valuable in detecting traumatic pericardial effusion, dyskinesis, akinesis, and valvular dysfunction. It should be used in patients with symptoms of cardiac tamponade, cardiac contusion, or penetrating injuries in the precordial box. As part of the focused assessment with sonography for trauma (FAST) examination, it is the first modality in detecting pericardial effusion. A 2.0 to 2.5 MHz transducer is used for large adults; a 3.5 MHz transducer in average-sized adults, and a 5 MHz transducer in the pediatric population. Three views are obtained: parasternal long axis view, subcostal four-chamber view, and the apical four-chamber view. Pericardial effusion appears as an anechoic rim between the heart and pericardium. A formal TTE using all three views should detect pericardial fluid, even in the presence of a hemothorax. If no pericardial fluid is observed on TTE, then tamponade can be ruled out. If pericardial fluid is present or if the study is equivocal, then subxiphoid pericardiotomy is required for definitive diagnosis, if clinically indicated.

D.   Pericardiocentesis

Diagnostic pericardiocentesis no longer plays a role in the evaluation of cardiac trauma. It has a high false negative rate because often pericardial blood causing tamponade is clotted and cannot be aspirated. Also, risk is seen of the pericardiocentesis needle being advanced too far, causing iatrogenic injury to the myocardium.

E.   Subxiphoid Pericardiotomy

Subxiphoid pericardiotomy (**Fig. 21-2**) or subxiphoid window is the gold standard in detecting occult cardiac injury. It is thought to have 100% sensitivity, with up to 92% specificity. The procedure should be done in the operating room (OR) under general anesthesia, because if it is positive for pericardial blood, the incision can be quickly extended as a median sternotomy. The entire chest, abdomen, and upper thighs are prepared and draped in standard trauma surgical fashion. A 6-cm vertical incision is carried over the xiphoid process down to linea alba, which is incised. The xiphoid process is retracted cephalad or is excised. Palpat-

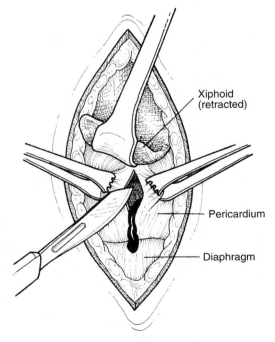

Xiphoid
(retracted)

Pericardium

Diaphragm

Figure 21-2.   Subxiphoid pericardiotomy.

ing the cardiac impulse identifies the pericardium. The pericardium is then grasped between two Allis clamps. Placing the patient in the reverse Trendelenburg position facilitates this maneuver. A 1-cm vertical incision is made through the pericardium. Once in the pericardium, copious clear straw-colored fluid will be released (a negative examination) or bloody fluid (a positive examination). If no fluid is released, then suction should be inserted into the pericardium to remove a clot that can be inhibiting the release of fluid. If a positive result is seen, then a median sternotomy should be performed to assess for cardiac injury.

IV.   Surgical Exposure

Median sternotomy is ideal for exposing the heart **(Fig. 21-3)**. The left anterolateral thoracotomy or emergency department (ED) thoracotomy, however, is the incision of choice for the unstable patient. Five incisions are commonly used in trauma surgery to expose the heart and mediastinum: (a) the left anterolateral thoracotomy, (b) bilateral anterolateral thoracotomy or "clam shell" thoracotomy, (c) the median sternotomy, (d) the "open book" or "trap door" incision, and (e) the left posterolateral thoracotomy.

A.   Left Anterolateral Thoracotomy or "ED" Thoractomy

Left anterolateral thoracotomy **(Fig. 21-4)** is often performed in the ED for a hemodynamically unstable patient with a bleeding cardiac tear or wound, or pericardial tamponade. Through this incision, the heart can be quickly exposed; blood can be evacuated from the pericardial sac relieving tamponade; direct bleeding from the heart or pulmonary hilum can be controlled; open cardiac massage can be performed; and the descending thoracic aorta can be cross-clamped, sending blood preferentially through the carotid and coronary arteries. The decision to do an anterolateral thoracotomy must be made quickly. Thoracotomy, with cross-clamping of the aorta followed by immediate cardiac repair and open massage results in a 10% success rate in patients in extremis after a cardiac wound. Patients with penetrating injury and pulseless electrical activity with closed cardiac massage initiated <5 minutes before arrival can benefit from ED thoracotomy. Patients with no electrical activity, >10-minute resuscitation time, or status after blunt chest wall trauma with no vital signs in the field, may not benefit from ED thoracotomy.

To perform the left anterolateral thoracotomy, elevate the left arm and prepare the chest wall quickly. Make an incision in the subpectoral crease in male patients and the inferior mammary crease in female patients and retract the breast up. Carry the incision from the edge of the sternum down to the border of the latissimus dorsi. Make the incision through skin, subcutaneous tissue, and serratus muscle until the intercostal muscle is reached. Divide the intercostal muscle with heavy scissors just over the rib up to the sternum and down to the latissimus. At this point, place a Finochietto rib spreader to spread the ribs apart. Retract the left lung medially. Palpate the descending thoracic aorta, which can be occluded by pressing against

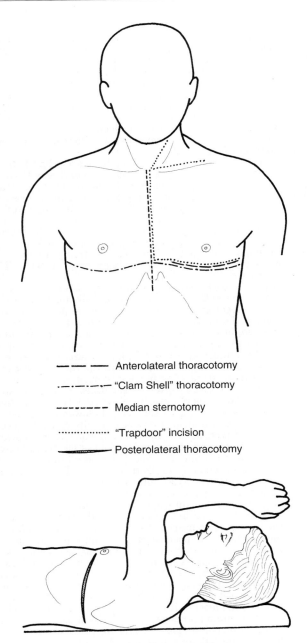

Figure 21-3.   Thoracic incisions.

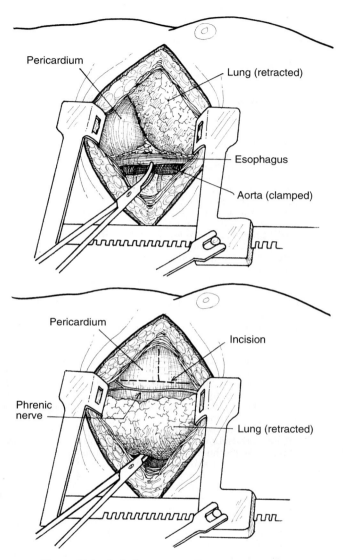

Figure 21-4.   Left thoracotomy. Top: Aorta exposed and cross-clamped. Bottom: Pericardium exposed.

the vertebral column, or can be completely cross-clamped after blunt dissection with fingers. Placement of an oro-gastric tube can facilitate distinguishing the aorta from the esophagus. At this time, a source of bleeding can be identified. If a penetrating wound to the heart is seen, the pericardium will seem tense with minimal movement. Grasp the pericardium with Allis clamps or Kelly clamps, and make a longitudinal opening anterior and parallel to the phrenic nerve. Remove clotted blood, and delineate the type and location of cardiac wound. In ventricular lac-erations, hemostasis is obtained by placing a finger over the wound, or alternatively, placing a Foley catheter through the injury and bringing the inflated balloon against the underside of the injury. Repair the injury with 3-0 or 4-0 pledgeted polypropylene sutures in inter-rupted horizontal mattress sutures. Placing the first suture in the middle of the wound often achieves enough hemostasis to make subsequent stitches easier. If the heart is in a malignant rhythm after repair, perform open cardiac massage until reaching the OR, or depolarize the heart with open paddles using 20 to 50 J. During this pro-cedure, the left internal mammary artery is often divided, and the surgeon must remember to tie off this artery in the OR or it will bleed profusely when the patient is vol-ume resuscitated.

B.   Bilateral Anterolateral or "Clam Shell" Thora-cotomy

The left anterolateral is the ideal incision for quickly exposing the heart and the aorta. An injury from a knife or missile, however, may traverse the mediastinum into the right chest. If this is the case, the left anterolateral incision can be carried to the right. This allows for com-plete exposure of the anterior mediastinum and both hemithoraces. Again, remember that the right internal mammary is divided and needs to be tied off in the OR after resuscitation.

C.   Median Sternotomy

Median sternotomy is the incision of choice for cardiac exposure in the hemodynamically stable patient. This inci-sion allows for adequate exposure of the heart, and proxi-mal control of the innominate and left carotid arteries.

D.   "Open Book" or "Trapdoor" Incision

The median sternotomy can be extended into the neck to further expose the carotid artery or it can be carried over the clavicle to expose the subclavian vessels. When this inci-sion is combined with the left anterolateral thoracotomy, it is called the "open book" or "trapdoor" thoracotomy. This incision often has a high morbidity. Alternatively, for left subclavian artery injuries, the vessel can be approached via a high left anterolateral thoracotomy through the third intercostal space. This approach allows for clamping of the subclavian artery at its origin from the aortic arch.

E.   Posterolateral Thoracotomy

The posterolateral incision exposes the descending tho-racic aorta as well as the esophagus, posterior hilum of the lung, mainstem bronchi, and carina. This incision will also expose the diaphragm, although a laparotomy is the preferred approach to evaluate an acute diaphragmatic injury.

V.   Blunt Cardiac Injury

As mentioned, the overall rate of cardiac injury in blunt chest trauma is 15%. Blunt cardiac injury occurs when the heart is compressed against the sternum and the thoracic vertebral column. Shear forces can cause the heart and thoracic aorta to tear at points of attachment (e.g., superior vena cava [SVC] and inferior vena cava [IVC], the pulmonary veins, aortic annulus, and arch vessels). Any type of blunt injury to the chest wall (e.g., precordial bruising, rib fractures, or fracture of the sternum) should alert the evaluating physician to injury to the heart. The major results of blunt cardiac injury are cardiac contusion and cardiac rupture.

A.   Cardiac Contusion

Cardiac contusion is a controversial entity that ranges in presentation from no symptoms or slight electrocardiographic (ECG) changes to major cardiogenic shock. Areas of myonecrosis followed by intramyocardial hemorrhage characterize cardiac contusion. Injury can impair ventricular contraction or induce arrhythmias. Injury to the coronary arteries can cause spasm or dissection, resulting in myocardial infarction. Failure secondary to traumatic aortic insufficiency or mitral regurgitation can appear acutely or in a few weeks after trauma, whereas tricuspid insufficiency can appear within a few days.

1.   Presentation

The patient can complain of anginalike chest pain or progressing dyspnea. Pericardial friction rub, an S_3 heart sound, or rales on auscultation should alert the evaluating physician to cardiac contusion. Elevated central venous pressure or systemic hypotension unresponsive to fluid resuscitation is also suggestive of cardiac contusion.

2.   Diagnosis

The baseline tests should be chest x-ray study, ECG, and cardiac enzyme testing. Chest x-ray film may reveal pulmonary failure. A negative ECG does not exclude cardiac contusion because small areas of injury may not lead to ECG changes. Common ECG changes range from nonspecific ST- and T-wave changes, minor arrhythmias such as sinus tachycardia, premature atrial complexes (PAC) and unifocal premature ventricular complexes (PVC) to complex arrhythmias such as conduction deficits (e.g., right bundle branch block, atrial fibrillation, multifocal PVC, and PVC couplets, and ventricular tachycardia. Also, cardiac contusion can result in ischemic changes (e.g., ST elevations and T-wave inversions). Abnormal cardiac enzymes (e.g., creatine kinase-MB [CK-MB] >50, with an index >5%) can represent myonecrosis secondary to cardiac contusion. Color flow echocardiography is the gold standard for diagnosis. Echocardiography can reveal dyskinesis or akinesis, pericardial effusion, and valvular dysfunction.

3. Management

Management of cardiac contusion should follow the algorithm (**Fig. 21-5**). Again, any patient with external evidence of blunt chest trauma, characterized by precordial ecchymosis, fractured ribs, or fractured sternum should be suspected of having cardiac contusion. A patient who is stable and whose ECG is normal or shows only nonspecific ST segment or T-wave changes, can be observed for several hours, then admitted to a regular surgical floor if other injuries permit. A patient who complains of anginal symptoms, has elevated cardiac enzymes with CK-MB >50 and CK index >5%, or minor arrhythmias (e.g., sinus tachycardia, PAC, or unifocal PVC) should be admitted to a monitored bed, followed by color flow echocardiography if symptoms persist after 12 hours. If the patient complains of dyspnea, has an ischemic ECG, or a complex arrhythmia (e.g., atrial fibrillation, multifocal PVC, or conduction delay), ICU monitoring is recommended, followed by TTE. Patients who demonstrate hypotension not responsive to fluid and not explained by bleeding should have urgent echocardiography to determine tamponade versus ventricular dyskinesia.

If pericardial fluid is seen on TTE, suggesting tamponade, then the patient should have subxiphoid pericardiotomy in the operating, if relatively stable, or anterolateral thoracotomy if in extremis. Severe akinesia if found should be treated by an inotropic agent or, on rare occasions, by intraaortic balloon pump. An aortic isthmus tear must be ruled out if a balloon pump is to be placed. Tachyarrhythmias (e.g., atrial fibrillation) can be controlled using diltiazem, which has no negative inotropic effects.

The natural history of cardiac contusion is that most arrhythmias resolve, and ventricular function returns usually in a few days, but can take up to 4 weeks. Care must be given to optimize pain control and normalize the serum potassium and magnesium.

B. Cardiac Rupture

Cardiac rupture after blunt trauma is rare. The RV is the most common chamber injured, followed by the LV, the left atrium, and the right atrium. The ventricles and interventricular septum are injured as a result of compressive forces during diastole, when the aortic and pulmonary valves are closed. The aortic and pulmonary valves are at risk of injury at end-diastole as well. Atrial tears occur during systole, when the atria are filled, and the tricuspid and mitral valves are closed. The mitral and tricuspid are also injured at end-systole. Shear forces at the SVC and IVC atrial junctions lead to atrial tears.

1. Presentation

Most patients die before arrival to the ED, although atrial ruptures have a higher survival rate secondary

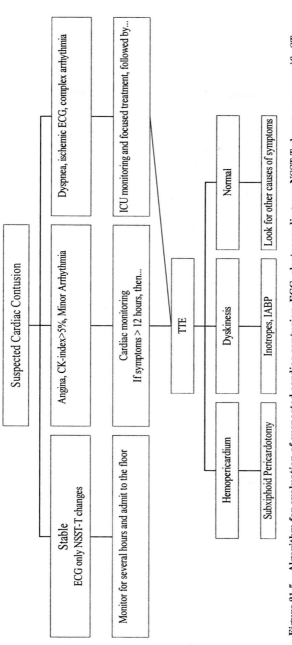

Figure 21-5. Algorithm for evaluation of suspected cardiac contusion. ECG, electrocardiogram; NSST-T changes, nonspecific ST and T wave changes; IABP, intraaortic balloon pump; TTE, transthoracic echocardiography; minor arrhythmia, sinus tachycardia, premature atrial complexes (PAC), or unifocal premature ventricle complexes (PVC); complex arrhythmia, atrial fibrillation, multifocal PVC, ventricular tachycardia.

to a low-pressure chamber. Patients, who survive the initial injury, present in either tamponade or shock. Symptoms include Beck's triad (hypotension, muffled heart sounds, and elevated neck veins) and Kussmaul's sign (increase in venous pressure with inspiration when breathing spontaneously) seen often, but not always, in tamponade. Also pulseless electrical activity (PEA) and hemothorax are suggestive of cardiac rupture. Presenting symptoms in acute valvular trauma include congestive heart failure (CHF) in mitral and aortic valve injuries, and right bundle branch block (RBBB) or right sided heart failure in tricuspid valve injury. Ventricular septal defects may present as a new holosystolic murmur, or CHF in severe shunt.

2. Diagnosis

A transesophageal echocardiography study may demonstrate pericardial fluid, septal defect, and ventricular or valvular dysfunction. Subxiphoid pericardiotomy will reveal pericardial blood and the patient should be followed by median sternotomy. Resuscitative ED thoracotomy in the appropriate patient will immediately expose the injury.

3. Management

a. Right and Left Ventricle Tears. The RV is the most likely chamber to rupture after blunt trauma. Tears in the right and LV are repaired with interrupted pledgeted polypropylene sutures as described in section **IV.A.**

b. Left and Right Atria Tears. Tears in the atria are grasped between Babcock or Allis clamps, and closed with a running polypropylene suture.

c. Ventricular Septal Defects. Often, a delay occurs in the diagnosis of traumatic ventricular septal defects, which tend to occur near the apex of the septum. Repair can often be delayed, allowing time for the surrounding septal tissue to heal from injury. Repair is indicated when the shunt is greater than 1.5:1, or the shunt leads to acute failure. For repair, place the patient on cardiopulmonary bypass and cover the defect with a Dacron patch. Close small lesions primarily. An intraaortic balloon pump (IABP) can be used to temporize the patient until urgent repair.

d. Aortic Valve Injuries. The aortic valve is the most common cardiac valve injured. The valve can be resuspended for commissure injuries or replaced for leaflet injuries.

e. Mitral Valve Injuries. Mitral valve injuries can occur as a result of papillary muscle rupture or, on rare occasions, chordae tendineae rupture or leaflet tear. If injured, the valve should be replaced.

f. Tricuspid Valve Injury. Mild lesions can be treated medically. Symptoms of right ventricle failure necessitate replacement.

VI. Penetrating Cardiac and Central Vessel Injury
Penetrating injuries to the heart and central vessels are primarily the result of assault. In the urban setting, gunshot wounds are the most common, followed by stab wounds. The RV is injured 43% to 51% of the time because of its anterior position. The frequencies of injury to the other chambers are LV 30% to 33%, RA 11% to 15%, and LA 4% to 6%.

A. Penetrating Cardiac Wounds

1. Presentation

Penetrating cardiac wounds present as either severe hemorrhage or pericardial tamponade, with 80% to 90% of stab wounds presenting as tamponade. Often, the thick myocardium of the ventricle seals the initial wound, presenting further extravasation of blood; pericardial fat seals the pericardial wound, leading to entrapped pericardial blood, limiting the mobility of the heart and causing tamponade.

2. Diagnosis

Echocardiography identifies pericardial fluid causing tamponade. Subxiphoid pericardiotomy in patients suspected of having penetrating cardiac injuries, will reveal pericardial blood. Emergent anterolateral thoracotomy in patients in shock will reveal exsanguinating injury.

3. Management

Management of suspected penetrating cardiac wounds should follow the algorithm seen in **Figure 21-6.** Patients with gunshot wounds or stab wounds to the chest should have emergent anterolateral thoracotomy if in extremis, and exploration of the heart and left chest. To evaluate missiles that traverse the mediastinum to the right chest, the excision may need to be extended to a bilateral anterolateral thoracotomy or *clam shell* incision. Patients who are stable and with gunshot wounds to the precordial box, should go emergently to the OR for median sternotomy and exploration. Stable patients with stab wounds to the precordial box should have an echocardiogram. Patients with a normal study should be observed, and patients with abnormal pericardial fluid should have a subxiphoid pericardiotomy in the OR. An examination positive for a penetrating cardiac injury necessitates a median sternotomy. To facilitate exposure and repair lateral wounds of the LV, LA, or circumflex coronary artery in the beating heart, the heart can be brought out anteriorly in the median sternotomy using retraction sutures characterized by Ricardo Lima in Brazil. Four 0 silk pericardial sutures are placed 2 cm anterior to the left superior and inferior pulmonary veins, near the aortapericardial reflection and halfway between the left inferior pulmonary vein and IVC.

a. Repair of the four chambers are as described in V.B.3.a–c.

b. Coronary Artery Injuries. The left anterior descending artery is the coronary artery most

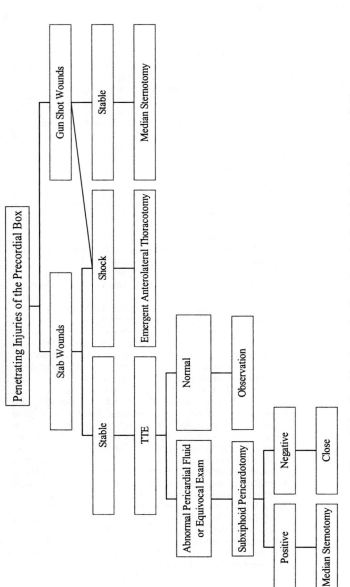

Figure 21-6. Algorithm for evaluation of penetrating injuries to the precordial box.

commonly injured. The right coronary artery and circumflex arteries are rarely injured. Distal lesions can be ligated without compromise of the myocardium. Proximal lesions should have bypass grafting.

B. Central Vessel Wounds

    1. Management

        a. Superior Vena Cava Lacerations. The SVC wound edges are approximated with Allis clamps and closed with a running 4-0 polypropylene suture.

        b. Pulmonary Artery Lacerations. Lacerations in the pulmonary artery are controlled with digital pressure, and closed with nonabsorbent mattress sutures.

SELECTED READING

Asensio JA, et al. Penetrating cardiac injuries. *Surg Clin N Am* 1996;76(4):685–724.

Baue AE, et al. *Glenn's thoracic and cardiovascular surgery.* Stamford, Connecticut: Appleton and Lange, 1995.

Chan D. Echocardiography in thoracic trauma. *Emerg Med Clin North Am* 1998;16(1):191–207.

Edmunds LH. *Cardiac surgery in the adult.* New York: McGraw Hill, 1997.

Feghali NT, et al. Blunt myocardial injury. *Chest* 1995;108(6):1673–1677.

Pretre R, et al. Current concepts: blunt trauma to the heart and great vessels. *N Engl J Med* 1997;336(9):626–632.

Vascular Trauma 1: Cervicothoracic Vascular Trauma

Luke Marone, MD, and Richard Cambria, MD

I. Introduction

Injury to the cervicothoracic vessels is largely an urban phenomena that presents both diagnostic and management dilemmas. These injuries are the result of either penetrating (gunshot wounds, stab wounds) or blunt trauma. They infrequently occur and are associated with significant morbidity and mortality. This chapter focuses on diagnostic modalities, operative exposure, and management of both penetrating and blunt injuries to the cervicothoracic vessels.

II. Penetrating Carotid Artery Trauma

Penetrating injury to the carotid artery occurs secondary to projectile, stab, and iatrogenic trauma (central venous catheter placement). The common carotid artery (CCA) is more frequently affected then the internal carotid artery (ICA) and injuries to these vessels are found in approximately 20% of all penetrating cervical vascular traumas. Patient presentation can range from hemodynamic shock with obvious hemorrhage to a complete absence of clinical signs in up to 30% of patients. In patients with "hard" signs of vascular injury (active bleeding, hypovolemic shock and expanding hematoma), immediate operative intervention is essential. Controversy exists, however, regarding the optimal diagnostic and treatment algorithm in patients with "soft" signs of vascular trauma (history of bleeding, stable neck hematoma, proximity injury) or without clinical indications of vascular injury.

Penetrating cervical neck trauma, which does not traverse the platysma, does not require further diagnostic or operative intervention. Considerable effort has been undertaken in an attempt to divide the neck into anatomic zones of injury to stratify patients into diagnostic and interventional categories. Debate surrounds this practice, with literature to support both mandatory surgical exploration as well as selective angiographic evaluation based on physical findings. Studies have revealed that physical examination alone can reliably exclude arterial injury in all zones of the neck (negative predictive value 100%).

Angiography is the accepted gold standard for evaluation of penetrating cervical vascular injuries and advances in endovascular intervention forecast continued applicability in this patient cohort. Recent prospective studies comparing color flow duplex with angiography have demonstrated the utility of duplex evaluation (sensitivity 95%, specificity 98%). This modality is efficient, inexpensive, and without the potential complications associated with invasive cerebrovascular angiography. Other modalities, including magnetic resonance angiography and spiral computed tomographic (CT) angiography are appealing; however, no prospective trials have been conducted testing these modalities.

Operative approach to the carotid artery is obtained via an oblique incision parallel to the anterior border of the sternocleidomastoid muscle (SCM) (**Fig. 22-1**). The chest should be prepared and draped in the event that proximal vessel control cannot be established through the cervical approach. Operative principles include the establishment of proximal and distal vascular control before entry into a contained hematoma, meticulous dissection to avoid injury to vital structures, and thorough exploration of the aerodigestive tract. All penetrating carotid injuries without concurrent neurologic deficit should be repaired. Controversy exists regarding the management of carotid injuries with concomitant neurologic deficit. Concern for the conversion of an ischemic stroke into a hemorrhagic stroke has not been substantiated and recent evidence supports the repair of these lesions. If thrombus is identified in the distal aspect of the traumatized

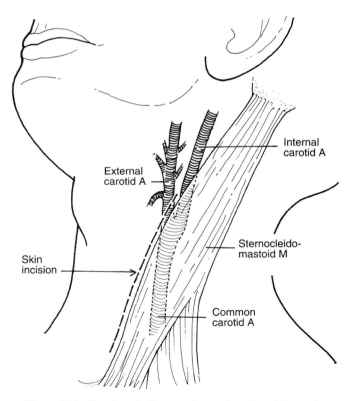

Figure 22-1.   Landmarks for vascular exploration of the neck.

carotid artery and back bleeding is not identified, consider ligation rather than repair, given the potential for embolic complication during thrombus extraction. In clinical scenarios that dictate carotid ligation, anticoagulation is recommended to prevent clot propagation and distal embolization. This is particularly important with ICA ligation because the risk of embolization is greater than that for ligation of the CCA. Repair techniques include primary repair with monofilament suture, vein patch angioplasty, resection and reanastomosis, external carotid artery (ECA) or ICA transposition, and interposition grafting (vein or prosthetic). The complexity of the injury dictates the type of repair applied (stab wounds are most often primarily repaired, whereas gunshot wounds often require interposition grafting). The use of cerebrovascular shunting during repair is generally not necessary because these injuries most often involve the common carotid artery and collateral circulation via patent ECA to ICA maintains prograde flow in the ICA. If concern over cerebral perfusion exists "stump" pressures can be monitored with a pressure >70 mm Hg, an indication of acceptable cerebral perfusion. Concomitant aerodigestive injury is frequent in this patient cohort and the surgeon must be aggressive in approach to detect these injuries (laryngoscopy, bronchoscopy, esophagoscopy and esophageal contrast radiography).

III.   Penetrating Vertebral Artery Trauma

Penetrating trauma to the vertebral arteries is exceedingly rare, secondary to their protected anatomic location. Most patients present without active hemorrhage or neurologic sequelae. The few patients who present with active hemorrhage should be brought to the operating room for immediate control of bleeding. The remainder of patients have an injury detected during angiographic evaluation initiated secondary to suspicious injury pattern or the proximity of the trauma. This cohort of patients can be treated with surgical or endoluminal modalities.

Operative exposure of the proximal vertebral artery can be achieved through a supraclavicular incision or via an incision that parallels the anterior border of the SCM. The supraclavicular incision allows excellent access to the proximal vertebral artery. It is most useful when exploration is directed at a confirmed vertebral artery injury (**Figs. 22-2 and 22-3**). During the exposure, take care to preserve the phrenic nerve (along the anterior scalene muscle), brachial plexus, and thoracic duct (left side) to avoid the morbidity associated with unrecognized injuries to these structures. Anterior exposure along the medial border of the SCM affords a more complete exploration of the neck, including the jugular vein, carotid artery, vertebral artery, and proximal aerodigestive structures. Medial retraction of the carotid sheath and removal of the supraclavicular fat pad facilitate exposure of the vertebral artery. Exposure of the distal vertebral artery is technically demanding and often complicated by venous bleeding secondary to the numerous veins surrounding the transverse foramen.

Current consensus is that all penetrating vertebral artery injuries should be treated by ligation or embolization. In the actively bleeding patient, emergent surgical intervention is warranted; however, in the remainder of patients, embolization or balloon

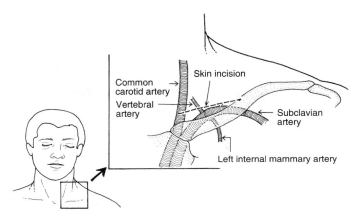

Figure 22-2.   Landmarks for vascular exploration of the thoracic outlet.

occlusion should be considered standard of care if experienced personnel are available. Despite the anatomic variability in the posterior circulation, a 1.5% to 3% incidence of brainstem ischemia has been reported with unilateral ligation of the vertebral artery. Concomitant injuries, rather than the specific vertebral artery lesion, influence the overall outcome of this patient cohort.

IV.   Blunt Cerebrovascular Trauma

The incidence of blunt carotid and vertebral artery injury is rare and ranges between 0.3% and 0.8% in all blunt trauma patients. Motor vehicle trauma is the most frequent mechanism, and associated injuries are common. The ICA is injured more frequently than the CCA because it courses over the lateral articular processes and pedicles of the upper three cervical vertebrae, producing a stretch injury during hyperextension and contralateral rotation of the neck. The vertebral artery is often stretched or disrupted as a consequence of fracture of the transverse foramen of the cervical spine) at the point of entry into the transverse foramen (C6) or while in the bony canal. Blunt trauma to these vessels is associated with specific injury patterns (**Table 22-1**). These lesions are frequently clinically silent and recognition of these patterns is crucial to diagnosis. Historically, most of these injuries are recognized after the appearance of neurologic deficits. Recent literature suggests that early recognition, diagnosis, and intervention are associated with improved outcome.

The gold standard of evaluation is angiography. Recently presented prospective data from Fabian et al. note sensitivities of 44% and 60% for computed tomographic angiography (CTA) and magnetic resonance angiography (MRA), respectively, when compared with cerebral angiography. Further studies are required; however, given these results, less invasive techniques should not be used for screening. Screening evaluation, which is recommended

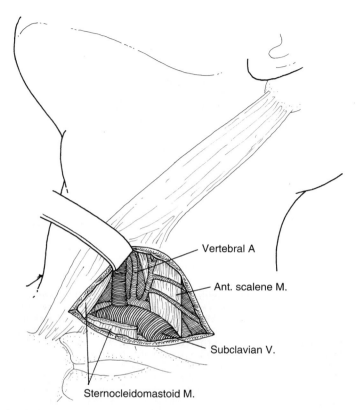

Figure 22-3.   Exploration of the vertebral artery.

in patient cohorts with suspicious injury patterns or neurologic changes incongruent with cerebral CT scans, has been associated with reduced stroke rates in patients with blunt vertebral artery injury.

Management of blunt cerebrovascular trauma is dependent on the type of injury identified as well as the anatomic location of the injury. Injuries include intimal tears, vessel dissection, occlusion, and formation of pseudoaneurysm or carotid-cavernous sinus fistulae. The most frequent site of blunt carotid trauma is the distal ICA. Given this location as well as the limited surgical exposure of the vertebral artery, operative intervention for blunt cerebrovascular trauma is often not feasible. Recent reports indicate the success of endoluminal intervention (balloon occlusion, coil embolization, or stent placement) in the treatment of fistulae, dissection, and pseudoaneurysm. The institution of heparin anticoagulation followed by warfarin therapy for 3 to 6 months has been

Table 22-1. Injury patterns associated with blunt cerebrovascular trauma

Carotid Artery	Vertebral Artery
Direct blow (strangulation)	Cervical spine fracture
Intraoral trauma	Midface fracture (Le Fort II/III)
Midface fracture (Le Fort II/III)	Chiropractic manipulation
Basilar skull fracture	Neck hematoma
(foramen lacerum)	Diffuse axonal injury
Neck hematoma	
Horner syndrome	
Diffuse axonal injury	

advocated for the treatment of intimal tears, pseudoaneurysm formation, vessel dissection, and occlusion. The rationale for this treatment is to minimize clot formation at the site of injury, decrease thrombus propagation, and prevent embolization. Although no prospective, randomized series exist, studies to date have demonstrated significant improvement in clinical outcome after anticoagulation therapy has been initiated. Long-term follow-up in this patient cohort is advocated to monitor for pseudoaneurysm expansion and formation because this is a frequent complication after vessel dissection.

V. Aortic Arch and Great Vessel Trauma

Trauma to the aortic arch and the great vessels is relatively uncommon. With the exception of deceleration injury-related aortic tears at the isthmus of the descending thoracic aorta, most great vessel injuries are secondary to penetrating trauma. Patients usually present in extremis with signs of exsanguinating hemorrhage and prehospital mortality is estimated to be as high as 50%. In this situation, diagnostic evaluation should not be pursued and patients should be brought to the operating room for emergent exploration. Concomitant aerodigestive and neurologic injury are discovered in 20% to 80% of patients at the time of exploration.

In hemodynamically stable patients, diagnosis is based on history and physical examination (**Table 22-2**). The identification of equal upper extremity pulses is often unreliable because pulse waves can be transmitted through injured vessels or via collateral circulation across the shoulder. An upright anteroposterior (AP)

Table 22-2. Clinical clues of great vessel trauma

History of significant hemorrhage at the scene of injury
Neck hematoma
Persistent hypotension
Horner syndrome
Vocal cord paralysis
Upper extremity limb pulse deficit?

chest radiograph often reveals signs of significant injury to the great vessels (**Table 22-3**). Chest tube thoracostomy should be performed for identified pneumothorax or hemothorax. The immediate drainage of 1500 mL of blood or >200 mL/hour of blood is an indication for operative exploration. Angiography is the gold standard for evaluation of penetrating trauma to the great vessels. In addition to the detection of clinically silent injuries, angiography can exclude the need for operative intervention in patients without other clear indications for surgery and can assist in operative planning.

Multiple operative approaches to injury of the great vessels have been described and a complete discussion of these is beyond the scope of this chapter. The most familiar and versatile of these approaches is the median sternotomy. This approach affords excellent exposure of the ascending aorta, aortic arch, and the innominate artery. Simple extension of this incision along the anterior border of the SCM provides access to the carotid artery and extension laterally in the supraclavicular space will provide excellent exposure to the subclavian artery. The one shortcoming of this incision is inadequate exposure of the origin of the left subclavian artery. This can be achieved through a separate anterior left thoracotomy in the third intercostal space. Isolated distal subclavian or proximal axillary arterial injuries can be adequately approached through combined medial supraclavicular and lateral infraclavicular incisions without the need for resection of the clavicle. Of note, the "trap-door" incision is often difficult to open and commonly results in posterior rib fractures, with added morbidity.

Surgical principles include control of hemorrhage (digital compression, packing, balloon occlusion) and meticulous dissection to establish proximal and distal vascular control before the removal of foreign bodies or exploration of a contained hematoma. In general, all arterial injuries should be repaired. Depending on the nature of the vascular injury, various methods of repair can be undertaken. Minor laceration type injuries of the ascending and arch aorta are often repaired with the use of a partial occlusion clamp and pledgeted monofilament suture. Inflow occlusion of the vena cava can assist both in lowering aortic pressure and in repair. Significant injury to the innominate or subclavian artery can be repaired via débridement with reanastomosis or with interposition grafting (vein or prosthetic). Major injuries to the aorta can require cardiopulmonary bypass (and systemic

Table 22-3.   Chest radiograph findings suggestive of great vessel trauma

Wide mediastinum
Loss of aortic contour
Left apical cap
Sternal fracture
First or second rib fracture
Hemothorax
Tracheal deviation

heparinization), which is associated with increased mortality. Despite frequent wound contamination from concomitant aerodigestive injuries, the use of prosthetic grafts has been reported with success. In cases of gross contamination, consider an extraanatomic revascularization procedure. As noted, isolated injuries to the carotid or the innominate artery do not require shunting for repair. Mortality ranges between 7% and 26% in patients who present to a trauma center with detectable vital signs.

Major venous injury often accompanies trauma to the great vessels and can complicate arterial repair. Exposure is identical to that for arterial injury. In general, ligation of the major brachiocephalic veins is associated with little morbidity. In scenarios in which significant damage to collateral venous structures has occurred, however, operative repair may prevent the development of extremity venous hypertension. In general, veins can be repaired by simple lateral repair with monofilament suture. Interposition grafting and resection or reanastomosis is often time consuming and unsuccessful.

VI. Endovascular Intervention in the Trauma Patient

Since the initial description of endovascular stenting by Dotter in 1969, continuing advances in technology have led to an expanding array of therapeutic indications. Use of this technology in the trauma patient is appealing because it is associated with decreases in anesthetic requirement, operative time, blood loss, and length of hospital stay. No randomized, prospective trials have been conducted to evaluate the success of endovascular therapy, although many case series describe applications in patients with penetrating and blunt arterial injuries.

Endoluminal devices can be delivered from remote access sites and, thus, are not associated with the attendant morbidity of cervicothoracic vessel exposure. Device choice is based on injury type and location. Devices can be either balloon expandable (increased radial strength) or self-expanding (increased flexibility); they can be bare metal stents or covered grafts (polytetrafluoroethylene, Dacron, polyester). Devices are available in an array of sizes to allow for application in a variety of anatomic locations.

Currently, this technology should be applied in stable patients in a controlled setting. Standard of care for the hemodynamically unstable patient remains emergent operative exploration. As noted, endoluminal therapy has been reported with both penetrating and blunt vascular trauma with various manifestations of injury (pseudoaneurysm, dissection, transection, arteriovenous fistula). Review of the current literature reveals successful therapy of blunt cerebrovascular pseudoaneurysms with covered self-expanding stents, successful treatment of carotid and vertebral dissection with bare stents, and successful treatment of penetrating injury to the subclavian and axillary artery through the deployment of both covered and bare stents. Although long-term follow-up is not available, short-term success gauged by accurate device deployment, PSA exclusion, and restoration of limb perfusion has been encouraging. Experience with this technology in the trauma patient is limited and randomized, prospective studies are required to determine the true benefits of this interventional approach.

SELECTED READING

Asensio J, Valenziano C, Falcone, et al. Management of penetrating neck injuries: the controversy surrounding zone II injuries. *Surg Clin North Am* 1991;71:267–296.

Ballard JL, McIntyre WB. Cervicothoracic vascular injuries. In: Rutherford RB, ed. *Vascular surgery.* Philadelphia: WB Saunders, 2000:893–900.

Brandt MM, Kazanjian S, Wahl L. The utility of endovascular stents in the treatment of blunt arterial injuries. *J Trauma* 2001;51(5): 901–905.

Bynoe RP, Miles WS, Bell RM, et al. Noninvasive diagnosis of vascular trauma by duplex ultrasonography. *J Vasc Surg* 1991;14(3):346–352.

Coldwell DM, Novak Z, Ryu RK, et al. Treatment of posttraumatic internal carotid arterial pseudoaneurysms with endovascular stents. *J Trauma* 2000;48(3):470–472.

Demetriades D, Theodorou D, Cornwell E, et al. Evaluation of penetrating injuries of the neck: prospective study of 223 patients. *World J Surg* 1997;21:41–48.

Fabian TC, Croce MA, Miller PR, et al. Prospective screening for blunt cerebrovascular injuries: analysis of diagnostic modalities and outcomes. Presented at the 122nd annual meeting of the American Surgical Association, 2002.

Ginzburg E, Montalvo B, LeBlang S, et al. The use of duplex ultrasonography in penetrating neck trauma. *Arch Surg* 1996;131(7): 691–693.

Marin ML, Veith FJ, Panetta TF, et al. Transluminally placed endovascular stented graft repair for arterial trauma. *J Vasc Surg* 1994;20(3):466–473.

McKinley AG, Carrim AT, Robbs JV. Management of proximal axillary and subclavian injuries. *Br J Surg* 2000;87(1):79–85.

Miller PR, Fabian TC, Bee TK, et al. Blunt cerebrovascular injuries: diagnosis and treatment. *J Trauma* 2001;51(2):279–286.

Ramadan F, Rutledge R, Oller D, et al. Carotid artery trauma: a review of contemporary trauma center experiences. *J Vasc Surg* 1995;21(1):46–56.

Thal ER, Eastridge B. Role of arteriography in penetrating vascular injuries. In: Ernst CB, Stanley JC, eds. *Current therapy in vascular surgery.* St. Louis: Mosby, 2001:584–586.

23

Vascular Trauma 2: Abdominal Vascular Injuries

Carrie Sims, MD, and David Berger, MD

I. Incidence

The incidence and mortality of major vascular injuries occurring in trauma patients varies considerably depending on the mechanism of injury. Abdominal stab wounds are associated with major vascular injury in 10% cases and carry an overall mortality rate of 32%. Approximately 25% of abdominal gunshot wounds will injure major abdominal vasculature, with an estimated mortality rate of 53%. Although patients sustaining blunt abdominal trauma injure major abdominal vessels in only 5% to 10% of the cases, these injuries are highly lethal and are associated with a 70% mortality rate.

II. Pathophysiology

A. Penetrating Trauma

Penetrating trauma to the abdomen causes direct damage the vessels encountered or is associated with collateral damage secondary to high-energy transfer. Knife wounds typically transect the vessel completely or create a lateral wall defect with free bleeding or hematoma formation. Gunshot wounds, on the other hand, are associated with a high-velocity injury and can damage a vessel several centimeters beyond the bullet track, even if the tissue appears grossly normal. This blast effect can lead to intimal flap formation with secondary thrombosis and requires a more extensive débridement to ensure viable tissue. Rarely, penetrating injuries are associated with the formation of arteriovenous fistulas.

B. Blunt Trauma

Abdominal vascular injuries resulting from blunt trauma with rapid deceleration have two different injury patterns. Deceleration leads to the avulsion of small branching vessels at sites of fixation (e.g., superior mesenteric artery). Vessels can also stretch or partially tear at points of fixation, resulting in an intimal injury with thrombosis or pseudoaneurysm formation.

Blunt trauma can also result in crush injuries. The "seatbelt aorta," which is a classic example of this injury, results when the abdominal aorta is crushed between the restraining seatbelt and the lumbar spine during deceleration. An anterior crush injury, or even a direct blow to the posterior spine, can create intimal disruption of the abdominal aorta that can progress to complete thrombosis. This injury may not cause significant signs or symptoms until the aorta is entirely thrombosed, making a high index of suspicion necessary for early diagnosis.

III. Diagnosis

A. Symptoms

Penetrating wounds to the trunk (i.e., the area between the nipples and the upper thighs) are the most common cause of abdominal vascular injuries. The track of the knife or bullet determines the extent of the injury. Patients can arrive in extremis or can complain of increasing abdominal pain or tenderness with or without hypotension.

With blunt trauma, injuries to the upper and mid-abdominal arteries and veins are more common. Injuries secondary to vessel avulsion will rapidly lead to intraperitoneal hemorrhage and hypovolemic shock. Vessel thrombosis, on the other hand, can present more insidiously with increasing abdominal or flank pain.

B. Signs

Physical findings will depend on whether the patient has a contained hematoma, frank hemorrhage, or vessel thrombosis. Patients with a contained hematoma will be hypotensive on transit but will respond rapidly to resuscitation. They may appear remarkably stable. Patients with free intraperitoneal hemorrhage, on the other hand, will be hypotensive and can present with a distended, firm abdomen. With vessel thrombosis, the patient's pain can be out of proportion to the examination. In addition to a thorough secondary survey, pay special attention to the vascular and neurologic examination. Femoral pulses can be absent in cases of aortic injury or lost on one side, which suggests a transected or thrombosed iliac artery. Lower extremity weakness may be found in patients with blunt infrarenal aortic injuries and neurologic findings can precede the development vascular deficits.

C. Diagnostic Tests

Diagnostic tests are generally more useful in the evaluation of blunt and crush injuries. Patients with penetrating abdominal vascular injuries require very little diagnostic workup other than a chest x-ray study before transfer to the operating room (OR). Available diagnostic tools include the following:

1. Focused Abdominal Sonography for Trauma Ultrasound

The focused abdominal sonography for trauma (FAST) examination is highly accurate in detecting free intraperitoneal fluid and can be used to quickly assess the abdomen in the unstable patient. Although the FAST examination is helpful in identifying the presence of hemoperitoneum, specific vascular injuries are difficult to detect.

2. Abdominal and Pelvic Computed Tomography Scan with Intravenous Contrast

An abdominal and pelvic computed tomography (CT) scan with intravenous contrast can provide rapid, noninvasive, and highly detailed information with little associated risk. The presence of contrast extravasation, contrast pooling, or the lack of vessel opacification suggests vascular injury.

3.   Abdominal and Pelvic Aortography

Although infrequently used as a primary diagnostic tool given the prevalence and excellent detail provided by CT scan, abdominal and pelvic aortography is particularly useful in diagnosing and treating deep pelvic arterial injuries.

4.   Renal Arteriography

If no renal function is seen on CT (or intravenous pyelogram [IVP]), arteriography may still be indicated. It may be possible to embolize actively bleeding vessels. If findings suggest major vascular injury on CT, however, it is prudent to go to the OR rather than delay with further diagnostic studies.

5.   Diagnostic Peritoneal Lavage

Although diagnostic peritoneal lavage (DPL) can readily reveal gross intraperitoneal blood, it cannot differentiate between solid organ trauma and vascular-specific injuries. Retroperitoneal injuries will also be missed because only the peritoneal cavity is surveyed during the lavage. Lastly, false positive results can occur in the setting of pelvic fractures if associated hematoma leaks into the peritoneum. Given these limitations, DPL is helpful in determining whether the abdominal cavity is a potential source of hemorrhage in a hemodynamically unstable patient, but it is not particularly helpful in specifically diagnosing abdominal vascular injuries.

6.   Intravenous Pyelogram

Before the emergence of the CT scan as a readily available diagnostic study, IVP was routinely used to evaluate the function of both kidneys. If the IVP demonstrated lack of contrast excretion, either the renal artery was thrombosed or the kidney was congenitally absent. Even today, some argue that it may be worthwhile to shoot a single shot IVP in the unstable patient to confirm the presence of renal function.

IV.   Surgical Evaluation

A.   Initial Management

In the emergency department (ED), the extent of resuscitation depends on the clinical status of the patient. Naturally, first attend to the basics of airway, breathing, and circulation. Perform the primary and secondary survey with special attention to the abdominal, vascular, and neurologic examination.

Obtain large bore intravenous access in the upper extremities. Lower extremity intravenous access should be avoided whenever the possibility of major abdominal vascular injury is suspected. In addition to the potential ineffectiveness of resuscitating via lower extremity access, there is a risk of forcing clot out of the venous injury into the chest. Once intravenous access has been established, a blood bank sample and basic laboratory studies, including a complete blood count and an arterial blood gas with base deficit, should be obtained.

As with all trauma patients, hypothermia should be avoided. Patients should be resuscitated with heated fluids and blood products should be warmed before infusion. The examination area should be heated and patients should be covered after the primary and secondary survey. If the patient is found to be hypothermic on arrival, external heating lamps or a Bair hugger should be used.

If the patient is hypotensive with a distended abdomen, the time in the ED should be minimized (e.g., 5 minutes) before transferring to OR. Stable patients with potential abdominal vascular injuries should have a CT scan with intravenous contrast as part of their trauma evaluation.

Patients who are agonal with a distended abdomen or those who have had a witnessed cardiac arrest in the emergency department may benefit from an emergent thoracotomy to cross-clamp the aorta. Although the mortality associated with this presentation is exceedingly high, an ED thoracotomy may be the only way to maintain perfusion to the heart and brain until definitive control can be obtained.

B. Operative Exploration
   1. Initial Moves
   The patient should be prepared and draped from the chin to knees while awake. Everything required for a successful operation, including blood products, should be in place before induction. Whenever possible, a cell-saver device should be used. A nasogastric tube and Foley catheter should be placed. A single dose of broad-spectrum antibiotics should be given before the incision.

   To decrease the risk of hypothermia, the OR should be heated and warming blankets should be applied to the patient's extremities. All fluids should be warmed and a heating cascade should be used in the anesthesia machine. Because hypothermia leads to coagulopathy, initiate aggressive maneuvers to rewarm the hypothermic patient. The nasogastric tube, thoracostomy tubes, and open body cavities can be irrigated with warm fluid to achieve normothermia.

   A role may be seen for thoracotomy before laparotomy in patients who are persistently hypotensive. In some centers, a lateral thoracotomy is performed to cross-clamp the descending thoracic aorta if systolic blood pressure is ≤70 mm Hg. If the descending aorta is cross-clamped, take care not to let the systolic blood pressure rise higher than 160 to 180 mm Hg. Sustained high pressures in the cross-clamped aorta will lead to left ventricular dilation and acute cardiac failure. When the bleeding site is controlled, the aortic cross-clamp can be gradually removed to prevent profound reflow hypotension.

   If a thoracotomy is not indicated, perform an exploratory laparotomy by making a generous midline incision. Take care not to violate the peritoneum until the fascia is divided over the entire length of the incision. The abdominal wall can serve as a tamponade and the release of the peritoneum can lead to rapid exsanguination and cardiac arrest. Communication with the anesthesiologist during this maneuver is critical. If the patient becomes hypotensive after the peritoneum is incised, compress the supraceliac aorta and allow the anesthetist to aggressively resuscitate the patient.

On entering the abdominal cavity, remove blood and clots that are readily visible and pack lap pads into areas of suspected injury. Control active hemorrhage before any further exploration. Packing typically controls solid organ injury hemorrhage. Continued bleeding despite adequate packing is suggestive of a major vascular injury. Use direct finger pressure, compression with sponge sticks, or vascular clamps to control vascular hemorrhage until formal proximal and distal control can be obtained. More definitive control may be needed if brisk hemorrhage continues. Compressing the aorta either above the celiac trunk or at the thoracic descending aorta is an effective means of abating the hemorrhage to identify and address the abdominal vascular injury.

Once temporary vascular control has been obtained concomitant gastrointestinal injuries can be expeditiously temporized. Rapidly apply Babcock noncrushing intestinal clamps or gastrointestinal staples to any intestinal perforations to prevent ongoing enteric contamination. Definitive vascular repair can then be performed. In the setting of a contained retroperitoneal hematoma, enough time generally exists to definitively repair the intestinal injuries, irrigate and then reapproach the vascular injury.

2. Operative Exposure

The abdomen can be divided into four anatomic vascular zones: the midline retroperitoneal area, the upper lateral retroperitoneum, the pelvic retroperitoneum, and the portal-retrohepatic area (**Fig. 23-1**). The Abdominal Vascular Injury Scale developed by the American Association for the Surgery of Trauma provides an objective method of rating the magnitude of injury (**Table 23-1**).

C. Injuries in Zone 1: Midline Retroperitoneal Area

It is useful to divide the midline retroperitoneal zone into two different anatomic areas: the supramesocolic area and the inframesocolic area. A hematoma or hemorrhage arising from the supramesocolic area suggests an injury to the suprarenal aorta, the celiac axis, the proximal superior mesenteric artery (SMA), or the proximal renal artery. Injuries arising in the inframesocolic area are secondary to trauma to the infrarenal abdominal aorta or the inferior vena cava (IVC).

1. Midline Supramesocolic Area

Penetrating injuries to the aorta as it enters the abdominal cavity carry an incredibly high mortality

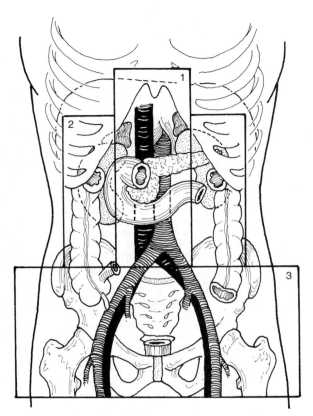

Figure 23-1.   Retroperitineal vascular injury zones: Zone 1 (midline retroperitoneal area), Zone 2 (upper lateral retroperitoneal area), Zone 3 (pelvic retroperitoneum).

rate (>60%), in part because of the difficulty in exposing and controlling an injury in this area. If a midline penetrating injury is found to have massive bleeding or a large midline supramesocolic hematoma is found on exploration, suspect an injury to the proximal aorta.

   a.   Exposure. A left medial visceral rotation will afford the best exposure to vessels within the supramesocolic area (**Fig. 23-2**). With this maneuver, all left-sided intraabdominal viscera, including the left colon, left kidney, spleen, tail of pancreas, and fundus of the stomach, are rotated medially. The abdominal aorta can be completely visualized from the diaphragmatic hiatus to the common iliacs. This exposure can take several minutes to complete, however, and a potential risk exists of damaging the spleen, kidney, and left renal artery during the rotation. This risk can

Table 23-1. AAST abdominal vascular injury scale

Grade	Injury Characteristics	OIS Grade	ICD-9	AIS-90
I	Unnamed superior mesenteric artery of superior mesenteric vein branches	I	902.20/902.39	NS
	Unnamed inferior mesenteric artery or inferior mesenteric vein branches	I	902.27/902.32	NS
	Phrenic artery or vein	I		NS
	Lumbar artery of vein	I		NS
	Gonadal artery or vein	I	902.89	NS
	Ovarian artery of vein	I	902.89	NS
	Other unnamed small arterial of venous structures requiring ligation	I	902.89 902.81/902.82 902.90	NS
II	Right, left, or common hepatic artery	II	902.22	3
	Splenic artery vein	II	902.23/902.34	3
	Right or left gastric arteries	II	902.21	3
	Gastroduodenal artery	II	902.24	3
	Inferior mesenteric artery, trunk, or inferior mesenteric vein, trunk	II	902.27/902.32	3
	Primary names branches of mesenteric artery (e.g., ileocolic artery) or mesenteric vein	II	902.26/902.31	3
	Other named abdominal vessels requiring ligation or repair	II	902.89	3
III[a]	Superior mesenteric vein, trunk	III	902.31	3
	Renal artery, vein	III	902.41/902.42	3
	Iliac artery or vein	III	902.53/902.54	3
	Hypogastric artery or vein	III	902.51/902.52	3
	Vena cava, infrarenal	III	902.10	3
IV[b]	Superior mesenteric artery, trunk	IV	902.25	3
	Celiac axis, proper	IV	902.24	3
	Vena cava, suprarenal and infrahepatic	IV	902.10	3
	Aorta, infrarenal	IV	902.00	4
V[b]	Portal vein	V	902.33	3
	Extraparenchymal hepatic vein	V	902.11	3 (hepatic vein)

continued

Table 23-1. *Continued*

Grade	Injury Characteristics	OIS Grade	ICD-9	AIS-90
	Vena cava, retrohepatic or suprahepatic	V	902.19	5 (liver)
	Aorta, suprarenal and subdiaphragmatic	V	902.00	5 4

[a] Increase one grade if multiple injuries involve >50% of vessel circumference.
[b] Reduce one grade if laceration is <25% of vessel circumference.
Note: This classification is applicable to extraparechymal vasular injuries. If the vessel injury is within 2 cm of the parechyma of a specific organ, refer to the injury scale for that organ.
AAST, American Association for the Surgery of Trauma; AIS, Abbreviated Injury Scale; ICD, International Classification of Diseases.

be minimized if the kidney is left in situ. Additionally, it can be helpful to transect the left crus at the 2 o'clock position to expose the distal descending thoracic aorta above the diaphragmatic hiatus.

With active hemorrhage, the supramesocolic area can be controlled temporarily by packing with laparotomy pads or by compressing the supraceliac aorta, either manually or with an aortic compression device.

b. Vascular Control. Proximal control of the aorta can be achieved in a number of ways. The abdominal incision can be converted to a thoracoabdominal incision by extending the midline into the left chest along the seventh or eighth interspace. The diaphragm is then divided from the ribs in a circumferential manner with at least 2-cm margins from the ribs to preserve blood and nerve supply. A left lateral thoracotomy can also be used to gain access to the descending thoracic aorta for proximal control. Lastly, a supraceliac clamp can be applied to the descending aorta. The lesser omentum is divided and the left crus of the diaphragm is incised at the 2 o'clock position. The stomach and esophagus are retracted to the left, exposing the aortic hiatus. The aorta is cleared using manual dissection and a supraceliac crossclamp is then applied.

Distal control of the aorta in the supramesocolic area can be difficult. The anterior location of the celiac axis and SMA, as well as the dense neural and lymphatic tissue surrounding these vessels, make exposure challenging. If necessary, the celiac axis can be ligated to better visualize the aorta and gain distal control.

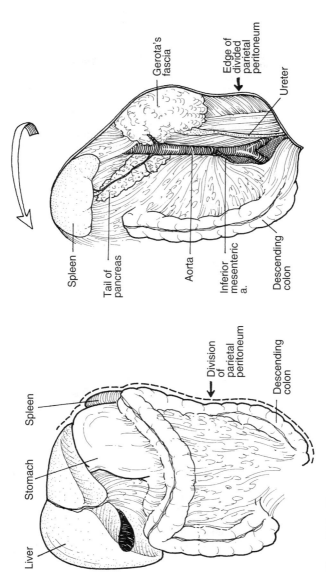

Figure 23-2. Mattox maneuver (left medial visceral rotation) exposes the midline retroperitoneal structures and affords excellent exposure of the abdominal aorta.

Close communication with the anesthesiologist throughout the operation is critical. The anesthesiologist should be alerted before applying and removing vascular clamps on major arteries. If an aortic cross-clamp has been in place for more than 30 minutes, the anesthetist should be forewarned 5 to 10 minutes before declamping to prepare for the possibility of hypotension by administering additional blood or fluids. If there has been a prolonged aortic cross-clamp time, the proximal clamp should be removed slowly and consideration should be given to prophylactically administering sodium bicarbonate to reverse the "washout" acidosis. Many surgeons will also administer mannitol for its antioxidant properties in cases of an extended aortic cross-clamp.

c. Specific Injuries in Zone 1: Midline Supramesocolic Area

(1) Supraceliac Aortic Injuries. Small wounds to the supraceliac aorta can be repaired with running 3-0 or 4-0 polypropylene suture. If two small injuries are adjacent, they can be connected and closed in a transverse fashion. If the closure results in excessive narrowing or a piece of aorta is missing, a patch aortoplasty with polytetrafluoroethylene (PTFE) can be used. If the aorta has been cleanly transected, an end-to-end anastomosis can be used. An end-to-end anastomosis should not be used in cases of extensive tissue loss. Instead, the damaged aorta should be resected and replaced. Even in the setting of gross enteric contamination, the most appropriate aortic conduit is a 12-mm or 14-mm Dacron or PTFE tube graft. Although, intuitively, concern is seen in placing a prosthetic graft in the setting of intestinal or gastric contamination, infectious complications are rare, provided the graft is covered appropriately and perioperative antibiotics are used. Vascular and intestinal injuries, however, should not be repaired simultaneously. Intestinal injuries should be rapidly controlled (e.g., closed with staples or Babcock clamps) and packed away. First, repair the vascular injuries. After changing gloves, copiously irrigate the abdominal cavity is copiously irrigated and address the intestinal injuries.

(2) Branches of Celiac Access. Injuries to the branches of the celiac access are difficult to repair secondary to the dense neural and lymphatic tissue found in this area. Excellent collateral blood supply exists to this area, however, making definitive repair less of a concern. In general, injuries to the left gastric artery or proximal splenic artery should be ligated. The common hepatic artery, however, is typically larger and often can be repaired by means of a lateral arteriorrhaphy, end-to-end anastomosis, or insertion of saphenous vein or prosthetic graft. The common hepatic artery can be ligated proximal to the origin of the gastroduodenal artery without hesitation, given the extensive collateral flow from the SMA. If the entire celiac access is injured, ligate all three vessels.

(3) Injuries to the Superior Mesenteric Artery. Injuries to the SMA are managed on the basis of their anatomic location. If injury is near the SMA origin, exposure can be obtained by performing a left medial visceral rotation (described above, zone 1 injuries). If the injury is beneath the pancreas, the pancreas may need to be divided to optimize exposure. Injuries between the origin of the SMA and the middle colic artery, however, are difficult to repair and a potential exists for pancreatic leaks near repair sites. Given these concerns, some authors have suggested that SMA should be ligated if there is extensive injury in this area. Theoretically, ligation of the SMA should be well tolerated, given the abundance of collateral vessels from the foregut and hindgut. Intense vasoconstriction of the distal SMA in the setting of shock, however, makes this unlikely. A temporary intraluminal shunt can be inserted into the débrided ends as a damage control maneuver. In the more stable patient or at the time of a second look laparotomy, the injured SMA can be bypassed to the aorta. A saphenous vein or PTFE graft is taken from the distal infrarenal aorta, tunneled through the posterior aspect of the small bowel mesentery and sutured to the underside of the proximal SMA. This avoids exposing the vascular anastomosis to possible pancreatic secretions. The aortic suture line should be covered with retroperitoneal fat or omentum to decrease the likelihood of an aortoenteric fistula.

If the SMA cannot be repaired, it can be ligated as a last resort. If the SMA is sacrificed, the distal midgut, especially the cecum and ascending colon, will be compromised. Postoperatively, the patient must receive enough fluid to ensure adequate collateral blood flow and the threshold for reexploration should be low.

Injuries beyond the middle colic artery and at the enteric branches of the SMA need to be repaired, given poor collateral blood supply. If the injured artery cannot be repaired, it may be necessary to resect the bowel supplied by the injured vessel. If bowel viability is questionable and resection is not performed, plan a second look laparotomy 24 to 48 hours later.

(4) Superior Mesenteric Vein. Given the close association to the overlying pancreas, uncinate process, and SMA, repair of superior mesenteric vein (SMV) injuries are difficult. The pancreas may need to be divided to better visualize and control the injury. If the injury is distal to the pancreas, the SMV can usually be manually compressed. Anterior injuries can be primarily repaired with a running 5-0 polypropylene suture. If a posterior injury is encountered, multiple collateral vessels that enter the vein at this level will need to be ligated to expose the injury adequately. In cases of multiple vascular and visceral injuries, the SMV can be ligated in the young trauma patient with good survivability, provided aggressive postoperative fluid resuscitation is administered. Small bowel congestion and discoloration often immediately follow SMV ligation. If this occurs, it is prudent to plan for reexploration within 24 to 48 hours to ensure that the venous congestion has not progressed to frank ischemia.

2. Midline Inframesocolic Area

The lower area of the midline retroperitoneum (zone 1) is considered the midline inframesocolic area. Injuries in this location can damage either the infrarenal abdominal aorta or the IVC.

a. Exposure. Injuries to the infrarenal aorta can be approached by retracting the transverse mesocolon superiorly, rotating the small bowel into the right upper quadrant, and then opening the midline retroperitoneum directly over the aorta. The aorta is exposed from the iliac bifurcation to the left renal vein, taking care not to injure the origin of the inferior mesenteric artery. An aortic cross-clamp is placed immediately inferior to the left renal vein. It may be necessary to divide the peritoneal attachments of the inferior duodenum and ligament of Treitz to more fully expose the left renal vein. If more exposure of the proximal aorta is needed, the left renal vein can be divided close to the IVC.

b. Specific Injuries in the Infrarenal Aorta

(1) Infrarenal Aorta. Penetrating injuries to the infrarenal aorta can be repaired using a lateral aortorrhaphy, patch aortoplasty, or end-to-end anastomosis, or by inserting a

prosthetic tube graft. In young trauma patients, it is rarely possible to place anything
larger than a 12- to 14-mm PTFE tube graft.
Following repair, cover the aortic injury with
healthy, viable tissue. In most young trauma
patients, the retroperitoneal tissue is rather
thin and not suitable coverage. If the retroperitoneal tissues are insufficient, the gastrocolic omentum can be mobilized into the
lesser sac and brought through the transverse
mesocolon to provide adequate coverage.

In patients with blunt trauma, the most
common injury to the infrarenal aorta is intimal disruption. As the intimal flap dissects
distally, aortic thrombosis can occur, leading
to acute arterial insufficiency. If the intimal
dissection is minimal, a thromboendarterec-
tomy can be performed and the intimal flap
can be sutured down. If the damage is extensive or if a false aneurysm has formed, an
interposition tube graft should be inserted.
Recently, however, this standard approach
has been challenged and there are several
case reports of endovascular stent placement.
Although long-term feasibility remains to be
determined, this minimally invasive approach
can provide a viable option for the repair of
infrarenal aortic injuries.

(2)   Inferior Mesenteric Artery. In general, if the inferior mesenteric artery is injured, it should be ligated as close to the aorta
as possible.

(3)   Inferior Vena Cava. An IVC injury
should be suspected if the aorta is intact but
a hematoma is present or active hemorrhage
coming from the base of the mesentery of the
ascending colon or hepatic flexure is discovered. The entire caval system can be examined by performing a Kocher maneuver in
conjunction with mobilization and medial
reflection of the right colon and mesentery.
This right medial visceral rotation maneuver
allows visualization of the entire infrahepatic
IVC down to the iliac veins (**Fig. 23-3**).

To adequately expose an injury to the IVC,
the loose overlying retroperitoneal fatty tissue must be stripped away. An injury to the
anterior surface is best controlled by applying a Satinsky-type vascular clamp. If this
proves challenging, the injury can be first
controlled with the application of Judd-Allis
clamps. With extensive injury, the vena cava
can be controlled proximally and distally
with sponge sticks, although extensive back-
bleeding can occur from lumbar veins. Occa-

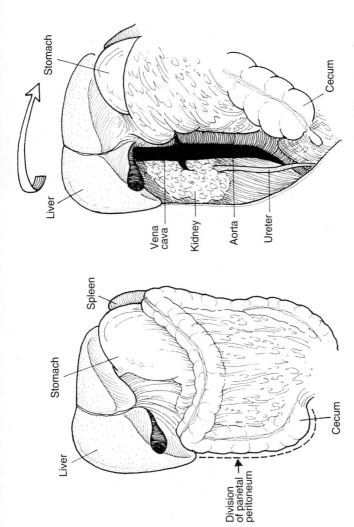

Figure 23-3.   Catell-Braasch maneuver (right medial visceral rotation) exposes the midline retroperitoneal structures and affords excellent exposure of the inferior vena cava.

sionally, the injury will be so extensive that it may be necessary to completely occlude the vena cava by applying large DeBakey aortic clamps above and below the IVC injury. Occluding the IVC can significantly reduce venous return and the patient can become profoundly hypotensive. If the hemorrhage can only be controlled by cross-clamping the inferior vena cava, the infrarenal abdominal aorta should be occluded simultaneously.

Particularly treacherous areas occur at the confluence of the iliac veins and at the renal junction because of the overlapping arterial structures. The right common iliac artery can be divided and reflected to the left to better visualize the proximal IVC and common iliac veins. Following the venous repair, the divided iliac artery is then reanastomosed in an end-to-end fashion. With injuries near the renal veins, the infrarenal and suprarenal vena cava are compressed with sponge sticks and the renal veins are isolated with vascular loops or clamps. Alternatively, the right kidney can be mobilized medially, exposing the junction of the IVC and right renal vein. A vascular clamp can then be applied, taking care to ligate and not avulse the first lumbar vein as it enters the junction of the IVC and renal vein. The left renal vein can be ligated and divided as it joins the IVC, given its extensive collateral vessels. A Foley catheter can also be used to tamponade caval hemorrhage. After inserting and carefully inflating a 5- or 30-mL Foley balloon into the caval laceration and carefully inflated, gently apply traction. Once the bleeding is arrested, place either vascular clamps or simple sutures. Deflate the balloon and remove the Foley catheter before completing the suture line

Anterior perforations of the IVC are best repaired transversely with a 4-0 or 5-0 polypropylene running suture, taking care to evert the edges. Everting the edges ensures intimal contact and decreases the risk of suture line thrombosis. Excessive efforts to mobilize the IVC to repair a small posterior wound can cause more harm than good. With large posterior perforations, the posterior injury can be repaired by extending the anterior laceration and repairing the posterior component from the inside of the cava. The patient can develop thrombosis and IVC occlusion if the repair excessively narrows the IVC. If the patient is unstable, make no attempt to revise the repair. If the patient is stable, consider applying a large PTFE venous patch to prevent postoperative venous occlusion.

Ligation of the IVC may be appropriate and necessary if the patient is exsanguinating and requires an extensive repair of the IVC. If the infrarenal IVC is ligated, the patient must receive aggressive resuscitation in the postoperative period to maintain adequate circulating intravascular volume. Additionally, bilateral below-the-knee, four-compartment fasciotomies should be performed at the first operation with an understanding that thigh fasciotomies may become necessary within the first 48 hours. Elastic wraps should be applied to the lower extremities, which should be continuously elevated for 5 to 7 days. The patient should continue to wear elastic wraps when ambulating in the postoperative period and full-length fitted support hose may be needed if residual edema is present at the time of discharge.

Ligation of the suprarenal vena cava is occasionally necessary in situations of life-threatening exsanguination. If the patient stabilizes in the early postoperative period, the vena cava should be reconstructed to prevent renal failure. The suprarenal vena cava can be repaired using either autogenous tissue or a PTFE graft. Occasionally, a vascular conduit cannot be placed. In these circumstances, manage the ligated suprarenal IVC either with a splenorenal or portocaval anastomosis.

D. Injuries in Zone 2: Upper lateral Retroperitoneum

A hematoma or hemorrhage found in zone 2 is suggestive of an injury to the renal artery, the renal vein, or the kidney itself. With blunt trauma, a perirenal hematoma should not be explored *if* a preoperative IVP, renal arteriogram, or CT scan has demonstrated *no* abnormality. The management of perirenal injuries secondary to penetrating trauma is controversial. Occasionally, a preoperative CT scan in stable patients with flank wounds will demonstrate an isolated minor renal injury. In stable patients without peritoneal signs, consider nonoperative management. In patients who have exploratory surgery, the management of a nonexpanding perirenal hematoma is open for debate. Some surgeons routinely explore these hematomas, but doing so can lead to a higher nephrectomy rate. If no free intraperitoneal blood is seen and the perirenal hematoma does not appear to be rapidly expanding, obtain proximal control. The renal vessels are located in the midline at the base of the mesocolon and can be isolated with silastic vessel loops. On the right, the duodenum will need to be reflected to control the renal vein as it enters the IVC. It is not necessary to obtain central control if active bleeding is seen from Gerota's fascia or from the retroperitoneum overlying the renal vessels. With active hemorrhage, incise the retroperitoneum lateral to the injured kidney incised and elevate the kidney into the wound. Apply a large vascular clamp proximal to the hilum.

1. Renal Artery

The renal artery can be difficult to repair because it is a small vessel that is deeply embedded. Simple lacerations can be managed with either primary repair or an end-to-end anastomosis. For more complex injuries, an interposition graft with saphenous vein or PTFE can be used if a reasonable hope exists for salvaging the kidney. In cases of multiple injuries with a long preoperative period of renal ischemia, a nephrectomy may be a more appropriate option provided the patient has another working kidney.

Management of renal artery deceleration injuries remains controversial. Intimal tears that do not compromise renal blood flow can be managed with anticoagulation therapy followed by an isotope renogram to document perfusion within the first several days. If the renal artery is totally occluded, the most important factor in terms of salvage is the total ischemic time. If the renal artery thrombosis is diagnosed within 6 hours of the injury, attempt revascularization. Mobilize the injured kidney medially and perform a limited resection of the renal artery with an end-to-end anastomosis. Until the period of acute tubular necrosis resolves (6 to 8 weeks), the success of the revascularization may not be known. For injuries that are identified >12 hours after the injury, the current trend is to recommend observation with or without anticoagulation. Although immediate nephrectomy has been advocated in the past, several reports have shown spontaneous recovery. Moreover, given the relatively low incidence of chronic hypertension in cases of renal artery thrombosis, prophylactic nephrectomy cannot be recommended.

2. Renal Vein

Patients with penetrating renal vein injuries are generally stable because the hemorrhage is tamponaded by the retroperitoneum. Renal vein avulsion, however, can result in exsanguination. In general, bleeding can be controlled with either manual compression or vascular clamps and the renal vein perforation can be repaired primarily. If ligation of the right vein is necessary, perform a right nephrectomy. If the left vein is ligated, the left kidney should remain viable if the left adrenal and gonadal veins are preserved.

E. Zone 3: Pelvic Retroperitoneum

Pelvic hematomas in the setting of blunt trauma are often secondary to bleeding from a pelvic fracture site and should not be explored. If such a hematoma continues to expand intraoperatively, the pelvis should be packed and the patient should be immediately transferred to interventional radiology for arteriography and embolization. Ligation of the internal iliac arteries in this situation is not helpful.

Hemorrhage or hematoma found in the pelvis following penetrating trauma, on the other hand, suggests an injury to the iliac artery or vein. Because significant bleeding can result from these injuries, the hematoma should not be opened until the patient is adequately resuscitated and vascular control has been obtained. If the hematoma is not actively bleeding or expanding, other intraabdominal injuries can be addressed first.

1. **Exposure**

Expose the proximal iliac vessels by packing the small bowel into the right upper quadrant and dividing the midline retroperitoneum over the aortic bifurcation. Obtain proximal control by passing silastic vessel loops around the iliac vein and artery. Distal control is easily obtained by isolating the external iliac vessels as they exit the abdomen just proximal to the inguinal ligament. Isolate and control bleeding in the internal iliac artery to prevent major back-bleeding. If bilateral iliac vessels are injured, total pelvic vascular isolation can be achieved by cross-clamping the aorta and IVC just above their bifurcations followed by the application of vascular clamps to the iliac artery and vein in the distal pelvis.

2. **Injuries to the Common or External Iliac Artery**

Injuries to the common or external iliac artery should be repaired because simple ligation leads to extremity ischemia and a 40% to 50% rate of amputation. The injured artery can generally be repaired with a lateral arteriorrhaphy, resection with end-to-end anastomosis, or with the insertion of a conduit. The saphenous vein provides an excellent conduit option, especially in the setting of gross contamination. If necessary, an intraluminal shunt can be inserted in the setting of a damage control laparotomy with the patient returning for definitive repair when stable.

Extensive injuries to common or external iliac in setting of significant enteric or fecal contamination, however, can be problematic. Both end-to-end repairs and vascular grafts can have late postoperative blowouts secondary to pelvic infection. In the setting of significant contamination, divide the iliac artery above the injury, oversew with a double row of running 4-0 or 5-0 polypropylene suture, and cover with uninjured retroperitoneum. If the devascularized limb looks threatened and the patient is stable, use an extra-anatomic femorofemoral bypass graft to reestablish blood flow. If the patient is not stable and revascularization is not an option, perform a four-compartment below-the-knee fasciotomy because the limb will go on to develop ischemic edema and a compartment syndrome. The patient should be aggressively resuscitated and revascularized with a femorofemoral bypass within 4 to 6 hours.

3. Injuries to the Internal Iliac Artery

The internal iliac artery can be ligated, if necessary. If fact, young healthy trauma patients have extreme pelvic collateral vessels and bilateral internal iliac artery ligation can be performed, if necessary.

4. Injuries to the Iliac Veins

Bleeding in the iliac veins can generally be controlled by compression and do not need to be isolated with silastic vessel loops. Significantly more damage can be caused with aggressive attempts at controlling the venous injury. Often, packing the injury coupled with patience is more effective. If necessary, the overlying right common iliac artery may be divided to expose an injury to the right iliac vein. Similarly, the internal iliac artery may be divided and ligated to expose an injury to internal iliac vein. The injured iliac vein can either be repaired primarily with 4-0 or 5-0 polypropylene suture or it can be ligated. If the vessel is ligated or appears narrowed after the repair, the lower extremities should be elevated and wrapped with elastic bands for the first 5 to 7 postoperative days.

F. Port Hepatis Zone

An injury to the porta hepatis should be suspected when a hematoma in the right upper quadrant is discovered. Before exploring the hematoma, apply a vascular loop or noncrushing vascular clamp to the proximal hepatoduodenal ligament (Pringle maneuver). An angled vascular clamp can be used to get distal control. If this is not feasible, it may be possible to get manual control with forceps until the bleeding site can be identified. Do not place sutures until the vascular injury is precisely defined in order to avoid damage to the common bile duct. The hepatoduodenal ligament should be carefully dissected to expose the hepatic artery, common bile duct, and portal vein.

1. Injuries to the Hepatic Artery

Injuries to the hepatic artery in this location can be difficult to repair, although occasionally the artery can be primarily repaired. In general, ligation beyond the origin of the gastroduodenal artery is generally well tolerated unless the patient has an associated hepatic injury that requires extensive suturing or débridement. If the right hepatic artery is ligated, a cholecystectomy should also be performed. Injuries that require ligation of both the hepatic artery *and* the portal vein as they enter one lobe, on the other hand, will lead to liver necrosis and mandate a hepatectomy.

2. Injuries to Portal Vein

Injuries to the portal vein are often lethal. To expose the portal vein above the pancreas, mobilize the common bile duct to the left and perform an extensive Kocher maneuver. Occasionally, the pancreas needs to be divided if the injury extends under the pancreas. The injured portal vein should be primarily repaired with a lateral venorrhaphy using a running 4-0 or 5-0 polypropylene sutures. Although other methods have been attempted for more complex injuries, including resection with end-to-end anastomosis, interposition grafting, transposition of the splenic vein, or end-to-side portocaval shunts, aggressive attempts at portal restoration are not appropriate in the hypovolemic patient. In the damage control setting, ligation of the portal vein is appropriate and is compatible with life, provided the patient is aggressively resuscitated.

3.   Retrohepatic Area

A hematoma or hemorrhage in the retrohepatic area is suggestive of an injury to the retrohepatic vena cava, hepatic vein, right renal vein, or overlying liver. If the hematoma is not expanding and has no clear association with the kidney, perihepatic packing around the right lobe of the liver for 24 to 48 hours has been shown to prevent further expansion of caval or hepatic vein injury. Frank hemorrhage that does not appear to be coming directly from the liver parenchyma will need further investigation. Compress the right lobe of the liver posteriorly to tamponade a caval injury while applying a Pringle maneuver. Mobilize the right lobe of the liver by dividing the anterior coronary and triangular ligaments. As the liver is rotated to view the IVC, grasp obvious injuries with a forceps or Judd-Allis followed by a Satinsky clamp. Injuries can be repaired with a running 4-0 or 5-0 polypropylene suture. If the hemorrhage cannot be controlled, an atriocaval shunt can be attempted by using a 36F chest tube.

V.   Complications

Major complications associated with the repair of injuries to the great vessels of the abdomen include thrombosis, dehiscence, and infection. Given the risk of occlusion in small vasoconstricted vessels, the patient must be aggressively resuscitated and a second look laparotomy should be considered within 12 to 24 hours if the patient's metabolic state suggests ischemia. Occasionally, vascular enteric fistulas occur following the repair of aortic or superior mesenteric artery injuries. These fistulas typically occur at suture lines and can be avoided by covering the suture lines with retroperitoneal tissue or viable omentum.

SELECTED READING

Asensio JA, Forno W, Roldan G, et al. Abdominal vascular injuries: injuries to the aorta. *Surg Clin North Am* 2001;81(6):1395–416.

Biffl WL, Burch JM. Management of abdominal vascular injuries. *Semin Vasc Surg* 1998;11(4):243–254.

Carrillo EH, Bergamini TM, Miller FB, et al. Abdominal vascular injuries. *J Trauma.* 1997;43(1):164–171.

Feliciano DV, Burch JM, Graham JM. Abdominal vascular injury. In: *Trauma,* 4th ed. New York: McGraw-Hill, 2000:783–785.

Feliciano DV. Injuries to the great vessels of the abdomen. In: *ACS surgery: principles and practice.* New York: WebMD, 2002:1–11.

Michaels AJ, Gerndt SJ, Taheri PA, et al. Blunt force injury of the abdominal aorta. *J Trauma.* 1996;41(1):105–109.

Mullins RJ, Huckfeldt R, Trunkey DD. Abdominal vascular injuries. *Surg Clin North Am* 1996;76(4):813–832.

Picard E, Marty-Ane CH, Vernhet H, et al. Endovascular management of traumatic infrarenal abdominal aortic dissection. *Ann Vasc Surg* 1998;12(6):515–521.

Thal ER, Eastridge BJ, Milhoan R. Operative exposure of abdominal injuries and closure of the abdomen. In: *ACS surgery: principles and practice.* New York: WebMD, 2002:1–8.

Voellinger DC, Saddakni S, Melton SM, et al. Endovascular repair of a traumatic infrarenal aortic transection: a case report and review. *Vasc Surg* 2001;35(5):385–389.

Wilson RF. Abdominal vascular injury. In: *Handbook of trauma: pitfalls and pearls.* Philadelphia: Lippincott, Williams & Wilkins, 1999:408–421.

Vascular Trauma 3: Peripheral Vascular Injuries

Steven M. Abbate, MD, and Susan M. Briggs, MD

I. Introduction and Epidemiology

Before World War II, peripheral vascular injuries were associated with a high field mortality rate. Those surviving to medical attention were treated with ligation and amputation. During World War II, improvements in evacuation and prehospital care resulted in fewer deaths from exsanguination, although ligation to control hemorrhage and amputation were frequently employed. Some series report amputation rates as high as 40%. The advent of modern vascular techniques has resulted in a significant decline in amputation rate to <10%.

Gunshot and stab wounds account for most injuries presenting to urban centers. A higher percentage of truncal injuries is seen in this population. Rural populations, on the other hand, have a higher percentage of blunt mechanisms and extremity injuries predominate. In addition, with the advent of catheter-based interventions, iatrogenic arterial injuries are becoming more common.

II. Patterns of Injury

Penetrating wounds cause vascular injury by several mechanisms (**Fig. 24-1**). The penetrating object can cause complete or partial vessel transection. In addition, the blast effect from a missile can result in vascular contusion and intimal disruption. Blunt forces generally result in vessel wall contusion or intimal disruption with thrombosis, although complete or partial transections can be seen with bony fractures and dislocations.

III. Presentation

Clinical manifestations of vascular trauma range from subclinical intimal tears to limb-threatening extremity ischemia or life-threatening exsanguination. Arterial lacerations can result in external hemorrhage, expanding hematoma, or pseudoaneurysm formation. The mass effect of the hematoma or pseudoaneurysm can cause compression on adjacent nerves, with associated neuropathy. Arterial contusion or intimal disruption can be clinically silent or result in thrombosis with distal ischemia. Up to 25% of patients with significant vascular injury will have normal distal pulses because of collateral circulation or incomplete occlusion of the vessel.

Clinical manifestations of vascular injury have been classified into *hard* and *soft* signs. Hard signs are diagnostic of vascular injury, whereas soft signs are suggestive of possible arterial injury. The incidence of injury seen in patients with soft signs depends on the intensity of the diagnostic evaluation. Reported incidence ranges from 10% to 35%.

A. Hard Signs of Arterial Injury

Hard signs of arterial injury include the following:

1. Pulsatile bleeding
2. Expanding hematoma

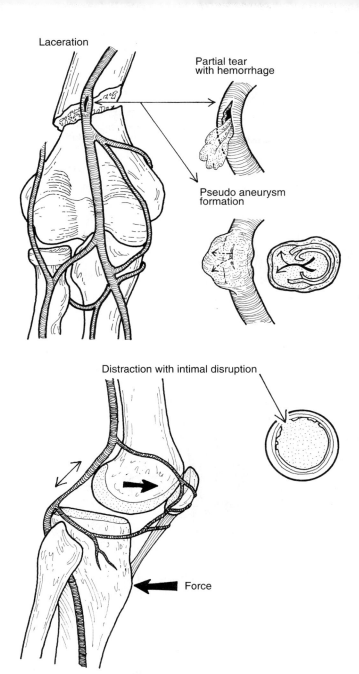

Figure 24-1. Patterns of extremity vascular injury. Top: Laceration. Bottom: Distraction with intimal disruption.

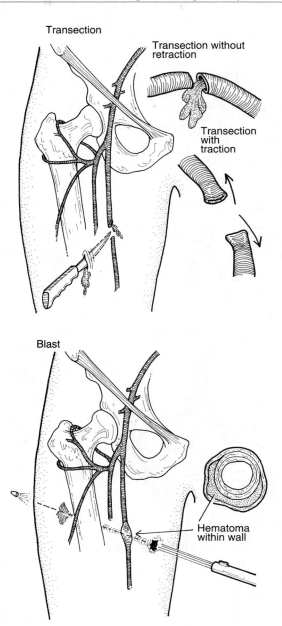

Figure 24-1. *(Continued)* Transection. D: Blast.

3. Palpable thrill or audible bruit
4. Distal ischemia: pain, paresthesia, pallor, paralysis, pulselessness, and poikilothermia

Hard signs are diagnostic of vascular injury and mandate either immediate operative exploration or further diagnostic imaging before surgical exploration.

B. Soft Signs of Arterial Injury
Soft signs of arterial injury include the following:

1. Diminished pulses
2. Fracture, dislocation, or missile in proximity to major artery
3. Peripheral nerve deficit in proximity to major artery
4. Nonexpanding, nonpulsitile hematoma

Soft signs can be suggestive of an arterial injury and merit either further diagnostic evaluation or careful clinical surveillance. Routine exploration for soft signs leads to a high negative exploration rate and is generally not recommended.

The restoration of a palpable pulse following fracture reduction does not mandate diagnostic evaluation. Similarly, proximity injuries without alterations in the quality of distal pulses or signs of ischemia no longer mandate angiography. An audible Doppler signal without a palpable pulse is abnormal and can be caused by systemic hypoperfusion, proximal arterial injury, vasospasm, or compartment syndrome and merits further evaluation.

IV. **Diagnostic Evaluation**
   A. Patients presenting with hard signs generally require no further diagnostic evaluation and can proceed directly to operative exploration. Angiography in this situation results in an additional delay to reconstruction and often does not significantly alter the surgical plan.
   B. Duplex Doppler Ultrasound
   The vascular supply to the extremities is anatomically accessible to Doppler examination, although the presence of open wounds, bone fractures, orthopedic splints, and bulky dressings can reduce the effectiveness of this modality. Ultrasound has a reported accuracy of 98% in diagnosing vascular injuries (e.g., thrombosis, pseudoaneurysm, intimal flaps, arteriovenous fistulas). The limitations of this technology are the skill required for interpretation and the availability of skilled personnel.
   C. Angiography
   Angiography is the gold standard diagnostic test for evaluating an arterial injury. It accurately defines the severity of the local injury as well as the status of the distal arterial tree. The complication rate from an angiogram is approximately 2% to 5%.
   The presence of hard signs of arterial injury mandates operative exploration. A diagnostic angiogram is not indicated for diagnosis unless it will assist in operative planning. Patients with antecedent peripheral vascular

disease or potential multilevel injuries can benefit from angiographic evaluation. A positive angiogram can be expected in 10% to 35% of patients with soft signs of arterial injury. When the indication is proximity alone without clinical signs of vascular injury, the rate drops to <10%. Most authors feel that proximity should no longer be an indication for diagnostic angiography.

Clinical and radiographic assessment of the arterial tree can be misleading in the presence of displaced extremity fractures or compartment syndrome. Patients should have bony reduction, fasciotomy, or both before any diagnostic evaluation, if possible. Intraoperative angiography can be a useful technique in some situations. The angiogram can be static or dynamic. A dynamic angiogram, which is done via a percutaneous approach, is best done with fluoroscopic assistance. A static angiogram, which can be done effectively without fluoroscopy, allows for the use of smaller volume of contrast. This technique requires a small open incision to isolate the artery proximal to the injury. An angiocatheter is used to puncture the vessel in an antegrade manner. The artery is clamped proximally. The radiographs are taken at the end of the contrast injection; 30 mL is used for the lower extremity and 15 mL for the upper extremity.

V.   General Principles of Management

Treat life-threatening injuries first. Avoid tourniquets in cases of suspected vascular injury with bleeding, if at all possible, because they will occlude collateral flow necessary to preserve limb perfusion. Clamp vascular structures under direct vision, not blindly. Intravenous lines should not be placed in extremities with suspected vascular injury because fluid extravasation can occur.

A.   Nonoperative Management

Selected individuals can be managed expectantly. An asymptomatic intimal flap with good distal perfusion can be treated with antiplatelet therapy and observed. Operative intervention would be warranted should evidence of distal ischemia develop. In addition, small (<2 cm), nonexpanding arterial pseudoaneurysm can be safely observed in patients not requiring anticoagulation therapy. Clinical resolution, as documented on vascular ultrasound, can be expected in most patients. Patients with severe injuries to their lower leg often have traumatic disruption of either a single tibial or peroneal vessel when examined angiographically. This most often occurs in the context of a severe crush injury or tibial fracture. The ultimate goal in the management of these injuries is to assure adequate vascular supply for wound healing and resting tissue oxygenation. In general, a single vessel run-off to the foot is sufficient to accomplish this objective. Delayed arterial reconstruction is acceptable if needed for wound healing or claudication.

B.   Operative Treatment

1.   Determination of the Extent of Injury

Obtain proximal and distal vascular isolation as the first steps in the repair of vascular injury. Then assess the extent of arterial injury. Some injuries are amenable to direct repair but many will require resection of the damaged arterial wall to uninjured artery with interposition graft (vein preferable). Before arterial repair, pass embolectomy catheters proximally and distally. The finding of backflow alone does not preclude the presence of distal thrombus. In addition, the patient should be systemically heparinized. If systemic heparin is contraindicated because of associated injuries, heparinized saline solution should be injected locally. After excision of an injured arterial segment, the length of the subsequent interposition graft is often two to three times the length of excision because of the elastic recoil of the artery.

2. **Types of Repair**

   a. **Primary Repair.** Lateral arteriorrhaphy is appropriate for injuries that involve a portion of the arterial wall without significant injury to the adjacent vessel. If primary closure would compromise the luminal diameter, then it is best to close with a vein or prosthetic patch. Excision of an injured segment with primary end-to-end anastomosis can be used in selected cases where the length of the injury is short and the two ends of the artery can be approximated without tension. The degree of arterial mobilization needed often makes this technique impractical, however.

   b. **Interposition Grafting.** Interposition grafting is the mainstay of managing extremity vascular trauma (**Fig. 24-2**). This technique allows for adequate débridement of the injured vessel with construction of a tension-free anastomosis.

3. **Choice of Conduit**

Contralateral greater saphenous vein (GSV) is the conduit of choice for interposition grafting. The advantages of the saphenous vein include long-term patency and lower incidence for infection in potentially contaminated wounds. In the setting of lower extremity arterial injury a high associated risk exists of injury to the deep venous system. Contralateral GSV harvesting preserves the superficial venous system in patients at risk for venous hypertension and insufficiency (i.e., patients with deep vein injury).

In managing vascular trauma to the extremities, use prosthetics sparingly. In general, they are reserved for patients without suitable autogenous conduit or in cases of a significant size discrepancy. Be cautious about using a prosthetic graft in a contaminated wound

4. **Management of Associated Injuries**

Soft tissue, orthopedic, and venous injuries often coexist with arterial injuries, making their management multidisciplinary, which requires coordination between the trauma, orthopedic, and plastic surgical services. The top priority is to achieve hemostasis and restore arterial flow to the distal extremity. Performing a vascular reconstruction in the setting of unstable

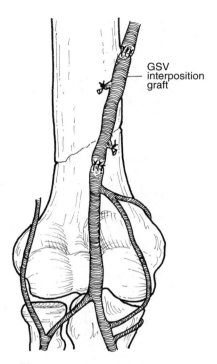

GSV
interposition
graft

Figure 24-2.   Interposition grafting.

bony injuries, however, can be very difficult. Accordingly, it is sometimes necessary to perform orthopedic stabilization before definitive vascular repair. In these situations, application of an external fixation device is generally the most expedient approach to obtain bony stability before vascular repair. More definitive orthopedic reconstruction can then be performed in the same setting or in an interval fashion. An alternative to this strategy, is placement of a temporary arterial shunt, followed by definitive orthopedic stabilization, and subsequent vascular repair.

Deep venous injuries frequently coexist with arterial injuries. These injuries can be the source of significant blood loss. Although generally managed with ligation, venous reconstruction should be attempted in injuries to major veins (e.g., femoral and popliteal) because the incidence of disabling venous insufficiency is significant.

Devitalized, contaminated soft tissue requires aggressive débridement following extremity trauma. Accordingly, large soft tissue defects are often seen in the surgical field. Perfused, healthy soft tissue coverage of any vascular reconstruction is necessary to help prevent graft infection and suture line dehiscence. This can usually be accomplished with advancement and rotation of adjacent soft tissue. In the situation where the local tissue is insufficient, plastic surgical consultation is required to assist with wound coverage.

5. Indications for Immediate Fasciotomy
Ischemia or reperfusion injury, deep venous injury, orthopedic fractures, and soft tissue trauma all place the patient with extremity trauma at risk for compartment syndrome. Furthermore, an altered mental status and associated nerve injuries can lead to delays in diagnosis of evolving compartment syndrome. Prophylactic extremity fasciotomy is recommended in patients with major venous injuries, severe soft tissue injury, distal ischemic times approaching 6 hours, and those with unreliable physical examinations (**Fig. 24-3**). If opting against prophylactic fasciotomy, then frequent clinical examinations and assessments of compartment pressures is warranted.

6. Indications for Early Amputation
Management of the mangled extremity is a challenging clinical situation. A strong desire exists by both the patient and the medical providers for limb salvage. It is, however, well documented that immediate amputation of mangled extremities results in shorter hospital stays, quicker return to normal activity, fewer operations, and less operative blood loss. Various extremity scoring systems have been developed to predict functional outcome after extremity salvage, all with varying degrees of success. These systems assess the severity of the local injury in association with the patient's clinical status and any medical comorbidity. Given the success of current vascular surgical techniques, the functional outcome after extremity salvage is governed by the severity of the associated soft tissue, nerve, and orthopedic injuries. Late amputation rates as high as 70% have been reported because of associated soft tissue, orthopedic, and neurologic injuries, despite successful vascular reconstruction. Accordingly, selected patients are often better served with immediate amputation, including the following:

1. Extensive soft tissue and orthopedic injuries
2. Tibial nerve injury, with loss of plantar sensation
3. Nonreconstructible vascular injury
4. Unstable patient with multisystem traumatic injuries
5. Noncorrectable metabolic *washout* following arterial reconstruction of a critically ischemic limb

C. Exposures
1. Axillary Artery
The axillary artery extends from the first rib proximally to the insertion of the teres major and latissimus

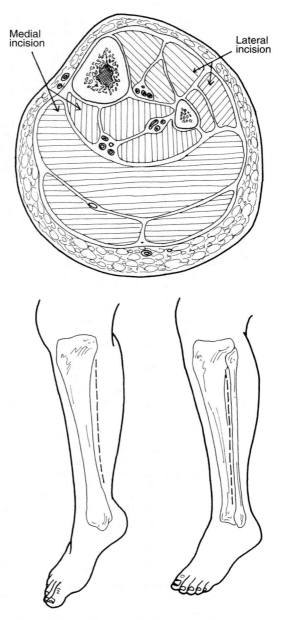

Medial incision

Lateral incision

Figure 24-3.   Indications for immediate fasciotomy.

dorsi distally. It is divided into three parts based on its relationship to the pectoralis minor muscle.

1. First part: medial to the pectoralis minor
2. Second part: underneath the pectoralis minor
3. Third part: lateral to the pectoralis minor

Topographically, the axillary artery is most easily identified in the infraclavicular fossa and in the deltopectoral groove.

Proximal axillary artery injuries may require control of the subclavian artery via a supraclavicular approach. The first portion of the axillary artery is the preferred site for control in distal axillary and proximal brachial artery injuries. This portion is readily accessible via an infraclavicular incision. Place the incision one fingerbreadth below the clavicle, starting at the midclavicle and extending laterally. Extend this incision through the pectoralis major muscle. Incise the clavipectoral fascia medial to the pectoralis minor muscle to expose the axillary sheath. Expose the artery by mobilizing the more superficial axillary vein. The brachial plexus will be deep to the artery in this location.

Distal axillary artery exposure is required for proximal to midbrachial artery injuries. A deltopectoral approach is often the most direct and it allows the flexibility for extension to an infraclavicular incision or for extension down the medial arm. Place the incision in the deltopectoral groove. Develop the dissection plane between the deltoid and pectoralis major muscle. Mobilize the cephalic vein and retract it laterally. Incise the clavipectoral fascia lateral to the pectoralis minor muscle to expose the distal axillary artery. The medial and lateral cords of the brachial plexus are superficial to the artery and require careful mobilization.

2. Brachial Artery

Exposure of the brachial artery in the arm is achieved via a medial incision oriented between the flexor and extensor compartments. The basilic vein lies superficial in the distal arm and penetrates the brachial sheath in the midbrachium to join the brachial vein. After incision of the deep fascia and the brachial sheath, the neurovascular bundle will be exposed. The median nerve lies superficial to the artery and requires careful mobilization. In addition, several venous branches connecting the two brachial veins will require ligation.

The distal brachial artery at the level of its bifurcation into the radial and ulnar arteries can be exposed in the proximal forearm. Place a transverse incision 1 cm below the antecubital crease. If more proximal or distal exposure is required, this incision can be easily extended to an S-shaped incision. The superior component extends into the medial arm, whereas the inferior component extends lateral to the biceps tendon. The brachial artery with its associated veins is identified medial to the biceps tendon after opening the bicipital aponeurosis. Continuing the dissection distally allows isolation of the proximal radial and ulnar arteries.

3.   Femoral Artery

The femoral artery originates at the level of the inguinal ligament. At this level, it is bound by the inguinal ligament anteriorly, the superior pubic ramus posteriorly, the femoral vein medially, and the femoral nerve laterally. For proximal femoral artery injuries, an oblique retroperitoneal incision placed 2 to 3 cm cephalad to the inguinal ligament affords access to the external iliac vessels. Direct exposure of the femoral artery is approached through a vertical inguinal incision. Center the incision over the femoral pulse with one third of the incision above the inguinal ligament. Early identification of the inguinal ligament is useful in that the vessel will lie deep to this level. After incising the femoral sheath, the common femoral artery is readily identified. Continuing this dissection inferiorly allows identification of the superficial and deep femoral arteries.

4.   Popliteal Artery

In the trauma patient, the popliteal artery is best approached through the medial thigh. The medial approach affords the greatest flexibility in accessing the artery more proximally and distally. The posterior or lateral approaches are best used in elective setting and are ill advised in the trauma patient.

The incision to expose the suprageniculate popliteal artery is placed one fingerbreadth below the femur along the anterior border of the sartorius muscle. The greater saphenous vein will lie within the subcutaneous tissue and should be identified and preserved. Then incise the fascia overlying the sartorius muscle. The plane between the adductor magnus and the sartorius is then easily dissected and the neurovascular bundle exposed. The two popliteal veins are intimately associated with the artery and require careful mobilization. If required, the adductor magnus tendon can be divided for additional exposure.

Exposure of the infrageniculate popliteal artery is analogous to its above-the-knee segment. The incision is oriented one fingerbreadth posterior to the tibia. The GSV is preserved and the fascia of the superficial posterior compartment is incised. The gastrocnemius muscle is then reflected posterior exposing the contents of the popliteal fossa. The semitendanosus tendon can be divided to facilitate exposure. Then separate the popliteal artery from its associated veins. More distal exposure of the trifurcation can be achieved by detaching the soleus muscle from the posterior tibia.

VI. Complications
A. Thrombosis
Causes of early graft thrombosis, which are multiple, include the following:

1. Technical error of the anastomosis
2. Distal dissection of the vessel
3. Kinking or twisting of the vein graft
4. Compression of the vein graft because of tissue edema or hematoma
5. Compromised distal outflow secondary to clot, compartment syndrome, or vasospasm

Once recognized, either by loss of pulse or Doppler signal, the patient should return to the operating room promptly. If the occlusion is related to external compression, then perfusion often returns after reopening the incision and evacuating any hematoma present. It is advisable to perform a fasciotomy or measure compartment pressures and to inspect the vein graft for evidence of kinking at this time. If no source to explain the graft occlusion can then be identified, an on-table angiography should be performed through the artery proximal to the anastomosis. This will detect anastomotic strictures, distal intimal dissection, and distal thrombosis.

B. Infection
Infection at the site of vascular reconstruction is a dreaded complication, often leading to graft thrombosis or suture line dehiscence. A small percentage of grafts can be salvaged with control of local sepsis, débridement of devitalized tissue, prolonged antibiotic therapy, and coverage of the artery or graft with a muscle flap. This management strategy is often unsuccessful and is ill advised in the patient presenting with hemorrhage. More often, the artery requires ligation and flow restored with an extraanatomic reconstruction through nonseptic tissue planes.

C. Pseudoaneurysm
Arterial pseudoaneurysm is a common late complication of vascular reconstruction and vascular trauma. Causes include the following:

1. Mechanical suture line stress from inadequate graft length or movement of the extremity
2. Degeneration of the native artery or vein graft
3. Missed arterial injury

Clinical manifestations include the presence of a pulsatile mass, arterial thrombosis, distal arterial embolization, or rupture with exsanguination. Once recognized a pseudoaneurysm should be repaired, either by open or endovascular techniques, especially if symptomatic or sizable.

VII. Summary
Extremity vascular injuries result from both blunt and penetrating mechanisms and often coexist with orthopedic, venous, and soft tissue injuries. The diagnosis is often established by physical examination and, when indicated, confirmed and defined by

angiography. The goal of surgical management is to restore normal arterial flow, either by local repair or interposition grafting. The importance of soft tissue coverage of all vascular repairs in preventing infection and dehiscence cannot be overemphasized. The mangled extremity is an especially challenging problem that requires a multispecialty approach. The functional outcome after limb salvage is governed by the severity of the orthopedic, soft tissue, and nervous injuries, and selected patients are best served with immediate amputation. The future role of vascular stents in patients with extremity vascular injury is unknown because of the limited clinical experience with these cases.

SELECTED READING

Briggs SE, Seligson D. Management of extremity trauma. In: *Trauma: clinical care and pathophysiology.* Chicago: Yearbook Publishers, 1987.

Caps M. The epidemiology of vascular trauma. In: Rutherford RB, ed. *Vascular surgery,* 5th ed. Philadelphia: WB Saunders, 2000.

Johansen KH, Watson JC. Compartment syndrome: pathophysiology, recognition, and management. In Rutherford RB, ed. *Vascular surgery,* 5th ed. Philadelphia: WB Saunders, 2000.

Shackford SR, Rich NH. Peripheral vascular injury. In: Mattox KL, Feliciano DV, Moore EE, eds. *Trauma,* 4th ed. New York: McGraw-Hill, 2000.

Weaver FA, Hood DB, Yellin AE. Vascular injuries to the extremities. In: Rutherford RB, ed. *Vascular surgery,* 5th ed. Philadelphia: WB Saunders, 2000.

Wind GG, Valentine RJ. Axillary artery. In: Wind GG, Valentine RJ, eds. *Anatomic exposures in vascular surgery.* Baltimore: Williams & Wilkins, 1991.

Wind GG, Valentine RJ. Brachial artery. In: Wind GG, Valentine RJ, eds. *Anatomic exposures in vascular surgery.* Baltimore: Williams & Wilkins, 1991.

Wind GG, Valentine RJ. Femoral vessels. In: Wind GG, Valentine RJ, eds. *Anatomic exposures in vascular surgery.* Baltimore: Williams & Wilkins, 1991.

Wind GG, Valentine RJ. Popliteal artery. In: Wind GG, Valentine RJ, eds. *Anatomic exposures in vascular surgery.* Baltimore: Williams & Wilkins, 1991.

Abdominal Trauma 1: Diagnostic Techniques

Ara J. Feinstein, MD,
and M. Charles Ferguson, MD

I. Introduction

Prior to World War I, the standard of care for abdominal wounds was observation. By the end of that war, it was apparent that survival improved for patients having laparotomy for abdominal injuries. During World War II, surgical exploration of all patients with suspected intraabdominal injury was the standard of care. This led to unnecessary and nontherapeutic laparotomies with high morbidity. It was not until the 1960s with the advent of diagnostic peritoneal lavage (DPL) that selective management of abdominal trauma became feasible. Since then, physicians have continued to adapt their diagnostic and therapeutic interventions according to available resources and injury patterns. The evaluation of patients with suspected abdominal trauma has evolved significantly, but still presents the physician with a diagnostic challenge. Missed abdominal injury is a frequent cause of preventable death in the trauma patient with multiple injuries. Once the ABCs have been addressed, the goal of the workup in patients with suspected abdominal trauma is to:

1. Quickly identify the presence of intraabdominal injuries
2. Determine if the injuries necessitate operative or nonoperative management
3. In patients with nonoperative injuries, provide definitive diagnostic evidence that injuries are stable over time

Although patients often do not present with these classic signs and symptoms, several indications still exist for immediate laparotomy after abdominal trauma: overt peritonitis, hemodynamic instability with obvious intraabdominal injury (evisceration), obviously penetrating abdominal gunshot wound, or progressive abdominal distention with hemodynamic instability in suspected blunt trauma.

II. Diagnostic Techniques

The diagnostic armamentarium continues to expand for clinicians dealing with abdominal trauma. Careful utilization of these techniques reduces morbidity from negative laparotomies by achieving a quick diagnosis of injuries and ensuring rapid intervention or observation.

A. Physical Examination

The physical examination is vital in the assessment of the patient with abdominal trauma. It remains the most important means of detecting the need for urgent laparotomy. In unstable patients, it can provide the only diagnostic information before operative intervention.

1. Indications

All patients with suspected abdominal trauma should have a complete physical examination during the secondary survey. Even when injuries are obvious, concomitant injuries that are less apparent can be elucidated by a thorough physical examination.

2. Limitations

The examination is often limited in patients who are intoxicated, those intubated in the field, those with head injuries or baseline impaired mental status, or children. Up to 25% of patients with blunt abdominal trauma can have associated head injury. Neurologic dysfunction presents the greatest compromise to the physical examination in patients with abdominal trauma.

3. Technique

The abdomen is defined as the area between the nipple line and the symphysis pubis and inguinal ligaments anteriorly, the scapula to the iliac crest posteriorly. The flank is the area between anterior and posterior axillary lines from the sixth intercostal space to the iliac crest. This area should be closely inspected for signs of trauma. Seatbelt marks are associated with an increased incidence of injuries to the duodenum, pancreas, and small and large bowel. Abrasions and penetrating wounds should be noted, as underlying organs are likely to be injured. Also, carefully inspect wounds for evisceration and foreign bodies. A rectal examination should be performed and a nasogastric tube placed. In the mentally and neurologically intact patient, severe pain, guarding, and tenderness are strong indications for operative intervention, especially in the setting of penetrating trauma or unstable vital signs.

B. Plain Films

The role of plain films in abdominal trauma is limited, but an upright chest x-ray study as part of the initial trauma series can be helpful, especially in the unstable patient.

1. Indications

All trauma patients should have a chest x-ray study as part of the initial trauma series.

2. Limitations

Minimal information regarding presence and location of injuries are obtained on plain films.

3. Technique

a. The chest should be visualized from the apices of the lungs to the costophrenic margins.

b. Free air under the diaphragm is an indicator of intraabdominal injury or possible diaphragmatic injury.

c. Rib fractures on can be highly suggestive of underlying organ damage, especially splenic injury.

d. A nasogastric tube with an abnormal path of lateral travel is suggestive of a diaphragmatic injury.

e. If the pleural cavity contains a significant amount of blood, it can raise suspicion that the hemodynamic instability may not be from an abdominal injury.

C. Ultrasound

Ultrasound (US) has evolved as a standard part of the diagnostic work-up in patients with abdominal trauma in recent years. Widely performed in Asia and Europe, North American trauma centers continue to increase their use of this technique. As part of the initial secondary survey, US has evolved as an extension of the physical examination. The best-studied technique for US is the focused abdominal sonogram for trauma (FAST) for blunt abdominal trauma. FAST is noninvasive, portable, and can be easily repeated. Although not specific, it is highly sensitive for intraabdominal injury and can be reliably performed by nonradiologist personnel, including house officers.

1. Indications

a. Examination of patients with suspected blunt abdominal trauma during the initial assessment

b. The amount of hemoperitoneum can be followed over time to decide if operative intervention may be needed

c. Because US is noninvasive and has no radiation risk, it is highly valuable in pregnant patients.

d. US can be used to examine the pericardium in penetrating wounds of the upper abdomen.

2. Limitations

a. US is somewhat limited by its sensitivity (80% to 95%), because missed injuries can cause significant morbidity and mortality.

b. Many patients will have little free intraperitoneal blood following blunt abdominal trauma. These patients mainly have contained liver and spleen injuries that are missed because US is best for detecting free fluid.

c. US is more operator dependent than other diagnostic modalities.

d. US is difficult to interpret in obese patients.

e. Subcutaneous emphysema obscures the US examination.

3. Focused Abdominal Sonogram Technique

Using a systematic approach, all areas should be evaluated in two planes, longitudinal and transverse. Direct localization and grading of organ injury (liver, spleen, or kidneys) by US is not possible in most cases, and time is usually not wasted in attempting to quantify the severity of detected injuries. The single most important criterion for proceeding to emergent laparotomy when using US for blunt abdominal trauma (BAT) is the quick and easy demonstration of a significant hemoperitoneum in a hemodynamically unstable patient (**Fig. 25-1**).

a. The pericardium is first visualized by longitudinal scanning in the midline under the xiphoid process, visualizing the left lobe of the liver. If the head of the transducer is directed toward the head

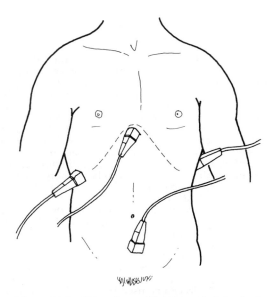

Figure 25-1.   Four views of the focused abdominal sonogram for trauma (FAST) examination.

of the patient, the pericardium and heart can be visualized. Transverse scanning in the midline under the xiphoid process visualizes the left lobe of the liver, the pericardium, and heart. This technique can be used in penetrating wounds of the upper abdomen to assess for hemopericardium.

b.   The transducer head is then placed over the intercostal space between the anterior and mid-axillary line at the level of the seventh or eighth ribs. Intercostal scanning is useful in trauma patients who cannot cooperate by holding their breath. Morison's pouch, the right kidney, and the posterior segments of the right lobe of the liver are clearly visualized by placing the transducer head in this position.

c.   The transducer head is then moved to the left subcostal margin in the left midaxillary line. In full inspiration, the spleen and the left kidney descend, allowing better visualization of these two organs by eliminating the interference of overlying ribs. A search for blood surrounding the spleen and the space between the spleen and the left kidney is best performed placing the transducer head in this position.

d.   Next, the transducer is oriented for transverse images using a midline reference point approximately 4 cm superior to the pubis. The urinary bladder should be distended for the sonographic examination of the pelvis. Longitudinal and transverse views are necessary to allow an accurate evaluation. If the urinary bladder is not distended at the time of evaluation, the bladder can be filled with sterile water through an indwelling catheter. Gross hematuria should first be excluded. Fluid will be identified posterior to the bladder or in the pouch of Douglas in female patients (posterior to the uterus). Fluid can also be detected within surrounding loops of bowel that are in the pelvis.

D. Diagnostic Peritoneal Lavage

In 1965 Root introduced diagnostic peritoneal lavage. This technique of paracentesis involves infusing normal saline into the abdomen and then analyzing the retrieved effluent. DPL is a relatively fast procedure that can be performed during trauma resuscitations with high sensitivity and specificity. The use of DPL has decreased with the increasing use of US and computed tomography (CT), but it can be extremely useful in several situations.

1. Indications

a.   In centers where US is reliably performed in the trauma bay, DPL is indicated in unstable blunt abdominal trauma patients with an indeterminate US.

b.   In centers where ultrasound is not used primarily, DPL should be used in unstable blunt abdominal trauma patients, especially those with multiple injuries.

c.   In the stable patient with penetrating trauma and peritoneal penetration by local exploration, DPL can help determine the presence of hollow organ injury, especially if tenderness develops during observation.

2. Limitations

a.   The procedure requires peritoneal puncture and is associated with a 1% incidence of significant complications.

b.   The exact red blood cell count that is considered to be *positive* is subjective.

c.   DPL cannot evaluate injuries in the retroperitoneum.

d.   DPL can be overly sensitive for small solid organ injuries.

e.   DPL is contraindicated in the settings of pregnancy, pelvic fractures, clotting disorders, and previous abdominal surgery.

f.   DPL compromises the information available by subsequent CT scans. Air and fluid introduced during DPL especially limit the ability to diagnose bowel injury by CT.

3. Technique

Although a closed technique has been described, the open technique is presented here because of its lower complication rate.

a. After sterile preparation and local anesthesia with 1% lidocaine with epinephrine, an infra-umbilical midline incision is made approximately one third of the length from the umbilicus to symphysis pubis. In patients with known pelvic fracture, some authors suggest an incision above the umbilicus.

b. Spread the soft tissues until the midline fascia is reached. Next, incise it with a 1-cm incision and grasp the edges with clamps. Then incise the peritoneum under direct visualization.

c. Place a dialysis catheter into the peritoneal cavity directed toward the pelvis. Aspirate and, if >5 mL of gross blood is returned, terminate the procedure; the study is considered positive.

d. If no blood is aspirated, instill a liter of normal saline into the abdomen. If possible, shift the patient from side to side, then lower the DPL infusion bag below the patient to siphon the fluid back into the bag to receive a representative aliquot (200 to 300 mL) for analysis (see below).

e. In addition to the aspiration of gross blood, the following criteria are considered a positive test result (these cutoffs can vary by institution).

1. Red blood cell count (RBC) >100,000/mm^3
2. White blood cell count >500/mm^3
3. Presence of bile, bacteria, or food particles
4. Presence of lavage fluid via urinary or pleural drainage
5. Presence of pleural effusion on chest x-ray film after lavage, which suggests diaphragmatic rupture.
6. In penetrating trauma, RBC >50,000/mm^3 is considered to be a positive test result.

E. Computed Tomography

Computed tomography came into wide use for abdominal trauma in the 1980s. It has significantly reduced the number of nontherapeutic laparotomies because of its ability to both diagnose and grade injuries. CT enabled physicians to noninvasively visualize injuries to the solid organs and retroperitoneum. More recently, helical CT scanners have improved the speed and contrast enhancement of abdominal studies. In combination with automated contrast injectors, optimal scans can be obtained in a short period of time. The ability to reconstruct injuries from multiple viewing angles also enhances the diagnostic ability of CT. Multidetector CT scanners are now being integrated into trauma centers and they will further decrease examination times.

1. Indications

Hemodynamically stable patients with an equivocal physical examination or US after blunt abdominal trauma should have a CT scan.

    a. CT should be performed on all patients with multiple trauma and an associated closed head injury or altered mental status.

    b. Patient with multiple trauma and an associated spinal cord injury should have a CT scan.

    c. Patients suspected of having pelvic fractures or gross hematuria should have a CT scan with cystogram to evaluate the genitourinary system and bony pelvis.

    d. Hemodynamically stable patients with posterior or flank stab wounds should have a triple contrast CT scan.

  2. Limitations

    a. Patients are relatively isolated and, therefore, resuscitation is difficult while the test is being performed.

    b. Patients may have renal failure or contrast allergy, limiting the use of intravenous (i.v.) contrast media.

    c. CT is relatively expensive and many favor using observation and FAST or DPL as screening tests to decide which patients should have a CT scan.

    d. CT is limited in its ability to diagnose bowel injury, especially immediately after perforation when little free fluid may be present.

    e. Diaphragmatic injury is difficult to visualize.

    f. CT is difficult to interpret after DPL has been performed because of the air and fluid introduced.

  3. Technique

To achieve optimal results, both oral and i.v. contrast medium should be used. The alert patient should drink 300 mL of contrast medium before scanning and then i.v. contrast medium should be administered just before scanning. Patients unable to drink should have a nasogastric tube placed to instill contrast medium. The CT images are taken from the level of the inferior lung fields to the inferior aspect of the ischia with 5- to 8-mm sections. Thinner sections of a certain region can be taken according to what injuries are suspected. In patients suspected of having colonic injury, rectal contrast medium should also be used. Reconstructions can be performed in coronal or sagittal planes to more closely examine an injured structure (**Table 25-1**).

F. Local Wound Exploration

Performed in the emergency department, local wound exploration in abdominal stab wounds can define the presence of peritoneal penetration, which requires further workup. If clearly negative, often patients can be discharged.

  1. Indications

    a. Anterior abdominal stab wounds in stable patients should be locally explored.

**Table 25-1.   Appearance of injured organs
by computed tomography (CT)**

Organ	Injuries seen on CT
SPLEEN	Contusion, laceration, subcapsular hematoma, vascular pedicle injury, pseudoaneurysms, active bleeding
BOWEL	Pneumoperitoneum with no other etiology (previous diagnostic peritoneal lavage, diaphragmatic injury with pneumothorax, air tracking in from penetrating injury), extravasation of oral or rectal contrast
VASCULAR	Aortic hematomas or dissections: blush appears with an active bleeding. Fresh blood has an attenuation of 30–45 Houndsfield Units (HF) Clot has attenuation of 70–90 HF. A sentinel clot can localize an injury because the densest portion of a clot is often adjacent to the injured organ
LIVER	Contusion, laceration, intraparenchymal hematoma, subcapsular hematoma, vascular pedicle injury, ischemia, intravenous contrast extravasation
GALLBLADDER	Collapse, gross displacement, intraluminal clot, wall thickening, wall continuity, pericholecystic fluid, mucosal irregularity
PANCREAS	Often appears normal by initial CT; when injured, the following signs may develop: focal or diffuse swelling, laceration appearing as a lucency, pancreatic fluid tracking along Gerrota's fascia, edema of the transverse mesocolon and peripancreatic fat, fluid collections in the anterior pararenal space, and peripancreatic hemorrhage. Injuries to the tail of pancreas should be investigated closely when the left kidney and spleen are injured

    b.   Flank stab wounds in stable patients can be locally explored but the technique is less reliable than when used in cases of anterior wounds.

2.   Limitations

    a.   Local wound exploration is only reliable in anterior wounds.

    b.   Local wound exploration is difficult to perform in uncooperative patients.

3.   Technique

After sterile preparation and draping, the wound and surrounding area are infiltrated with 1% lidocaine. Enlarge the wound until the posterior fascia unequivocally intact. If this cannot be verified, the wound must be considered intraperitoneal.

G. Laparoscopy

Similar to its use in general surgery, the use of laparoscopy in abdominal trauma continues to evolve. Currently, the indications for laparoscopy in abdominal trauma are largely related to penetrating injuries. Diagnostically, it can be used instead of laparotomy in limited situations. Laparoscopy has the advantage of being less invasive than a traditional laparotomy. Therapeutic laparoscopy has resulted in injuries to the spleen, diaphragm, liver, gallbladder, and bowel, according to reports. In all cases, operator experience is vital in the use of laparoscopy for trauma. More established diagnostic and therapeutic interventions should be used in the absence of extensive laparoscopic expertise.

1. **Indications**

   a. Identification and possible repair of diaphragmatic injury in stable patients with stab wounds with a likely thoracoabdominal trajectory has been shown to be effective. The pericardium can be evaluated with a transdiaphragmatic pericardial window.

   b. In anterior or flank stab wounds, stable patients with no peritoneal signs with questionable peritoneal penetration seen by local exploration can be managed without laparotomy if no peritoneal penetration is seen by laparoscopy.

   c. In gunshot wounds, stable patients without peritoneal signs that have doubtful transperitoneal trajectory can have the peritoneum examined using the laparoscope. Patients without evidence of peritoneal penetration can be managed without laparotomy.

2. **Limitations**

   a. Compared with traditional diagnostic techniques and laparotomy, laparoscopy is relatively expensive.

   b. Insufflation can cause pneumothorax if a diaphragmatic injury is present.

   c. The bowel is difficult to examine and some studies have shown that laparoscopy has a sensitivity as low as 18% for detecting bowel injury.

   d. The retroperitoneum is difficult to evaluate.

   e. Carbon dioxide (CO_2) insufflation can cause pneumothorax if diaphragmatic injury is present. It can lower cardiac output and increase intracranial pressure in patients with closed head injury.

   f. Techniques require significant operator experience.

3. **Technique**

Although local anesthesia and sedation has been reported, general anesthesia allows more complete examination of the abdomen. The chest should be prepared with the abdomen in case of the need for chest tube placement. A 10- to 12-mm port is placed at the umbilicus for introduction of the laparoscope. CO_2 insufflation or an abdominal retraction system can be used. Meticulously examine the peritoneal wall, solid organs, and bowel. Examine the pelvis for blood or enteric contents. Inspect the lesser sac for blood in cases of anterior stomach injury.

H. Exploratory Thoracoscopy

In stable patients with wounds that may traverse the abdominal and thoracic cavities, the role of thoracoscopy is evolving. Experienced surgeons can evaluate the pleura, pericardium, and diaphragm. It is possible to control hemorrhage, evacuate a clot, and repair small diaphragmatic hernias. Larger hernias or those containing viscera necessitate laparotomy. Thoracoscopy has less morbidity than thoracotomy.

1. **Indications**

Thoracoabdominal stab wounds in stable patients with evidence of hemothorax or pneumothorax by chest x-ray study

2. **Limitations**

a. Requires an experienced operator.

b. The patient must be stable.

c. The patient must be able to tolerate single lung ventilation.

d. Some diaphragmatic injuries can be diagnosed, but cannot be repaired.

3. **Technique**

a. After placement of a chest tube, bring the patient to the operating suite where general anesthesia is induced and a double-lumen endotracheal tube is placed to allow selective left lung ventilation. Place the patient in the lateral decubitus position according to the side of injury. Insert the scope into the pleural space through the ninth intercostal space in the medial axillary line. Two instrumentation ports can be placed, as necessary.

III. Integration and Approach

The approach to the patient with abdominal trauma first requires strict adherence to the primary survey. It must first be determined whether a patient is hemodynamically stable or unstable (systolic blood pressure <90, ongoing fluid requirement, obvious ongoing hemorrhage).

A. Unstable Patients

After ABCs, a thorough physical examination and plain film trauma series and laboratory studies, further workup should be confined to tests that will not delay resuscitation or operative intervention. With obvious abdominal injury (gunshot or stab wound, increasing abdominal distention, peritoneal signs, evisceration), the focus should be on preparation for transport to the operating room. In patients with multisystem blunt trauma and no obvious signs of abdominal injury, US and DPL can help to quickly determine the presence of intraabdominal hemorrhage. If these tests are negative, other areas can become the focus of the workup (**Fig. 25-2**).

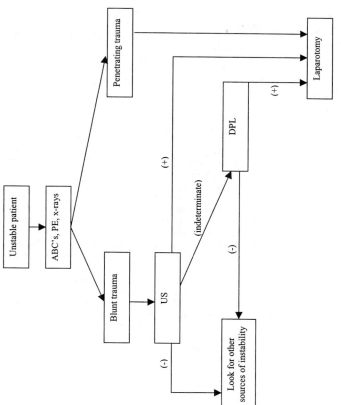

Figure 25-2. Evaluation of the unstable patient with abdominal trauma (algorithm).

B.   Stable Patients

Careful workup can help clearly define injuries and optimize treatment. Always carefully monitor all patients who are initially stable for signs of shock until the workup is finished. For diagnostic purposes, stable trauma patients can be categorized according to whether the injuries are blunt or penetrating.

1.   Blunt Abdominal Trauma

Blunt trauma is caused in descending frequency by motor vehicle crashes, assaults, falls, and pedestrian injuries. The liver and spleen are the most frequently injured organs, with bowel injury several times less frequent. In most centers, patients with blunt abdominal trauma have US in the resuscitation area as part of the secondary survey (**Fig. 25-3**).

a.   If the patient is hemodynamically unstable, US can give immediate information on the presence and degree of intraabdominal hemorrhage. If the US is positive, the patient should be prepared for transport to the operating room. If the US is negative in the hemodynamically unstable patient, turn attention to other sources of hemorrhage (thighs, pelvis, thorax). If the US is indeterminate and hemodynamic instability can be caused by other sources (thigh, chest, neurologic injury), a DPL can be performed in the trauma bay.

b.   In the hemodynamically stable patient, if the US examination is negative, the patient can be observed. If a patient with a reliable physical examination shows no further abdominal signs or symptoms (hypotension, abdominal pain, hematuria) during observation, the assessment can be terminated.

c.   Hemodynamically stable patients who have significant mechanism of injury or develop hematuria, transient hypotension, or abdominal pain during observation should have a CT scan.

d.   If a patient under observation becomes hemodynamically unstable, a repeat US should be performed and preparations made for laparotomy.

e.   If the initial US studies are positive, stable patients should have a CT examination to further evaluate and grade the injury.

f.   If the US is deemed indeterminate and the patient is stable, a CT scan should be performed.

2.   Penetrating Abdominal Trauma

Penetrating abdominal trauma is almost inevitably caused by gunshot or stab wounds. The approach to these types of injuries differs because of the differences in type and severity of injury. The organs most likely to be injured in penetrating abdominal trauma in decreasing frequency are small intestine, liver, colon, stomach, and spleen.

a.   Stab Wounds. The severity of stab wounds depends on the number, depth, angle, and path

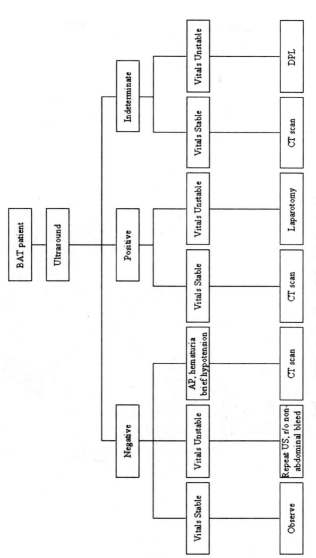

Figure 25-3.   Evaluation of blunt abdominal trauma.

of the wound. Approximately one third of stab wounds to the abdomen penetrate the peritoneal envelope. All hemodynamically unstable patients with abdominal stab wounds should be prepared for exploratory laparotomy. The management of hemodynamically stable abdominal stab wounds often depends on the region of the wound.

(1) Anterior stab wounds are located ventral to the midaxillary lines, from the subcostal region to the inguinal ligaments. Because the peritoneum is relatively superficial, local wound exploration has been used to determine peritoneal penetration. If findings are negative, the patient can be discharged. If positive, the patient can be observed for development of symptoms. Some centers will perform DPL or exploratory laparoscopy. Exploratory laparotomy based solely on peritoneal penetration has a false negative finding rate as high as 50% (**Fig. 25-4**).

(2) The flanks are the area between anterior and posterior axillary lines, from scapular tip space to the iliac crest. Local wound exploration is difficult and less reliable than in anterior wounds. Unless the wound is obviously superficial, triple contrast CT, observation, or laparoscopy is indicated because both peritoneal and retroperitoneal injuries can be present (**Fig. 25-5**).

(3) Posterior stab wounds are between the scapular tip and the iliac crest, between the posterior axillary lines. Because of the relative mass of the back musculature, local wound exploration is not useful. Because retroperitoneal injury is a significant risk, many advocate triple contrast CT. Observation with low rates of delayed surgery has also been reported (**Fig. 25-6**).

(4) Thoracoabdominal stab wounds are in the region of the nipple line to the subcostal margin. Even if a chest tube has been placed to treat a thoracic injury, take care to evaluate the abdomen. If a thoracic injury is present on chest x-ray film and the patient is stable, many advocate thoracoscopy. In patients without hemothorax or pneumothorax, laparoscopy or laparotomy may be indicated to evaluate the diaphragm. Some surgeons base their decision to operate on the results of DPL or observation (**Fig. 25-7**).

b.   Gunshot Wounds

Because of the high incidence of intraabdominal injury (80%), abdominal gunshot wounds in stable patients are typically explored. A recent exception is tangential gunshot wounds where the trajectory

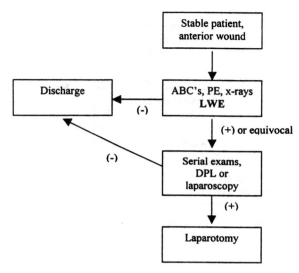

Figure 25-4. Stable patient, anterior stab wound. LWE, local wound exploation.

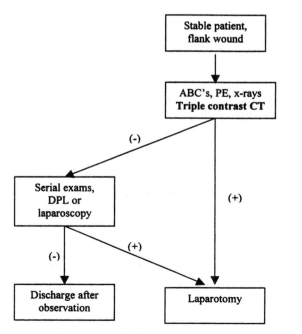

Figure 25-5. Stable patient, flank stab wound.

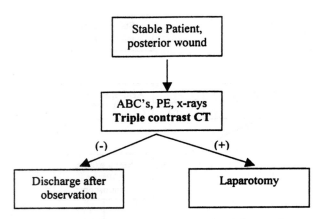

Figure 25-6. Stable patient, posterior stab wound

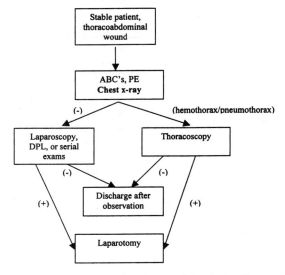

Figure 25-7. Stable patient, thoracoabdominal stab wound

suggests questionable peritoneal penetration. An entrance and exit wound must be observed. In this situation, some centers advocate CT scan, whereas others recommend laparoscopy. Management with either modality requires significant surgical experience with abdominal gunshot wounds.

V. Summary

In summary, the following points should always be kept in mind:

1. Always look at abdominal CT scans in lung windows to examine for free air.
2. Do not order tests that will not change your management.
3. Always personally look at tests you order because the radiologist cannot correlate the test with the patient's examination findings.
4. Never send an unstable patient to the CT scanner.
5. Pay special attention during the secondary survey to locate all penetrating wounds, including the perineal and buttock areas.
6. The more severely injured a patient is, the fewer tests they need in the emergency department.

SELECTED READING

Fabian TC. Abdominal trauma including indications for celiotomy. In: Feliciano DV, Moore EE, eds. *Trauma,* 4th ed. New York: McGraw-Hill, 1999.

Fernandez L, McKenney MG, McKenney KL, et al. Ultrasound in blunt abdominal trauma. *J Trauma* 1998;45(4):841–848.

Hoff WS, Holevar M, Nagy KK, et al. Eastern Association for the Surgery of Trauma: practice management guidelines for the evaluation of blunt abdominal trauma: the East practice management guidelines work group. *J Trauma* 2002;53(3):602–615.

Root HD, Hauser CW, McKinley CR. Diagnostic peritoneal lavage. *Surgery* 1965;57:633.

Shatz et al. Manual of trauma and emergency surgery. Philadelphia: WB Saunders, 2000.

Abdominal Trauma 2: Diaphragm and Abdominal Wall

Sharon L. Stein, MD,
and John T. Schulz III, MD, PhD

I. Diaphragmatic Injury: Introduction

Injury to the diaphragm is estimated to occur in 5% of patients with blunt trauma and 10% to 15% of patients with penetrating trauma of the chest or upper abdomen. Acutely, diaphragmatic injury can lead to hemodynamic instability and respiratory compromise. Long-term sequelae from undiagnosed injuries include bowel herniation, visceral infarction, sepsis, and death. Morbidity from diaphragm injury is caused by bowel herniation, displacement of lung parenchyma, increased thoracic pressure, and hemorrhage. In this section is reviewed the basics of evaluation, diagnosis, and treatment of traumatic injuries to the diaphragm.

A. Anatomy and Epidemiology of Injuries

The diaphragm separates the thoracic and abdominal cavities. It serves as the major muscle of respiration and is responsible for attaining negative intrathoracic pressure in the thorax during inspiration. During respiration, the excursion of the diaphragm varies from the fourth or fifth rib during expiration to the seventh or eighth intercostal space during inspiration. Any penetrating injury of the thorax or upper abdomen throughout this region should raise the possibility of diaphragmatic injury.

1. Diaphragmatic injury has been found to occur in 10% to 15% of penetrating wounds to the chest. If the wound is located in the anterior chest, below the nipple line, several studies have shown an incidence of diaphragmatic injury as high as 50%. A gunshot can have an unpredictable trajectory, which can result in diaphragmatic injuries, even if both entrance and exit wounds are identified. A diaphragmatic injury must always be suspected.

2. Approximately 3% to 5% of patients with blunt trauma are noted to have diaphragmatic injury. Suspect both diaphragmatic and abdominal wall injuries in cases of high-pressure blunt trauma that causes bruising from seatbelts, pelvic fractures, or broken ribs. In addition, history of side impact has been correlated with increased incidence of diaphragmatic injury.

3. Of diaphragmatic injuries, 1% are bilateral. Injuries occur three times more frequently on the left side in both penetrating and blunt trauma. In penetrating trauma, this tendency is attributed, in part, to the fact that right-handed assailants are more common. In blunt trauma, both an apparent inherent weakness in the left hemidiaphragm and the protective effect of the liver to the right hemidiaphragm are believed to account for the higher incidence of left hemidiaphragm herniation.

4. Injury patterns are different for penetrating and blunt trauma. Penetrating trauma most often leaves a small rent in the diaphragm. Blunt trauma is more likely to cause a large radial tear, most frequently in the central tendinous portion of the diaphragm.

B. Initial Evaluation

1. Initial evaluation of the trauma patient should adhere to advanced trauma life support (ATLS) guidelines with appropriate evaluation of airway, breathing, and circulation. Large-bore intravenous access should be established.

2. Diaphragmatic injuries can produce difficulties with breathing and circulation, which should be noted during the primary survey.

   a. Respiratory distress and hypotension can result from herniation of abdominal contents into the thorax and displacement of lungs and mediastinum. This can mimic pneumothorax or tamponade, causing collapse of the ipsilateral lung or twisting of the mediastinum.

   b. Cardiac output can be affected. As thoracic pressure increases, venous return attenuates, reducing diastolic filling pressures and leading to decreased stroke volume and cardiac output.

   c. Abdominal contents migrate cephalad into the thoracic cavity through the disrupted diaphragmatic barrier.

3. Bag-mask ventilation can distend the intrathoracic stomach and intestines, compromising ventilation. Pneumatic antishock garments can increase abdominal pressure further, forcing abdominal contents cephalad. In contrast, positive pressure ventilation can reduce the pressure gradient between the two compartments and prevent further herniation.

C. Diagnostic Methods

1. History

Mechanism of injury is a crucial component of a trauma evaluation. A high level of suspicion for injury can help the caregiver make a correct diagnosis, particularly in the case of diaphragmatic and abdominal wall injuries.

   a. Any blunt trauma to the abdomen or chest forceful enough to cause markings on the body surface or other associated injuries suggests diaphragmatic injury. A motor vehicle accident, in which the patient was improperly wearing a seatbelt or in which a side impact was sustained, is also indicative of a possible injury.

   b. Penetrating trauma between the nipple line and umbilicus must be evaluated for diaphragmatic injury even if entrance and exit wounds are established.

    c.   Generally, patients report nonspecific symptoms of dyspnea, orthopnea, and chest pain. Occasionally, a patient will present with a positive Kehr's sign (shoulder top pain).

2. Physical Examination

Classical physical examination findings of diaphragmatic injury include diminished anterior chest wall excursion, diminished breath sounds ipsilaterally, dullness to percussion, ectopic sounds in the thorax (e.g., borborygmi), cardiac displacement, circulatory collapse, cyanosis, and dyspnea. A scaphoid abdomen should also raise suspicion, especially in the obese patient. Patients with penetrating trauma anywhere on the trunk below the nipple line anterior, lateral, or posterior must be examined for diaphragmatic injury. Findings of seatbelt marks, especially at the waist rather than lap, should raise suspicion. Broken ribs or pelvic fractures have been correlated with an increased incidence of diaphragmatic injury.

3. Nasogastric Tube Placement

Nasogastric tubes are frequently placed in trauma patients to decompress the stomach and rule out intraluminal hemorrhage. In a patient suspected of having a diaphragmatic injury, take extreme care while placing the tube because thoracic herniation of abdominal contents can grossly distort the gastroesophageal junction. Should resistance be met while placing the tube, leave the tube in place in the esophagus to evacuate swallowed air and prevent further gastric distension.

4. Chest Radiography

Of patients with a diaphragmatic injury, 25% have chest x-ray studies diagnostic of their injury; 50% have a chest x-ray study that is not conclusively diagnostic, but has some finding consistent with diaphragmatic hernia; and 25% have completely normal findings on chest x-ray film. Findings diagnostic of diaphragmatic injury include nasogastric tube in the thorax, liver in the thorax, curvilinear shadows, or air fluid levels above the diaphragm (**Fig. 26-1**). Findings suggestive of diaphragmatic injury include abnormally high diaphragm, small pneumothorax, hemothorax or atelectasis, and displacement of heart and mediastinum. Because positive pressure ventilation can push herniated bowel back into the abdomen, end-expiratory films are those most likely to show bowel herniation in a ventilated patient. Sensitivity is also increased with Trendelenburg positioning, over penetration of the film to highlight bowel markings, and serial films. Nonetheless, in at least 25% of patients with a diaphragmatic injury, the chest x-ray study is completely normal.

5. Computed Tomography

Computed tomography (CT) is not sensitive for diaphragmatic injuries secondary to poor visualization

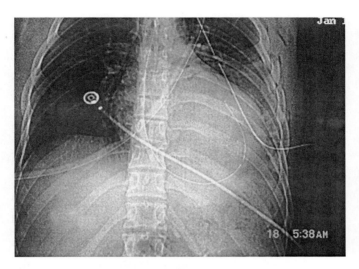

Figure 26-1.   Chest x-ray image consistent with diaphragmatic hernia.

and localization of the level of the diaphragm. The diaphragm is often tangential to the scanning plane and no fat or air distinguishes the diaphragmatic tissues from other soft tissue structures. If protrusion of abdominal contents occurs above the level of visualized diaphragm (collar sign), the study may be diagnostic. Most studies show sensitivity of approximately 50% to 80% in blunt trauma, with decreased sensitivity in the case of penetrating trauma. Reformatting films for coronal views has improved sensitivity, but CT examinations still remain reader dependent.

6.   Magnet Resonance Imaging
Initial evaluations appear promising, but insufficient evidence demonstrates reliable sensitivity and specificity of magnetic resonance imaging (MRI) for diagnosing diaphragmatic injury. Patients with hemodynamic instability should not have this examination.

7.   Chest Tube Placement
Digital exploration should always precede placement of a chest tube in a trauma patient. Palpation of a free pleural space and the collapsed underlying lung ensures that the chest tube is placed in the pleural space, and not into the herniated abdominal contents.

8.   Diagnostic Peritoneal Lavage
Diagnostic peritoneal lavage (DPL) is a poor predictor of diaphragmatic injury. Typically, red blood cell (RBC) count is the variable most indicative of diaphragmatic injury. Even with RBC counts as low as $5,000/mm^3$, 20% to 25% false negative rates have been reported. If a chest tube has been placed before

lavage, clear-colored high-output drainage from the chest tube during lavage can be diagnostic (although this could also indicate a transdiaphragmatic chest tube). Increasing dyspnea during DPL can be suggestive of diaphragmatic injury.

D. Surgical Exposure

An algorithm for patients with penetrating lower chest wounds is outlined below.

1. Thoracoscopy

In the setting of a negative DPL and penetrating chest trauma, thoracoscopy can be pursued for excellent visualization of the diaphragm and surgical repair. The peritoneal cavity is unexplored, however, and intraperitoneal injuries can be missed.

Thoracoscopy must be performed in the operating room with the patient intubated with a double lumen endotracheal tube to allow for deflation of the ipsilateral lung. Patients should be continually monitored and on ventilation throughout the procedure. A lateral decubitus position allows improved exposure as the mediastinum shifts away from the diaphragm and provides adequate visualization of the entire hemithoracic cavity. The patient should be prepared and draped appropriately. A 12-mm trocar is typically placed in the fifth intercostal space in the midaxillary line, depending on the location of the injury. To allow for retraction of the lung, one to two additional trocars can be placed, typically at the seventh or eighth intercostal space in the posterior axillary line. Insufflation is generally not necessary. Yankauer suction or sponge sticks can be used to evacuate hemothorax and manipulate the lung.

Should an injury be discovered, additional ports can be placed to facilitate surgical thoracoscopic repair or trocar sites can be enlarged for a traditional thoracoabdominal incision and open repair.

2. Thoracotomy

In the case of penetrating trauma, if the entrance and exit wounds are both intrathoracic, a thoracotomy incision can be selected for repair of the diaphragm. In addition, a right anterolateral or posterolateral thoracotomy may be required for occasional defects (e.g., a posterior defect in the region of the bare area of the liver). The thoracotomy is the preferred method of repair when the diagnosis of the injury has been delayed or in cases of chronic presentation.

3. Laparoscopy

Laparoscopy has been used successfully to diagnose left diaphragmatic hernias in penetrating trauma, but is dependent on technique and experience of the surgeon. The role of laparoscopy in blunt trauma is increasing as surgeons become more experienced in exploratory laparoscopy and bowel exploration.

   a. First obtain adequate monitoring of vital signs, control of the airway, and appropriate anesthesia. Following preparation of skin and creation of a sterile field, pneumoperitoneum is established by CO_2 insufflation to 15 mm Hg via a Hassan trocar (open placement). A 10-mL trocar is generally placed into the initial incision and one or more additional 5- or 10-mL trocar is placed to provide adequate retraction. A 30- to 45-degree scope, visceral retraction, and steep reverse Trendelenburg with right lateral tilt all increase the sensitivity of laparoscopy and ability to visualize the entire left hemidiaphragm. A systematic exploration of the abdomen ensues, including adequate visualization of the peritoneal cavity, solid organs, bowel and diaphragm. Hemoperitoneum can be evacuated using laparoscopic irrigation and suction.

b. Tension pneumothorax and transient hypotension can occur during insufflation if a diaphragmatic hernia exists. The chest should always be aseptically prepped and the surgeon prepared for rapid decompression of the pleural space via thoracostomy and subsequent conversion to open procedure.

D. Midline Celiotomy

A midline incision provides excellent exposure to either diaphragm. An abdominal incision is preferable to thoracotomy for acute presentation of the diaphragmatic herniation because it allows for full exploration of the abdominal cavity and reduction of herniated viscera. A full exploratory laparotomy should be performed, allowing adequate visualization of both hemidiaphragms, including the posterior leaflets. Many chest injuries can be handled nonoperatively and this approach avoids the need for two operations. Phrenic nerve injuries can be missed using this approach, however.

a. After control of the airway and anesthesia have been attained, the patient is prepared from proximal thighs to the neck to ensure an adequate surgical field is accessible in case of urgent thoracotomy. Next, make a midline incision from xiphoid to below the umbilicus. Evacuate any intraperitoneal blood and place packs to secure temporary hemostasis. Then systematically explore the abdomen using both visual inspection and palpation.

b. Visual inspection of the right diaphragm usually requires transection of the falciform ligament and release of the triangular and coronary ligaments. Manual assessment (palpation) of the diaphragm is very sensitive. Unless there is good evidence of a laceration requiring visualization for repair, do not mobilize the suspensory ligaments of the liver.

c. Caudad retraction of the stomach and spleen allows for inspection of the left hemidiaphragm.

E.   Treatment

A basic tenet for management of diaphragmatic hernias is that no injury is small enough to be free from sequelae. The negative intrathoracic pressure and constant motion of the diaphragm prevent spontaneous healing of the injury and allow the injury to increase in size over time, resulting in herniation and strangulation.

1.   Once adequate exposure and exploration have been completed, the next step is to reduce herniated viscera. Avoid the use of nitrous oxide because it can distend visceral organs and make reduction more difficult. The stomach is found intrathoracic in 50% of cases with herniation. The colon, small intestine, and omentum can also herniate, although less frequently. The liver can herniate into the right side of the diaphragm. Use gentle traction to reduce the herniated organs; if resistance is met, place a sterile nasogastric tube through the site of herniation, which may facilitate the reduction by alleviating the vacuum from the chest. If unsuccessful, it may be necessary to extend the diaphragmatic defect a short distance.

2.   Take care to avoid the phrenic nerves during extension of the incision. For anterior medial and parahiatal defects, extend the incision anteriorly if extension is required. In ruptures of the central tendon, avoid the phrenic nerves by lateral extension.

3.   After reduction of the abdominal contents, the chest cavity should be well irrigated with warm saline to prevent formation of empyema. A chest tube can be left through the defect at the time of closure to allow for adequate irrigation.

4.   Diaphragmatic defects <2 cm in length and linear defects can be closed using 1-0 or 2-0 nonabsorbable suture in running or interrupted horizontal mattress for a tension-free repair. In defects >2 cm, a layered closure is recommended to ensure a watertight closure and decrease the chances of a subphrenic abscess. An inner layer of interlocking horizontal mattress sutures everts the diaphragmatic edges and is reinforced with a running layer of 3-0 polypropylene sutures. If it is difficult to visualize posterior aspects of the defect, traction on anteriorly placed sutures can provide improved exposure.

5.   Complex repairs rarely require the use of synthetic material to create a tension-free repair. Tenuous tissue occasionally can be supported by pledgets. When the diaphragm has been avulsed from the rib margin, paracostal sutures can be used to reattach the diaphragm to the chest wall. It may be necessary to attach the diaphragm one to two ribs superior to the original attachments to ensure a tension-free repair. Figure-of-eight sutures are place around the corresponding rib (taking care to avoid the neurovascular bundle inferior to each rib) and into the lateral leaf of the diaphragm.

6. A chest tube or red rubber catheter can be left through the defect into the chest cavity while completing the repair. This allows air and fluid to be evacuated from the chest cavity as the lung is reexpanded. Remove the chest tube during full expiration to complete the diaphragmatic closure. Alternatively, insert a conventional chest tube on the side of the repair.

7. A postoperative chest x-ray study should be done and a chest tube should remain if significant pneumothorax persists, typically for 24 to 72 hours. The injured diaphragm tends to remain elevated with paradoxic movement for several weeks after the repair. Eventration can occur if phrenic nerve has been severly damaged. Ventilatory support may be required for significant injures. Common postoperative complications include atelectasis, pneumonia, and empyema. Aggressive chest physiotherapy should be pursued.

VI. Delayed Diagnosis

If initial diaphragmatic injury is missed, a patient can present weeks, months, or even years after the initial incident with chronic diaphragmatic hernia. Frequent complaints are progressive dyspnea, chest pain, and signs of abdominal obstruction. Abdominal contents can become strangulated, ischemic, and perforated, all of which increase mortality. A chest x-ray study is typically diagnostic with air fluid levels above the diaphragm. An upper gastrointestinal series may definitively make the diagnosis. If a diaphragmatic hernia is found, the treatment is surgical repair. Because of chronic adhesions and muscle atrophy, a thoracotomy is recommended for repair. Often, nonabsorbable, bioprosthetic material is required to provide a tension-free repair of a chronic injury. Up to 30% of patients who present with strangulation develop sepsis and die of their injury.

VII. Abdominal Wall Herniation: Initial Presentation

Abdominal wall herniation is a rare consequence of abdominal trauma. Abdominal wall herniation is typically secondary to a deceleration injury with shearing stress to the abdominal wall. It has been strongly associated with the use of seatbelts in motor vehicle accidents. An approximate 30% chance exists of associated injuries.

A. Epidemiology

Abdominal wall herniations are rare but morbid conditions resulting from blunt abdominal trauma. The umbilicus appears to serve as a source of attachment, creating increased tension on the inferior aspect of the abdominal wall.

1. Impact from small blunt objects (e.g., a bicycle handle bar) that do not penetrate the skin surface can cause shearing stress on muscles and fascia. The skin is more mobile than underlying fascia and typically remains intact. Defects caused by these injuries typically occur in lower quadrants in the regions of the inguinal canal.

2. Larger objects and deceleration forces (e.g., from improperly placed seatbelts) cause transverse tears in the abdominal wall, typically along the borders of the rectus abdominus or at the site of muscle insertions into the pelvis. The classic description of seatbelt injuries includes abdominal wall trauma, bowel injury, and lumbar spine fractures.

B. Generally, three criteria must be met to qualify a traumatic abdominal wall hernia.

1. A history of injury significant enough to cause abdominal wall herniation.

2. Immediate appearance of the defect with intact skin

3. Absence of a peritoneal sac on exploration, indicating acute presentation

VIII. Diagnosis

A. History

Any injury to the abdominal wall involving an acute elevation in abdominal pressure can cause abdominal wall herniation. Use of seatbelts, force sustained by handlebars, deceleration injuries, crush injuries, and falls can cause this type of injury. Patients are often entirely asymptomatic. They can complain of abdominal pain or a bulge in abdominal wall.

B. Physical Examination

Examination alone can be diagnostic. Full-thickness defect with hematoma or ecchymosis or reducible hernia with abdominal contents that is new in onset is diagnostic. A mass may be palpable in the anterior abdominal wall. Typically, this worsens when patient strains to sit up or tenses the rectus sheath. The mass is frequently reducible, but does not move from side to side with palpation or positioning. It may be possible to auscultate the bowel within the subcutaneous tissue. Peritoneal signs can herald associated injuries.

C. Computed Tomography

Computed tomography has been very useful in the diagnosis of abdominal wall herniation. Defects in the abdominal wall fascia can be seen on soft tissue windows. Particular attention must be paid to the muscle walls and their insertions to avoid missing subtle injuries. CT is also instrumental in separating abdominal wall herniation from rectus sheath hematoma.

IX. Management

As with repairs of all hernias, the goal of treatment is a tension-free repair.

A. Exploratory laparotomy and repair of associated injuries occurs first. A midline incision allows for exploration and visualization of the extent of defect after the abdomen has been explored. Although a transverse incision can decrease tension, it does not allow adequate exposure for the repair of associated injuries.

B. After visceral issues have been addressed, direct attention to proper débridement of affected tissues.

C. Immediate repair is generally possible. If primary tension-free repair is possible, use a running closure of nonabsorbable monofilament. A no. 2 nylon suture is generally acceptable. Use the basic techniques of tension-free hernia repair.

D. Contraindications for immediate repair are secondary to high rate of repair failure in the following scenarios.

    1. If areas of further ischemia exist, delay primary repair until viability of tissues has been established.

    2. In cases of significant muscle damage, approach the muscle remnant with caution because suture may fail to hold in the remnant.

    3. Associated intraabdominal injury with spillage of abdominal contents is a contraindication for immediate repair because of the possibility of contaminating the closure and causing a larger defect in the abdomen.

    4. Large gunshot wounds or areas with indistinct border of injury should encourage delayed repair.

E. Delay in repair requires surgical sterile packing of wound and treatment of pain issues. In cases of associated intestinal injury requiring creation of an ostomy, some recommend delay of closure for periods of up to 1 year secondary to a high rate of complications.

F. If tension-free repair is not possible secondary to the size or location of tissue loss, options exist for using autologous graft or artificial graft materials.

    1. Autologous graft possibilities include vascularized skin, fascia, and muscle flaps, including tensor fascia lata, latissimus dorsi, rectus abdominus, and rectus femoris, which provide strong material for replacement of the traumatic injury, often with the patient's own blood supply to enable survival. Disadvantages of using autologous graft material include donor site morbidity, seroma, hematoma, scars, and possible muscle weakness.

    2. Artificial graft options include Gortex and polypropylene mesh. Advantages include the inert nature, pliability, and resilience of the graft. Complications can include mesh extrusion, need for removal in case of infection, and bowel fistula formation. In addition, mesh is contraindicated in the acute setting in cases of any soilage of the peritoneal cavity by abdominal contents.

X. Rectus Sheath Hematoma

    A. Presentation

Rectus sheath hematomas are caused by injuries to the inferior or superior epigastric arteries, which are contained within the posterior aspect of the rectus sheath. Injuries are usually self-contained and limited, unless comorbidity exists or anticoagulation therapy is being used.

    B. Diagnosis

        1. History and Physical Examination

Rectus sheath hematoma can present similarly to abdominal wall herniation with palpable central mass. The mass increases in size with tension of the abdominal wall. The mass is palpable in the central portion of the abdominal wall but is neither mobile nor reducible.

    2. Computed Tomography findings suggestive of rectal sheath hematoma include Hounsfield units consistent with hematoma or blood and containment of hematoma by the rectus sheath.

C. Management

Observation of the mass is typically sufficient. Most rectus sheath hematomas are generally self-contained and self-limited. Anticoagulants and antiplatelet agents can be withheld if a patient's medical conditions can tolerate. Should the mass continue to expand, the patient can be surgically explored for evacuation of the hematoma and ligation of the offending vessel(s).

SELECTED READING

Brenneman FD, Boulanger BR, Antonyshyn O. Surgical management of abdominal wall disruption after blunt trauma. *J Trauma* 1995;39(3), 539–544.

Carrico CJ, Thal ER, Weigelt JA. *Operative trauma management: an atlas.* Norwalk, Connecticut: Appleton and Lange, 1998.

Moore EE, Mattox KL, Feliciano DV. *Trauma,* 2nd ed. Norwalk, Connecticut: Appleton & Lange, 1991.

Thal EW, Provost DA. Traumatic rupture of the diaphragm. In: *Mastery of surgery,* 3rd ed. Boston: Little, Brown and Company, 1996.

Wilson RF, Walt AJ. *Management of trauma: pitfalls and practice,* 2nd ed. Baltimore: Williams & Wilkins, 1996.

27

Abdominal Trauma 3: Hepatic and Biliary Tract Injuries

Jennifer A. Wargo, MD, Ruben Peralta, MD, and Robert L. Sheridan, MD

I. Introduction

The liver is the most commonly injured intraabdominal organ. Over the past few decades, management strategies for injuries to the liver and biliary tree have changed significantly, largely because of improvements in diagnostic imaging and innovative nonoperative techniques.

II. Epidemiology and Mechanisms

Penetrating injuries to the abdomen most often involve the liver and account for 37% of all intraabdominal injuries. Gunshot wounds typically cause more damage than stab wounds because they are associated with cavitation and further tissue destruction. Blunt injury to the abdomen frequently results in injury to solid organs (e.g., the liver and spleen) because they are unable to tolerate the sudden application of pressure to the abdominal cavity. Hollow viscera (e.g., the intestine) are more likely to tolerate such an insult. Furthermore, points of attachment (e.g., the ligamentum teres) make the hepatic parenchyma susceptible to tearing from shear strain during blunt injury. The liver is also susceptible to compressing injuries owing to its proximity to structures such as the rib cage and vertebral column.

Two types of blunt liver trauma that have been described include those induced by deceleration injuries or by direct blows to the abdominal cavity. These distinct mechanisms of blunt injury yield significantly different patterns of injury. In a deceleration injury, such as encountered with motor vehicle crashes and falls from significant height, expect to find injuries that include lacerations between the anterior (segment VI and VII) and posterior portions (segments V and VIII) of the liver. This is in sharp contrast to injuries produced by crush injuries often seen in segments I, IV, V, and VII (**Fig. 27-1**).

Although injuries to the biliary tree do not occur as frequently as injuries to the liver parenchyma, they remain a significant cause of morbidity and mortality from intraabdominal injury. Injuries to the portal triad occur in <1% of traumatic injuries, but are associated with a mortality rate of >50%.

III. Initial Evaluation

A. Examination and Diagnostic Modalities

Even before the patient's arrival in the tertiary care setting, the potential for serious intraabdominal injury can be suspected based on the mechanism and pattern of injury as well as the prehospital vital signs and physical findings. An injury to the liver should be suspected in a victim of

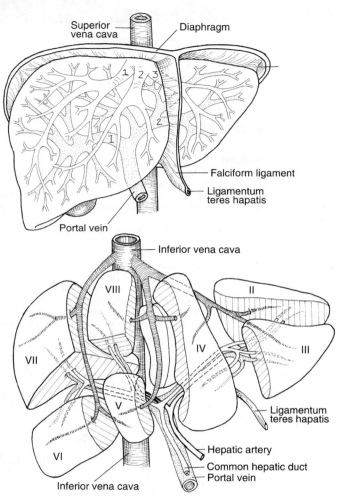

Figure 27-1.   Liver anatomy.

blunt trauma that involves the epigastrium or right upper quadrant, and must be highly considered in deceleration injuries such as motor vehicle crashes and falls from significant height. In penetrating trauma, injury to the liver or biliary tree must be considered even if the entry wound is relatively distant from these organs because the trajectory and other details (e.g., length of penetrating object, caliber of the bullet) are often not known.

Initial evaluation of injured patients should ensue based on the recommendations of the Advanced Trauma Life

Support guidelines. Physical examination should be performed; however, even in an alert patient the false positive and false negative rates can be as high as 56% and 46%, respectively. Any patient who is hemodynamically unstable should be considered for emergent laparotomy. During the secondary survey, the abdomen should be fully inspected and bowel sounds auscultated, although the absence of bowel sounds does not necessarily indicate intra-abdominal injury. During percussion and palpation, tympany in the left upper quadrant caused by a largely dilated stomach or guarding may be found. Voluntary guarding is not dependable, although involuntary guarding and rebound tenderness are reliable signs of peritoneal irritation.

Special attention must be given to patients in whom concurrent neurologic injury is suspected, as general anesthesia can induce significant changes in intracranial pressure and prohibit timely identification of progressive neurologic deficits. Traditionally, diagnostic peritoneal lavage (DPL) was recommended for such patients, although this modality has largely been replaced by ultrasound (US) assessment and abdominal computed tomography (CT) in most major centers. Patients who are hemodynamically unstable and either have a stab wound to the abdomen or have a blunt trauma injury and have peritoneal signs should be considered for immediate laparotomy. A gunshot wound to the abdomen is typically considered a clear indication for laparotomy in a hemodynamically unstable patient regardless of physical findings.

B. Ultrasound and Computed Tomography

Ultrasonography and computed tomography have become significant assets in the evaluation and management of trauma patients. In many institutions, US assessment in the trauma bay using the focused abdominal sonography for trauma (FAST) approach has significantly improved timely identification of intraabdominal injuries. This technique involves assessment of four regions in the abdomen: Morison's pouch, splenic and left pararenal space, pelvis and paravesical space, and pericardium. Prospective studies performed during recent years have yielded values of sensitivity and specificity for US to be 88% and 99%, respectively.

Computed tomography yields the most complete noninvasive evaluation of soft tissues of the abdomen and pelvis, although its use must be cautioned against in the hemodynamically unstable patient.

The diagnosis of intraabdominal injuries using CT has improved since its inception with the development of spiral and helical CT, which greatly improve the speed, resolution, and image reconstruction capabilities. Traditionally, oral contrast medium has been used to better delineate the small and large bowel and to identify possible sites of intestinal injury by evidence of extravasation. Its use, however, has several disadvantages, including a side effect of vomiting with a risk of aspiration and, possibly, requiring nasogastric tube placement. More recently, the use of oral contrast media has been disputed and several series suggest that it is not essential.

Intravenous contrast is highly recommended because it allows visualization of the great vessels as well as yielding valuable information regarding the presence or absence of active hemorrhage, hematoma, and organ contusions. Use of a noncontrast scan can result in missed injuries because hematomas can be isodense when compared with surrounding tissue.

Hemoperitoneum can be quantified using the value for Hounsfield units (HU) on a CT image, with 25 HU representing fresh blood and 60 HU representing hematoma. A high value of 150 indicates rapid extravasation of intravenous contrast and suggests active hemorrhage from a major vessel. The extent of blood in the abdomen can be quantified by assessing seven intraabdominal areas. Hemoperitoneum is considered to be *mild* if blood is localized to the perihepatic, subphrenic, and subhepatic space; *moderate* if localized to the above areas and to the paracolic gutters; and *large* if localized to these areas along with the pelvis. The classifications of mild, moderate, and large hemoperitoneum correspond to approximate volumes of 250, 250 to 500, and >500 mL. Indications for laparotomy have changed over the past several years, and it is now generally accepted that a patient with a 500-mL hemoperitoneum who is hemodynamically stable may indeed tolerate nonoperative management, although anyone with hemoperitoneum of >500 mL should be strongly considered for laparotomy. CT with intravenous contrast is helpful in deciding whether a patient should be considered for observation, angiography, or laparotomy.

C. Angiography

Consider angiography for any hemodynamically stable patient in whom CT or US suggests a significant vascular injury.

Angiography has the advantage of being both diagnostic and potentially therapeutic because the actively bleeding vessels can be embolized. Other potential applications of angiographic embolization following trauma include its use for the treatment of pseudoaneurysms and hemobilia.

The sensitivity of angiography in the diagnosis of hepatic injuries is high and can help predict which patients will fail nonoperative management. Several studies have demonstrated that the most likely predictors of failure in nonoperative management include the presence of extravasation on CT or angiography and the presence of a pseudoaneurysm.

Use caution, however, in patients who require vigorous fluid resuscitation to maintain hemodynamic stability. Consider laparotomy for these patients rather than angiography.

D. Diagnostic Peritoneal Lavage

Before the advent of CT and the common use of US in the evaluation of trauma patients, diagnostic peritoneal lavage (DPL) served as the standard means of evaluating for hemoperitoneum or bowel injury following blunt abdominal trauma. DPL can be done quickly and relatively easily, but it is invasive and cannot assess for the presence of a retroperitoneal hematoma. DPL still plays a role in the evaluation of patients with abdominal trauma in selected circumstances.

E. Laparoscopy

Over the past several years, the use of diagnostic laparoscopy has broadened to include evaluation in trauma. Its use is established for penetrating trauma. Its use in the evaluation of injuries caused by blunt abdominal trauma, however, is clearly emerging, with some institutions using laparoscopy in the trauma bay of the emergency department to evaluate patients with suspected intraabdominal injury. Its use can be helpful in reducing the number of nontherapeutic laparotomies as well as decreasing length hospitalization and overall treatment costs. Although minor interventions can often be performed at the time of diagnostic laparoscopy, an open procedure is usually required if significant injuries are identified.

IV. Treatment

A. Hepatic Anatomy

Although the shape and specific dimensions of the liver are somewhat variable, the organ generally lies in the right upper quadrant with the apex extending across the midline into the left upper quadrant. It is enveloped by peritoneal folds consisting of the falciform ligament, two triangular ligaments, and two coronary ligaments. The dome of the liver lies within close approximation of the right hemidiaphragm and is typically located at the level of the fifth rib.

The left and right lobes are divided by the incisura, or portal fissure, in which lies the middle hepatic vein. This area can be identified by picturing a line drawn from the gallbladder fossa to the inferior vena cava. The left lobe is further divided by the falciform ligament into a medial segment (representing the quadrate lobe) and a lateral segment. The right lobe is divided into anterior and posterior segments by an indistinct intersegmental line (**Fig. 27-1**).

Using the French system, the liver may also be divided into eight segments. This anatomic division of the liver parenchyma is based on the supply of portal and hepatic branches to each of the segments. In this system, the right and left paramedian sectors are divided centrally by the main portal fissure, or scissura. These are separated from the lateral sectors by lateral fissures. Collectively, these four sectors are further divided by the right and left portal veins into a total of eight hepatic segments. On the left, the sectors are divided into anterior and posterior, whereas on the right they are divided into anteromedial and posterolateral. The segments are enumerated from left to right, starting with segment I (representing the caudate lobe). Segments II and III represent the superior and inferior segments of the left lateral lobe. The fourth segment represents the quadrate lobe, and can be further divided into segments IVa and IVb. Segments V and VIII represent the inferior and superior segments of the anteromedial sector, whereas segments VI and VII represent the inferior and superior segments of the posterolateral sector.

B.   Grading of Liver Injuries

The severity of injury to the liver following trauma can be graded using the Hepatic Injury Scale (**Table 27-1**). Grade I and II account for most injuries and are considered relatively minor, rarely requiring operative intervention. Grade III, IV, and V injuries are considered increasingly severe and often require laparotomy, whereas grade VI injuries (complete avulsion of the liver) are incompatible with survival.

C.   Nonoperative Management

Proponents of nonoperative management of selected patients with penetrating trauma cite that most small-caliber penetrating wounds and stab wounds to the liver

Table 27-1.   Grading of liver injuries

Grade[a]	Injury	Description
I	Hematoma	Subcapsular hematoma (<10% of surface area)
	Laceration	Capsular tear (<1 cm in depth)
II	Hematoma	Subcapsular hematoma (10% to 50% of surface area) OR Parenchymal tear (<10 cm in diameter)
	Laceration	Parenchymal tear (1–3 cm in depth, <10 cm length)
III	Hematoma	Subcapsular hematoma (>50% of surface area) Ruptured subcapsular or parenchymal hematoma Parenchymal hematoma (>10 cm in diameter)
	Laceration	Parenchymal tear (>3 cm in depth)
IV	Laceration	Parenchymal disruption (25% to 75% of lobe) OR One to three segments within a single lobe
V	Laceration	Parenchymal disruption (>75% of lobe) OR > Three segments within a single lobe
	Vascular	Juxtahepatic venous injuries
VI	Vascular	Avulsion of the liver

[a]Advance one grade for multiple injuries, up to grade III.

are not found to be actively bleeding at the time of laparotomy. Additionally, less concern is seen for a concomitant diaphragmatic injury than when the injury is on the left.

Appropriate patient selection for nonoperative management is based on several factors. Above all, patients with evidence of hepatic injury must be hemodynamically stable after adequate fluid resuscitation to be considered good candidates for nonoperative management. In addition, the injury to the hepatic parenchyma should not involve major vascular structures or be actively bleeding (as evidenced by a blush of contrast or contrast pooling on CT). The volume of hemoperitoneum based on CT evaluation should be <500 mL and no other abdominal injuries present that require laparotomy. The patient should have minimal requirement for replacement of blood from hepatic losses and should not have evidence of peritoneal findings if neurologically intact. The strongest predictors for failure of nonoperative management include hemodynamic instability, advanced grade of liver injury, contrast pooling on CT, and periportal tracking.

Patients who are selected for nonoperative management must be monitored closely using frequent vital sign monitoring, repeat physical examination, and serial measurement of the hemoglobin and hematocrit. It is difficult, however, to predict which patients will fail nonoperative management based on their presentation and initial CT scan appearance. Therefore, they should be carefully monitored, ideally in a tertiary care facility where an interventional radiologist is available should the need for embolization arise.

Follow-up CT scans were once standard in the nonoperative management of patients with liver trauma. Recent studies, however, suggest that this practice does not affect outcome and, therefore, is not indicated routinely. Follow-up CT scan after liver injury typically demonstrates resolution of the hemoperitoneum within 1 week, resolution of a laceration within 3 weeks, resolution of a subcapsular hematoma within 8 weeks, and hematomas and biloma sometimes persisting for months to years. The incidence of rebleeding following hepatic injury is much lower than that for splenic injury, occurring in less that 2% of all patients managed nonoperatively. Additionally, rebleeding following liver trauma does not follow the pattern of catastrophic bleeding seen in splenic trauma. Thus, follow-up CT for patients with liver trauma is recommended only for those patients who have a change in clinical status or a drop in hematocrit, suggesting possible continued bleeding or development of another complication (e.g., bile leak).

Potential complications of nonoperative management are serious. Associated bowel injuries occur at an overall rate of up to 63% in penetrating trauma and up to 15% in blunt trauma to the liver. Bowel injuries can be missed in these patients because they may not be fully evident on CT. The incidence of missed intraabdominal injury when

CT is used ranges from 0.5% to 12% and 5% to 15% when CT is not used. Some advocate the use of diagnostic peritoneal lavage in patients with equivocal physical findings and isolated hepatic injuries on CT because this can increase the diagnostic yield in deciding whom to treat nonoperatively.

Delayed hemorrhage is the most common complication of nonoperative management of liver trauma, occurring in approximately 2% of all patients so managed. Rebleeding following traumatic liver injury, however, does not follow the catastrophic pattern of that following splenic injury, and is typically illustrated by gradual drop in hematocrit as well as an ongoing fluid or transfusion requirement. A recent review cited the most common treatment errors in patients with delayed hemorrhage: (1) assuming that the bleeding is not from the liver and overestimating blood loss from other injuries; (2) treating ongoing hemorrhage with multiple (>4) units of blood; and (3) misreading the abdominal CT scan regarding the amount of hemoperitoneum or the presence of active bleeding. Although often requiring laparotomy, delayed hemorrhage can be managed nonoperatively in selected circumstances.

Biliary tract injuries can also complicate nonoperative management of these patients because their reported incidence is between 1% and 5% in patients with abdominal trauma. The incidence may be even higher, reported as high as 21.4% in one series. The gallbladder and the common bile duct are the most frequently injured structures, and these injuries are often associated with liver, gastric, colon, and pancreatic injuries. Biliary fistulas and biloma can also occur, with a reported incidence between 0.5% and 20%. Most biloma (70%) can be managed nonoperatively. Liver abscess, which can also occur, can be treated with percutaneous drainage and antibiotics, although surgical intervention should be considered in any patient with fungemia or bacteremia.

Hemobilia and bilhaemia are conditions that occur when there is fistulous connection between a vascular structure and the biliary system. The constellation of symptoms, including upper abdominal pain, jaundice, and gastrointestinal hemorrhage, first described by Quinke in 1871, serves as a useful diagnostic tool in hemobilia. All three are present in 22% of patients, with abdominal pain or bleeding alone in 10% and 32% of patients, respectively. Following trauma, hemorrhage can be immediate or delayed, presenting as hematemesis or melena if bleeding is brisk. Slower bleeding into the biliary tract causes clots to form in the biliary radicals, causing bilie stasis and resultant jaundice. Endoscopy may reveal a blood clot at the ampulla of Vater, but this finding is rare. Angiography is now recognized as the diagnostic method of choice, and can be potentially therapeutic with the intervention of embolization. Operative intervention is indicated when embolization fails, when associated cholecystitis is present, or in cases of sepsis from an undrained biliary tree. Bilhaemia is a rare complication of hepatic trauma that occurs when there is a fistulous connection between the biliary tract and a hepatic venous structure *and* the physiologic pressure difference of these structures exceeds 15 cm of water. This condition is heralded by profound jaundice following abdominal trauma, usually occurring within 48 and 72 hours. If patients are on ventilatory support with positive pressure ventilation, the jaundice may not appear until this support is withdrawn and the pressure differential is established. Suspect bilhaemia in any patient with abdominal trauma and a markedly elevated serum bilirubin, as renal excretion usually prevents levels above 500 µmol/L when caused by biliary obstruction. Transaminase level can be normal or slightly elevated, depending on the presence of associated injuries to the hepatic parenchyma.

The diagnosis can be confirmed using several diagnostic modalities, including endoscopic retrograde cholangiography, percutaneous transhepatic cholangiography, or biliary scintigraphy. The aim of surgical management for this condition is biliary decompression with repair of the biliary and venous structures if the injury is apparent. If the injury cannot be identified, T-tube drainage (without negative pressure) can be used. Some have reported success with nonoperative management using endoscopic stents and nasobiliary drainage, but experience is limited.

D. Operative Management

Any patient with an abdominal injury who is hemodynamically unstable, despite adequate fluid resuscitation, should have emergent laparotomy. Additional indications for laparotomy in patients with hepatic trauma include any evidence of peritonitis or frank evisceration, hemoperitoneum >500 mL, evidence of associated intraabdominal injuries, significant transfusion requirement (>4 units of blood), or clinical deterioration during observation.

Patients who are deemed operative candidates should receive appropriate resuscitation in the emergency ward; however, efforts to obtain hemodynamic stability should not prevent their timely transfer to the operating room. Patients should be in a facility where an experienced surgeon familiar with hepatic anatomy can care for them. Access should be available to interventional radiology should the need arise, as well as adequate blood products and intensive care monitoring. If any of the above is not available, consider transfer to the nearest specialized facility once the patient is stabilized.

E. Anatomy and Exposure

Once the patient is in the operating room, the patient should be prepared and draped from the midneck to the midthighs and fully side to side. If the patient's hemodynamic status is particularly tenuous, prepare the skin before induction of anesthesia because this often causes a significant drop in blood pressure and operative intervention may be required immediately. A wide preparation allows for extension of the midline abdominal incision to a median sternotomy or right thoracotomy to help provide exposure if a posterior liver injury is encountered.

After the patient has been prepared, make a generous midline skin incision, extending from the xiphoid to below the umbilicus. An alternative approach if a through-and-through liver injury is suspected is a bilateral subcostal incision. Do not complete the incision in the peritoneum until the full skin incision is made. Be fully prepared to act once the tamponade effect of the intact peritoneum is breached. If a midline incision is used, this then can be extended to the pubis, followed by removal of all blood and clots with an estimation of initial blood loss. Then pack the abdomen in all quadrants to stop bleeding temporarily while injuries are evaluated and the anesthesiology team is allowed to replace fluids or blood products and assure that the patient is being properly warmed. Hemostasis can also be obtained via Pringle maneuver or bimanual compression of the liver if severe liver injury is encountered.

The packs can then be removed sequentially, starting with the lower quadrants to assess for associated injuries, particularly those that can cause fecal contamination. Any injury leading to fecal contamination should be excluded at this time, either with staple devices or umbilical tape, until they can be definitively repaired. With no evidence of fecal contamination, use autotransfusion, if available. Packs should then be removed from the left upper quadrant with assessment of the spleen, and splenectomy, if indicated. Finally, remove the packs in the right upper quadrant and assess the extent of hepatic injury. The liver can be gently rotated cephalad to determine any injury to the hepatic vein by assessing for a gush of blood when this maneuver is performed. If an injury to a hepatic vein is suspected, decide whether to pack and reexplore at a later time or address the vascular injury, depending on the stability of the patient and the extent of the injury.

Portal triad compression (Pringle maneuver) can be used both diagnostically and therapeutically during laparotomy for hepatic injury. If digital compression of the portal triad controls hemorrhage, it heightens the suggestion of an injury to the portal venous or hepatic arterial structures. If it does not control hemorrhage, suspect injury to the vena cava or the presence of aberrant anatomy. If bleeding is controlled, a vascular clamp can be applied to the structures, taking care to compress the clamp just enough to occlude blood flow but not cause injury to the common bile duct. Atraumatic vascular clamping of the portal triad for up to 1 hour is considered safe by many, although others discourage clamp times of > 30 minutes. Intermittent clamping, which has also been advocated, can be performed for up to 15 minutes at a time, repeated as often as required. If bleeding has been controlled and adequate resuscitation and warming has been accomplished, proceed to mobilization of the liver by dividing the falciform, coronary, and triangular ligaments. The avascular region of the gastrohepatic ligament can then be incised to allow access to the lesser sac. Place packs posteriorly, taking care not to cause excessive compression of the inferior vena cava. Should the patient become coagulopathic at any point during the procedure, consider packing and returning in 48 to 72 hours.

Hepatorrhaphy, initially described in 1897, involves the use of large horizontal mattress sutures to compress bleeding liver parenchyma. Hepatorrhaphy alone in severe liver injuries has been discouraged because it can lead to extensive necrosis and can predispose to sepsis. Its use may be more appropriate in less severe liver injuries (grade I or II) and in the management of critically ill patients when a timely procedure with planned reoperation is required.

In severe liver injuries, hepatotomy with suture ligation is often performed. This procedure involves extending the tear in the hepatic parenchyma using a "finger fracture" technique, electrocautery, or ultrasonic scalpel to expose hepatic vessels and ducts in close proximity to the injury. Injured structures can then be repaired or suture ligated under direct vision, with a low incidence of rebleeding and sepsis. The use of vascular clips has been discouraged because they can become dislodged with the motion of respiration.

Resection can be performed for traumatic liver injury, either following the line of injury or tissue viability (débridement resection) or via anatomic resection. In débridement resection, the devitalized hepatic parenchyma is removed using a finger fracture technique or the blunt end of a scalpel with suture ligation of any vessels or ductal structures. The advantage of this method is that it can be performed rapidly, with the caveat that a complete resection of all involved tissue should be done even in the event of an isolated disruption to a segmental bile duct to prevent the development of a biliary fistula. True anatomic resection requires significantly more time and identification of portal structures, and has an associated mortality rate nearing 50%. Therefore its use is reserved for those cases of severe injury (e.g., deep lacerations involving major structures) and extensive areas of devitalized tissue, provided that more conservative methods have failed.

Selective hepatic artery ligation was previously used frequently, but has fallen out of favor because bleeding from most injuries can be controlled by other means. Its use is warranted when the Pringle maneuver is successful in controlling the bleeding but the site cannot be identified during hepatotomy or perihepatic packing is ineffective. It is contraindicated in patients with cirrhosis.

Perihepatic packing was used frequently in the early 20th century but its use has been largely abandoned because of the reported high rates of infection and associated complications. More recently, its use has been reevaluated in selected circumstances of severe liver injury with planned reoperation and in those instances where patients become hypothermic and develop coagulopathy and acidosis intraoperatively. Packing can even serve as definitive treatment for certain hepatic injuries.

Laparotomy sponges are ideal for packing hepatic parenchyma and should be placed so that they compress the wounded liver edges together. Pay careful attention not to compress the diaphragm or inferior vena cava unduly. Do not place packs within the wound because this can cause further tissue destruction and hemorrhage. Controversy still exists over when perihepatic packing should be used, but solid indications include uncontrollable coagulopathy, bilobar injury, and a large nonexpanding capsular hematoma with capsular avulsion. Many feel that packing should be performed when the body temperature is <32°C, pH <7.2, transfusion requirement of >10 units of blood, or the patient demonstrates any evidence of coagulopathy. Close the abdomen following placement of packs, using mesh if the abdominal closure proves difficult from edema and pack placement. Patients with packs in place should be on broad-spectrum antibiotics to reduce the risk of sepsis, and packs should be removed when coagulopathy, acidosis, and hypothermia are corrected typically within 12 to 72 hours. A relatively new technique involves the use of a synthetic, absorbable mesh to wrap the liver parenchyma in the case of a substantial laceration or intraparenchymal hemorrhage. The advantages of this technique are that a second laparotomy is not necessarily required and compression of surrounding structures is rare. It cannot be used, however, with concurrent hepatic vein injury.

An adjunct to the methods discussed above, is the use of fibrin glue. Fibrin glue contains a mixture of calcium chloride, fibrinogen, and thrombin. It can be applied to raw surfaces of liver parenchyma to control venous oozing and to prevent postoperative hemorrhage and bile leaks by sealing small blood vessels and biliary ductules. Potential complications with the use of fibrin glue include hypotension, if it gains access to the circulation, and possible transmission of blood-borne disease.

Liver transplantation has been described in the treatment of severe liver trauma, although donor organs are not often readily available.

V.   Retrohepatic Vena Cava and Juxtahepatic Venous Injuries

Injuries to the retrohepatic vena cava and juxtahepatic venous structures pose significant challenges for trauma surgeons caring for patients with hepatic injuries. They occur in up to 15% of patients with liver injury and are most often associated with blunt abdominal trauma, although they can be seen in cases of penetrating trauma as well. Mortality rates when these injuries are present are exceedingly high, ranging from 50% to 70%. The cause of death in these instances are typically from exsanguinating hemorrhage, either before the venous injury can be exposed or during exposure and attempted repair. These injuries should be suspected if Pringle maneuver fails to control hemorrhage intraoperatively.

The retrohepatic vena cava is typically 8 cm long, its limits being defined by the phrenic veins superiorly and the right adrenal vein inferiorly. It lies within the bare area of the liver and is frequently surrounded by hepatic parenchyma. Its posterior aspect is in close association with the inferior surface of the diaphragm. The inferior vena cava joins the right atrium approximately 3 cm from the most superior portion of the retrohepatic vena cava. Three major hepatic veins (right, left, and middle) have long intrahepatic courses and join the retrohepatic vena cava, where accessory (dorsal hepatic) veins may also be found. The suspensory ligaments of the liver (triangular, falciform, and coronary) surround the bare area of the liver and the retrohepatic cava and veins and, therefore, are significant when dealing with hemorrhage from any of these structures.

Injury to the hepatic veins can occur throughout their length both in their intraparenchymal segments or closer to the retrohepatic vena cava. Injury to these veins or to the retrohepatic vena cava is often accompanied by disruption of the tissues surrounding these structures, leading to hemorrhage into either the chest or abdomen. In selected circumstances, the integrity of the surrounding structures (i.e., hepatic parenchyma, suspensory ligaments, diaphragm) remains intact, preventing hemorrhage, unless they are breached, and even allowing for nonoperative management in some patients.

Two patterns of injury have been described in the context of these injuries and are designated type A and B. In type A injuries, the venous injury is intraparenchymal and hemorrhage occurs *through the wound* in the hepatic parenchyma. In contrast, type B injuries involve venous injuries *outside* the hepatic parenchyma with associated disruption of the diaphragm or suspensory ligaments, leading to hemorrhage around the liver parenchyma. Although type A injuries are reported to occur more frequently, combinations of the two can also be seen in both blunt and penetrating trauma to the liver.

More patients with these injuries are actually making it to tertiary care facilities because of advances in prehospital care. In addition, adjunctive intraoperative techniques, including atriocaval shunting, venovenous bypass, and total vascular exclusion, have been devised in an attempt to aid in repair and reduce the high mortality rates associated with these injuries.

Minor injuries to the retrohepatic vena cava or hepatic veins can be repaired by direct suture of the venous injury. Most of these injuries require the use of adjunctive techniques to control venous bleeding and allow adequate and full visualization of the injury. This technique involves the use of Pringle maneuver and the application of vascular clamps to the suprahepatic and infrahepatic inferior vena cava. Although it was used successfully in elective resections in patients with adequate circulating blood volume, it was noted to cause profound hypotension in hypovolemic patients on application of the clamps to the vena cava, as well as cardiac arrhythmias on their release. Its use, therefore, has become infrequent in the acute trauma setting.

Another method of hepatic isolation is atriocaval shunting. To use this technique, access to the right atrial appendage must be gained through a median sternotomy. A shunt is then created between the right atrium and the inferior vena cava, classically using a 36F chest tube with an extra side port created 20 cm from the most proximal side port. Use of the atriocaval shunt in conjunction with clamping of the portal triad provides vascular exclusion, theoretically providing a bloodless field. When a chest tube is used, control of the suprarenal vena cava must be obtained to prevent back-bleeding. A more recent modification to the technique involves the use of a cuffed endotracheal tube as a shunt to potentially avert the need to provide suprarenal control externally. Complications of this technique include air embolism and venous perforation. The mortality rate associated with atriocaval shunting, however, approaches 90%, often attributable to delays in diagnosis of vena caval injuries, inexperience in inserting these shunts, and the intraoperative complications of hypothermia, acidosis, and coagulopathy. More recently, shunts inserted via the femoral vein have been developed to provide balloon occlusion of the inferior vena cava while allowing venous return to the heart from below the renal veins through a series of proximal side ports. This method allows shunting without sternotomy; however, experience with this technique is limited. Potential complications of this catheter-based device include dislodgement as well as the possibility of thrombus formation.

Venovenous bypass is another technique that has been used during operative management of injuries to the retrohepatic vena cava and hepatic veins. This method was initially pioneered for hepatic transplantation and involves the Pringle maneuver, combined with vascular clamping of the suprahepatic and infrahepatic vena cava. A shunt is then used to bypass venous flow from the left common femoral vein to either the left axillary vein or left internal jugular vein using a centrifugal vortex pump. Several advantages of this method include no requirement for heparinization and preserved venous return. Although initially described, the placement of a cannula into the inferior mesenteric vein to provide portal venous drainage is not felt to be necessary.

Other reported means of repair of juxtahepatic venous injuries include the use of anatomic resection as well as tamponade and containment. Anatomic resection is typically not advocated for the treatment of these conditions because the mortality rate associated with this modality in the trauma setting is exceedingly high.

Although no controlled, randomized trials currently suggest that control of hemorrhage from juxtahepatic venous injuries through tamponade and containment is plausible, historical controls suggest that it may have a role in these injuries. This method of hemorrhage control may be preferable to direct venous repair with hepatic isolation in patients with type A injuries. Advocates of direct venous repair suggest that rebleeding may complicate this approach, although no recent clinical evidence supports this and experimental evidence suggests that repair of the cava is not necessary. Given the improved operative strategies using tamponade and containment and the high mortality rates associated with direct repair using hepatic isolation, the issue of which procedure is best in the acute trauma setting clearly needs to be readdressed. It is possible that prompt control of venous hemorrhage from juxtahepatic venous injuries can best be accomplished through methods of containment through reinforcement or repair of surrounding structures.

VI. Extrahepatic Biliary Tract Injuries

Injuries to the extrahepatic biliary tract are estimated to occur at a rate of between 1% and 5% in blunt and penetrating abdominal trauma. Before the increase in penetrating abdominal injuries seen in trauma centers over recent years, most of these injuries were reported to occur following blunt abdominal trauma. Although blunt abdominal trauma still accounts for most of the injuries in the pediatric population, penetrating trauma is now responsible for the bulk of these injuries in adults. The typical mechanism resulting in blunt injury to the biliary system involves either compression or a direct blow to the upper abdomen. The gallbladder is the biliary structure most commonly injured, followed by the common bile duct, the confluence of hepatic ducts, and the left hepatic duct. Patients with these injuries tend to be young and are often male. A significant proportion of the blunt injuries to the extrahepatic biliary tract occurs in children.

Injuries to the bile ducts can be classified as complete or incomplete transections and by their location in the biliary tree. The most frequent sites of bile duct injury following blunt abdominal trauma include the confluence of hepatic ducts and at its point of attachment as it enters the head of the pancreas. The classification of injuries to the gallbladder is more complex, owing to the wider range of injury patterns associated with this structure. Injuries to the gallbladder can range from contusion to laceration or even complete avulsion. Other constellations that have been described include traumatic cholecystitis related to hemobilia or associated acalculous cholecystitis as well as biliary peritonitis without perforation.

Most patients with injury to the extrahepatic bile duct have associated injuries, typically to the liver, duodenum, stomach, or pancreas. If no indication is seen for emergent laparotomy, many of these injuries go undiagnosed for hours, days, or even weeks after the initial traumatic event. A review in 1985 revealed that over half of these injuries were delayed (>24 hours) in their presentation and diagnosis. With the increasing move toward treating hepatic injuries nonoperatively, it is estimated that even more of these injuries will be diagnosed late.

Early symptoms of bile leakage are rare, and patients with injury to the extrahepatic biliary ducts can have a completely benign abdominal examination on presentation to the emergency department. Even during laparotomy for associated injuries, injuries to the bile duct can be missed. Some intraoperative signs of injury to the biliary tract include free bile or bile staining of the peritoneum or retroperitoneum, as well as associated injury to the other structures of the portal triad. If bile staining is noted in the region of the duodenum, perform the Kocher maneuver to assess for possible injury to the extrahepatic biliary tract. Intraoperative cholangiography can be performed with a high index of suspicion for such an injury and careful inspection has revealed no overt evidence of injury.

If the patient does not have an indication for emergent laparotomy and an indication exists for DPL, the presence of bile in the effluent is pathognomonic of a biliary injury. Absence of bile, however, does not exclude the possibility of injury to the extrahepatic biliary tract, and is rare even in the presence of a confirmed injury because these injuries often occur in the region of the lesser sac or retroperitoneum. Initial abdominal CT is not very sensitive for injuries to the extrahepatic bile ducts, and specific signs for these injuries are frequently not found on CT scans shortly after blunt or penetrating trauma to the abdomen. Peritonitis from bile leakage often does not develop for several days following the injury because bile is only moderately toxic and can be absorbed through the peritoneum.

Patients who have a delayed diagnosis of injury to the extrahepatic bile typically present with jaundice, abdominal distention from bile ascites, abdominal pain, low grade fever, and weight loss. Abdominal CT or US at this point typically demonstrates a fluid collection, which can then be aspirated and analyzed for the presence of bile as well as sent for culture, amylase, and other studies, as indicated. If the presence of bile is confirmed, endoscopic retrograde cholangiopancreatography or ^{99m}Tc dimethyl iminodiacetic acid (HIDA) radionuclide scanning can be performed to help localize the injury. Angiography can also be used in patients with suspected hemobilia. If presentation is particularly delayed and symptoms of obstructive jaundice are present, percutaneous transhepatic cholangiography can be useful in the diagnosis of injury and preoperative planning.

Cholecystectomy is used to manage injuries to the gallbladder. The caveat with this recommendation is to be certain that no associated ductal injury exists because the gallbladder can be used to repair a defect in the bile duct. Some have advocated suture repair or observation in the case of a small laceration or partial avulsion, although most agree that bile leakage from repair of a distended gallbladder far outweighs the benefits of preserving this structure. Hemobilia with subsequent biliary colic has also been described.

An incomplete bile duct injury can be managed using several different techniques, depending on the extent of the injury and the degree of damage to surrounding tissue. Small lacerations can be repaired primarily, with subsequent placement of a T-tube stent above or below the area of primary repair. Others have described the use of a Heineke-Mikulicz type repair if concern exists for narrowing of the duct. Patch repair using gallbladder wall, intestinal wall, or saphenous vein patch have been described, although formal biliary enteric anastomosis should be considered if a significant defect is seen in the duct wall. With extensive damage to surrounding structures (e.g., the hepatic or pancreatic parenchyma) in addition to the bile duct, the patient can best be served by resection (e.g., hepatic débridement resection or pancreaticoduodenectomy) rather than complex reconstruction.

Complete bile duct injuries typically necessitate biliary enteric anastomoses because the stricture rate is high for end-to-end anastomoses for complete transections. This is often best accomplished using a 75- to 80-cm long Roux-en-Y limb of jejunum. End-to-end anastomoses are generally discouraged because the rate of stricture with this method of repair is as high as 55%, but drops to 4% when a biliary enteric anastomosis is performed. End-to-end anastomosis of the common bile duct can be performed, however, in the rare instance of a clean transection.

One of the challenges of biliary enteric anastomoses in the trauma setting is that the ducts are typically not dilated and relatively small. Methods that can be used to widen the anastomosis include incorporating an oblique angle at the terminal duct, incising the common duct along its length, and proximal dissection if the injury occurs near the hepatic confluence. Pay special attention to preserving the blood supply to the common duct, as excessive dissection can disrupt the vasculature. Another option in repair of injuries to the common bile duct injury is choledochoduodenostomy, although this method has not been used frequently owing to undue tension on the anastomosis and concern for fistula formation. Synthetic grafts are not considered suitable, as rejection rates are high.

Injury to the common bile duct along its intrapancreatic course poses a challenging problem. Options for repair in this scenario include formal resection (pancreaticoduodenectomy), "diverticularization" procedure, or duodenal diversion. Duodenal *diverticularization* involves gastric antrectomy, gastroenterostomy, and duodenostomy tube placement. Duodenal diversion is accomplished by gastroenterostomy with oversewing of the pylorus. Roux-en-Y choledochojejunostomy, using the proximal duct with distal duct ligation, can be used in the rare instance of an isolated injury to the intrapancreatic bile duct.

Significant injury to the extrahepatic bile ducts at the level of the left and right hepatic duct is also best managed with biliary enteric anastomosis because the complication rate with this repair method is associated with fewer complications than primary repair. Primary repair can be used with minor tears of either the left or right hepatic ducts, although division of the peritoneum between the duct and liver capsule may be required for adequate exposure. Hepatic duct ligation has also been described as a means for treating these injuries, although atrophy of the involved segments is known to occur and this technique is generally discouraged unless absolutely necessary. Hilar injuries are best treated with Hepp-Couinaud approach, using a sutured mucosa-to-mucosa anastomosis to the left hepatic duct. As with associated pancreatic injuries, if extensive damage has occurred to surrounding structures (e.g., the hepatic parenchyma) in addition to the bile duct, the patient can best be served by resection (e.g., hepatic débridement resection or formal resection) rather than complex reconstruction. With little experience with these repairs and no assistance available, a viable option is T-tube drainage with planned repair or reconstruction. Repeated attempts at reconstruction are discouraged because the number of reconstructive attempts has been shown to correlate inversely with the percentage of patients with good results. Cholecystectomy is recommended in patients requiring operative intervention for injury to the extrahepatic bile ducts because concern for traumatic cholecystitis and delayed gallbladder perforation.

VII.   Postoperative Care

Abnormal liver function tests are to be expected following major hepatic trauma, particularly if resection débridement is required. Transaminases and bilirubin are likely to rise with a concomitant fall in serum albumin. Jaundice, which is not unexpected, can either be a manifestation of resorption of hepatoma or signify hepatic dysfunction.

Between 5% and 10% of patients who have laparotomy for blunt hepatic injuries have leakage of bile from closed suction drains that typically resolves within 3 weeks. If drainage of bile continues beyond this time period, consider endoscopic retrograde cholangiopancreatography. If a leak from a major bile duct is identified, it can be treated with stent placement, although surgical intervention is sometimes required. If hemobilia is suspected, angiography is the diagnostic method of choice; it can be potentially therapeutic with the intervention of embolization.

Septic complications, which occur in 7% to 12% of cases following major hepatic trauma, consist mainly of pneumonia, acalculous cholecystitis, intraabdominal abscess, and ischemic bowel. Associated injury to the bowel puts patients at a much higher risk of developing intraabdominal abscesses. Other factors that increase the risk of intraabdominal sepsis are packing of the liver to control hemorrhage, associated splenectomy, advanced grade of injury, injury to the large intestine, and significant transfusion requirement.

VIII.   Rehabilitative Issues and Delayed Complications

The natural history of healing occurring in both nonoperative and operative management of blunt hepatic trauma remains largely unknown. Accordingly, no hard and fast rules exist to when patients can resume their usual activity. It is generally recommended, however, that patients refrain from heavy physical activity for at least 8 weeks following the initial injury. Overall, the patient's clinical status is the most important indicator of recovery and of the possible development of delayed complications.

As noted, patients with blunt abdominal trauma may not develop symptoms from an associated biliary injury for days, weeks, or even months. Even those patients who are identified as having an injury to the extrahepatic biliary tree who have had definitive repair can develop biliary stricture. The rate of stricture formation is significantly lower in patients treated with biliary-enteric bypass.

Hemobilia can also occur days to weeks after the initial injury, typically presenting with symptoms of gastrointestinal bleeding (hematemesis or melena) or biliary stasis and jaundice. It is best treated angiographically.

Late infectious complications are typically manifested by fever, abdominal pain, and weight loss. When suspecting biloma or fluid collection, use CT or US with percutaneous drainage, if necessary.

A.   Common Traps and Decision Dilemmas

Little argument is seen that patients who have had abdominal trauma and are hemodynamically unstable should be considered for emergent laparotomy. Yet, often patients respond initially to resuscitation with crystalloid solution, then later have evidence of tachycardia or transient hypotension. These patients often have multiple associated injuries including long bone fractures, to which some degree of blood loss may be attributed. A recent review, however, cited the most common treatment errors in patients with hemorrhage from hepatic trauma are (1) assuming that the bleeding is not from the liver and overestimating blood loss from other injuries; (2) treating ongoing hemorrhage with multiple (>4) units of blood; and (3) misreading the abdominal CT scan regarding the amount of hemoperitoneum or the presence of active bleeding.

Another area of caution is in the use of radiologic studies in the marginally stable trauma patient. Although life-saving procedures can be performed in the radiology suite, a patient who remains unstable despite adequate fluid resuscitation should likely be taken to the operating room rather than the radiology suite.

Even after the decision to perform laparotomy has been made, diagnostic dilemmas exist in the realm of the operating room. Often, if an injury to the hepatic parenchyma or biliary tract is evident, it is tempting to perform definitive repair at the time of first laparotomy. If the patient is hypothermic and coagulopathic, however, the best decision may be to pack for hemorrhage control and return the patient to the intensive care unit to be rewarmed and coagulopathy can potentially be corrected. Many feel that packing should be performed when the body temperature is <32°C, the pH <7.2, transfusion requirement >10 units of blood, or the patient demonstrates any evidence of coagulopathy.

Management of blunt and penetrating abdominal trauma poses challenging problems to the trauma surgeon, particularly in cases of injury to the liver, retrohepatic veins, and extrahepatic biliary tree. As indications for operative intervention continue to change and the role of nonoperative management broadens, the trauma surgeon must have an ever-present familiarity with the available means of diagnosis and treatment of these injuries.

SELECTED REFERENCES

American College of Surgeons Committee on Trauma. *Advanced trauma life support manual,* 5th ed. Chicago: American College of Surgeons, 1995.

Bade PG, Thomson SR, Hirsberg A, et al. Surgical operations in traumatic injury to the extrahepatic biliary tract. *Br J Surg* 1989;76:256.

Carillo EH, Platz A, Miller FB, et al. Non-operative management of blunt hepatic trauma. *Br J Surg* 1998;85:461–468.

Knudson MM, Lim RC Jr, Oakes DD, et al. Nonoperative management of blunt liver injuries in adults: the need for continued surveillance. *J Trauma* 1990;30:1494–500.

Knudson MM, Lim RC, Oakes DD, et al. Nonoperative management of blunt liver injuries in adults: the need for continued surveillance. *J Trauma* 1990;44:1494.

Moore EE, Coghill TH, Jurkovich GJ, et al. Organ injury scaling: spleen and liver (1994 revision). *J Trauma* 1995;38:323–324.

Ochsner MG, Jaffin JH, Golocovsky M, et al. Major hepatic trauma. *Surg Clin North Am* 1993;73:337–352.

Ochsner MG. Factors of failure for nonoperative management of blunt liver and splenic injuries. *World J Surg* 2001;25:1393–1396.

Pachter HL, Feliciano DV. Complex hepatic injuries. *Surg Clin North Am* 1996;76:763–782.

Pachter HL, Hofstetter SR. The current status of nonoperative management of adult blunt hepatic injuries. *Am J Surg* 1995;169:442.

Pachter HL, Knudson MM, Esrig B, et al. Status of nonoperative management of blunt hepatic injuries in 1995: a multicenter experience with 404 patients. *J Trauma* 1996;40:31–41.

Parks RW, Chrysos E, Diamond T. Management of liver trauma. *Br J Surg* 1999;86:1121–1135.

Parks RW, Diamond T. Non-surgical trauma to the extrahepatic biliary tract. *Br J Surg* 1995;82:1303–1310.

Sonderstrom CA, Mackawa K, DuPriest RW, et al. Gallbladder injuries resulting from blunt abdominal trauma: an experience and review. *Ann Surg* 1981;193:60.

Strong RW. The management of blunt liver injuries. *Aust N Z J Surg* 1999;69:609–616.

Abdominal Trauma 4: Splenic Injuries

Douglas R. Johnston, MD,
and Robert L. Sheridan, MD

I. Introduction

Its location, fragility, and copious blood supply make the spleen a primary consideration in the evaluation of patients sustaining abdominal or low thoracic trauma. The first splenectomy for trauma was performed in 1678, and by 1928 William Mayo had published a series of 500 splenectomies with a mortality rate of 10%. Reports of healthy survivors, coupled with a high success rate, established splenectomy as the primary surgical therapy for splenic trauma. Despite a long history of successful operation for the injured spleen, however, several considerations have dictated a shift in approach to these injuries over the last two decades. First, a greater awareness of the lifelong susceptibility to infection that occurs after splenectomy has established splenic preservation as the ideal in management. Second, cumulative experience has demonstrated the safety and efficacy of nonoperative management for many patients who would earlier have had laparotomy for splenic injury. Third, the development of innovative approaches to splenic salvage surgery, along with increasing surgical experience with these techniques, has led to wider use of partial splenectomy or splenorrhaphy for patients with more severe injuries. Fourth, the use of less-invasive therapeutic modalities (e.g., angiography and laparoscopy) has widened the scope of potential interventions. This chapter presents an approach to splenic trauma that takes into account the current state of the art in trauma diagnostic strategies. Considered are both operative and nonoperative management and the long-term complications of splenic trauma.

A. Presentation

Rapid intraperitoneal hemorrhage in a patient who arrives at the hospital hypotensive and tachycardic and remains unstable, despite initial resuscitation, is the most acute presentation. Alternately, the spleen can bleed more slowly, such that patients initially respond to fluid therapy, but become tachycardic when the fluid rate is slowed. A third presentation is a slow or intermittent bleeding that can manifest 24 to 48 hours after injury, when other injuries have been addressed, which often manifests as a drop in hematocrit in an otherwise relatively stable patient. Hypotension after blunt or penetrating trauma to the abdomen must always raise the question of spleen injury.

Initial symptoms of splenic injury can be minimal or absent. Some authors believe only 15% of patients present with left-sided abdominal pain or shoulder pain. Many patients in whom splenic injury is being considered have sustained trauma in multiple locations after major mechanism blunt impact (e.g., a fall or motor vehicle crash). In such patients, symptoms directly attributable to the spleen are unreliable. In all cases, evaluation should proceed according to advanced trauma life support (ATLS) guidelines, establishing airway, breathing, and circulation (ABCs). The first indication of splenic injury can come during the "C" phase (establishing circulation), presenting as tachycardia or hypotension initially responsive to fluids. Significant intraabdominal hemorrhage will be evident as failure to respond to fluid resuscitation, potentially with distended abdomen. Focused abdominal sonogram for trauma (FAST) evaluation is useful in the differential diagnosis of splenic injury in the unstable patient, as discussed below.

B.   Anatomy

The spleen, the largest lymphoid organ in the body, is composed primarily of sinusoidal vessels and lymphoid cells, the red and white pulp seen on gross examination, all of which is encased in a fibrous capsule. The splenic capsule is thickest in children. Unlike the spleens of lower mammals, which can contract vigorously and serve as a reservoir for blood in the event of injury, the human spleen has only minimal contractile ability secondary to a lack of muscle fiber investing the capsule. This is greatest in children, who have a thicker, more elastic capsule. With age, the splenic capsule becomes thinner and more fragile. A normal-sized spleen in an adult lies mostly within the bony thorax, and is protected by the left ninth, tenth, and eleventh ribs. Its location also makes it susceptible to injury secondary to rib fracture in high-impact, blunt trauma. The spleen is primarily an intraperitoneal organ, lying in the left upper quadrant superior and to the left of the fundus of the stomach, supported by the phrenocolic ligament. It is connected to the greater curvature of the stomach superiorly via the gastrosplenic ligament, to the splenic flexure of the colon inferomedially via the splenocolic ligament, and to the Gerota's fascia of the kidney posteriorly via the splenorenal ligament. The hilum of the spleen contains the splenic artery and vein and is contiguous with the tail of the pancreas.

The primary blood supply to the spleen is via the splenic artery. Collateral circulation via the left gastric artery is supplied through the gastrosplenic ligament via the short gastric arteries, which anastomose richly with the splenic branches. The splenic vessels divide at variable positions within the hilum to form individual branches, separating the organ into functional vascular segments. Most commonly, these form at least three major branches feeding the upper, middle, and lower poles of the spleen, but they can form a greater number of discrete branches, dividing the spleen into roughly horizontal vascular segments in what has been called a "pancake" distribution. Minimal communication exists between vascular segments within the parenchyma, allowing for successful partial splenectomy with preservation of the remaining segments.

Accessory spleens are found in 15% to 30% of people. Although they can remain after splenectomy for trauma, their volume is seldom enough to compensate for loss of the spleen proper.

C. **Physiology**

The spleen serves several important functions in immune surveillance and, in the developing fetus, it serves as a major site of extramedullary hematopoiesis. In certain hematologic conditions, the spleen can again become a source of red cells; however, in most patients this is not an important function of the spleen. As mentioned, the human spleen is differentiated from that of some other mammals by the lack of a fully formed contractile capsule, which means the human spleen cannot serve a significant reservoir function. It is primarily a filter for blood-borne antigens and abnormal red blood cells, and a major site for antigen presentation to immune effector cells. This filtration function is of greatest physiologic importance for the trapping and processing of encapsulated bacteria and subsequent production of pathogen-specific IgM antibody. Animal studies have demonstrated that both volume of blood flow and microvascular anatomy of the native spleen are important for the trapping of encapsulated organisms and production of IgM. Implantation of homogenates of spleen cells or slices of spleen tissue into the omentum (splenic autotransplantation) results in viable spleen tissue, but these implants seem unable to recapitulate the antibody response of the native organ.

II. **Initial Evaluation of Spleen Injury**

A. **Examination**

It should be emphasized that examination of the patient with suspected splenic injury should take place in the context of a thorough trauma evaluation focusing on the ABCs. In many patients, tachycardia or mild hypotension secondary to hypovolemia is the only manifestation of splenic injury on physical examination. Mild left upper quadrant pain and tenderness can accompany splenic injury. In a small percentage of patients, irritation of the left hemidiaphragm produces shoulder pain, but this sign is neither sensitive nor specific, especially in the blunt-injured patient. Hematoma or ecchymosis of the anterior abdominal wall, the so-called "seatbelt sign," is an indication of the extent of direct energy transfer to the abdomen and, as such, indicates a greater likelihood of splenic injury. In many patients, the abdominal examination may be unrevealing because of altered mental status or concomitant extremity injury. Direct attention to left-sided rib fractures that suggest the severity of impact and also correlate with splenic injury. Risk factors that correlate with spleen injury in the blunt trauma patient are those that suggest a high-energy impact: long bone fracture, pelvic fracture, or major chest injury. Penetrating wounds above or below the diaphragm can injure the spleen. Direct attention to the point of entry, the likely track of the weapon, and the presence of accompanying peritonitis or hemodynamic instability.

B. Focused Abdominal Sonogram for Trauma

The FAST examination, involving surgeon-performed bedside ultrasound as part of the initial trauma workup, is quickly becoming the standard of care, and should be performed as part of the examination for splenic trauma. The utility of FAST is primarily in the unstable patient, in whom a FAST positive for intraperitoneal fluid likely indicates an intraperitoneal source for the patient's hypotension. Ultrasound is clinically of lesser utility in evaluating the extent of injury to the spleen, for which computed tomography (CT) scan remains the most effective tool.

C. Computed Tomography

Abdominal CT scanning is an accurate and specific modality for the detection of splenic injury. Its importance in the initial evaluation of injuries to the spleen is increasing along with the widespread adoption of emergency department CT scanners. CT-based grading of splenic trauma has allowed a convenient categorization of injury severity, which facilitates triage of patients and comparison of results among trauma centers. The splenic organ injury scale, based on CT criteria for extent of injury and presence of viable splenic parenchyma, is presented in **Table 28-1**. Intravenous (i.v.) contrast is essential to the proper evaluation of the spleen by CT. Direct attention to the pres-

Table 28-1. Spleen injury scale

Grade		Injury Description
I.	Hematoma	Subcapsular, <10% surface area
	Laceration	Capsular tear, <1 cm parenchymal depth
II.	Hematoma	Subcapsular, 10% to 50% surface area; intraparenchymal, <5 cm diameter
	Laceration	Parenchymal depth (1–3 cm) that does not involve a parenchymal vessel
III.	Hematoma	Subcapsular, >50% of surface area or expanding, ruptured subcapsular or parenchymal hematoma
		Intraparenchymal hematoma >5 cm or expanding
	Laceration	Parenchymal depth (>3 cm) or involving trabecular vessels
IV.	Laceration	Laceration involving segmental or hilar vessels producing major devascularization (>25% of spleen)
V.	Laceration	Completely shattered spleen
	Vascular	Hilar vascular injury that completely devascularizes spleen

From Moore EE, et al. Advance one grade for multiple injuries, up to grade III. *J Trauma* 1995;38:323–324, with permission.

ence of hilar injury, the extent of subcapsular or intra-parenchymal *hematoma, the remaining viable splenic tissue, and the amount of intraperitoneal fluid. These criteria allow for the assignment of an injury grade, which, in conjunction with a thorough evaluation of the other intraabdominal organs for injury, will guide further intervention on the spleen. An additional finding on CT scan has received increasing attention. Active extravasation of contrast material, referred to as* pooled contrast *or* contrast blush, may suggest arterial bleeding and the need for more urgent intervention. Such injuries may need immediate surgery, while some can be amenable to catheter-based intervention (see below). The utility of follow-up CT scanning as part of a nonoperative management strategy is controversial. In general, follow-up CT scan is not necessary in hemodynamically stable patients with grade I or II injury. Repeat CT scan can be most useful in patients with multiple injuries in whom ongoing blood loss cannot be confidently attributed to the spleen.

In the patient with stab wound to the flank or back, triple contrast CT scan is often used to evaluate colon injury and, as such, provides excellent imaging of the spleen. Isolated stab wounds to the spleen without intraperitoneal blood can often be managed nonoperatively in the stable patient.

D. Catheter Angiography

Given the primacy of CT in current protocols for trauma evaluation, catheter angiography is now more likely to be performed as a therapeutic rather than a diagnostic procedure. Because it provides realtime images of blood flow, angiography can illuminate the extent of remaining vasculature in a damaged spleen, and, therefore, can guide resection. The real utility of angiography, however, is in the documentation of ongoing arterial bleeding, which may be amenable to catheter-based embolization. Active extravasation of contrast during angiography suggests failure of nonoperative management if it cannot be controlled with intravascular means.

E. Laparoscopy

Whereas laparoscopic splenectomy is now firmly established in the armamentarium of general surgery for elective splenectomy, laparoscopic surgery in splenic trauma is a young and evolving technique. In practice, laparoscopy for splenic trauma is done most often in a patient with a stab wound to the anterior abdomen in which violation of the peritoneum is suspected. Small injuries to the spleen, without hemorrhage, can be managed with topical hemostatic agents with little difficulty. Although laparoscopic splenorrhaphy has been reported, some authors have reported difficulty assessing the depth of injury with the laparoscope.

III. Management of Splenic Injuries

A. Techniques of Nonoperative Management

Criteria for nonoperative management of splenic injuries are listed in **Table 28-2.** It has been reported that 50% of adults and 60% to 70% of children with blunt splenic injuries can be managed without operation. The failure rate of initial nonoperative management may be 5% to

Table 28-2. Criteria for nonoperative management of blunt splenic injury

1. Hemodynamic stability
2. Documentation of injury by CT scan
3. Absence of active contrast extravasation on CT scan
4. Absence of other indications for laparotomy
5. Limitation of spleen-related blood transfusions (<2 U).

CT, computed tomography.

10%. The mainstays of nonoperative management of the injured spleen are adequate imaging of the initial injury to allow for triage, and frequent reassessment once the decision has been made to observe rather than operate. Patients to be considered for nonoperative management should have an abdominal CT scan with i.v. contrast as part of the trauma evaluation. A spleen does not enhance with i.v. contrast material points to a proximal injury to the splenic blood supply and a devascularized spleen. These patients should not be considered for nonoperative management, even with no active extravasation and minimal hematoma, because little point is seen in maintaining a totally necrotic spleen.

Once the extent of injury is graded based on radiographic criteria, a decision to proceed with nonoperative management should be made based on an overall assessment of the patient's condition. If other indications are seen for surgery (e.g., injury to other abdominal viscera, diaphragm), this should direct the focus to splenic salvage surgery. Other potential sources of hemorrhage (e.g., pelvic fracture, long-bone injury, or chest injury) can complicate the use of hemodynamic parameters or hematocrit measurements to detect ongoing bleeding from the spleen, and may suggest the need for exploration and splenorrhaphy. In many patients with blunt abdominal trauma and multisystem injury, abdominal examination is unavailable (intubated patient) or unreliable as a measure of ongoing bleeding. Experience has shown that patients with grade I and II injuries can be safely observed in other than an intensive care unit (ICU) setting, depending on the extent of other injuries. Patients with grade II or IV injuries should be managed in an ICU setting with more frequent and intensive monitoring. Hemodynamic parameters should be measured continuously in the intubated patient or no less than every 4 hours in the awake patient with isolated splenic injury. Hematocrit is measured every 4 hours. Blood, fresh frozen plasma, and platelets can be given, as needed. In general, a blood transfusion requirement of >2 units, attributable to ongoing bleeding from the spleen, is taken as failure of nonoperative management. The most common reason to proceed to laparotomy is ongoing blood loss in the early observation period. Later complications are discussed below.

B. Indications for Surgery

Evolving experience with nonoperative management of the injured spleen has led to a trend toward accepting more exclusive criteria for operating on the spleen for trauma. In general, younger patients do better with nonoperative management than do older patients. In the pediatric population, in which the techniques of nonoperative management were pioneered, grade III and IV splenic lacerations are often successfully managed, sometimes with larger than normal transfusion thresholds, with a low rate of conversion to laparotomy. The primary indications for surgery are hemodynamic instability with a high suspicion of intraabdominal source. In the early period after blunt trauma, positive FAST examination or diagnostic peritoneal lavage in a hypotensive patient can mandate laparotomy without a clear preoperative diagnosis of the source of hemorrhage. In patients who are stable enough to have a CT scan and do not have another indication for laparotomy, the operative decision can be based on the grade of spleen injury and response to a nonoperative approach. Devascularized spleens should proceed to laparotomy. Patients initially triaged to nonoperative management who subsequently develop hypotension or need >2-unit transfusion can be evaluated by repeat CT scan. If this indicates worsening spleen injury, operation is warranted.

C. Surgical Anatomy

The surgical anatomy of the spleen, as with that of the liver, relates primarily to vascular supply. The splenic artery courses superiorly and posteriorly to the tail of the pancreas before dividing into the segmental arteries of the spleen. This vascular division can occur a variable distance away from the hilum, up to 10 cm away in a small percentage of cases. The most common arrangement of splenic vessels involves a superior, middle, and inferior pole artery. **Figure 28-1** depicts the normal distribution of the splenic arteries. Segmental resection of the spleen can be performed along these natural divisions. Note, the short gastric vessels that tie the upper pole artery and

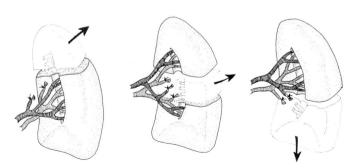

Figure 28-1.   Vascular anatomy of spleen.

vein to the greater curvature of the stomach can preserve vascular supply to the upper pole, even in cases of an injury to the splenic artery. Approach to the spleen should take into account the attachments of the spleen to the colon and diaphragm, which must be divided before adequate exposure can be obtained. The tail of the pancreas lies within the splenic mesentery, and great care must be taken when clamping the vessels in the splenic hilum not to injure the pancreas. Once the spleen is freed from its peritoneal attachments and elevated into the wound, the vessels can safely be visualized on the posterior aspect of the pancreatic tail.

D.   Exposures

The stomach should be decompressed with a nasogastric or orogastric tube to facilitate identification and control of the short gastric vessels. In most cases, carry out the approach to the spleen in trauma through an upper midline incision, which can easily be extended to gain access to the entire abdomen. With the surgeon on the patient's right, the lateral attachments of the spleen are identified and the spleen is retracted medially with the surgeon's open hand. Divide the splenocolic and splenorenal ligaments to free the inferior pole and the splenophrenic ligament to free the superior pole. In cases of a significant perisplenic hematoma, blood may have dissected the spleen free from its attachments and facilitated this process. In most cases, the short gastric arteries can be preserved while the spleen is dissected free and elevated into the wound. Gently lift the spleen anteromedially and place at least two folded laparotomy pads behind it to facilitate access positioning and examination of the spleen.

E.   Splenic Repair

1.   Indications

Once a decision to proceed with laparotomy is made, whether for failure of nonoperative management or for access to other intraabdominal organs, consider splenic salvage surgery. Successful splenic salvage has been described in all injuries except a completely devascularized spleen. Indications for splenic salvage after failure of nonoperative management are less clear. Few such cases have been described in the literature, and some authors advocate splenectomy in the case of failed observation to avoid the possibility of a second surgery should bleeding recur after splenorrhaphy. As techniques for splenic salvage are increasingly refined, however, it is likely that repair will be attempted on more patients who initially fail nonoperative management.

2.   Techniques

Splenic repair should only proceed after the organ is fully mobilized. Approach to repair of the traumatically injured spleen should be directed by a careful evaluation of the location of injury and an understanding of splenic anatomy. Small lacerations can be controlled with compression and the use of hemostatic agents (e.g., Gelfoam and oxidized cellulose). Areas of denuded capsule with raw surface oozing are well controlled with electrocautery at higher voltages or with an argon beam coagulator if available. Fibrin glue, especially in combination with Surgicel as a reinforcement, can be effective at controlling bleeding from raw surfaces or deep lacerations. Limited areas of injury can be débrided and the defect closed. Horizontal mattress sutures of 0 chromic with blunt hepatic needles can be used. Alternatively, some surgeons prefer to use a straight Keith needle to pass through thicker pieces of parenchyma. Folded Surgicel pads can be used as pledgets (**Fig. 28-2**). Figure-of-eight sutures can also be used. Alternatively, larger repairs can be buttressed with strips of polytetrafluoroethylene (PTFE) or omentum.

If a large area of one pole of the spleen is devascularized, a partial splenectomy can be performed, preserving the vascular supply to the uninjured portion. The segmental anatomy of the spleen is essentially divided into several "pancakes" of variable extent (**Fig. 28-1**). Although not as consistent as the segments of the liver, they are nonetheless present in most patients. Often, hematoma secondary to splenic injury will have begun the process of dissection. The vessels feeding the involved pole can be identified at the hilum and encircled with vessel loops, which allows for better confirmation of the vascular supply to the involved segments by temporary occlusion. Division of the parenchyma may be accomplished with blunt finger dissection or electrocautery. The resulting raw surface can be controlled with argon beam, and patched with omentum.

For the shattered but still viable spleen, several salvage techniques have been described. The spleen can be wrapped in an absorbable mesh (Vicryl), which is formed into a bag to hold the fragments of spleen in place. Take care that the edge of the mesh does not abrade or compress the vessels at the hilum. Autotransplantation of splenic tissue into the omentum

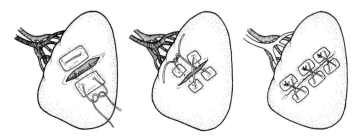

Figure 28-2. One method of splenic repair.

does result in some neovascularization and viable splenic tissue; however, this neovascularized tissue does not seem to recreate adequately the antigen-trapping functions of the spleen, such that it does not confer protection against postsplenectomy sepsis.

F. **Splenectomy**
   1. **Indications**
   Although the indications for splenectomy are narrowing, still a number of patients are seen in whom splenectomy will be the most appropriate treatment. Splenectomy is indicated for the devascularized spleen not amenable to splenic salvage. In cases of gross fecal contamination, especially in high-energy projectile injuries with a significant amount of devitalized tissue, splenic salvage can increase the risk of infection and splenectomy may be desirable. In the unstable patient with multiple intraabdominal injuries, splenectomy can be the best option for rapid hemorrhage control. Significant ongoing bleeding during attempt at splenorrhaphy can also necessitate splenectomy. In no case should a desire to preserve the spleen put the patient at significant additional risk from hemorrhage.
   2. **Techniques**
   With the spleen delivered into the wound as described above, the splenic arterial branches are identified in the hilum. Dissection should be as close to the spleen as possible to avoid injury to the tail of the pancreas. The splenic artery is controlled with suture ligature, and the splenic vein is doubly ligated and divided. After removal of the spleen, careful attention to hemostasis should be directed toward the greater curvature of the stomach, the ligated splenic hilum, and undersurface of the diaphragm.

G. **Angiographic Embolization**
   1. **Indications**
   Indications for an angiographic approach to the injured spleen are controversial. Most authors have suggested that the presence of a *contrast blush* on contrast CT scan of the abdomen is indicative of arterial injury amenable to angiographic control if the patient is stable. Consider other injuries and the need for additional interventions, given the time a blunt trauma patient necessarily will spend in angiography. Thus, the greatest likelihood of success is in the hemodynamically stable patient with no other major intraabdominal injury, who demonstrates pooling of contrast by CT on initial scan, or worsening hematoma on subsequent CT scan, suggesting ongoing hemorrhage. Other patients who can benefit from angiography are those with injuries to the splenic hilum because these have been found to have a high failure rate with nonoperative management.
   2. **Caveats**
   One significant question that remains to be answered is whether embolization affects the immune function

of the remaining spleen. Animal studies suggest that at least 30% of the spleen must remain intact, with functional vascular supply, to preserve immune function. If the splenic artery is embolized, it is not yet clear whether the splenic microvasculature remains intact or whether the resulting parenchyma function analogous to autotransplanted splenic tissue, in which immune function is compromised.

H. Postoperative Care

Postoperative care for the patient having splenectomy or splenorrhaphy is similar to that for any intraabdominal operation. The question of whether to leave drains in the left upper quadrant is often debated. Unless an associated injury to other abdominal viscera is present, drains are not needed. If circumstances dictate that a drain would be useful, use closed suction drains to minimize the chance of contamination and remove them as soon as possible. Postoperative complications specific to splenectomy or splenorrhaphy, including recurrent bleeding, should be of minimal concern if adequate hemostasis is maintained during the operation. This most often presents as unexplained tachycardia or a drop in hematocrit. Left lower lobe atelectasis can occur secondary to diaphragmatic irritation, and responds to appropriate respiratory care. Gastric ileus may require nasogastric tube drainage for some period after operation. Pancreatitis can present as persistent fever or prolonged ileus. Poor visualization of the pancreatic tail in a patient with brisk bleeding or multiple abdominal injuries should raise the question of pancreatic tail injury. Gastric fistula has been reported secondary to clamping of the short gastric arteries too close to the stomach. If gastric injury is suspected, the area of injury can be oversewn with inverting silk Lembert sutures at the time of operation.

IV. Rehabilitation Issues and Delayed Complications

A. Delayed Bleeding

Delayed bleeding most often occurs hours to days after injury, but has been reported up to weeks later. More severe (grade III or IV) injuries are at greater risk. Some authors advocate follow-up CT scanning before discharge to evaluate the extent of healing. Because of the risk of delayed bleeding with activity, especially sports, patients have traditionally been prohibited from such for as long as 6 months (see below).

B. Thrombocytosis

The platelet count often increases to 600,000 to 1,000,000 following splenectomy, normally peaking during the second week. An elevated platelet count can persist as long as 3 months after operation. Aspirin is recommended if the platelet count increases to >750,000 to prevent deep venous thrombosis (DVT), although no good evidence quantifies the risk of DVT according to degree of thrombocytosis.

C. Posttraumatic Splenic Pseudocyst

Posttraumatic splenic pseudocyst seems to have increased in prevalence since more splenic injuries have been managed nonoperatively. Pathogenesis is likely secondary to liquefaction of a large subcapsular hematoma. Splenic pseudocyst can present as epigastric fullness or discomfort or be found incidentally on follow-up imaging. Some are amenable to US-guided percutaneous drainage.

D. Prevention of Overwhelming Postsplenectomy Sepsis

Overwhelming postsplenectomy sepsis (OPSS), the much-feared complication of splenectomy, might affect as many as 2.5% of patients after splenectomy for trauma. The possibility of OPSS is the primary impetus for the push toward splenic salvage surgery rather than splenectomy for those patients requiring laparotomy. The organisms that cause OPSS are encapsulated bacteria, primarily neisseria, pneumococcus, and *Haemophilus influenzae,* which require adequate filtration function of the spleen, and circulating IgM, for clearance.

E. Antibiotics

No clear consensus exists whether treatment of splenectomized patients with antibiotics reduces the risk of post-splenectomy sepsis. Although oral penicillins have been widely used for prophylaxis, many of the organisms that cause OPSS are resistant to penicillin. The standard of care is shifting toward providing patients with oral antibiotics to take at the first sign of infection, rather than as a daily dose. Amoxicillin is generally chosen because of its activity against *H. influenzae.* Prophylactic antibiotics should also be given before any invasive procedures or teeth cleaning.

F. Vaccination

Vaccination against pneumococcus, *H. influenzae,* and meningococcus is recommended for all splenectomized patients. In a trauma patient having urgent or emergent splenectomy, vaccination can be given postoperatively. Protective levels of antibody are usually achieved, even though the titers can be lower than when given to a patient with an intact spleen.

G. Return to Activity

Experimental evidence in animal models suggests that splenic wound strength returns to normal as early as 3 weeks after injury. Recent trends have been to allow a return to activity in 6 to 8 weeks, rather than the traditional 6 months, after the event. This time period can be modified, based on the grade of injury, especially in the case of large intraparenchymal hematomas.

H. Common Traps and Decision Dilemmas

Often, the difficult decision in management of patients with blunt splenic injury is when to proceed to laparotomy. This is especially true in the polytrauma patient in whom multiple potential sources of hemorrhage may be present. In these cases, a follow-up CT scan can provide valuable information. If the grade of injury has not changed over several hours despite ongoing transfusion requirement, be reasonably confident that the spleen is not the source. A change in the radiographic appearance of the spleen with increasing hematoma, or a contrast blush or pooling, should tip the balance toward laparotomy. If pooling contrast is observed, these patients can be best managed by angiography and attempted embolization. Splenic preservation should be the goal in the management of all patients with trauma to the spleen. It cannot be overemphasized, however, that splenectomy remains a safe and expeditious option in patients with other injuries in which the time necessary to perform splenorrhaphy would unnecessarily prolong the operation or subject the patient to additional blood loss.

SELECTED READING

Cocanour CS, et al. Delayed complications of nonoperative management of blunt adult splenic trauma. *Arch Surg* 1998;133:619–625.

Godley DT, Warren RM, Sheridan RL, McCabe CJ. Nonoperative management of blunt splenic injury in adults: age over 55 years as a powerful predictor of failure. *J Am Coll Surg* 1996;183:133–139.

Hagiwara A, et al. Nonsurgical management of patients with blunt splenic injury: efficacy of transcatheter arterial embolization. *AJR Am J Roentgenol* 1996;167:159–166.

Pachter HL, et al. Changing patterns in the management of splenic trauma. The impact of nonoperative management. *Ann Surg* 1998; 227(5):708–719.

Zantut LF, et al. Diagnostic and therapeutic laparoscopy for penetrating abdominal trauma: a multicenter experience. *J Trauma* 1997;42(5):825–831.

Abdominal Trauma 5: Injuries to the Pancreas and Duodenum

Matthew M. Hutter, MD,
and Andrew L. Warshaw, MD

I. **Introduction**
   A. **Background and Epidemiology**
   The pancreas and duodenum reside in a protected anatomic area, near the midpoint of the body in the retroperitoneum. As such, the incidence of damage to these structures is low; each is diagnosed in only 1% to 4% of blunt abdominal trauma cases. Because of this anatomic location, injuries to the pancreas and duodenum are rarely isolated. They are commonly associated with hepatic, gastric, vascular, splenic, renal, or cardiothoracic injuries. In fact, the aorta, portal vein, or vena cava is injured in >75% of cases of penetrating pancreatic trauma. Of pancreatic injuries, 90% are linked with at least one associated injury. Most of the deaths do not result from the injuries to the pancreas or duodenum per se, but from the associated vascular or hepatic injuries. Missed or mismanaged injuries to the pancreas or duodenum can lead to devastating septic and inflammatory complications. With careful identification of injuries and adherence to technical principles in their repair, mortality and morbidity specific to pancreatic and duodenal injuries can be minimized.

   B. **Mechanisms**
   Blunt mechanisms for pancreatic and duodenal injuries result from a blow to the epigastrium. Seatbelt or steering wheel injuries are common in adults (and children can develop similar injuries from bicycle handlebars). Penetrating wounds traversing the epigastrium or entering through the back are also associated with injuries to these retroperitoneal structures.

   C. **Overall Management**
   Management of injuries to the pancreas and duodenum relies on the following:

   1. Prompt diagnosis of injuries
   2. Adequate intraoperative exposure
   3. Recognition of major pancreatic duct injuries and associated injuries
   4. Appropriate intraoperative management decisions regarding resection and repair
   5. Adequate peripancreatic drainage
   6. Appropriate enteric and biliary diversion, when necessary.

Because of the fragility of the nondiseased pancreas and the amount and nature of the fluids that pass through the duodenum, undiagnosed or mishandled injuries to the pancreas or duodenum can lead to devastating morbidity and mortality in these cases.

II. Initial Evaluation and Diagnosis

Early identification of injuries is crucial because of a well-documented delay-induced escalation in morbidity and mortality specific to the pancreas and duodenum.

A. Examination

A history or examination consistent with a significant force impacting the epigastrium should raise clinical suspicion for a pancreatic or duodenal injury. Although peritonitis can result, even vague abdominal pain and an unimpressive physical examination can occur with a full-thickness duodenal perforation confined to the retroperitoneum. Vomiting can indicate duodenal hematoma with gastric outlet obstruction. Physical examination otherwise is not specific for determining the severity of the underlying injury.

B. Computed Tomography

In the stable patient, abdominal computed tomography (CT) with oral and intravenous contrast material is helpful in identifying pancreatic and duodenal injuries, as well as other intraabdominal solid organ injuries. Oral contrast, which is not routinely used in many trauma CT protocols, distends the duodenum, increasing the ability to diagnosis duodenal injuries. (Oral contrast media is routinely used for the Massachusetts General Hospital trauma protocoled abdominal CT.) Intravenous contrast is essential in assessing pancreatic injuries, as it is for all other solid organ evaluations. CT scans done shortly after the time of the trauma might not identify pancreatic injuries because the evolving nature of pancreatic injury. Patients with persistent abdominal pain or persistently elevated amylase and lipase need to have repeat imaging to allow time for pancreatic injuries to become evident. The sensitivity and specificity of CT scan to identify the severity of pancreatic injury, specifically the integrity of the major pancreatic duct, is thought to be very low. As studies are done with the present and future generations of CT scans, the usefulness of CT may change, but currently CT findings are not reliable for recognition or grading of pancreatic injury, especially major pancreatic duct integrity.

C. Diagnostic Peritoneal Lavage

Diagnostic peritoneal lavage (DPL) with positive results can mandate a surgical exploration, during which the pancreas and duodenum can be explored. Even with significant pancreatic or duodenal injuries, DPL can be completely negative because the lesser sac is somewhat inaccessible to lavage fluid. The retroperitoneal location of these organs shields them from the lavage fluid unless the peritoneum is disrupted.

D. Serum Amylase and Lipase

High serum amylase levels suggest pancreatic injury and cannot be ignored. Because false-positives findings related to salivary gland injuries can be seen, serum lipase levels are thought to be more specific to the pancreas. Even without salivary gland injury, a false-positive finding from these biochemical markers is common.

Although elevated levels suggest damage, pancreatic injury cannot be ruled out with normal serum amylase or lipase levels. Levels need to be redrawn in several hours after an injury to allow these chemical markers of pancreatic damage to be evident systemically. The actual amylase level does not correspond with the degree of pancreatic injury, but is simply a marker for injury to the pancreas. An elevated serum amylase level serves as an indication for further determination of the integrity of the duct to prevent the delay-induced escalation in pancreatic-specific morbidity and mortality related to major pancreatic duct injuries.

E.   Endoscopic Retrograde Cholangiopancreatography

Endoscopic retrograde cholangiopancreatography (ERCP) is helpful in an otherwise stable patient, who has no other operative indications and for whom concern for a major pancreatic duct disruption exists. This modality, however, has been underutilized in the management of pancreatic trauma. The sensitivity and specificity of diagnosing major pancreatic duct disruption is excellent with ERCP. Because the integrity of the duct is of paramount importance for determining pancreatic-specific morbidity and mortality, ERCP should be considered in patients with hyperamylasemia who are being considered for nonoperative management. A magnetic resonance cholangiopancreatogram (MRCP) can also be used to diagnose pancreatic ductal injury in hemodynamically stable patients.

III.   Pancreatic Injuries

A.   Injury Grade

A pancreatic organ injury scale as described by the American Association for the Surgery of Trauma is shown in **Table 29-1.**

B.   Indications for Surgery

Surgical exploration of the pancreas is indicated during laparotomy for other intraabdominal injuries, when an appropriate mechanism for pancreatic injury is suggested. In the hemodynamically stable patient with no other indications for laparotomy, pancreatic exploration is warranted if CT suggests transection, hemorrhage, or pancreatic fluid collection consistent with major pancreatic duct disruption. The patient with persistent or developing abdominal pain, nausea, and vomiting with high amylase or lipase level warrants a CT scan, and subsequent exploration for positive findings.

C.   Nonoperative Management

Nonoperative management of pancreatic injuries can be undertaken if no other associated injuries require exploration and if imaging studies do not suggest major pancreatic duct disruption. ERCP should be considered in the hemodynamically stable patient, with hyperamylasemia,

Table 29-1. American Association for the Surgery of Trauma pancreas organ injury severity scale

Grade		Injury Description
I	Hematoma	Minor contusion without duct injury
	Laceration	Superficial laceration without duct injury
II	Hematoma	Major contusion without duct injury or tissue loss
	Laceration	Major laceration without duct injury or tissue loss
III	Laceration	Distal transection or parenchymal injury with duct injury
IV	Laceration	Proximal (to the right of the superior mesenteric vessels) transection or parenchymal injury involving the ampulla
V	Laceration	Massive disruption of pancreatic head

being considered for nonoperative management. Gastrografin upper gastrointestinal (GI) study should also be done to rule out an associated duodenal injury.

D. Intraoperative Management

1. Damage Control

Because of the high incidence of associated injuries, the first priority is to control hemorrhage and bacterial contamination. Pancreatic injuries can be drained and readdressed at a later time once life-threatening injuries are managed and the cold, coagulopathic patient has been adequately resuscitated.

2. Principles of Intraoperative Management

a. Achieve Adequate Exposure for a Thorough Exploration. As with most abdominal trauma, a generous midline incision is preferred. The anterior portions of the head, body, and tail are explored by taking down the gastrocolic ligament and entering the lesser sac. The uncinate process is evaluated with a wide Kocher maneuver, releasing the lateral and posterior attachments of the duodenum. The inferior aspect of the pancreas can be explored after incising the peritoneum along the inferior aspect of the body and tail of the pancreas and finger palpation posterior to the gland. The tail of the pancreas can be explored with the Aird maneuver, in which the spleen is mobilized from its bed, and the plane posterior to the pancreas is mobilized, elevating the tail of the pancreas for evaluation. Fluid collections and hematomas need to be cleared to allow adequate evaluation (**Fig. 29-1**).

b. Débride Devitalized Tissue. Tissue that is clearly devitalized must be débrided, although with extreme care to avoid troublesome bleeding.

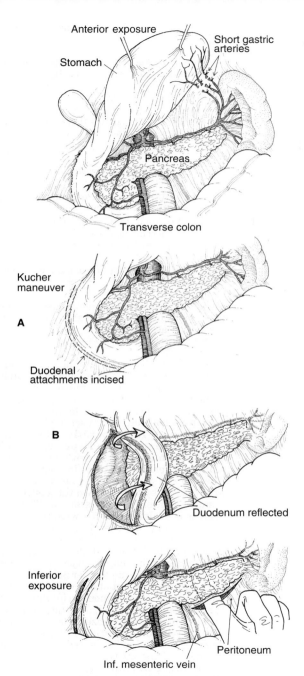

Anterior exposure

Stomach

Short gastric arteries

Pancreas

Transverse colon

Kucher maneuver

A

Duodenal attachments incised

B

Duodenum reflected

Inferior exposure

Inf. mesenteric vein

Peritoneum

Figure 29-1. Exposure of the pancreas: anterior, Kocher, inferior, Aird.

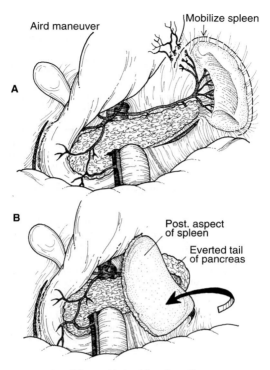

Figure 29-1. (Continued).

c. **Determine the Presence or Absence of Major Pancreatic Duct Disruption.** Major duct disruption can be determined by the following.

(1) CT findings of pancreatic transection or large peripancreatic fluid collections.

(2) Direct visualization of duct transection intraoperatively. Identification of the small, normal caliber ducts may be assisted with loupe magnification. Secretin can also be used to stimulate exocrine function of the gland, increasing the possibility of seeing the ductal injury.

(3) ERCP can be performed preoperatively in the stable patient. Sphincterotomy and pancreatic stent placement can assist with draining minor injuries.

(4) Intraoperative pancreatography is appropriate only if concern exists over the integrity of the major pancreatic duct to the right of the superior mesenteric vessels. With adequate concern for a duct injury to the left

of the superior mesenteric vessels, a distal pancreatectomy is recommended. The techniques of pancreatography include transcholecystic cholangiopancreatogram, distal pancreatogram, and transduodenal pancreatography.

A transcholecystic cholangiopancreatogram provides an adequate study only 25% of the time. A 16-gauge catheter is inserted in the gallbladder fundus and 20 to 30 mL of half-strength contrast medium is injected under pressure, while the second portion of the duodenum is compressed and 5 mg MSO4 is given intravenously to induce spasm in the sphincter of Oddi.

If the distal pancreas is involved and concern exists for a proximal injury, perform a distal pancreatogram by doing a distal pancreatectomy, cannulating the duct with a 5F pediatric feeding tube, and then injecting contrast material antegrade for the pancreatogram to rule out a more proximal injury.

A transduodenal pancreatograph should only be done if absolutely necessary. Try to avoid turning an isolated pancreatic injury into a combined pancreatic and duodenal injury. Make a longitudinal lateral duodenotomy (after a Kocher maneuver). Cannulate the ampulla with a 5F pediatric feeding tube and inject 2 to 5 mL of contrast material under gravity pressure only, and take radiograph. Close the duodenotomy.

d.   Operative Management. Operative management depends on the anatomic location of the injury and the status of the main pancreatic duct. The operative plan, therefore, corresponds with the grade of injury (**Table 29-2**).

(1)   Grade I and II Injuries. Simple contusions and superficial lacerations are best treated by placing adequate soft, closed-suction drains (no. 10 flat JP or Blake drains) in the areas of suspected injuries.

(2)   Grade III Injuries. Injuries to the left of the superior mesenteric vein (SMV) are consider grade II injuries. Distal pancreatectomy is recommended in cases of a major pancreatic duct injury to the left of the SMV. Do not try to rule out a major pancreatic duct injury to the left of the SMV with a pancreatogram. If adequate concern for such an injury exists, a distal pancreatectomy is appropriate. The spleen should usually be resected with the distal pancreas, although it can be salvaged in the young stable patient with a defined penetrating injury (**Fig. 29-2**).

Table 29-2. Grade of pancreatic injury correlates with operative plan

Injury Grade	Operative Plan
I	Place drains
II	Place drains
III	Distal pancreatectomy
IV	Subtotal pancreatectomy or Whipple procedure
V	Whipple procedure

(3) Grade IV and V. Try to manage these injuries to the right of the SMV conservatively. ERCP with sphincterotomy and temporary pancreatic stent can be a conservative option. Disruptions of the pancreatic substance, significant edema, or hematoma to the right of the SMV is an indication for pancreatography to confirm major duct disruption. If injury is *just* to the right of the SMV, such that >20% of the gland remains, then an extended distal or subtotal pancreatectomy is a good option.

A Whipple procedure is indicated for extensive devitalizing injuries to the pancreatic head (or duodenum) (**Fig. 29-3**). Experience of the individual surgeon must be taken into account. If the trauma surgeon does not feel comfortable with this procedure, it may be best to leave adequate drains and get out.

A normal soft, friable pancreas and non-dilated ducts make biliary and pancreatic anastomoses technically challenging. Given this "normal" anatomy, it may not be possible to perform a mucosa-to-mucosa anastomosis. Rather, it may be necessary to place the

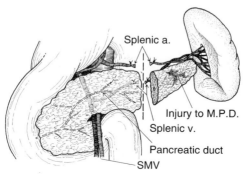

Figure 29-2. **Distal pancreatectomy.**

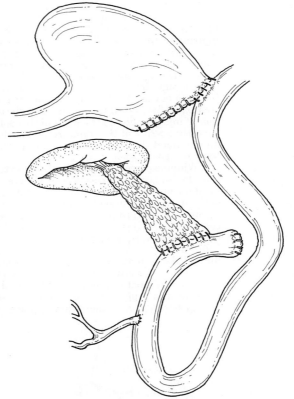

Figure 29-3.   Whipple procedure.

pancreas end into the jejunum, with a two-layer serosal, jejunum-to-pancreatic capsule anastomosis, thereby invaginating the pancreas into the jejunal limb.

For combined injuries of the pancreas and duodenum, multiple surgical options can be considered and will be discussed below.

e.   Closed Suction Drains. All suspected injuries or repairs should have adequate placement of closed suction drains. A no. 10 flat Jackson Pratt or Blake drain is appropriate.

f.   Feeding Jejunostomy Tube. Think of placing a feeding jejunostomy tube for extensive injuries or repairs, to allow early postoperative enteral feeding.

IV. Duodenal Injuries

A. Presentation

As with pancreatic injuries, blunt duodenal injuries can occur with any significant blow to the epigastrium, including seatbelt or steering wheel injuries, or in handlebar injuries in children on bicycles. Any penetrating injury that transverses the epigastrium, either from the front or from the back, can cause a duodenal injury.

B. Indications for Surgery

Duodenal exploration is indicated in cases of other injuries requiring exploration and a mechanism for possible duodenal damage has been identified. Surgical exploration is also warranted for CT findings that suggest extravasation from the duodenum, with either leaking of oral contrast material, fluid collections, or retroperitoneal or intraabdominal air. Patients with persistent abdominal pain, nausea, or vomiting warrant a repeat CT and exploration for positive findings.

The American Association for the Surgery of Trauma has created a duodenum organ injury scale (**Table 29-3**).

C. Techniques of Nonoperative Management

Duodenal hematomas do not necessarily require exploration. Most will resolve on their own with the patient kept off oral intake, with nasogastric tube decompression. Total parenteral nutrition may be necessary if the hematoma and inflammation cause gastric outlet obstruction for more than a week. An upper GI Gastrografin swallow should be done to rule out a leak. If seen intraoperatively, methylene blue can be used to rule out a leak (see below).

D. Intraoperative Exposures

As with all abdominal trauma explorations, a generous midline incision is the most versatile. Adequate exploration requires visualization of the anterior and posterior surfaces of the first through fourth portion of the duodenum. Bile staining, periduodenal crepitance, fluid collections, gastric contents or succus, and hematoma are signs of injury.

1. Wide Kocher Maneuver

Incision of the lateral and posterior peritoneal attachments of the second portion of the duodenum is necessary for a complete exploration (**Fig. 29-1**).

Table 29-3. American Association for the Surgery of Trauma duodenum organ injury severity score

Grade		Injury Description
I	Hematoma	Involving single portion of duodenum
	Laceration	Partial thickness, no perforation
II	Hematoma	Involving more than one portion
	Laceration	Disruption <50% of circumference
III	Laceration	Disruption 50% to 75% of D2
		Disruption of 50% to 100% circumference of D1, D3, D4
IV	Laceration	Disruption of >75% circumference of D2
		Involving ampulla or distal common bile duct
V	Laceration	Massive disruption of duodeno-pancreatic complex
	Vascular	Devascularization of the duodenum

2. Explore through the lesser sac to visualize the posterium proximal duodenum.

3. Mobilize the duodenum at the ligament of Treitz (LOT) to visualize the fourth portion of the duodenum.

4. Rule Out a Perforation.

Methylene blue via the nasogastric tube can be used to find occult perforation. Inject diluted methylene blue through the tube while compressing proximally and distally to distend the duodenum. Adequate exposure of the duodenum is necessary and clean white packs should be placed posterior to identify any staining signifying a leak.

Hematomas in the *duodenal wall* should not be débrided, as full-thickness injuries are likely to result. If the wall is necrotic, then débridement is necessary. Hematomas over the pancreas or over the central vessels require intraoperative débridement to explore underlying injuries.

E. Intraoperative Management

1. Principles

a. Damage Control. In the unstable, coagulopathic patient, it may be best to staple or oversew any obvious injury, and repair and restore intestinal continuity with a staged procedure.

b. Factors Determinant of Optimal Operative Management

(1) Extent of the injury

(2) Presence of associated injuries

(3) Time from injury to repair

(4) Condition of the patient

c. Duodenal Decompression. All repairs require appropriate duodenal decompression, with either of the following:

(1) Extended nasoduodenal decompression
(2) Tube duodenostomy through a site not involved in the injury or repair (antegrade or retrograde tubes)
(3) Adjunctive procedures: pyloric exclusion or duodenal diverticularization

2. **Operative Repairs**
   a. Simple two-layer closure, is possible in the following instances:
      (1) No extensive devitalizing injury. The extent of injury must be assessed by débriding injured tissues to viable edges.
      (2) The injury can be closed while maintaining adequate lumen diameter, without tension.
      (3) The ampulla and common bile duct are not obstructed with the repair. Avoid oversewing of the ampulla or the common bile duct as it courses behind the duodenum. A temporary antegrade stent can be placed to assist in identifying their location. Perform a cholecystectomy and pass a pediatric feeding tube through the cystic duct, the common bile duct, and into the duodenum. This stent can be palpated while the repair is done, and removed only after all sutures are placed. If any concern exists, an intraoperative cholangiogram can be performed.
   b. **Resection and Anastomosis.** The fourth portion of the duodenum can be treated as is other injured small bowel, and resection and anastomosis after mobilizing the LOT can be an option.
   c. **Duodenal Augmentation.** Duodenal augmentation is an option in cases where viable healthy edges to the duodenal wound remain after débridement, yet primary closure is not an option because of tension or narrowing of the lumen. A Roux-en-Y or loop jejunal graft is brought up and a two-layer, mucosa-to-mucosa anastomosis is performed. A serosal patch (in which serosa of the loop is sewn to the duodenum) is *not* effective.
   d. **Whipple Procedure.** A Whipple procedure may be necessary for extensive devitalizing injuries to the duodenum (or head of the pancreas).

3. **Diversion Procedures**
Once the injury is oversewn, appropriate diversion of gastric, pancreatic, and biliary contents is necessary to allow the injury to heal.
   a. **Three Tube Drainage (Fig. 29-4)**
      (1) **Retrograde Duodenal Decompression.** An external tube is placed distally through healthy jejunum and fed back retrograde to decompress in the area of injury.
      (2) **G-tube**
      (3) **Feeding J-tube**

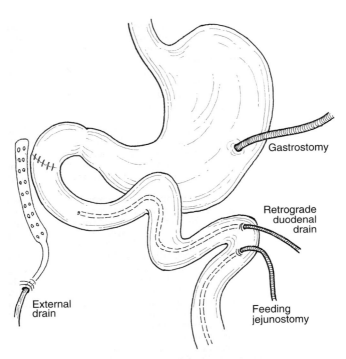

Figure 29-4.   Three-tube drainage of duodenal repairs.

b.   Pyloric Exclusion (Fig. 29-5). After the duodenal injury has been repaired, a gastrotomy is
made in the area of the eventual gastrojejunostomy, and the pylorus is occluded with intraluminal sutures (either PDS or permanent sutures).
Stapling is an option. Even closure with permanent sutures or staples is thought to be temporary because the mechanical action of the pylorus
eventually leads to recanalization. Intestinal continuity is maintained with a gastrojejunostomy.
Tube duodenostomy, external drainage, or T-tube
biliary decompression can also be performed, depending on the extent and nature of the injury.
c.   Duodenal Diverticularization. The duodenum is permanently diverted from enteric
contents with an antrectomy and gastrojejunostomy. Oversew the duodenal wound and divert
pancreatic and biliary contents with tube duodenostomy, T-tube biliary decompression, and
external drainage to contain a possible leak or
fistula.

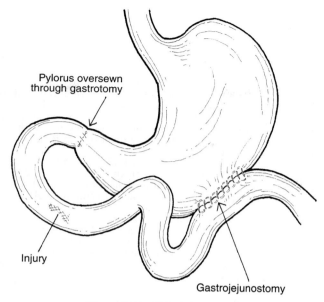

Figure 29-5.   Pyloric exclusion.

V.   Combined Pancreaticoduodenal Injuries

The presentation, evaluation, and indications for surgery for combined pancreaticoduodenal injuries are the same as for pancreatic or duodenal injuries as listed above. The principles for intraoperative management, likewise, are the same, including adequate exposure for a thorough exploration, débridement of devitalized tissue, assessment of major pancreatic duct integrity, appropriate resection and repair, and adequate diversion and drainage. Each injury must be appropriately identified, and handled according to the principles detailed earlier. The key point is: *when an injury to the duodenum is identified, have a high index of suspicion for injury to the pancreas, and vice versa.*

A Whipple procedure is indicated for extensive devitalizing injuries to the pancreatic head or duodenum. Experience of the individual surgeon must be taken into account. If the trauma surgeon does not feel comfortable with this procedure, it may be best to leave adequate drains and get out. A normal soft, friable pancreas and nondilated ducts make biliary and pancreatic anastomoses technically challenging. Given this "normal" anatomy, it may not be possible to do a mucosa-to-mucosa anastomosis. Rather, it may be necessary to place the pancreas end into the jejunum, with a two-layer serosal, jejunum-to-pancreatic capsule anastomosis, thereby invaginating the pancreas into the Roux limb.

VI.   Postoperative Care

The trauma patient with pancreatic or duodenal injuries has the potential to become very sick, from either septic or inflammatory complications. Adequate monitoring and resuscitation will depend on the extent of the injury. Postoperative care issues specific to pancreatic and duodenal injuries include the following:

A. Drains

1. On POD no. 4 to 5, peripancreatic drains should have fluid amylase levels sent.

2. Drains with low output (<15 to 30 mL/day, regardless of amylase levels) can be removed. Drains with low amylase levels (less than, or equal serum amylase levels) can be removed (if contents are not enteric, not bilious, or not in the area of a difficult duodenal closure that may need to be left until oral intake is started.)

3. Drains with output >30 mL/day and significant amylase levels (in the thousands) can be inched back once or twice. If output decreases to <30 mL/day, the drain can be removed. If output remains high, leave it in to control the fistula.

B. Nasogastric Decompression

If a duodenal repair or injury is not otherwise protected with a pyloric exclusion or duodenal diverticularization, then extended nasogastric tube decompression is warranted. Suturing a nasogastric tube in position or placing a bridle can possibly ensure that it is not removed prematurely. The duration of suction depends on the injury and the surgeon's satisfaction with the repair. An upper GI Gastrografin study can be done before removal, to assess for leak.

C. Feeding Jejunostomy

Early enteral feeding is of vital importance, and a feeding jejunostomy should be placed for extensive injuries, if an anatomic bypass is not performed (i.e., gastrojejunostomy).

D. Complications

Complications occur in 25% to 30% of patients with pancreatic injuries.

1. Bleeding

Bleeding complications can be disastrous. Pseudoaneurysms are not uncommon, and angiography and embolization can be life saving.

2. Pseudocysts

Unlike pseudocysts that develop in chronic pancreatitis or after acute pancreatitis, external drainage of pseudocysts from trauma can lead to complete resolution. If the output after external drainage of a pseudocyst persists for > 2 weeks, then a drain study or ERCP can be performed to assess for major pancreatic duct disruption.

3. Pancreatic Fistulas

Of pancreatic injuries, 25% to 35% lead to pancreatic fistula. A low-fat diet or keeping the patient off oral feeding (through jejunal feeds) is beneficial, and ERCP with sphincterotomy and stent can help to decrease fistula output and lead to eventual closure. Persistent fistulae that are controlled may have to be addressed at a later date, once the initial inflammation has subsided and tissues have softened up.

4. Duodenal Fistulas
  a. Duodenal fistulas occur in up to 10% of duodenal injuries.
  b. Fistulas after duodenal diverticularization or pyloric exclusion are usually end fistulas, many of which will close with time.
5. Pancreatic Bed Infection
Pancreatic bed infection may require débridement of infected or devitalized tissue.

SELECTED READING

Asensio JA, Demetriades D, Berne JD, et al. A unified approach to the surgical exploration of pancreatic and duodenal injuries. *Am J Surg* 1997;174:54–60.

Bradley EL III, Young PR, Chang MC, et al. Diagnosis and initial management of blunt pancreatic trauma. Guidelines from a multiinstitutional review. *Ann Surg* 1998;227:861–869.

Jurkovich GJ, Carrico CJ. Pancreatic trauma. *Surg Clin North Am* 1990;70:575–593.

Mackersie RC. Pancreatic and duodenal injuries. In: Cameron JL, ed. *Current Surgical Therapy,* 7th ed. St. Louis: Mosby, 2001:1104–1110.

Patton JH, Lyden SP, Croce MA, et al. Pancreatic trauma: a simplified management guideline. *J Trauma* 1997;43:234–241.

Weigelt JA. Duodenal injuries. *Surg Clin North Am* 1990;70:529–539.

Wisner DH, Wold RL, Frey CF. Diagnosis and treatment of pancreatic injuries. An analysis of management principles. *Arch Surg* 1990;125:1109–1113.

Abdominal Trauma 6:
Hollow Viscus Injuries

Ruben Peralta, MD, Alexander Iribarne, MS,
and Oscar J. Manrique, MD

I. Introduction

The use of exploratory laparotomy for suspected intestinal injury was not practiced routinely until late in World War I. Exploratory laparotomy for intestinal perforation at that time carried a 75% to 80% mortality rate, almost equal to that of nonoperative management. Currently, the mortality rate has been reduced as low as 1%, primarily because of advances in prehospital transport, resuscitation, antibiotics, and anesthesia care.

II. Epidemiology and Mechanisms

Gastric and small bowel injuries together comprise the third most common type of blunt abdominal injury. In addition, they are the most common types of injury seen in penetrating abdominal trauma. The incidence of intestinal injury secondary to penetrating trauma of the abdomen, especially from gunshot wounds, may exceed 80%. The incidence of hollow viscus injury secondary to stab wounds that have penetrated the peritoneum is approximately 30%. The mechanism of injury is classified in two groups: penetrating and blunt injuries. Stab and gunshot wounds are the most common causes of penetrating injuries.

A. Penetrating Wounds

1. Stab Wounds

Stab wounds are often singular and seldom accompanied by any significant area of tissue damage. In many cases, however, the signs and symptoms can be minimal for a number of hours, even days until peritonitis or abscess develops.

2. Gunshot Wounds

In general, gunshot wounds are paired perforations and often associated with some surrounding tissue damage. Lesions caused by high-velocity missiles not only cause damage by direct contact, but also by the blast effect, primarily from dissipation of energy through its pathway. High-velocity missiles can also be powerful enough to necrose bowel wall several inches from its original path.

B. Blunt Injuries

Bowel rupture secondary to blunt abdominal trauma is uncommon, and the injury mechanisms remain controversial. Some reports have shown that proximal jejunum and terminal ileum are the areas of small bowel most likely to be injured by blunt trauma. In addition, a propensity exists for blunt large bowel injuries to occur in the cecum, the midtraverse colon, and the sigmoid colon because the colon in these areas can be squeezed between the seatbelt or shoulder harness and the spine and pelvic brim. Studies have shown that the intraluminal bursting pressure required for rupture of the small intestine ranges between 140 and 150 mm Hg.

Blunt rupture of the stomach is rare, unless is distended with food or weakened by preexisting pathology. Blunt gastric perforations in adults most commonly occur on the lesser curvature. An explanation of this phenomenon is that gastric tissue has less elasticity, a limited muscular layer, and a paucity of mucosal folds.

III. Diagnostic Evaluation
A. Examination
Physical examination can be extremely helpful for diagnosing intraabdominal injuries in patients who are awake and alert. The early signs of peritoneal irritation, however, are often variable and nonspecific, especially after blunt intestinal trauma.

Patients with stab wounds and very carefully selected patients with gunshot wounds, who are hemodynamically stable with no signs of peritoneal irritation, may be eligible for further radiography studies, including computed tomography (CT) scans, exploration of the wound, or laparoscopy.

B. Computed Tomography Scan
In many cases, CT scans are replacing diagnostic peritoneal lavage (DPL) in the diagnosis of intraabdominal trauma, especially for retroperitoneal injuries. CT scanning has reduced the incidence of negative laparotomy by allowing the identification of certain injuries of solid organs, especially spleen and liver, which can be treated nonoperatively. In addition, the CT scan is an excellent tool in the evaluation of penetrating injury of the flank and posterior torso in hemodynamically stable patients using a triple contrast protocol. CT can evaluate the bony pelvis, lumbosacral spine, and upper femurs. A CT scan performed for possible abdominal trauma requires a combination of oral and intravenous contrast media (see Chapter 42, *Trauma Radiology,* section V, "Abdominal Trauma" for details). Abdominal CT scans, however, cannot be solely relied on to detect small injuries, especially to the small intestine distal to the ligament of Treitz.

C. Laparoscopy
The use of laparoscopy for diagnosing abdominal trauma has increased over the last several years. The effectiveness of laparoscopy for blunt abdominal trauma is still not clear. It can be effective, however, in some cases for identifying hollow viscus injuries. Contrary to blunt trauma, laparoscopy seems offers a greater scope for penetrating trauma, especially when the thoracoabdominal area is involved, because of the difficulty in evaluating the structures of this area. In addition, laparoscopy is extremely useful in determining peritoneal penetration. Previous studies have shown that 30% to 50% of asymptomatic patients have no peritoneal penetration and can be managed non-

operatively. In addition, other studies have shown that 60% to 70% of patients with questionable peritoneal penetration will have no peritoneal penetration on laparoscopic examination and avoid a laparotomy. In the evaluation of flank and back wounds, laparoscopy has not been effective because of the difficulty in evaluating bowel perforations and the inadequate visualization of the retroperitoneum.

IV. **Management**
A. **Nonoperative management**
With the availability of a CT scanner in most hospitals, nonoperative management of solid organ injuries in hemodynamically stable patients has replaced the more traditional surgical approach of mandatory exploration. With the new generation, high-resolution scanner, accuracy rates of 92% to 98% have been reported. Evaluation of hollow viscus and pancreatic injuries is inadequate with this technique and a high index of clinical suspicion should dictate the surgical management.

In the past, most penetrating abdominal wounds were strictly evaluated by laparotomy. Currently, however, hemodynamically stable and alert patients with some of these same injuries can be managed by selective observation.

Depending on the mechanism of injury, some patients with penetrating abdominal injury can be observed for the development of any peritoneal signs, taking into consideration the mental status of the patient and that no distracting injuries are encountered. Penetrating wounds to the flank or back, however, can inflict occult injuries to the retroperitoneal right or left colon. Some studies have shown that stab wounds of the flank have a 15% to 25% incidence of causing an intraabdominal organ injury, whereas wounds in the back have a 5% to 10% incidence of such injuries. Anatomically, the more posterior a wound goes from the anterior midline, the less threatening it is, because structures such as the spine and paraspinous muscles provide a thicker defense. A wounding agent would have to penetrate 8 cm or more to cause significant organ damage. We use a triple contrast CT protocol to evaluate penetrating injury to the flank and posterior torso in hemodynamically stable patients.

B. **Indications for Surgery**
Indications for operative management are hemodynamic instability, clinical signs and symptoms of peritoneal irritation, an anterior penetrating wounds with evisceration, gunshot wounds, and radiographic evidence of free air or bullets below the diaphragm.

V. **Gastric Injuries**
A. **Anatomy**
Because of high intraluminal acidity, the normal stomach is relatively free of bacteria and other microorganisms. Most victims of trauma have normal gastric physiology,

and the risk of bacterial peritoneal contamination with gastric perforation, therefore, is low. Preexisting diseases alter gastric physiology, increasing the risk of peritoneal contamination.

B. Exposure

Several aspects of the initial exploration are specific to patients suspected of having gastric injury. Exposure is generally easier if a nasogastric tube is in place. Exploration is facilitated, especially in obese patients and those with narrow costal flare, by extending the midline laparotomy incision to the left of the xiphoid process. The aorta and celiac trunk, which lie just posterior to the gastroesophageal junction, sometimes have missed, especially in victims of stab wounds. With penetrating trauma in the proximity of the gastroesophageal junction or distal esophagus, an esophagogastroduodenoscopy (EGD) is recommended in that same operative setting to avoid intraoperative missed injuries. Division of the left triangular ligament and mobilization of the lateral segment of the left lobe of the liver are helpful during exploration. When the stomach has been injured, the diaphragm should be closely inspected for an associated injury. An important aspect of the intraoperative diagnosis of gastric injury is close inspection of the greater and lesser curvatures. If necessary, segments of the gastrocolic or gastrohepatic ligaments should be divided to provide better exposure. The Kocher maneuver and entry into the lesser sac helps to avoid missed injuries in these areas as well as the pancreas, duodenum, or major vasculature. Exploration of the lesser sac also exposes injuries to the posterior wall of the stomach and is mandatory in all patients with anterior gastric trauma.

C. Management

Regardless of the means of diagnosis of gastric injury, patients in whom such injury is known or suspected should have exploratory surgery (**Fig. 30-1**). A nasogastric tube is sometimes useful diagnostically if blood is seen in the nasogastric aspirate. Lesions should be addressed in the order of their potential lethality. Injuries to major blood vessels should be dealt with first. Major vascular injury is particularly likely in cases of a central hematoma of the upper abdomen. In such circumstances, the gastroesophageal junction should not be approached directly without first ensuring that vascular control is possible. Major hemorrhage from solid abdominal viscera is the next priority. For the occasional lesion in which mucosal bleeding is a major problem, place an atraumatic clamp to control hemorrhage. Stapling and suturing is another rapid means by which contamination of the peritoneal cavity can be immediately controlled. Also, when the stomach has been injured, the diaphragm should be explored for associated injuries. Diaphragmatic injuries in association with gastric injuries are of

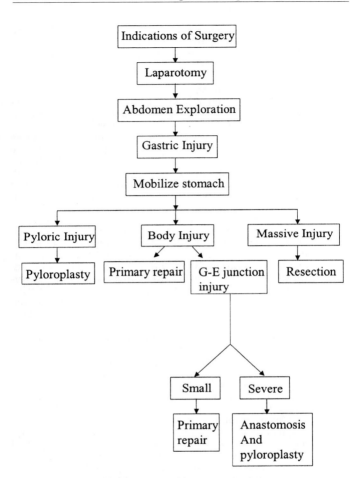

Figure 30-1.   Gastric injury algorithm.

particular significance because of potential contamination, not only of the peritoneal cavity but also of the
pleural cavity (usually on the left side). An early focus on
the stomach, without a thorough examination of the rest
of the peritoneal cavity is a mistake, however.

VI.   **Small Bowel Injuries**

A.   **Anatomy**

The length of the small intestine averages 6.5 m in the
adult. Approximately, the first 40% of the small bowel is
jejunum and the remainder is ileum, and this transition
from jejunum to ileum is gradual. The distinction between
jejunum and ileum is of clinical importance if bowel resection is necessary. Because of the increase in bacterial load

from the proximal to the distal end of the small bowel, the likelihood of intraabdominal or wound infection is greater when the distal bowel is perforated.

B. Intraoperative Evaluation and Exposures

Injuries to the mesentery of the small bowel are sometimes associated with massive bleeding. In a patient with hemoperitoneum in association with small bowel injury, direct initial attention to the possibilities of major vascular or solid viscus injury. If these are not present or not serious enough to account for the amount of hemoperitoneum, or if they have been temporarily controlled and bleeding continues, the mesentery should be rapidly inspected. The key to rapid and complete mesenteric inspection for ongoing bleeding is complete evisceration of the small bowel. The bowel is then run from the ligament of Treitz to the ileocecal valve, paying special attention to spreading out the mesentery and examining both sides. The direction of inspection is unimportant, as long as the inspection is systematic, but many surgeons find it more convenient and slightly easier technically to go in a proximal to distal direction. It is easy to miss small injuries of the bowel. No assumptions should be made about the course of the knife or bullet. Injuries to the most proximal portion of the jejunum are particularly easy to miss, especially if they are small. Medial visceral rotation, in conjunction with division of the ligament of Treitz, improves exposures of this area. The distal ileum close to the ileocecal valve is another area in which injuries can be missed. Small injuries on the mesenteric surface of the small bowel can be obscured by the mesentery, particularly if it is thick or fatty. Mesenteric injuries can also be missed if examination is too rapid or cursory. If such lesions are bleeding significantly, they are usually picked up by the inspection done at the beginning of the abdominal exploration.

C. Management

During exploration, if serious ongoing bleeding is discovered, it should be controlled either with clamps on the ends of bleeding vessels or with rapid, shallow whip stitching of the edge of the mesenteric rent. Once other bleeding and bowel leakage has been controlled, the bowel should be carefully inspected throughout its length. As mentioned, it is important to eviscerate the small bowel during inspection. No injuries should be definitively repaired until the entire length of both the small and large bowel has been inspected. The small bowel has a good blood supply, and division of short segments of the mesentery immediately adjacent to the bowel surface is well tolerated. Mesenteric bleeding should be definitively controlled by the suture ligation of large bleeding points. Mesenteric hematomas that follow penetrating trauma should be explored and any active sites of bleeding controlled. When large serosal tears are found, they should be closed because of the possibility of delayed mucosal breakdown and postoperative leakage. An algorithm for management of small bowel injury is shown in **Figure 30-2.**

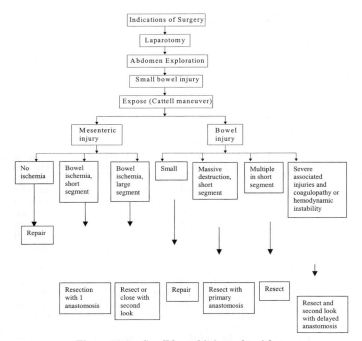

Figure 30-2.   Small bowel injury algorithm.

VII.   Colon Injuries

A.   Anatomy

The presence of the colon in all quadrants of the abdomen places it at risk with almost all penetrating abdominal wounds, and the high concentration (10^9 to 10^{12} per mL) of bacteria in the colon make sepsis an ever-present threat with colonic trauma.

B.   Intraoperative Evaluation and Exposures

Colonic injuries are readily diagnosed at the time of laparotomy. They can be identified preoperatively with good accuracy with the use of triple contrast CT, especially in penetrating injuries of the flank or back. Injuries in areas that are difficult to examine are the splenic flexure and rectosigmoid portion. If a perforation is not obvious, a feculent odor, blood staining of the colonic wall or mesentery, or a suspicious trajectory of the wound indicates that the area in question requires more evaluation. As with other bowel injuries, the key for diagnosis is to mobilize the suspected area. All bloodstaining or hematomas of the colonic wall must be explored. It may be necessary to divided one or two terminal mesenteric vessels at the junction of the mesentery and colon to adequately expose potential injuries of the mesenteric border. A final diagnostic maneuver in equivocal circumstances is to grasp the colon on both sides of the area in question and gently milk the luminal contents toward the presumed injury. The extrusion of fecal material or gas is diagnostic, and the absence of fecal discharge eliminates the possibility of a missed injury.

C. Management

In addition to any resuscitation management, patients with suspected colon or rectal injuries should receive preoperative parenteral antibiotics to cover gram-negative aerobes and anaerobes. Most colon injuries are at high risk of complications, especially those related with inection (e.g., intraabdominal abscess, peritonitis, sepsis). Broad-spectrum antibiotic use has contributed to the decrease any kind of infection related to colon trauma.

Once the bleeding has been controlled and hemodynamic stability established, perform a rapid examination of the bowel. Such injuries should be identified and controlled early to prevent further contamination. If the injury found is big enough that resection is required, proximal and distal occlusive clamping of the bowel with Kelly or Kocher clamps will help prevent further fecal contamination.

Other colon injuries difficult to find are those located in the retroperitoneum. Any hematoma, staining or air in this area is an important indication of a possible retroperitoneal colonic injury. As a general rule, extend the colon examination distally down to the peritoneal flexion. Dissecting deeply into the pelvis to search for rectal injury is generally not recommended, however, and should only be performed after considering the possible risks and benefits. In severe trauma cases with exsanguinating hemorrhage, coagulopathy, acidosis, and hypothermia, the colon can be stapled, dropped in to the peritoneal cavity, and packed, as needed, for hemostatic control.

Appropriate management of most colon injuries is primary two-layer closure except in cases of extensive blood loss, shock, or serious rectal trauma. Proximal diversion is indicated for unstable patients, when operation has been delayed, or massive contamination occurred.

VIII. Rectal Injuries

A. Anatomy

Rectal anatomy is key for the differential diagnosis and treatment of colon and rectal injuries. Approximately two thirds of the rectum is extraperitoneal and cannot be mobilized into the peritoneal cavity. Much of the rectum is surrounded by the rigid body pelvis, which makes direct access to extraperitoneal injuries difficult. In addition, the rectum is readily accessible via the anus. This fact has both etiologic and diagnostic implications. Due to these anatomic differences, wounds of the extraperitoneal rectum cannot be reliably managed by primary repair. Resection or proximal diversion with or without presacral drainage is recommended for extra peritoneal rectal injuries. Recent reports have demonstrated that in selected patients, small extraperitoneal rectal injuries could be managed by trans-anal repair and antibiotics without proximal colonic diversion or drainage.

B. Endoscopic and Intraoperative Evaluation

Rectal injury is less common than intraabdominal hollow viscus injury because of the relatively protected position of the rectum within the bony pelvis structure. Rectal injury, however, more often results in significant morbidity and mortality because of misdiagnosis or mismanagement. Suspected rectal injury should prompt rigid proctosigmoidoscopy. Rigid sigmoidoscopy is the diagnostic study of choice because it can be done with minimal insufflation, aids in the evacuation of stool and blood from the lumen of the rectum, and more accurately assess the level of rectal injury than does flexible sigmoidoscopy. Previous studies have shown that rigid sigmoidoscopy identifies the presence and site of rectal injury in 90% of the cases. A careful vaginal examination, anoscopy, and abdominal and pelvic radiographic studies complete the evaluation of such patients. Visualization of the injury itself is not always possible and is not necessary to make the diagnosis.

C. Exposures and Management

Diverting colostomy and presacral drainage are the cornerstones of management of rectal injuries. Repair of the rectal injury itself is not mandatory and should be done only if it can be visualized and performed easily, either transanally or at laparotomy without extensive dissection. Thus, attempts to achieve initial definitive repair can be hazardous and can lead to excessive morbidity. Four different types of colostomies have been advocated for the treatment of rectal injuries: (1) loop colostomy; (2) loop with the distal stoma closed, colostomy and mucous fistula; and (3) Hartmann's procedure (**Figs. 30-3, 30-4, and 30-5**). The loop colostomy is the most commonly used procedure. The advantages of this technique are the rapidity of its construction and its ease of closure. Whatever technique is used, the colostomy should be located as close to the injury as possible, usually in the sigmoid colon.

Saline irrigation of the nonfunctional rectum to wash out the feces is not absolutely necessary, but, theoretically, it should reduce the amount of continuing contamination of perirectal tissues. Adequate drainage of the presacral space posterior to the rectum is often desirable. The optimal style of drain has not been established, yet most surgeons prefer Penrose drains because they are comfortable for the patient, provide dependent drainage when placed through a retroanal incision, and are inexpensive. Drains are usually removed when the drainage becomes serous and the volume minimal. This change usually occurs between the fourth and seventh postoperative days (**Fig. 30-6**).

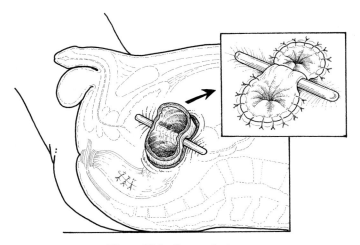

Figure 30-3.   Loop colostomy.

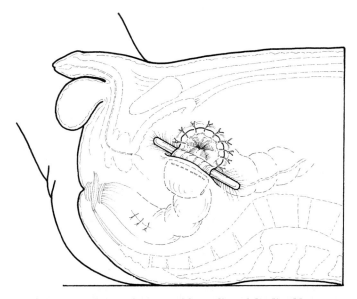

Figure 30-4.   Loop colostomy with stapling of the distal lumen.

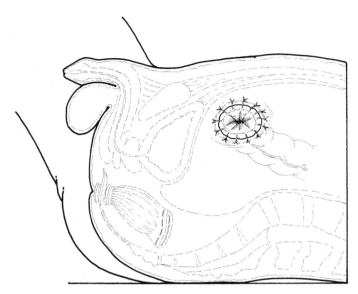

Figure 30-5. Hartmann's procedure.

IX. Postoperative Care

Postoperative care is generally based on associated injuries. Parenteral nutrition is not needed in most patients with isolated gastric or small bowel injuries. Depending on the kind of injury, enteral nutrition is preferred, when feasible. If the patient has an injury to the proximal jejunum, the creation of a feeding jejunostomy, is helpful in instituting early enteral feeding. The postoperative use of nasogastric tubes in patients who have had small bowel surgery is still controversial. Gastric decompression, however, is generally continued until good bowel sounds are heard, the abdomen is not tender except at the incision site, little or no distension is present, and the patient is passing flatus or has had bowel movements. If contamination has been severe, the key of avoiding infection is adequate abdominal irrigation, the removal of any intraperitoneal food particles, and a full course of therapeutic antibiotics. Depending on the case, however, prolonged courses of antibiotics have not been shown to be beneficial and can promote the growth of resistant bacterial strains in subsequent nosocomial infections.

X. Delayed Complications and Rehabilitation Issues

The most important postoperative complications specific to gastric and small bowel injuries are bleeding, suture line disruption, and infection and formation of abscesses. Metabolic or nutritional complications are rare, except in cases of massive small bowel resection, in which short bowel syndrome can ensue. Postoperative bleeding complications can occur when gastric repair is done under prolonged traction to enhance exposure. The single most

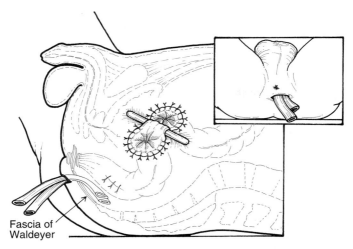

Figure 30-6.   Presacral drainage of rectal injuries.

Fascia of Waldeyer

common site of postoperative intraabdominal bleeding after gastric surgery is an injury to the spleen. Postoperative gastric bleeding from the stomach can also occur from stress gastritis.

Because of the wide lumen and the ability of the stomach to stretch, postoperative stenosis in the cardia or the body of the stomach is rare. If the injury is near the esophagogastric junction or the pylorus, however, stenosis can easily develop.

Small bowel obstruction is a common complication, especially after intestinal injuries. Most of the obstructions are caused by adhesions; however, edema at anastomosis or intussusception can also occur. Suture line disruption occurs much more commonly in the small bowel than in the stomach. Prompt recognition is necessary, and the treatment consists of aggressive resuscitation, intravenous antibiotics, and prompt reexploration and surgical correction. Occasionally, a suture line disruption is not recognized until an enterocutaneous fistula presents.

Malabsorption syndrome results from a loss of absorptive segments and alterations in bacterial flora after resection of large amounts of small bowel, as in the short bowel syndrome. If large amounts of small bowel need to be removed, however, special efforts should be made to preserve the distal ileum.

Colon and rectal injuries are associated with a relatively high incidence of complications, including peritonitis or abscess formation, fever of unknown origin, fecal fistula, and wound infection. Abdominal abscess can occur in 5% to 17% of the cases, especially in those treated with colostomy. Drainage of most postoperative abscesses can be done percutaneously. Wound infection following rectal injuries have a frequency of about 5% to 15%, but can be prevented by leaving the skin and subcutaneous tissue open. Complications with colostomy closure in trauma patients can range between 5% to 27%. Fever, leukocytosis, or abdominal pain within 2 weeks of a colostomy closure should be considered to be caused by a leaking anastomosis until such is proved otherwise.

SELECTED READING

Asensio JA, Chahwan S, Forno W, et al. Penetrating esophageal injuries: multicenter study of the American Association for the Surgery of Trauma. *J Trauma* 2001;50:289–296.

Burch JM. Injury to the colon and rectum. In Mattox KL, et al., eds. *Trauma,* 4th ed. Vol. 1. New York: McGraw-Hill, 2000:763–782.

Chiu WC, Shanmuganathan K., Mirvis, SE, et al. Determining the need for laparotomy in penetrating torso trauma: a prospective study using triple-contrast enhanced abdominopelvic computed tomography (CT). *J Trauma* 2000;49:1164.

Dumire DR, Doriac WC, Roth BJ, et al. Comparison of a hand portable ultrasound instrument to standard ultrasound for emergency department FAST exam. *J Trauma* 2000;49:1174.

Eggenberger JC. Rectal injury. In: Cameron J, ed. *Current therapy of trauma,* 4th ed. Vol. 1. St. Louis: Mosby, 2001:247–249.

Fabian TC, Croce MA. Abdominal trauma, including indications for celiotomy. In: Mattox KL, et al. eds. *Trauma,* 4th ed. New York: McGraw-Hill, 2000:583–602.

Hoyt DB. What's new in general surgery: trauma and critical care. *J Am Coll Surg* 1994;194:335–351.

Ivatury, MR, Nallathambi MN. Colon. In: Ivatury RR, Cayten CG, eds. *The textbook of penetrating trauma.* Baltimore: Williams & Wilkins, 1996:657–668.

Killeen, KL, Shanmuganathan K, Poletti PA, et al. Helical computed tomography of bowl and mesenteric injuries. *J Trauma* 2001; 51: 26–36.

Patton JH. Small bowel and colon injuries. In: Trunkey DD and Lewis FR, eds. *Current therapy of trauma,* 4th ed. Vol. 1. St. Louis: Mosby, 1999: 243–246.

Stassen NA, Lukan JK, Carrillo EH, et al. *Abdominal seatbelt marks in the era of the FAST scan.* San Antonio: Western Trauma Association, 2001.

Velmahos GC, Demetriades D, Toutouzas KG, et al. Selective non-operative management in 1,856 patients with abdominal gunshot wounds: should routine laparotomy still be the standard care? *Ann Surg* 2001;234:395–403.

Wilson RF, Walt AJ, Dulchavsky S. Injuries of the colon and rectum. In: Wilson RF and Walt AJ, eds. *Management of trauma: pitfalls and practice,* 2nd ed. Vol. 1. Baltimore: Williams & Wilkins, 1996:534–553.

Wilson RF and Walt AJ. Injury to the stomach and small bowel. In: Wilson RF and Walt AJ, eds. *Management of trauma: pitfalls and practice,* 4th ed. Vol. 1. Baltimore: William & Wilkins, 1996:497–509.

Wisner DH. Stomach and small bowel. In: Mattox KL, ed. *Trauma,* 4th ed. Vol. 1. New York: McGraw-Hill, 2000:713–734.

Abdominal Trauma 7: Damage Control and the Abdominal Compartment Syndrome

Glenn Egrie, MD, Ruben Peralta, MD, and Robert L. Sheridan, MD

I. Introduction

In contrast with the controlled setting of an elective celiotomy, a trauma laparotomy often occurs under suboptimal conditions. Difficult exposures, unstable hemodynamics, unclear anatomy, and systemic physiologic derangement resulting from profound injury that may have occurred minutes before presentation often characterize the trauma laparotomy. The administration of blood and crystalloid, used to treat hypovolemia, leads to hypothermia and resultant platelet dysfunction and cardiac instability. Depletion coagulopathy results from dilution of coagulation factors and leads to nonsurgical bleeding. Metabolically, hypothermia, acidosis, and coagulopathy characterize the patient. Successful and safe completion of the operation becomes extremely difficult under these conditions. The phrase "damage control laparotomy" has been coined to describe an alternative approach to this situation, where the laparotomy is rapidly terminated after bleeding and contamination are controlled in the unstable patient.

II. Damage Control Concept

Damage control involves three phases of therapy, first surgical control of hemorrhage and contamination, followed by abrupt termination of the laparotomy. The abdominal cavity is packed and the abdomen is temporarily closed. Subsequently, the patient is brought to the intensive care unit (ICU) for rewarming, and to have coagulopathy corrected and normal hemodynamics restored. Lastly, when normal physiology is restored, the patient is returned to the operating room for definitive repair of injuries and closure of the abdomen.

III. Organ System Injuries

A. Hepatic Injuries

Although the liver is the abdominal organ most commonly injured after blunt trauma, most injuries are relatively minor. Fortunately, 70% to 90% of blunt liver injuries are not severe and are treatable with simple operative management: superficial suture ligation, use of hemostatic agents, or application of manual pressure. Most of these injuries stop bleeding because of the liver's low-pressure portal venous system. As many as 50% of patients having damage control laparotomy will have hepatic injuries and half of these will be grade IV.

The goal of treatment of the hepatic injuries is to reduce the morbidity of hemorrhage and sepsis. A complex liver injury is explored through a midline incision and seldom requires extension into the thorax. The first effort is directed at controlling further blood loss and resuscitating the patient. Manual pressure is applied to the liver while the anesthesia team corrects the metabolic and hemodynamic derangement. Subsequent examination of the liver for injuries may require portal triad occlusion, which can be accomplished with a vascular clamp or by placing a Penrose drain around the structures in the hepatoduodenal ligament.

Damage control uses perihepatic packing to control persistent bleeding. This is necessary in ~5% of patients having laparotomy for hepatic injuries. Perihepatic packs are required for:

1. Failure to control bleeding when definitive surgery is precluded by metabolic derangement
2. Development of intraoperative coagulopathy
3. Severe hemorrhage from bilobar injuries
4. Presence of a large and expanding subcapsular hematoma

The packs are removed at reoperation 48 to 72 hours later, after the metabolic alterations and hemodynamic instability are treated in the ICU. Rebleeding at that time is unusual. The use of an absorbable Dexon mesh has been advocated to compress the liver to achieve hemostasis, similar to perihepatic packing, but experience with this is limited.

Use of hepatic artery angiography and embolization as adjuncts to damage control surgery has recently been shown to be effective and safe. Usually implemented in the immediate perioperative period, with appropriately selected patients, hepatic angiography can help identify and treat bleeding hepatic vasculature not controlled with packing.

B.   Splenic Injuries

Because of the lifelong susceptibility to encapsulated organisms after splenectomy, splenic preservation is desirable when safe and feasible. Splenic injuries in patients having damage control laparotomy are primarily treated by splenectomy, with the exception of minor splenic injuries, which may be amenable to simple suture repair. Splenic conservation techniques are time consuming and usually not warranted in the setting of damage control. The time used to perform the splenectomy incurs minimal additional morbidity compared with the potential blood loss from the injured spleen that would likely persist in the setting of coagulopathy.

C.   Pancreatoduodenal Injuries

The posterior and protected location of the pancreas and duodenum make injury to these structures uncommon. When injury does occur, however, it is usually associated with concomitant organ injuries because of the force required for pancreatoduodenal injury in blunt trauma and the path usually needed in penetrating injury. Most pancreatoduodenal injuries will be diagnosed at laparotomy. Mortality from these injuries is usually related to associated injuries. Late mortality is primarily the result of pancreatic sepsis or multisystem organ failure precipitated by sepsis. Therefore, prioritization during damage control laparotomy requires control of hemorrhage and control of contamination from duodenal injury. Definitive surgery for major injuries, however, is usually not accomplished in the damage control procedure.

Most minor injuries not involving the duct require no treatment. If possible, a closed suction drain can be placed alongside the injury, but this is not necessary if the abdomen is packed and left open. If the injury is more extensive and to the left of the superior mesenteric vessels, it may be possible to perform a rapid distal pancreatectomy.

Massive injuries to the pancreaticoduodenal complex are almost always associated with injuries to the surrounding structures. Patients will not survive complex operations such as pancreaticoduodenectomy at the first setting. The common bile duct and pancreatic duct can be ligated if injured and not amenable to simple repair. Reconstruction can be carried out in the next 48 hours, if absolutely necessary. Otherwise, wide drainage, total parenteral nutrition, and careful overall care may be most appropriate. Small duodenal injuries can be repaired with a single layer suture, but large duodenal injuries should be débrided and the ends closed temporarily with suture or umbilical tape to be dealt with at the second procedure. At the second procedure, repair the larger duodenal injuries, and perform pyloric exclusion and gastrojejunostomy.

D. Hollow Viscus Injuries

Hollow viscus injuries (e.g., stomach, intestine, bladder) remain a challenge of the trauma surgeon; they are a risk of the nonoperative management strategies adopted for solid organ injuries. Repeat clinic examinations, a high index of suspicion, and follow-up imaging will help detect these injuries early and minimize associated morbidity. Free intraperitoneal fluid on computed tomography (CT) scan, without evidence of an associated solid organ injury, can be the result of a hollow organ injury. In addition, the presence of lower abdominal wall ecchymosis in a seatbelt-restrained passenger (seatbelt sign) or a handlebar mark should raise concerns for hollow viscus injury. Overall, hollow viscus injuries are present in relatively few blunt abdominal injuries. The risk for hollow visceral injuries increases significantly with a pancreatic injury or when multiple intraabdominal organs (e.g., liver and spleen) are affected. Once detected, all hollow organ injuries require operative intervention, except for some bladder injuries.

The small bowel is the most commonly injured intraabdominal organ in penetrating trauma. The most common sites of perforation from blunt injury are at the ligament of Treitz, ileocecal valve, midjejunum, or in areas of adhesions. Small bowel injury, however, is often not diagnosed on initial presentation, which can contribute significantly to mortality. Diagnostic peritoneal lavage findings commonly reveal blood, whereas CT can show fluid collections without solid viscus injury, free intraperitoneal air, mesenteric infiltration, and bowel wall thickening. Note, however, that CT has a significant false negative rate in the diagnosis of small bowel injury. Colonic injuries may be indicated on examination if blood is seen on rectal examination. Moreover, gross blood on rectal examination with a penetrating abdominal, buttock, or pelvic wound is pathognomonic of colorectal injury.

After control of hemorrhage, the primary priority in damage control surgery is control of spillage from the gastrointestinal tract or urinary system. It is important to accomplish this control while avoiding time-consuming reconstructions. A simple, small bowel injury can be repaired with a single layer continuous suture. A more extensive injury should be excluded using a linear stapler or umbilical tape. Reconstruction of the bowel can be carried out at subsequent procedures. Injury to the colon can be managed with distal stapling and exteriorization of the proximal segment. The colostomy can be matured or left stapled. In the early postoperative period, the patient can have extensive abdominal wall edema, which could compromise the ostomy or cause it to retract. Therefore, leaving the colostomy stapled or in the abdomen is simpler and probably safer.

E.   Vascular Injuries

Vascular injuries in patients having damage control surgery can be intraabdominal or peripheral. The former are often life threatening and the latter often present with severe external bleeding or threatening limb ischemia.

The primary objective during management of vascular injuries is to perform maneuvers to prevent exsanguination and maintain perfusion to distal organs. Within the scope of damage control surgery, vascular injuries are challenging because of the need to balance between performing a complex vascular reconstruction and an expeditious procedure to avoid irreversible physiologic insult. Within this operative setting, vascular bailout procedures can be used to maximize the patient's survival from complex injuries.

Control of external hemorrhage is the first priority in the presence of peripheral injuries. Direct focal pressure is the most effective way to control external bleeding. The hand of the person applying pressure should be prepared into the operative field and should remain until adequate proximal and distal control is obtained. Do not attempt to blindly clamp the bleeding structure. This will often lead to further bleeding and cause iatrogenic injury to other structures.

Damage control principles to manage vascular injuries require the use of simple versus complex vascular repair techniques. Simple techniques include primary repair, ligation, and temporary intraluminal shunt. These techniques are recommended in the cold, coagulopathic patient. Complex repairs, vascular reconstructions, are more time consuming and often are inappropriate during the initial operation. They are generally undertaken during secondary operations, after resuscitation is conducted.

Primary repair can often be used for larger vessels of the proximal extremities and trunk. This is appropriate for clean penetrations of arteries and veins when the surrounding tissues are not devitalized and a complete transection has not occurred.

Vessel ligation is a valid technique in damage control procedures. It is useful if the damaged vessel is inaccessible or a complex repair is required. All limb veins can be ligated with impunity. No role exists for limb vein reconstruction in damage control surgery. If necessary, the subclavian, iliac, and inferior vena cava can be ligated. Postoperative limb edema can result. Portal vein ligation can be performed.

IV. Abdominal Compartment Syndrome

Abdominal compartment syndrome (ACS) is organ dysfunction attributable to increased intraabdominal pressure. Other criteria that have been used to define ACS include high peak inspiratory pressure and development of oliguria. ACS can develop in a wide variety of situations. It can occur secondary to accumulation of fluid or gas in the abdominal cavity and can have many different causes: intraabdominal bleeding after blunt and penetrating abdominal trauma, particularly after abdominal packing for uncontrollable bleeding; aggressive fluid resuscitation with the resultant bowel edema; retroperitoneal edema or bleeding; pancreatitis; ascites; and liver transplantation. Although the incidence of ACS is hard to determine, it has been observed in 10% to 15% of patients who have sustained severe abdominal trauma (injury severity score >15).

The classic scenario is the patient who has had trauma surgery with intraabdominal hemorrhage, particularly after damage control laparotomy. The factors that contribute to ACS are accumulation of blood and clot, bowel edema or congestion from mesenteric injuries or crystalloid resuscitation, or from packing. Closure of a noncompliant abdominal wall under tension can also exacerbate ACS. ACS has been described in patients after liver transplantation because of intraabdominal bleeding and in critically ill cirrhotic patients with ascites. Other causes described include retroperitoneal edema after aortic surgery or retroperitoneal bleeding. ACS has also occurred after other types of abdominal surgery (e.g., gynecologic and urinary tract surgical procedures). More recently, attention has been drawn toward the development of ACS in patients with multiple trauma, who do not have any intraabdominal injury. These patients develop abdominal compartment syndrome secondary to massive bowel edema and ascites. The mechanism involved is still subject to speculation, but might be caused by shock with associated bowel hypoperfusion. Secondary reperfusion injury, capillary leak, and tissue swelling follow the correction of the hypovolemia. This reperfusion injury is probably partly responsible for the increased abdominal pressure as described in the "classic" ACS.

Intraabdominal pressure (IAP) can be monitored directly or indirectly. Direct monitoring can be done by placing a catheter in the peritoneal cavity and connecting it to a pressure transducer. Indirect methods measure pressure inside accessible abdominal organs. Most commonly, bladder pressure is measured as an indirect technique. Changes in bladder pressure directly reflect changes in IAP. This technique involves connecting a transurethral catheter to a T connector and one arm to a collection bag. The other arm is connected to a pressure transducer through saline-filled tubing. Using the symphysis pubis as a reference point, the collection bag arm is clamped and the bladder pressure is measured. The level at which IAP causes ACS is not well defined. IAP between 20 to 35 mm Hg has been suggested to cause ACS and require intervention. Splanchnic hypoperfusion has been observed experimentally at an IAP of 15 mm Hg. IAP can be measured in millimeters of mercury or centimeters of water. It is important to remember the conversion factor when comparing values of IAP (1 mm Hg = 1.36 cm of H_2O).

Elevated IAP and ACS cause significant changes in most organ systems. The cardiovascular effects present as decreased cardiac output, leading to hypotension, is caused by obstruction of venous return through the vena cava. ACS can also decrease splanchnic bold flow greater than can be attributed to diminished cardiac output. This can lead to bowel ischemia, which may be, at least partially, responsible for the increased rate of anastomotic breakdown seen in trauma patients with ACS. Renal effects of ACS are manifested by oliguria and are related to inadequate renal perfusion from low cardiac output, direct compression of the kidney, obstruction of renal venous outflow, or compression of ureteral outflow. Because correction of cardiac output may not improve renal function, the compressive effects on the kidney parenchyma or renal veins can the major cause of renal dysfunction in ACS.

The pulmonary effects of ACS present as hypercarbia and decreased compliance with elevated peak airway pressures and low tidal volumes. The poor compliance results from upward movement of the diaphragm and compression of lung parenchyma. This compression of the alveoli leads to alveolar hypoventilation with increased ventilation of death space and hypercarbia. Chest radiographs in these patients typically show clear but small lung fields and elevated hemidiaphragms. Positive end-expiratory pressure is required to maintain oxygenation, further complicating the hemodynamic stability.

Of particular concern in patients with head injury and elevated intraabdominal pressure is a worsening of the intracranial pressure (ICP) with an associated decrease in cerebral perfusion pressure (CPP). Abdominal decompression has been reported to decrease the ICP in patients with multiple trauma with head injury and ACS. This effect of the increased intraabdominal pressure on the ICP seems to be mechanically mediated by the diaphragmatic elevation, reduced chest compliance, and increased central venous pressure with decreased of ICP.

A. Operative Techniques and Management

The first part of damage control consists of emergency laparotomy and evacuation of hematoma. Four-quadrant packing to control hemorrhage, including clamping or ligation of vascular injuries, and control of contamination follows this. Ligation, staples, or running sutures are used temporarily to control spillage from hollow viscus injuries. Definitive vascular repair can then be completed, if warranted. Perform rapid surgical closure of the abdominal or thoracic wound by placing a large adherent plastic drape over the abdomen or chest over closed suction drainage. A similar closure can also be achieved with closure of the skin or skin and fascia if ACS is not present, with a running nonabsorbable suture (e.g., 2-0 nylon). We discourage the use of towel clips closure of the abdomen, which has been previously advocated. One of the reasons is that the towel clips can interfere with subsequent diagnostic and therapeutic radiological intervention (i.e., angiographic embolization).

Extensive edema and distention of the midgut, the presence of a multitude of intraabdominal packs, or cardiac edema after a major cardiac procedure can make closure of an abdominal or thoracic wound with suture impossible. In this situation, closure with a silo is performed. A variety of materials and techniques can be used. Small thoracic or abdominal wall defects can be closed with an esmarch bandage sewn with a continuos 2-0 nylon or polypropylene stitch to the skin edges. A larger silo can be created with a 3-L bag of irrigating solution cut open and then gas sterilized or used not sterile, if necessary. Reinforced silastic sheet is ideal, as it drapes well and holds sutures securely. Revision of the closure is based on the patient's recovery from physiologic dysfunction and resolution of midgut edema. In most patients, primary fascial closure is possible.

Absorbable meshes can be used to close abdominal wall defects; however, once these are absorbed and granulation has occurred on top of the mesh, a ventral hernia is created. This type of closure is used when the decision is made to allow the wound to close by secondary intention or when a septic process exists in the abdominal cavity. Absorbable mesh allows drainage of contaminated abdominal fluid and is less likely to erode into bowel or get infected compared with permanent mesh. An alternative to mesh closure, if primary fascial closure is not possible, involves component release of the lateral abdominal wall fascia. This is generally very well tolerated and provides several centimeters of additional laxity.

Reoperation is ideally performed in the patient who is normotensive, without a coagulopathy, and has stable renal function. This will often occur within 48 to 72 hours of the original surgery. After the towel clips, sutures, or silos are removed, clots and packs are removed and the abdomen explored for missed injuries. Next, perform resection, bowel anastumosis, vascular reconstruction, or maturation of colostomies. The abdomen is copiously irrigated, drains inserted and the abdomen closed primarily. If the wound cannot be closed, reapply a silo and reattempt at closure within several days. We recommend the use of vacuum-assisted closure device in the management of open abdomen. In a recent retrospective review study, the rate of fistula and abscess formation did not differ from that of the traditional ventral hernia creation and the hernia recurrence rate was approximate 9%.

V.   Complications

Management of complex trauma patients has a series of expected complications, which include the onset of recurrent ACS and bleeding in the immediate and late postoperative period.

Perihepatic packing can cause clinically significant recurrent ACS because of compression of the suprarenal vena cava leading to renal dysfunction and hemodynamic derangement, including decreased preload and decreased cardiac output. The patient should be returned to the operating room for decompression of the abdomen.

Infections, including wound infections and abscess formation have been well documented in the setting of multiple abdominal operations. For example, perihepatic and intrahepatic sepsis are the most common long-term complications of complex liver injuries. Their incidence can be decreased by débriding nonviable hepatic tissue and proper hemostasis. A pedicle omental graft is placed in the débrided area.

Abdominal complications are frequently encountered in patients who require damage control. These complications include recurrent ACS; the formation of intraabdominal abscess; biliary, gastrointestinal, and pancreatic fistula; bowel obstruction; hepatic necrosis; anastomotic disruption; and intraabdominal and abdominal wall hernias.

Primary repair of larger vessel injuries can result in stenoses when these repairs are conducted rapidly with the aim of getting the patient out of the operating room to complete resuscitation in the ICU. Early postoperative evaluation or secondary exploration is important for detecting and revising initial repair, if necessary.

Mortality rate has been described in the range of 12% to 67% in a recent collective review for which the development of multiple organ dysfunction syndrome was a significant factor. The specific timing and the optimal criteria to guide the use of this maneuver, as well as the use of adjunctive procedures during damage control, requires further evaluation.

SELECTED READING

Carvillo C, Fogler RJ, Shafton GW. Delayed gastrointestinal reconstruction following massive abdominal trauma. *J Trauma* 1993;34: 233–235.

Cue JI, Cryer HG, Miller FB, et al. Packing and planned reexploration for hepatic and retroperitoneal hemorrhage—critical refinements of a useful technique. *J Trauma* 1990;30:1007–1013.

Hirshberg A, Mattox KL. Planned reoperation for severe trauma. *Ann Surg* 1995;222:3–8.

Johnson JW, Gracias VH, Schwab WC, et al. Evolution in damage control for exsanguinating penetrating abdominal injury. *J Trauma* 2001;51(2):261–271.

Miller PR, Thompson JT, Faler BS, et al. Late fascial closure in lieu of ventral hernia: the next step in open abdomen management. *J Trauma* 2002;53:843–849.

Moore EE. Staged laparotomy for the hypothermia, acidosis and coagulopathy syndrome. *Am J Surg* 1996;172:405–410.

Morris JA, Eddy VA, Blinman TA. The staged celiotomy for trauma—issues in unpacking and reconstruction. Ann Surg 1993;217:576–586.

Peralta R, Hojman H. Abdominal compartment syndrome. Int Anesthesiol Clin 2001;39(1):75–94.

Reilly PM, Rotondo MF, Carpenter JP, et al. Temporary vascular continuity during damage control—intraluminal shunting for proximal superior mesenteric artery injury. *J Trauma* 1995;39:757–760

Richardson JD, Bergamini TM, Spain DA, et al. Operative strategies for management of abdominal aortic gunshot wounds. *Surgery* 1996;120:667–671

Rotondo MF, Schwab CW, McGonigal MD, et al. Damage control—an approach for improved survival in exsanguinating penetrating abdominal injury. *J Trauma* 1993;35:375–382.

Schein M, Wittman DH, Aprahamian CC, et al. The abdominal compartment syndrome–the physiological and clinical consequences of raised intra-abdominal pressure. *J Am Coll Surg* 1995;180:745–753.

Shapiro MB, Jemkins, DH, Swab CW, et al. Damage control: collective review. *J Trauma* 2000;49:969–978.

Velmahos GC, Baker C, Demetriades D, et al. Lung-sparing surgery after penetrating trauma using tractotomy, partial lobectomy, and pneumonorrhaphy. *Arch Surg* 1999;134:86–89.

Wall MJ Jr, Villavicencio RT, Miller CC, et al. Pulmonary tractotomy as an abbreviated thoracotomy technique. *J Trauma* 1998;45:1015–1023.

32

Genitourinary Trauma

Adam S. Feldman, MD, Patricio C. Gargollo, MD, and Joseph A. Grocela, MD

I. Introduction

Genitourinary (GU) injuries frequently occur in the setting of multiple organ system trauma and, although other life-threatening injuries must be addressed first, the treating physician must be alert to clues pointing to the presence of these injuries.

II. Epidemiology and Mechanisms

Urologic injuries, which occur in 10% to 20% of major trauma patients, can be the result of either blunt or penetrating trauma. Upper tract injuries usually result from significant force, whereas lower tract injuries occur after less forceful, localized injury. Fractures of the lower ribs, vertebral bodies, or transverse processes can be associated with renal injuries. Pelvic fractures are often accompanied by urethral or bladder injuries.

III. Important Surgical Anatomy

The GU system is divided into three regions, each with its own pattern of injury. The upper tract includes the renal arteries, the kidneys, and the ureters. The lower tract consists of the bladder and the posterior portion of the urethra. The external portion is composed of the anterior urethra, penis, scrotum, and testicles in men and the labia, clitoris, hymen, and urethral meatus in women.

IV. Upper Urinary Tract: Renal Injuries

A. Presentation

Traumatic injury to the kidney should be suspected in any case of trauma to the back, flank, lower thorax, and upper abdomen. Renal trauma is present in approximately 3% of all hospitalized trauma patients and accompanies 8% to 10% of all significant intraabdominal trauma. Renal injuries are commonly associated with injuries to adjacent organs, including the liver, spleen, small bowel, colon, stomach, and pancreas, as well as fractures of inferior ribs or lumbar vertebrae. In the general population, blunt trauma is much more common than penetrating trauma, accounting for up to 90% of renal injuries. Most renal injuries requiring surgical intervention, however, are those secondary to penetrating trauma. Renal injury is also more likely to occur in patients with preexisting renal structural abnormalities, including hydronephrosis, cysts, tumors, renal calculi, vascular malformations, and congenital abnormalities.

Classification of the renal injury is important in approaching the management of renal trauma, especially in the patient with complex multiple trauma. The American Association for the Surgery of Trauma has developed a staging system that classifies traumatic renal injuries into five grades, ranging from least to most severe (**Table 32-1**). This system can be classified into two broad categories. *Minor*

Table 32-1. American Association for the Surgery of Trauma renal injury scale

Grade	Injury Description
I	Renal contusion with microscopic or gross hematuria and no renal injury injury on radiographic studies Nonexpanding subcapsular hematoma without parenchymal laceration
II	Nonexpanding perirenal hematoma confined to the renal retroperitoneum Renal cortex laceration <1 cm with no urinary extravasation
III	Renal cortex laceration >1 cm with no urinary extravasation
IV	Renal laceration extending through renal cortex into medulla and collecting system with positive urinary extravasation on renal imaging Segmental renal artery or vein injury indicated by a segmental parenchymal infarct on renal imaging Renal artery or vein injury with a contained hematoma Thrombosis of the main renal artery
V	Completely shattered kidney Avulsion of the renal pedicle

From Moore EE, Shackford SR, Pachter, et al. Organ injury scaling: spleen, liver, and kidney. *J Trauma* 1989;29:1664, with permission.

injuries (grades I and II) include contusions, superficial lacerations, and small subcapsular hematomas. *Major injuries* (grades III, IV, and V) include deep parenchymal lacerations, involving the corticomedullary junction and collecting system; renovascular pedicle injuries; and shattered kidney. Qualifying the extent of the renal injury is important in evaluating the trauma patient. Determining whether to follow the path of *conservative* management versus *aggressive* intervention, however, is not "cut and dry" along these grades of injury, but requires careful clinical judgment.

B. Diagnosis

   1. Physical Examination

   As in any trauma patient, hemodynamic stability should be assessed. Hypotension and tachycardia can indicate active hemorrhage and, in the patient with suspected renal trauma, suggest a possible severe parenchymal or renovascular injury. In the patient subjected to blunt trauma, large flank ecchymosis, crepitation, or a lower rib fracture raise the suspicion for a renal injury. Stab wounds or bullet entry and exit wounds with trajectory through the flank, back, lower chest, or upper abdomen suggest penetrating renal trauma.

   2. Urinalysis

   Although gross hematuria is generally associated with a more severe renal injury than is microscopic hematuria, the degree of hematuria does not necessarily predict the nature of the injury. Hematuria can be absent in 0.5% to 25% of all renal trauma and in up to 40% of injuries to the renal pedicle.

3. Renal Imaging

Computed tomography (CT) scan is a sensitive and efficient mechanism for evaluating the trauma patient. In many emergency departments, is seen a low threshold to evaluate abdominal trauma with a CT scan. Nevertheless, if renal trauma is to be considered alone, renal imaging may be unnecessary in the adult with blunt trauma and microscopic hematuria alone, unless the history, mechanism of injury, or physical examination suggests an increased risk of injury. Adult patients with penetrating trauma to the back, flank, or abdomen; blunt trauma with gross hematuria; or blunt trauma with microscopic hematuria plus shock should be imaged. Children with blunt trauma and hematuria should be imaged regardless of hemodynamic instability or degree of hematuria.

    a. Intravenous Pyelography. Excretory urography was once the first-line radiographic study for renal injury; however, with the accessibility and greater diagnostic sensitivity of the CT scan it now has a more limited role. The intravenous pyelogram (IVP) is used to evaluate for the presence and function of both kidneys and to assess the renal parenchyma and collecting system. Poor visualization suggests a major parenchymal injury. No visualization can result from congenital or surgical renal absence, renal ectopia, shock, renovascular spasm secondary to severe contusion, renal artery thrombosis, avulsion of the renal pedicle, or high-grade obstruction of the collecting system. The unstable patient with multiple trauma who is taken to the operating room for exploration without the opportunity for abdominal imaging may have an intraoperative "one-shot" IVP taken to assess for a present and functioning noninjured kidney. It can be argued, however, that the absence of a second kidney would unlikely alter the management of renal trauma if nephrectomy is performed only for the most severe renal injuries.

    b. Computed Tomography. The CT scan with intravenous (i.v.) contrast and appropriate delayed images is an extremely sensitive tool in the evaluation of renal trauma with a diagnostic accuracy of up to 98%. In addition to assessing for parenchymal contusion or laceration, hemorrhage, and urinary extravasation, the CT scan can also demonstrate evidence of vascular injury and avascular segments. Parenchymal hematomas typically appear as a nonenhancing, round, poorly marginated lesion, whereas perinephric hematomas often exhibit a bubbly or streaked appearance in the perinephric fat. Segmental devascularization or arterial spasm may be indicated by sharp parenchymal margins on the contrast-enhanced scan. The CT scan also elucidates valuable information about the remainder of the abdomen and retroperitoneum, which helps determine management decisions for the trauma patient.

c. Arteriography. As a diagnostic tool, arteriography is uncommonly used, given the availability and accuracy of the CT scan. Given the ability to perform therapeutic embolization of areas of persistent hemorrhage, however, angiography is used for diagnosis and intermediate intervention in renal trauma.

d. Ultrasound. The initial evaluation of all trauma patients in the trauma bay includes an ultrasound-focus abdominal sonogram for trauma (FAST) scan of the abdomen, pelvis, and pericardial space. In skilled hands, the scan may reveal a perinephric fluid collection or renal laceration. The FAST scan, however, has a low diagnostic sensitivity compared with CT scan and should not preclude the decision to obtain an abdominal CT scan. Formal ultrasound examination has little, if any, role in the evaluation of the trauma patient.

e. Radionucleotide Imaging. Radionucleotide imaging has a limited, if any, role in assessing the acute trauma patient because of the duration of the examination. Isotope flow scanning can be used to assess vascular patency in follow-up after a renovascular repair or in a patient with a severe allergy to i.v. contrast media.

C. Nonoperative Management

With the development of minimally invasive techniques, the term "nonoperative management" has expanded far beyond observation. The use of selective conservative management of renal trauma and nonoperative interventional techniques (e.g., angiographic embolization, percutaneous drainage, ureteral stenting) allows for successful treatment of renal trauma without surgical exploration in up to 80% of patients.

1. Observation

All patients with minor renal injuries who remain clinically stable and have no other injuries that would require intervention should be managed conservatively. Patients with more severe renal injuries consisting of deep parenchymal lacerations with possible urinary extravasation can often also be conservatively managed, given that hemorrhage and extravasation are not extensive, hemodynamic parameters remain stable, and no additional injuries require exploration. Avascular, nonfunctional renal fragments can also be amenable to nonoperative management if no associated hemorrhage or urinary extravasation exists.

A risk is seen, however of delayed bleeding or extravasation secondary to necrosis of this segment. Some would argue that early exploration and débridement of the necrotic tissue is advisable, given that the inflammatory response present at the time of a delayed exploration can increase the risk of nephrectomy.

Clinical observation involves admission to the hospital, confinement to bedrest until gross hematuria resolves, and limited activity until microscopic hematuria is no longer present. Gross hematuria should resolve within a matter of hours; however, microscopic hematuria can remain present for up to 3 to 4 weeks following the injury. Serial hematocrit levels should also be followed to ensure that hemorrhage has stabilized. Remain aware that injuries requiring intervention may not present themselves at the time of the initial trauma evaluation. Delayed gross hematuria can indicate arteriovenous fistula or vascular fistula with the collecting system, which would require intervention.

Minor injuries and uncomplicated deep lacerations should resolve within 4 to 8 weeks. Clinical follow-up with a repeat urinalysis should occur within this time period and should not require any repeat imaging, unless indicated by a change in clinical status. Urinary extravasation managed with observation alone should have repeat imaging with a CT scan within 3 to 5 days to evaluate for resolution or persistence of the leak.

2. **Minimally Invasive Intervention**

    a. **Angiographic Embolization.** In an effort avoid surgical exploration and the risk of nephrectomy, angiographic embolization becomes a valuable tool in the hemodynamically stable patient with grade III and IV renal injuries. As mentioned, patients with deep parenchymal lacerations, with or without minor urinary extravasation, can be amenable to observation alone. Angiographic evaluation and embolization, however, offer early intervention and can decrease the risk of delayed surgical exploration. Retroperitoneal hematomas that clearly extend beyond Gerota's fascia should be managed more aggressively than with observation alone. Therefore, angiography with embolization should be the next step in the management of a patient who is hemodynamically stable without associated intraabdominal injury demanding surgical exploration. In general, the use of angiographic embolization applies mainly to blunt renal trauma. In penetrating renal trauma of grade III or higher, surgical exploration is most often advisable to rule out an associated intraabdominal injury. Although these penetrating injuries can be controlled by embolization, the risk of an adjacent liver, splenic, duodenal, or pancreatic injury often warrants operative investigation.

b. **Percutaneous Drainage and Ureteral Stenting.** Deep parenchymal lacerations can involve the collecting system and, thus, result in urinary extravasation. A small amount of extravasation can be managed by observation alone and it often spontaneously resolves as long as ureteral drainage is not impeded. Larger persistent extravasation or urinoma development, however, often can be successfully treated with percutaneous drainage combined with ureteral stenting. Extravasation extending medially from the hilum suggests a renal pelvic defect and, possibly, ureteral avulsion from the renal pelvis. A small defect can be successfully treated with percutaneous drainage and stenting; however, a ureteral avulsion demands operative repair. Failure to drain a urinoma successfully can result in the development of a pseudocyst within a month to several years after the injury. These can often also be successfully treated with percutaneous drainage combined with instillation of sclerosing agents.

D. **Indications for Surgery**
   1. **Absolute Indications**
      a. **Grade V Injury.** Most grade V injuries are life threatening. They include avulsion of the renal pedicle (artery, vein, or both) or the severely shattered kidney. At times, however, the shattered kidney has been managed nonoperatively. The kidney can fracture along planes in between the arterial distributions, resulting in segments that are well vascularized. When imaging demonstrates a shattered kidney with major tissue destruction or devascularization, however, exploration is indicated.
      b. **Hemodynamic Instability.** Persistent hypotension and tachycardia are clinical indications that traumatic renal hemorrhage is severe, persistent, and potentially life threatening. The unstable trauma patient may require operative exploration before imaging can be obtained. Such a patient becomes an "unstaged" trauma patient in whom renal exploration may or may not be indicated following celiotomy.
   2. **Relative Indications**
      a. **Urinary Extravasation.** In most cases with urinary extravasation, the patient can be managed nonoperatively with observation alone or minimally invasive techniques. When a large amount of extravasation is present, however, surgical exploration should be considered. Occasionally, percutaneous drainage, ureteral stenting, or nephrostomy will be unsuccessful. In this scenario of persistent urinary leak, operative repair is required. When imaging demonstrates

major extravasation and no visualization of the ureter, surgical exploration is necessary to rule out and, possibly, repair a complete disruption of the ureteropelvic junction (UPJ). The same is true for blunt trauma and stab wounds; however, gunshot wounds with any degree of urinary extravasation should be explored surgically.

b.   Devascularized or Devitalized Parenchyma. An injury resulting in a large devascularized or devitalized segment of renal tissue should be managed with early operative exploration. Eventual necrosis of this segment presents a significant risk of delayed bleeding or urinary extravasation, which would demand surgical intervention. At the time of delayed exploration, an intense inflammatory response occurs in the area of injury, making the possibility of repair much more difficult and, thus, increasing the risk of nephrectomy. The ability to perform a partial nephrectomy and repair a large injury in a nephron-sparing manner is markedly improved when exploration occurs closer to the time of injury.

c.   Gunshot Wounds. Nearly all gunshot wounds to the kidney should be explored surgically. Gunshot injuries with any degree of extravasation, a significant perinephric hematoma, or devascularized tissue must be explored. Because of the blast effect of the bullet, a higher risk exists for delayed complications (e.g., bleeding or urine leak). Therefore, the injury should be explored, injured tissue should be débrided, and the parenchyma and collecting system should be formally repaired. In the case of a superficial and peripheral small laceration from a bullet that has not entered the peritoneum, nonoperative management can be considered. On our trauma service, however, it would be unusual *not* to explore a gunshot renal injury, given the risk of injury to associated organs (e.g., duodenum, bowel, pancreas, liver, spleen, large vessels).

d.   Arterial Thrombosis. Thrombosis of the main renal artery or one of its major segments can occur in blunt trauma when the artery is stretched, resulting in an intimal tear. The goal of repairing such an injury is the salvage of kidney function; however, the main barrier to this task is the limit of warm ischemic time of the renal parenchyma. The limits of warm ischemic time can vary, depending on a number of clinical factors including age, preexisting vascular or renal pathology, and serum creatinine level, with the absolute maximum being 4 to 12 hours if any significant renal function is to be recovered. The function of the contralateral kidney is a crucial factor in the decision to attempt revascularization or manage the patient nonoperatively and allow the ischemic kidney to slowly atrophy. In the case of a solitary kidney or bilateral renal artery thrombosis, the surgical approach should be much more aggressive to preserve renal function.

3. Intraoperative Indications for Renal Exploration

When a trauma patient is taken to the operating room because of hemodynamic instability or for exploration and management of an associated injury, renal exploration may or may not be performed. The presence of a pulsatile, expanding, or unconfined retroperitoneal hematoma demands intraoperative renal exploration. In the patient with a visible retroperitoneal hematoma at the time of laparotomy, renal exploration can be avoided only if the injury was adequately staged with preoperative imaging demonstrating that it is an injury that can be safely observed. If urinary extravasation is suggested, then renal exploration should be performed. Any penetrating renal trauma, including gunshot and stab wounds, with an associated significant retroperitoneal hematoma should be explored when preoperative staging was not possible. If the injury has not been staged, an intraoperative one-shot IVP performed at 10 minutes after contrast medium injection will provide valuable information about the nature of the renal injury in addition to the presence or absence of a functioning contralateral kidney. An intraoperative one-shot IVP which demonstrates urinary extravasation or a nonfunctioning contralateral kidney, serves as an indication for renal exploration.

E. Operative Exposure and Technique
1. Exposure and Primary Vascular Control

In the trauma scenario, the patient should be explored through a standard midline incision extending from xiphoid to pubis symphysis. This allows for systematic examination of the entire abdomen for any associated intraabdominal injury. Examine and repair associated injuries before exploration of the kidneys unless renal bleeding is massive or life threatening. The first step in exploring the kidney should be to obtain primary vascular control. This proves to be a valuable step, given that Gerota's fascia serves as a tamponade mechanism. Once Gerota's fascia is incised, significant hemorrhage can result and temporary occlusion of the renal artery may be necessary. Displace the transverse colon and small bowel anteriorly to expose the root of the mesentery and great vessels. Then incise the posterior peritoneum medial to the inferior mesenteric vein from the inferior mesenteric artery to ligament of Treitz. Identify the left renal vein with a vessel loop as it crosses anterior to the aorta. Rarely, the left renal vein will cross posterior to the aorta. As the left renal vein is retracted cephalad, the left renal artery should be exposed and isolated and the right renal artery can be identified with dissection in the interaortocaval space. The right renal vein can then be identified and isolated lateral to the vena cava, at the same level as the left renal vein. To improve exposure of the vena cava and renal vessels, a Kocher maneuver can be performed to reflect the duodenum and the head of the pancreas medially. Once vascular control is obtained, turn attention to exposing the kidney by first mobilizing the ipsilateral colon along the white line of Toldt and reflecting it medially. Gerota's fascia can then be incised longitudinally, hematoma and fat evacuated, and the entire kidney, renal pelvis, and upper ureter can be exposed with blunt and sharp dissection. Preserve the renal capsule as best as possible and begin dissection away from the site of injury to avoid subcapsular dissection. In a situation where immediately life-threatening hemmorhage is encountered, access to the kidney through the colonic mesentery may be performed.

2.   Debridement of Devitalized Parenchyma
Débridement begins with evacuation of intrarenal hematoma and continues with sharp excision of nonviable tissue. In injuries from high velocity missiles, aggressive débridement helps to avoid complications from residual devitalized tissue resulting from blast effect. Inadequate débridement can result in delayed bleeding or urinary extravasation. When the injury is to the interpolar aspect of the kidney, the débridement will result in a wedge-shaped parenchymal defect; however, major polar injuries are most effectively managed by partial nephrectomy. Take care to preserve the renal capsule, which will be used in the closure.

3.   Hemostasis
Once adequate débridement is performed, suture-ligate all bleeding arterial vessels with 4-0 chromic figure-of-eight sutures. Venous bleeding should stop once the parenchymal defect is closed; however, thrombin-soaked absorbable gelatin sponge can be used as bolsters in between cut parenchymal edges.

4.   Repair of the Collecting System
Close tears in the collecting system in a watertight fashion with continuous 4-0 chromic catgut suture. The integrity of this repair and less discrete injuries can be evaluated with the injection of 2 to 3 mL of indigo carmine into the renal pelvis while digitally occluding the ureter distally. Place a double-J ureteral stent in the case of significant renal pelvic or ureteral injuries.

5.   Repair of the Parenchyma
a.   Primary Repair. Smaller parenchymal defects in which the capsule is well preserved can be repaired primarily. The capsular edges should be reapproximated with 3-0 Vicryl suture in an interrupted horizontal mattress fashion. Vicryl

pledgets can be used at either edge to prevent the suture from pulling through the capsule and thrombin soaked absorbable gelatin foam bolsters in the parenchymal defect aid in hemostasis while decreasing tension on the suture line.

b.   Coverage of Large Defects. In polar injuries or larger defects in which the capsule cannot be reapproximated primarily, the defect must be covered. A pedicle flap of omentum serves as the ideal coverage because of its vascular supply and lymphatic drainage. The omentum is also ideal for placement between the injured kidney and an associated colon, pancreatic, or vascular injury. This interposition helps to prevent formation of abscess or fistula. If the omentum is not available, perinephric fat, a free graft of peritoneum, or a Vicryl patch can be used to cover the defect. The flap, graft, or patch is tacked down to the capsular edges with 3-0 Vicryl sutures. For coverage of large defects or in the case of multiple lacerations or shattered kidney, a large sheet of Vicryl mesh can be wrapped around the kidney like an envelope and sewn into place to approximate the multiple parenchymal edges.

6.   Repair of Injuries to the Renal Vasculature
    a.   Renal Artery. Lacerations to the renal artery can be closed primarily with 5-0 polypropylene suture. Avulsion or thrombosis of the main renal artery requires primary reanastomosis or bypass with an interposition graft using the hypogastric artery and, in the case of arterial thrombosis, the injured arterial segment should be excised. Successful repair resulting in normal renal function is rare and after 12 hours is futile. During the repair, the kidney can be perfused with a cold hypertonic solution to improve viability. Injured segmental arteries should be ligated unless primary repair is simple. If the area of ischemic parenchyma is small and the capsule is intact, the segment may be allowed to atrophy. A significant devitalized segment should be excised, however.

    b.   Renal Vein. Lacerations to the main renal vein should be closed primarily with 5-0 polypropylene suture, whereas segmental veins can be ligated with adequate intrarenal collateral drainage. Complete avulsion of the main renal vein typically demands ligation. The left renal vein, typically, can be ligated because of collateral drainage through the adrenal, lumbar, and gonadal veins. Ligation of the right main renal vein, however, typically requires nephrectomy.

7.   Retroperitoneal Drain Placement
A retroperitoneal Penrose drain should be placed behind the kidney after all repairs. Closed suction drains can keep an injured collecting system open

through negative pressure. A urostomy bag can be placed over the Penrose to quantify output and maintain a relatively clean environment. Unless drainage is high, the drain is removed within 48 hours. A large amount of drainage should be tested for creatinine level to identify serum or lymph from a urine leak. Manage persistent urinary drainage with the placement of a ureteral stent and continued drainage with the Penrose until output ceases. If the drainage is serum or lymph, the Penrose drain can be removed regardless of output. If an associated pancreatic injury is present, drain the kidney and pancreatic beds separately to avoid abscess or fistula formation.

F.   Postoperative Care

Postoperatively, the patient should remain on bedrest until gross hematuria resolves. A Foley catheter should remain in place until the patient is hemodynamically stable, the urine is clear, and the patient is ambulatory and able to void. Serial hematocrit and creatinine levels should be followed to ensure that they remain stable. Retroperitoneal drains should be removed by 48 hours postoperatively unless a persistent urine leak is indicated. At about 3 months postoperatively, the patient should have repeat imaging with CT, IVP, or radionuclide scan to evaluate renal function and to ensure no silent obstruction is present.

G.   Potential Complications

Indications of a possible postoperative complication include a new onset in flank pain, fever, mass, sudden hematocrit drop, or rise in creatinine. Most postoperative complications, including delayed bleeding, perinephric abscess, urinoma, fistula formation, and hydronephrosis, will become evident within a month. A patient with any of the above signs or symptoms should be evaluated by CT scan. Most complications can be managed with minimally invasive techniques, including percutaneous drainage, ureteral stenting, or both. Delayed bleeding can be secondary to a segmental renal artery injury with false aneurysm development and subsequent rupture. Such delayed hemorrhage can be effectively treated with selective angiographic embolization. Hypertension is a common complication following renal injury and typically resolves spontaneously within 6 weeks.

V.   Upper Urinary Tract: Ureteral Injuries

A.   Presentation

Ureteral injuries from external trauma are relatively rare, occurring in approximately 3% of all urologic trauma. Most of these injuries result from penetrating trauma, particularly from gunshot wounds. Blunt trauma resulting in ureteral injury is rare, usually the result of a rapid acceleration or deceleration injury causing hyperextension of the spine and avulsion of the UPJ from the ureter. These injuries more commonly occur in children because of their greater degree of vertebral column flexibility. Penetrating ureteral injuries nearly always coexist with associated organ injuries, including trauma to the small bowel, colon, liver, and ileac vessels. Ureteral injuries can also be graded on a scale from I through V, ranging from hematoma or contusion to complete transection with surrounding area of devascularization (**Table 32-2**).

B. Diagnosis

  1. Physical Examination

  Penetrating wounds with apparent trajectory through the path of the ureter should raise suspicion for ureteral injury. Direct flank tenderness or ecchymosis can also be suggestive of ureteral injury. These physical findings, however, are nonspecific and other clinical signs of ureteral or renal pelvis trauma are typically delayed in their manifestation.

  2. Urinalysis

  Microscopic or gross hematuria may not be present in 25% to 45% of ureteral injuries and, therefore, is an unreliable indicator for ureteral trauma.

  3. Radiographic Imaging

    a. Intravenous Urography. In the recent past, intravenous urography (IVU) was the primary imaging study to evaluate for ureteral injury with an accuracy as high as 95%. Contrast extravasation is a clear finding demonstrating ureteral injury; however, often the radiologic signs, including slight dilation or deviation of the ureter or delayed function, are less obvious.

    b. Computerized Tomography. The most common CT finding in a proximal ureteral injury is the extravasation of contrast medium into the medial perirenal space. In the case of a complete ureteral transection, the absence of contrast in the distal ureter can be observed on delayed images. Given the high speed of helical CT scanners, the collecting system can be poorly opacified unless delayed images are specifically requested.

Table 32-2.   American Association for the Surgery of Trauma ureter injury scale

Grade	Injury Description
I	Contusion or hematoma without devascularization
II	Laceration with <50% transection
III	Laceration with >50% transection
IV	Laceration involving complete transection with 2 cm of devascularization
V	Laceration involving complete transection with >2 cm of devascularization Avulsion of the ureteropelvic junction

From Moore EE, Shackford SR, Pachter, et al. Organ injury scaling: spleen, liver, and kidney. *J Trauma* 1989;29:1664, with permission.

Without a delayed sequence of imaging, the overall sensitivity of CT scanning for ureteral injury therefore is reduced. Furthermore, hypotension can also lessen the opacification of the collecting system, thus also decreasing the sensitivity of the CT scan.

4. Intraoperative Diagnosis

Most ureteral injuries are diagnosed intraoperatively during exploratory laparotomy for investigation and management of associated injuries. In the case of penetrating trauma from high-velocity missiles, all efforts should be made to trace the bullet's path and directly inspect the ureter in that region. In addition to obvious urinary extravasation, contusion, discoloration, or decreased peristalsis can indicate ureteral injury or devascularization from blast effect. The presence of peristalsis, however, cannot exclude devascularizing injury. Incision and observation for a bleeding edge may be the only reliable method of effectively ruling out devitalizing trauma. Intravenous or intraureteral injection of indigo carmine or methylene blue can aid in the identification of urinary extravasation.

5. Delayed Diagnosis

Despite efforts to promptly diagnose an acute ureteral injury, occasionally these injuries are missed and a urinoma or, occasionally, a fistula develops. The most common symptoms of a missed ureteral injury are abdominal or flank pain, fever, ileus, and eventually sepsis. Radiologic imaging (e.g., abdominal and pelvic CT scan) should be used to evaluate such a patient.

C. Management

1. Delayed Diagnosis

In the case of a delayed diagnosis of a ureteral injury, the patient can be treated with percutaneous drainage of the urinoma and nephrostomy placement or ureteral stenting. Stent placement may allow complete healing of the ureter if the injury is minor; however, with a large amount of extravasation of urine and a large suspected ureteral defect is suggested, then the patient should have exploratory surgery and the injury repaired at that time.

2. Low Grade Injuries

At intraoperative inspection, ureteral injuries classified as grade I and select grade II can be treated by ureteral stenting and retroperitoneal drainage without the need for surgical repair. This includes ureteral hematoma or contusion and selected lacerations of <50% of the ureteral circumference. It is wise practice to place a ureteral stent and retroperitoneal drain for even minimal evidence of ureteral injury.

3. The Unstable Patient

In the patient with multiple trauma and a concomitant ureteral injury, the patient's clinical condition and urgency of associated injuries take precedence to surgical repair of the ureteral injury. A time-consuming,

complex ureteral repair may not be best for the critically ill patient. Depending on the severity of the
injury, ureteral stenting with retroperitoneal drain
placement or ureteral ligation with percutaneous or
open nephrostomy tube placement can serve as a temporizing measure in the acute setting. Definitive surgical reconstruction can then be planned for after the
patient has recovered from nonurologic injuries and
the periureteral inflammatory process has resolved.

4. Surgical Repair

Most ureteral injuries require surgical repair. The surgical approach, typically through the midline laparotomy, most often has been performed in the acute
trauma patient for the exploration of associated injuries. In the case of a delayed repair, the approach
can be modified, based on the location of the injury. A
subcostal incision can be used for a proximal injury or
a Gibson incision for a distal injury. The foundation
for successful ureteral repair lies in adequate ureteral
mobilization without devascularization; débridement
of devitalized tissue to a bleeding cut edge; formation
of a tension-free, water tight, spatulated mucosa-to-
mucosa anastomosis; and protection of the anastomosis from any associated bowel, pancreatic, or vascular
injury with an omental wrap. All repairs should be
performed over a ureteral stent and a retroperitoneal
drain should always be placed.

The choice for surgical repair depends on the anatomic location of the injury in either the upper, middle, or lower portion of the ureter. To avoid vascular
compromise during dissection, the blood supply to
these segments must be respected. The upper ureter
is supplied by the renal arteries, the midureter from
ileac and aortic branches, and the lower ureter from
uterine, vaginal, superior vesical, and middle hemor-
rhoidal arteries. The adventitia of the ureter contains
an anastomotic network of vessels directly supplying
the ureter and, therefore, this layer must be carefully
preserved during any repair.

> **a. Primary Closure.** Some grade II ureteral
> injuries from stab wounds or blunt trauma can be
> managed by primary closure of the injury with
> little or no débridement of devitalized tissue.
> Renal pelvic and ureteropelvic tears from stab
> wounds and blunt trauma can also be treated with
> primary repair. If the surrounding tissue appears
> compromised in any way, however, primary clo-
> sure should not be attempted and the appar-
> ently devitalized tissue should be adequately
> débrided. In this regard, injuries from gunshot
> wounds should never be treated with primary clo-
> sure, given the high risk of surrounding tissue
> destruction from the blast effect of the bullet.
> Primary repairs of lacerations >50% of the ure-
> teral circumference should be accompanied by the
> placement of a ureteral stent. All primary clo-

sures should have a retroperitoneal drain placed adjacent to, but not touching, the repair.

b.   Ureteroureterostomy. Most complete ureteral transections, lacerations >50% of the ureteral circumference, partial transections with compromised surrounding tissue, or any ureteral injury secondary to a gunshot wound can be treated with a direct spatulated end-to-end anastomosis over a ureteral stent using 4-0 or 5-0 interrupted absorbable suture. Most traumatic injuries involving the upper and midureteral segments can be treated in this manner. After adequate débridement of all devitalized tissue, the repair should be tension free. Occasionally, if a large segment of ureter needs to be débrided, the kidney can be mobilized caudally, thus allowing for a tension-free repair. The repair can be protected by wrapping an omental flap around the anastomosis. With all repairs, a retroperitoneal drain is placed and removed within 48 hours in the absence of any leaks. The ureteral stent is left in place for 4 to 6 weeks.

c.   Ureteroneocystostomy. Any injury to the distal third of the ureter should be managed by ureteral reimplantation into the bladder. This repair is performed using a combined extra- and intravesical approach, necessitating the formation of an anterior cystotomy. After the end of the ureter is débrided and spatulated, it is then brought through the bladder wall medial and superior to the original ureteral hiatus. A submucosal tunnel is then developed toward the bladder neck using the nonrefluxing principle of an at least 3:1 ratio of tunnel length to ureteral diameter. The ureteral end is anastomosed to the bladder mucosa and the mucosal defect is closed with interrupted 4-0 absorbable sutures. A double-J ureteral stent and Malecot suprapubic tube are placed and the bladder is closed in two layers.

(1)   Psoas Hitch. When concerned that the anastomosis of the ureter to the bladder will not be tension free, the bladder can be partially mobilized and elevated to meet the compromised ureter. The bladder fundus is dissected at the peritoneal reflection. The superior vesical pedicle vessels contralateral to the injury are ligated and divided. If needed, the ipsilateral superior vesical pedicle vessels can also be ligated and divided for further mobilization. An anterior longitudinal cystotomy is then made; the bladder is shifted superiorly and laterally and then sutured to the psoas minor tendon with interrupted monofilament nonabsorbable sutures. Take care not to penetrate the bladder mucosa nor entrap the genitofemoral nerve.

(2) Boari Anterior Bladder Wall Flap.
When the psoas hitch cannot adequately mobilize the bladder to meet the viable edge of a
severely injured ureter, a Boari flap can be
fashioned to provide the additional length
needed for a tension-free anastomosis. Make
a long U-shaped incision in the anterior bladder wall and raise the flap cephalad toward
the ureteral edge, which can then be reim-
planted submucosally into the flap. The flap
is then tubularized around the ureter and
the bladder wall defect is closed in two layers. In the acute trauma setting, perform this
procedure only in the most stable patient
because it is time-consuming. It is an excellent tool, however, in a delayed, well-planned
reconstruction.

d. Transureteroureterostomy. An alternative reconstruction when the distal to mid ureter
is severely injured is to implant the injured ureter
into the contralateral healthy ureter in an end-to-
side fashion. This repair is useful in cases of associated extensive bladder, rectal, or pelvic vascular
trauma. Mobilize and extend the affected ureter
across the midline through a window in the colonic
mesentery. Its course should run superior to the
inferior mesenteric artery in a gradual arc to avoid
sharp angulation. Perform an end-to-side anastomosis with 4-0 interrupted absorbable suture and
leave a stent in place across the anastomosis. This
procedure risks the compromise of the normal contralateral ureter and is contraindicated in a
patient with a history of nephrolithiasis, chronic
pyelonephritis, and upper tract transitional cell
carcinoma. This procedure should be considered as
an elective repair, rather than emergent.

e. Ileal Interposition. When the entire ureter
is irreversibly traumatized, an option for a delayed reconstruction is to use a segment of ileum
as a ureteral substitution. Do not perform this
procedure in the acute setting, however, because
a standard antibiotic and mechanical bowel preparation should be performed preoperatively.
This repair should also be reserved for patients
with normal renal function. A segment of ileum
approximately 20 to 25 cm in length is identified
at least 15 cm proximal to the ileocecal valve.
Next, divide and mobilize the bowel by incising
the mesentery to a point above the vascular pedicle. Reanastomose the bowel and position the ileal
neoureter posteriorly in an isoperistaltic fashion.
Perform an end-to-end pyeloileal anastomosis
and anastomose the distal ileal end to the posterior bladder wall in an end-to-side fashion. This
is usually performed as a reconstructive stage.

f.   Renal Autotransplantation. In a patient with compromised renal function or a solitary kidney, a reconstructive option when the entire length of the ureter is traumatized is to perform a renal transplantation. If possible, this procedure should be reserved for a delayed reconstruction and not performed in the acute setting. The affected kidney is dissected, mobilized, and transplanted into the iliac fossa. The renal vessels are anastomosed with the ileac vessels and a pyelovesicostomy is performed to restore continuity of the collecting system.

D.   Postoperative Care

For all ureteral reconstructions a ureteral stent, retroperitoneal drain, and a Foley catheter, with or without a Malecot suprapubic tube, are all left in place. The ureteral stent, usually an internal double-J, is typically removed in 4 to 6 weeks. For the retroperitoneal drain, use a Penrose passive drain to avoid negative pressure on the suture line, which can occur with closed suction drains and result in a prolonged leakage from the ureteral injury. The drain is typically removed after 48 hours, except in cases of significant drainage with a measured creatinine level consistent with urine, suggesting extravasation. With evidence of a urine leak, the drain is left in place and treated as a controlled fistula. If the fluid creatinine level is consistent with serum, remove the drain, regardless of its output. As long as the urine is clear, the Foley catheter and suprapubic tube are removed in 2 to 7 days, depending on the extent of bladder dissection and type of repair.

As part of the follow-up evaluation, routine IVP are performed after 1 month and 1 year to rule out any silent ureteral stenosis or hydronephrosis and to evaluate renal function. Also check serum chemistries after ileal interposition to rule out any metabolic complications.

E.   Potential Complications

When a ureteral injury is recognized and treated acutely, morbidity is low. Potential postoperative complications include ureteral stricture, anastomotic leak, urinoma, and fistula formation. Most complications after ureteral trauma, however, occur because of delayed diagnosis. Urinoma, abscess formation, ureteral scarring, obstruction, fistula formation, sepsis, loss of renal function, and death can occur in up to 50% of patients. Delayed diagnosis is also associated with an increased risk of nephrectomy. If an injury is diagnosed within 1 week of injury and no associated infection is seen, perform surgical exploration and repair. After 10 to 14 days, an intense inflammatory response is present, which makes dissection extremely difficult and dangerous. These patients, therefore, require percutaneous nephrostomy for urinary diversion and delayed reconstruction after 3 months.

VI.   The Lower Urinary Tract: Bladder Injuries

A.   Presentation

Injuries to the urinary bladder can be secondary to blunt or penetrating trauma with blunt injuries resulting in

60% to 85% of cases. These injuries should be suspected in all cases of blunt abdominal trauma, especially in cases of a pelvic fracture, because concomitant bladder injury occurs in 5% to 10% of these patients. The most important initial diagnostic clue in evaluating bladder injuries is the quality of the urine because 98% of patients with a bladder injury will have gross hematuria. Microscopic hematuria in the setting of a pelvic fracture should raise the suggestion that a bladder injury has occurred. Other indicators of possible bladder trauma include blood at the urethral meatus, inability to void, a high palpable intraabdominal bladder, suprapubic tenderness, or no urine output with Foley catheter placement. Bladder rupture resulting from trauma can be classified into intra- or extraperitoneal injuries.

In intraperitoneal bladder rupture, the peritoneal surface is disrupted and there is urinary extravasation into the abdomen. This type of rupture involves a high degree of force and, because of this, it is usually associated with other severe injuries. Because of the severity of these injuries, patients with intraperitoneal rupture have a high mortality risk (20% to 40%). Injury usually occurs when blunt force is extrinsically applied to a full and distended bladder. If the intraluminal bladder pressure exceeds 300 mm Hg, the bladder can rupture. This usually occurs at the dome, which is the weakest part of the bladder wall. Because the peritoneum is adherent to the dome, lacerations here extend through the peritoneum and result in extravasation of urine into the abdominal cavity. The most common presentation of intraperitoneal bladder rupture is the trauma patient involved in a motor vehicle accident who has extrinsic force applied to the bladder by a seatbelt. Intraperitoneal bladder rupture is more likely to occur in women and children who have thinner musculature in their bladder wall. Furthermore, the bladder in children is located higher in the abdomen than in adults, which also predisposes them to bladder injury.

Extraperitoneal bladder rupture results in leakage of urine into the perivesicular space and is almost universally associated with fractures of the pelvis. Lacerations to the bladder are thought to occur from fragments of bone or from tears at ligamentous attachments secondary to the force of blunt trauma. These tears usually occur at the lateral aspect of the bladder neck, either ipsilateral or contralateral to the pelvic fracture.

B. Diagnosis

Injuries to the bladder can be well visualized using either CT or conventional cystography. The decision which to use relates to available equipment (CT scanner) and to the need to evaluate other organ systems. Before cystography is performed, urethral injury must be ruled-out. A Foley catheter is placed and 200 to 300 mL of water-soluble contrast media is infused into the bladder. When full, a small contraction of the bladder will cause a brief rise in the level of the contrast media in the syringe. The Foley catheter is then clamped and the radiograph or the CT is obtained. With plain film cystograms, it is imperative to obtain postdrainage films because a full bladder can hide small anterior or posterior extravasations. An intraperitoneal bladder rupture (**Fig. 32-1A**) will show the contrast material extending into the abdomen and pooling around loops of bowel. By contrast, extraperitoneal ruptures (**Fig. 32-1B**) will have contrast contained within the soft tissues of the pelvis anterior and lateral to the bladder.

C. Management

The initial treatment of a patient with bladder rupture involves stabilization of all life-threatening injuries. After the patient is stable the decision regarding operative management is made in conjunction with the trauma and orthopedic teams (if pelvic injuries are present). If the

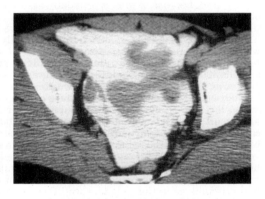

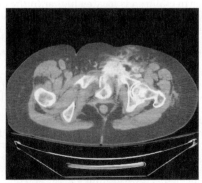

Figure 32-1.   A: Intraperitoneal bladder rupture on CT-cystogram. B: Extraperitoneal bladder rupture on CT-cystogram. CT, computed tomography. Courtesy of Dr. Thomas Ptah and Dr. James Rhea, Department of Radiology, Massachusetts General Hospital.

patient has had penetrating trauma and is to have surgical exploration, the bladder can be visually inspected. Extra- or intraperitoneal bladder ruptures discovered during an exploratory laparotomy are usually repaired primarily through a layered closure. In the case of blunt trauma, intraperitoneal bladder ruptures usually require operative exploration and repair through a layered closure. Extraperitoneal injuries can be managed by primary closure, delayed closure, or nonoperatively with a suprapubic tube or a Foley catheter. Pelvic fractures extending into and causing injury to the bladder require primary repair. If no injury by bony fragments is found, conservative treatment with catheter drainage will result in closure of 75% of extraperitoneal bladder lacerations within 1 to 2 weeks. In all cases, long-term complications can include stricture formation, vesicular fistulas, and infection. Patients with traumatic bladder injuries, therefore, require close follow-up with a urologist.

VII. The Lower Urinary Tract: Urethral Injuries
   A. Presentation
   Urethral injuries are almost always seen in male patients. The female urethra is rarely injured because of its short length. Traumatic injuries in these patients, therefore, occur almost exclusively in conjunction with pelvic fractures. The male urethra is anatomically divided into four segments: the prostatic, membranous, bulbous, and pendulous urethra. Urethral trauma is classified into posterior (prostatic and membranous) and anterior (bulbous and pendulous) injuries, with the urogenital diaphragm representing the anatomic division between these two segments. Posterior urethral injuries are most commonly seen with pelvic ring fractures, whereas anterior injuries are usually caused by external blunt or straddle injuries.

   1. Posterior Urethral Injuries
   Posterior urethral injuries involve separation of the prostate from the urogenital diaphragm and the bulbous urethra. A significant amount of force is required to cause posterior urethral injuries and, because of this, these injuries are often associated with abdominal visceral injuries and pelvic fractures. In fact, 10% to 25% of pelvic ring fractures have associated posterior urethral disruptions and 80% to 90% of posterior urethral injuries occur in conjunction with some type of pelvic fracture. Bladder injuries are seen in up to 35% of posterior urethral injuries. Injury to the posterior urethra is thought to occur secondary to shearing forces applied to the puboprostatic ligaments.

   Posterior urethral injuries can be classified according to the degree of separation of the prostatic from the bulbous urethra.

   Type I: elongation of the urethra without disruption
   Type II: laceration occurring above the urogenital diaphragm with extravasation of urine exclusively into the pelvis

Type III: disruption of the urogenital diaphragm and extravasation below *and* above the diaphragm

Type IV: posterior urethral injury involving the bladder neck

The diagnosis of posterior urethral disruption should be suspected in any patient who presents with gross hematuria after pelvic trauma. Symptoms can include lower abdominal pain and urinary retention, in assition to the sensation of a full bladder. The GU examination may demonstrate blood at the meatus, gross hematuria, and, in some cases, a perineal hematoma. Rectal examination typically reveals a high-riding prostate, which is caused by the shearing of the prostate from the pelvis with subsequent migration of the prostate superiorly. In female patients, the principal sign is blood at the urethral meatus with or without urinary retention.

Any patient suspected of having a urethral injury should be evaluated by a retrograde urethrogram. This should be done before placement of a Foley catheter because urinary catheterization can convert a partial tear to a complete tear.

2. Anterior Urethral Injuries

Anterior urethral injuries, which are more common than those of the posterior urethra, result most often from blunt trauma, owing to straddle, or from blunt trauma with a direct blow to the perineum. Other causes of anterior urethral injury include penetrating wounds from gunshots, stabs, sexual intercourse, or iatrogenic instrumentation. These types of injuries, in contrast with those of the posterior urethra, usually occur in isolation. Anterior urethral injuries can produce partial or complete disruption of the integrity of the urethra and its fascial coverings. Buck's fascia surrounds the erectile bodies and the corpus spongiosum of the urethra from the suspensory ligament proximally to the coronal sulcus distally. Extravasation of blood and urine confined to Buck's fascia will appear as a "sleeve" of ecchymosis and edema on the penis. Rupture of the urethra or corpora cavernosa through Buck's fascia will lead to extravasation of blood and urine to an area bound by Colles' fascia. Colles' fascia fuses posteromedially with the fascia of the superficial and deep transverse perineal muscles and laterally with the fascia lata of the thigh. Superiorly, Colles' fascia continues on the abdominal wall as Scarpa's fascia. Extension of urethral rupture into Colles' fascia will result in a characteristic "butterfly" perineal hematoma. As with posterior injury, urethral injury should be suspected in any patient presenting with an appropriate mechanism of injury and gross hematuria, inability to void, or blood at the urethral meatus.

B. Diagnosis

Both anterior and posterior urethral injuries should be evaluated by retrograde urethrography. If a Foley catheter has inadvertently been placed, it should be left in and contrast material injected around the catheter with a 16-gauge angiocatheter to obtain a urethrogram. Extravasation of contrast at any point in the urethra confirms the presence of urethral disruption. If the bladder fills with contrast material, the injury is classified as partial. In complete tears, no communication will be seen between the urethra and the bladder. A normal urethrogram excludes a urethral injury and a Foley catheter can be placed. Diagnosing urethral injuries in female patients is more challenging, given that urethrography is of limited value in evaluating the short female urethra. These injuries must be suspected when vaginal examination demonstrates a hematoma on the urethra or urine leak into the vagina.

C. Management

    1. Posterior Urethral Injuries

    Type I injuries are usually treated with urethral catheterization for 3 to 5 days. These mild injuries usually heal without significant complications. The management of patients with complete or partial rupture of the posterior urethra (types II and III) is still controversial. Suprapubic cystotomy is the preferred initial treatment for posterior urethral rupture. A urethral catheter can be passed by a urologic surgeon into the bladder in many patients with small, partial tears of the posterior urethra. The catheter is maintained for 1 to 2 weeks, and a voiding cystourethrogram is obtained when the catheter is removed. If passing of a catheter is deemed unsafe by the urologic consultant, a suprapubic catheter should be placed.

    Delayed versus primary repair of posterior urethral injuries remains controversial. In most cases, a delayed repair is preferred. This allows for a decrease in the swelling and absorption of the pelvic hematomas that accompany these injuries. Initial realignment of the urethra is possible in almost all cases, given recent advances in endoscopic techniques. This can be accomplished by passing cystoscopes from the urethral meatus and the suprapubic cystotomy and then threading a flexible guidewire under direct vision. A catheter is then threaded over the wire into the bladder. Primary repair is recommended with severe prostatomembranous dislocation, major bladder neck laceration, and concomitant pelvic vascular or rectal injury. Late complications from posterior urethral injuries include stricture formation, impotence, urinary retention, and urinary incontinence.

    2. Anterior Urethral Injuries

    Anterior urethral injuries are usually treated with long-term catheter drainage to allow for primary healing of the urethra. In cases of penetrating anterior injuries, surgically explore the area, débride, and perform a primary reanastomosis. Urethral strictures and impotence are common complications from anterior injuries.

VIII.   External Genitalia: Penile Injuries

Injuries to the penis can occur from blunt or penetrating trauma, as well as during sexual activity. The most common blunt injury to the penis is a "penile fracture," which is a rupture of the corpus cavernosum. This type of injury occurs after sudden flexion of an erect penis. The patient may hear an audible snap, usually accompanied by severe pain and loss of erection. Physical examination reveals swelling, tenderness, and ecchymosis. Treatment involves exploration and surgical repair of the ruptured portion of the corpora. In some cases of downward flexion, the suspensory ligament of the penis will be torn. In contrast with penile fractures, usually no visible hematoma is seen. Surgical repair should be done to provide future stability during intercourse.

Penetrating penile injuries can occur from stab or gunshot wounds. All wounds should be explored and signs of urethral injury (e.g., blood at the meatus or inability to void) should be investigated with a retrograde urethrogram. Surgical exploration, débridement, and repair are indicated for patients with injury to the corpora, persistent bleeding, or urethral injury. Good results can be expected in most cases of penetrating penile trauma and patients with these injuries can expect potency rates of >70%. Degloving injuries to the penis usually occur in industrial and farm accidents. These patients will usually require surgical débridement and skin grafting.

Penile amputations can result from assault, accident, or self-mutilation. In these cases, if the amputated penis is located it should be cleaned, wrapped in sterile gauze, and placed in a bag with sterile saline. This bag is then kept in ice. Reattachment is possible using microsurgical techniques and should be undertaken as soon as possible

Strangulating lesions of the penis can occur when self-mutilation or masturbation is carried out by the patient and objects are placed around the shaft of the penis. Accidental strangulation can occur in the pediatric or elderly population from hair or condom catheters wrapped too tightly. Solid objects around the penis usually are removed by applying a lubricant or by using a string or latex tourniquet wrapped around the distal penis to decrease swelling. If these methods fail, removal will need to be done using a ring cutter, hacksaw, or other tools

IX.   External Genitalia: Testicular Rupture
A.   Presentation

Testicular trauma can result from blunt or penetrating trauma. Testicular rupture is uncommon because of the size, location, and mobility of the testes. Gunshot or stab wounds, however, can penetrate the testicle and blunt force can isolate the testis against the ischial ramus or the symphysis pubis. More than half of testicular ruptures occur in younger patients during sporting events. Up to approximately 15% occur during motor vehicle collisions and the remainder occur during falls, straddle injuries, penetrating wounds, and other miscellaneous events. Testicular rupture involves a tear in the tunica albuginea, which permits the formation of a hematocele when the seminiferous tubules extrude into the tunica vaginalis. When the rupture involves the tunica vaginalis at its junction with the tunica albuginea, a scrotal hematoma develops by the extension of bleeding into the scrotal sac. Traumatic testicular rupture is an immediate and extremely painful event and can often be associated with nausea and vomiting.

B. Diagnosis

1. Physical Examination

Examination of the genitalia often reveals exquisite tenderness, hematoma formation, ecchymosis, and a variable amount of scrotal edema.

2. Scrotal Ultrasonography

Ultrasound can reliably diagnose the presence of a testicular rupture in approximately 70% to 90% of cases. Seminiferous tubule extrusion creates an abnormal parenchymal echo pattern and intraparenchymal hemorrhage and contusion can also be identified. Ultrasound, however, should never delay surgical exploration when the clinical presentation is concerning.

3. Intraoperative Diagnosis

Surgical diagnosis is the gold standard for a definitive diagnosis of testicular rupture and a low threshold for exploration should be used if concern for such exists.

C. Management

1. Nonoperative Management

Conservative management consisting of ice packs, scrotal elevation, and antiinflammatory medications can be used when ultrasound demonstrates a small hematocele, epididymal hematoma, or testicular contusion and no clinical concern exists for testicular rupture. Expansion of the hemiscrotum, however, would warrant delayed exploration.

2. Surgical Management

Scrotal exploration is indicated in cases of clinical or sonographic evidence of testicular rupture or ultrasound evidence of a large hematocele. Make a midline longitudinal or transverse incision in the scrotum, incise the tunica vaginalis and albuginea, evacuate any hematocele, and deliver the testis into the surgical field. Intratesticular hematomas can also be evacuated and any necrotic parenchyma should be débrided. Hemostasis can be achieved with electrocautery or 4-0 chromic suture. The tunica albuginea is reapproximated with 3-0 running chromic suture, a Penrose drain is left in place through a separate stab incision, and dartos fascia and the skin are closed in layers with chromic suture. Perform orchiectomy only when multiple injuries to the testicle make repair impossible or when the testis is infarcted. Broad-spectrum oral antibiotics should be prescribed for 7 days.

X.   External Genitalia: Scrotal Skin Loss

Avulsion injuries can occur in high-speed motor vehicle collisions or from farm or industrial machinery. Copiously irrigate the wound and débride any obviously necrotic tissue. If possible, primary closure is performed in layers with chromic suture. Because of the flexibility and regenerative ability of the scrotal skin, primary closure under tension may be attempted. If skin loss is excessive and primary closure is not possible, then treat the wound with normal saline wet to dry dressings twice a day. Once the scrotal granulation tissue is adequate, a split-thickness skin graft can be performed to cover the defect. The testes can also be temporarily positioned subcutaneously in the thigh, groin, or abdomen until the scrotum has regenerated sufficiently to allow for a delayed grafting and closure.

SELECTED READING

Armenakas NA. Current methods of diagnosis and management of ureteral injuries. *World J Urol* 1999;17:78–83.

Bonder DR, Selzman AA, Spirnak JP. Evaluation and treatment of bladder rupture. *Semin Urol* 1995;13:62–64.

Brandes SB, McAnnich JW. Reconstructive surgery for trauma of the upper urinary tract. *Urol Clin North Am* 1999;26:1;183–199.

Haas CA, Brown SL, Spirnak JP. Penile fracture and testicular rupture. *World J Urol* 1999;17:101–106.

Hagiwara AH, et al. The role of interventional radiology in the management of blunt renal injury: a practical protocol. *J Trauma* 2001;51;3:526–531.

Sagalowsky AI, Peters PC. Genitourinary trauma. In: Walsh PC, Retik AB, Vaughan ED, et al., eds. *Campbell's urology,* 7th ed. Philadelphia: WB Saunders, 1998:3085–3120.

Skinner EC, Parisky YR, Skinner DG. Management of complex urologic injuries. *Surg Clin North Am* 1996;76:4;861–878.

Velmahos GC, et al. Angiographic embolization for intraperitoneal and retroperitoneal injuries. *World J Surg* 2000;24;5:539–545.

Wessells H. Genital skin loss: unified reconstructive approach to heterogeneous entity. *World J Urol* 1999;17:107–114.

Orthopedic Trauma 1: Spine Fractures

Raymond Malcolm Smith, MD

I. Introduction

Spinal fractures are frequently seen in patients with major trauma. They are a common source of significant disability and, occasionally, of death. Overall, spinal fractures remain a source of fear and poor understanding for most medical staff receiving trauma patients. Most medical staff, even in orthopedics, are not specifically trained in spinal surgery. No doubt, significant neurologic damage carries more serious consequences for the patient than any other survivable injury. The dominating feature of spinal injuries is that of a secondary loss of neurologic (spinal cord) function because of inadequate control of an unstable spinal column injury. In truth, most spinal cord injury is defined at the time of injury and the ability of medical staff to influence the outcome is currently extremely limited. Secondary injuries are very rare but can and must be avoided. The principles of the assessment and management of spinal injuries are as follows:

1. A basic understanding of the bony stability conferred by normal spinal anatomy
2. A concept of how this stability is changed by injury
3. Ability to decipher how and when to provide stability by external support or surgery

II. Definitions

The spinal column extends from the foramen magnum to the tip of the coccyx. Although injuries to the sacrum and coccyx are usually considered with pelvic fractures, they are not considered in this chapter. Although initially spanning the whole length of the spinal column, differential growth of the bony and neural elements brings the adult spinal cord to finish at the level of L1. The cauda equina extends below this level, but represents part of the peripheral nervous system and, as such, is more resilient to injury. Throughout their length, however, the neural elements are at risk of direct trauma, traction, or damage to their blood supply. The result can produce a variety of clinical pictures of neurologic damage (specifically considered elsewhere). From the practical point of view, a spinal column injury is considered stable or unstable, and the neurologic injury is distinguished as none (intact), incomplete (partial), complete, or progressive. The overall effect of large forces applied to the spine is often focused at multiple sites. The identification of any spinal injury makes it mandatory to assess fully the whole spine because often a second or further injury has occurred that can be more important clinically.

Throughout the spine, stability is defined as "the ability of the spinal column to withstand normal physiologic forces without significant deformity."

III.   Assessment and Diagnostic Methods

As with all clinical situations, the overall management of the injured patient follows accepted advanced trauma life support (ATLS) guidelines. Whenever a mechanism or presentation suggests the possibility of a spinal injury, full manual cervical protection with manual inline immobilization or collar, bolsters and tape, or strapping is essential. The specific assessment of a spinal injury then follows standard clinical methods involving a history, examination, and special tests. The technical nature of modern medicine emphasizes the latter with early provision of computed tomography (CT) and even magnetic resonance imaging (MRI) scans in many centers. These special tests, however, cannot be interpreted out of the clinical context. A history of the mechanism of injury and local spinal symptoms is essential, as is a history of transient and permanent neurologic symptoms. On examination, a documented initial neurologic assessment is invaluable as is an assessment of local tenderness or even frank deformity. The posterior aspect of the spine should be examined when the patient is log rolled to determine the presence of local tenderness or even a gap or step in the spinous processes. The latter will indicate posterior ligamentous damage that is often part of the major injury pattern and poorly assessed by plain radiographs. Plain x-ray films provide invaluable information on spinal alignment and go a long way to exclude major injury. The films of the cervical spine, however, must include the C7-T1 junction. This often proves difficult to obtain in the clinical setting. Pull-down x-ray study, swimmer's views, and oblique views that show the facet joint alignment are all useful. In practice, injuries in the C1/2 region and cervicothoracic junction are difficult to define without CT scanning. Today, access to a fully reconstructible fine section CT scan of the entire cervical spine is the gold standard for bony injury. On occasion, assessment of the spine to exclude a ligamentous or disk injury becomes important. On these occasions, stress screening by an experienced surgeon or MRI scanning is of great value, although it can produce practical difficulties in the acute situation.

IV.   Spinal Clearance

The most common critical issue is clearance of the cervical spine so that the protection of the collar, bolsters, and tape initially applied can be removed. Early removal is desirable because collars and backboards themselves cause significant morbidity. This ranges from inconvenience to dangerous. A poorly applied collar, on rare occasions, can increase intracranial pressure (ICP), whereas pressure effects commonly can produce sores on the scalp or chin. Leaving patients on a backboard for protracted periods can easily produce sacral sores that cause significant morbidity. Many protocols for cervical spine clearance have been published. In the conscious patient with no distracting injury and a normal clinical examination, the spine can be easily cleared and protection removed. If clinical clearance is not possible, radiologic examination should follow the scheme described above with CT scanning of C1-2 and C7-T1 as a minimum. Each radiologic investigation reduces the chance that a spinal injury is present but often the risk of ligamentous instability in the presence of normal radiographs is raised. This is rare and often the patient can be clinically cleared when able to be cooperative. If this is not a short-term prospect, additional investigation may be required by screening traction radiographs using an image intensifier or an MRI scan to exclude ligamentous instability (**Table 33-1**).

V. Indications for Surgery

Surgical management of spinal injuries is primarily directed at restoring mechanical stability to the spinal column. This has major advantages for nursing and mobilization of the seriously injured patient and facilitates healing of the spine in a close to anatomic position. In most cases, neurologic issues are determined at the time of injury and the presence of a neurologic defect is not in its own right an indication for surgery unless it is progressing.

Table 33-1. Simplified cervical spine clearance protocol in patients with multiple trauma

---

This protocol only applies to patients with no signs or symptoms of possible spinal cord injury. Both bones and ligaments must be cleared, but not necessarily at the same time. Often, the ligaments can be cleared by a negative clinical examination (**NCE**) when the patient has become sober or has recovered sufficiently from a concussion.

TO CLEAR THE BONES

NCE[a]

All others

–Spiral computed tomography with or without of collar lateral[b]

OR

–Adequate five-view cervical spine series[b]

TO CLEAR THE LIGAMENTS

Patient is awake, alert, and sober and without significant distracting injury:

–NCE[a]

OR

–Active flexion-extension views (typically, with pain or distracting injury in those whose bones have been cleared).

All others

If clinical suspicion is high: passive flexion-extension views under floroscopic control by attending surgeon, orthopedist, or radiologist[b]

If clinical suspicion is low: neck magnetic resonance imaging[b]

---

[a] A NCE can only be performed if the patient is sober, awake, alert, and without significant distracting injuries. It requires that the alert patient deny significant neck pain, physical examination reveal no significant tenderness of the cervical spine, and the patient is able to move the neck through a full voluntary range of motion without significant pain.

[b] NO radiology study of the cervical spine is considered normal until an interpretation is signed by an attending on the CAS system or on the chart. Until such is available, the cervical spine is considered NOT clear and immobilization should be continued.

NOTE: When evaluating seriously injured multiple trauma patients, it is reasonable to forgo the in-collar lateral (part of the traditional "trauma series") if a helical computed tomography scan of the cervical spine and subsequent out-of-collar lateral is planned.

Spinal stabilization will usually significantly improve the overall management of the patient with spinal cord injury, but the neurologic injury itself is rarely influenced. The only hard indication for surgery is the presence of secondary deterioration of neurologic function associated with mechanical instability (**Table 33-2**).

VI.   Cervical Spine

The cervical spine is essentially divided into two regions: C1 and C2 are referred to as the *axial* cervical spine because of their unique anatomy, whereas the segment from C3 to C7 represents the *subaxial* cervical spine. The axial segment has a special articulation based on the odontoid peg that confers a large range of rotation but also produces characteristic injuries including the C1 ring fractures, (Jefferson), specific patterns of odontoid peg fractures, and specific pedicle (Hangman's) fractures of C2. The subaxial cervical spine has common features along the whole length from C3 to C7 and then blends into the upper thoracic area. It is essentially built as three columns of bone: the vertebral bodies, articulating through the intervertebral disks, and two lateral columns, articulating with the obliquely orientated facet joints. The whole structure is held together by the intervertebral disks and by strong ligaments. These include the anterior and posterior longitudinal ligaments at the front and back of the vertebral bodies, the interspinous and supraspinous ligaments between the spinous processes, and the capsule around the facet joints. Different degrees and directions of trauma produce particular injuries, based on the local anatomy and intrinsic stability of the spine. Understanding any injury depends on knowledge of the position and function of the ligaments and bony structure together with an assessment of the deforming forces and what may then have failed. With all cervical spine injuries, especially with high axial injuries, it is essential not to miss an associated second injury because this may be the site of the more important instability.

VII.   Cervical Spine Injury Patterns
A.   Axial Cervical Spine
1.   Jefferson Fractures
Axial force on the head is often transmitted to the upper cervical spine, where the shape of the occipital

Table 33-2.   Indications for surgical management of spinal injuries

Nerve Injury Bony Injury	Intact	Partial	Complete	Progressive
Stable	Non-operative	Non-operative	Non-operative	Non-operative
Unstable	Operative (general care issues)	Operative (general care issues)	Operative (general care issues)	Operative (for neurologic function)

and C1-2 condyles convert this to a force that can explode the ring of C1 away from the spinal cord. Major spinal cord injury at this level is not survivable because the essential central centers are damaged and respiration compromised. Unless devastating force is applied, however, the spinal cord elements are normally uninjured and the issue is the common association with other injuries in the spine and local stability. Normally, a halo orthosis is applied to hold position during the healing process, which likely takes approximately 3 months. As this is a bony injury, however, healing is normally reliable without surgical intervention.

2.   Odontoid Peg Fractures
The odontoid peg is the body of C1 that has become fused to the body of C2 during development. It is susceptible to injury by angular forces that are often concentrated at its base. These fractures have been classified into type 1, 2, and 3. Type 1 is extremely rare and represents a fracture of the very tip of the peg. Stability and treatment usually are associated with other related injuries. Type 2 and 3 injuries are formally differentiated on a CT scan. The type 2 injury is the greater problem because the local forces are concentrated at the fracture site and considerable risk of avascular necrosis exists because of the limited local blood supply to the small peg fragment. Surgical treatment is indicated for displaced type 2 odontoid peg fractures. Surgical stability can be accomplished with direct screw (anterior) or indirect atlantoaxial fusion (posterior) techniques. The space available for the cord is maximal at C1-C2 to accommodate the normal range of rotational motion, so some degree of neurologic protection is available.

3.   Hangman's Fractures
The other well-recognized fracture of the axial cervical spine is commonly known as a "Hangman's fracture." This is a pedicle fracture of the posterior arch of C2. If displaced, specific stability issues rely on the integrity of the C2-C3 disc and associated facet joints, further classifying Hangman's fractures into types 1 through 3, the latter being the most unstable. Initially, this injury should be considered unstable and referred for appropriate stabilization, usually with a halo ring and vest. If minimally displaced, simple reduction and reduction and stabilization will be adequate treatment. As a bony injury, the pedicle fracture should heal with immobilization, although this can take 3 months. Displaced grade 2 or 3 Hangman's fractures are often made worse by traction and may need open reduction.

B. Subaxial Cervical Spine Injuries
1.   Cervical Body Fractures
The cervical bodies, which comprise the main axial structure of the spine, can be fractured by axial or angular forces. Isolated fractures (no posterior ligament

injury) without significant displacement are usually treated nonoperatively in a collar. A common trap is the teardrop fracture of the anterior margin of the body. This can be part of a bursting injury associated with pure axial compression but more often is associated with distraction of the anterior column. As such, it represents instability or the anterior longitudinal ligament complex and, possibly, a subtle sign of significant instability. Further assessment with scans or dynamic tests (e.g., flexion-extension views) should be considered.

2. Lateral Mass Fractures

The lateral masses are essentially the two columns of bone associated with the relatively horizontally orientated facet joints. Isolated fractures of the lateral masses are common but difficult to define without CT scanning. Although the facet joints are often involved, they are usually stable and can be treated in a hard collar alone.

3. Facet Joint Dislocations

Instability of the cervical spine is often associated with dislocations of one or both facet joints. As these are more horizontally orientated than in lower areas of the spine, dislocation without fracture is often seen. On occasion, facets partially dislocate or "perch" on the top of the inferior facet. Single facet dislocations are associated with a rotational and flexion force. They are usually initially suggested by the appearance of a small step in the anterior vertebral line (approximately one third the width of a vertebral body) and differential rotation of the facet joints will be seen on both anteroposterior (AP) and lateral x-ray films. The oblique views, which show the facet alignment, are diagnostic as are CT scans. Bifacet dislocations are more pure flexion injuries. On x-ray film, they are identified by the presence of a forward step of approximately half the width of a vertebral body on the lateral x-ray. Both injuries are considered unstable and require reduction. Manipulation can be performed with or without anesthesia. The latter is preferable because it allows direct communication with the patient to assess neurologic function during reduction. Under anesthesia, monitoring is limited before recovery. Occasionally, these injuries are associated with damage to the intervertebral disc that can then be prolapsed posteriorly by reduction and cause additional neurologic damage. Accordingly, MRI scanning is indicated before reduction and is mandatory if a general anesthesia is planned. I prefer to reduce these injures with traction applied through a halo orthosis and without anesthesia. Flexion and rotation can be applied progressively until the dislocated facet is distracted and then lifted back into place. Stability can then be maintained with the halo orthosis or by operative means.

C. Instability with Minimal or No Bony Injury

A rare potential exists for normal radiologic investigations with ligamentous instability in the cervical spine. This possibility is accommodated in spinal clearance protocols by an emphasis on clinical examination of the conscious patient and MRI scanning or flexion-extension views when it is not possible to clear the spine clinically.

D. Thoracic Spine

The thoracic spine tends to sustain simple wedge fractures or complex complete fracture dislocations with significant spinal cord compromise. The more simple injuries are additionally splinted by the ribs and usually need symptomatic support only. The overall structure of the chest wall creates a clear association between sternal fractures, thoracic spine injuries, and aortic injuries, such that a high index of suspicion is essential. Complete dislocations are significant injuries that are often associated with serious neurologic injuries. Surgical management follows the basic principles outlined above.

E. Thoraco-lumbar Spine

Thoracolumbar fractures occur at the high-risk area between the relatively stiff thoracic spine and the more flexible lumbar segment. Here, the segments become more lumbar, the overall shape is lordosis with a posterior axis of rotation, the bodies become larger, and the facet joints change to a more vertical orientation. The common fracture mechanisms, fall (axial compression), acute flexion or flexion and rotation, and the local bony and ligamentous anatomy produce well-recognized failure patterns. Some controversy continues to exist among spine surgeons with regard to the functional mechanics of failure, essentially whether the spine should be considered as a two- or three-column structure. It is essential, however, to fully assess both sides of an injury by clinical or radiologic means. An x-ray study (or CT scan) produce the best assessment of the anterior vertebral bodies and allow definition of the specific bony anatomy as well as overall spinal alignment. To complete an evaluation of the local structures, however, a clinical assessment of the posterior ligaments is essential. Posterior injury can be identified by careful palpation of the posterior elements and supraspinous ligaments when the patients is log rolled; local swelling, a step, gap, or focal tenderness may be identified. The essential fracture patterns are wedge, burst, flexion or seatbelt (chance), or fracture dislocations.

1. Wedge Fractures

Wedge fractures represent failure of the anterior column of the vertebral body without other damage. No loss of posterior body height and no injury to the posterior ligaments are seen. The force applied is axial, with forward flexion, and results in a kyphotic angulation. The limited damage to one column means that acceptable stability remains and symptomatic treatment with an orthosis designed to resist forward flexion is all that is required.

2. Burst Fractures

The burst fracture represents the next stage of fracture after the wedge. Usually after a fall, the whole vertebral body fails in compression. The feature defining a wedge from a burst fracture is damage to the posterior wall of the vertebral body (middle column). In a wedge fracture, the height of the posterior body is maintained (same as adjacent vertebrae), whereas in the burst fracture it is reduced. In a burst fracture, the bony failure is usually focused on the superior endplate where flexion and compressive forces push the disk into the vertebral body below it. The result is a posterior-superior body fragment, which is retropulsed back into the spinal canal and can cause neurologic damage. This fragment can usually be seen on a lateral x-ray study, but is more clearly seen on the axial cuts on the CT scan. The way the vertebral body explodes in a burst fracture is also seen in the posterior elements when a vertical split in the lamina and widening of the pedicles (seen on the AP x-ray study) also are seen. The association of burst fractures with neurologic damage is variable and associated with the initial energy of injury rather than the recoil position of the fragments seen on the presenting x-ray study. These fractures are relatively unstable, but all of the ligamentous elements are intact.

Burst fractures can be managed either nonoperatively in a thoracolumbar-sacral orthosis (TLSO) or by direct operative means. The individual indications in the absence of neurologic issues are controversial. The advantages of operative stabilization are early mobility and healing in a better anatomic position. It is assumed that this will produce earlier mobilization and less long-term discomfort but is unproved. Operative management usually involves posterior instrumentation and distraction of the burst level. This produces tension on the intact longitudinal ligaments and realigns the body fragments. Distraction also produces a bony defect where the body was crushed. Grafting of this defect via the pedicle is often performed in an attempt to resist late kyphotic collapse. The development of more functional implants to replace the anterior column of the spine has allowed direct anterior surgery addressing the bony defect itself and even the development of less-invasive (laparoscopic) techniques for their insertion. Initial results from these techniques are promising, but many surgeons prefer to avoid the less familiar anterior approaches. If direct canal clearance before stabilization is required, then an anterior approach is indicated. Following surgical stabilization, the patient usually still wears a TLSO as a postural reminder, but is able to mobilize as pain allows. From the general trauma care and nursing point of view, operative stabilization has a great advantage, particularly in a polytrauma patient.

3. Flexion or Seatbelt (Chance) Injuries

Acute spinal flexion can both disrupt the posterior tension structures as well as the anterior compression structures. When this happens, the spine is unstable in flexion because an opening posteriorly can occur. The fracture plane can be variable at the extremes, passing entirely through bone or entirely through soft tissue. The instability is the same but, rarely, the latter can be a diagnostic problem if the injury recoils back to the normal position. In this situation (comparable to the purely ligament instability in the cervical spine), the clinical identification of posterior signs is essential. This injury is stable in extension; if displaced and associated with significant loss of the anterior column or predominately through ligament, it should be treated operatively. The primary aim of surgery is to replace the posterior tension band. The term "seatbelt fracture" is also applied to these flexion injuries and refers to the injury associated with the use of a lap strap only seatbelt.

4. Fracture Dislocations

Complete disruption of all three spinal columns results in multidirectional instability, often with facet dislocation and significant neurologic compromise. As the spinal cord ends at the thoracolumbar segment, some neurologic function in the cauda equina can be maintained but significant instability is produced. In the acute situation, general care dominates the clinical picture with log roll precautions before surgical stabilization. Facet joint dislocations carry significance in the lumbar area because the vertical facets cannot dislocate or be reduced without significant distraction occurring. Surgical reduction is achieved by facet resection to avoid additional distraction and stabilization is usually achieved by a "rod long, fuse short" philosophy. In many cases, anterior and posterior stabilization are required.

SELECTED READING

Anderson LD, D'Alonzo TR. Fractures of the odontoid process of the axis. *J Bone Joint Surg* 1974;56A:1663.

Denis F. The three-column spine and its significance in the classification of acute thoracolumbar spinal injuries. *Spine* 1988;8:817–827.

Holdsworth SF. Review article. Fractures, dislocations, and fracture-dislocations of the spine. *J Bone Joint Surg* 1970;52A:1534–1551.

Levine AM, Edwards CC. The management of traumatic spondylolisthesis of the axis. *J Bone Joint Surg* 1985;67A:217–226.

Orthopedic Trauma 2: Pelvic Fractures

Mark Vrahas, MD, and David Joseph, MD

I. Introduction

Pelvic fractures are a harbinger of high-energy trauma. The normal young pelvis is structurally stable and substantial energy is required to disrupt it. In an elderly person, however, the bones are often much weaker and low-energy fractures do occur. A disrupted pelvis in a young person should warn the trauma team that the patient has incurred a substantial impact. The pelvic fracture itself can result in exsanguinating blood loss and can also give clues to what else might be injured.

II. Anatomy

To understand pelvic injuries, consider the pelvis a ring. The pelvis is stable when the ring is intact and unstable when it is disrupted. The degree of instability depends on the structures that have been disrupted.

The pelvis ring is composed of three bones (two innominate bones and the sacrum) connected by strong ligamentous structures. Anteriorly, the pubic symphyseal ligament connects the bones. Posteriorly, several strong ligaments connect the ilia to the sacrum. Together, these are called the "posterior sacroiliac complex." The ligaments that connect the ilium to the sacrum are sometimes called the strongest ligaments in the body. The ligaments that maintain the posterior sacroiliac complex are critical for pelvic stability because they are necessary for weightbearing.

It is instructive to consider what happens to the pelvis as these ligaments are sequentially divided. If the pubic symphyseal ligaments are cut, the pelvis can open like a book gapping at the symphysis. Traditionally, the limit of opening is thought to be approximately 2.5 cm. The anterior sacroiliac ligaments prevent further opening. Because the entire posterior sacroiliac complex is intact, no translation can occur at the sacroiliac joint. Cutting the anterior sacroiliac ligaments allows the pelvis to open even further—to approximately 8 cm. With the anterior sacroiliac ligaments disrupted, the sacroiliac joint can spread open anteriorly, but because the posterior sacroiliac ligaments are still intact, no vertical displacements are possible. Finally, cutting the posterior sacroiliac ligaments completely destabilizes the pelvis.

Pelvic stability is generally discussed by considering which ligaments have been disrupted. Keep in mind, however, that a ligament can be functionally disrupted by breaking the bone next to it. For example, a complete sacral fracture does not disrupt the ligamentous posterior complex, but it does make the posterior pelvis unstable. More importantly, remember that progressive disruption of the pelvic ring requires progressively increasing energy. Thus, the more unstable the pelvis, the higher the injury's energy.

III. Mechanism of Injury

It is often difficult to know the exact mechanism of injury. A patient thrown from a car can incur forces from multiple different directions. Nevertheless, assumptions about the predominant vector are based on pelvic displacements. When the pelvis is collapsed, it is assumed to have been hit from the side, creating a lateral compression injury. When the pelvis is open like a book, disrupting force is assumed to have come in the anterior posterior direction. When one or both of the ilia is displaced superiorly, a vertical sheer mechanism is assumed to have caused the displacement. When no predominant pattern of displacement is seem, the injury is categorized as a combined mechanical injury.

IV. Classification

All current classification systems are based on pelvic stability as originally purposed by Tile. A fractured pelvis is classified by type:

Type A: completely stable
Type B: partially stable
Type C: completely unstable

Type A fractures (completely stable) are most common. Usually, they result from a lateral compression force, which causes rami fractures and a compression fracture of the sacrum posteriorly. In type B fractures (partially stable), a disruption of the anterior pelvis and a partial disruption of the posterior pelvis are seen. The pelvis can open and close like a book, but because the posterior sacroiliac ligaments remain intact, no vertical displacements are possible. In type C fractures, both the anterior pelvis and the entire posterior sacroiliac complex are disrupted. The disrupted pelvic bones are free to displace in any direction.

The Young Burgess classification, which considers both pelvic stability and mechanism of injury, can be useful in predicting the patient's associated injuries and potential to bleed. In this system, pelvic injuries are classified by mechanism of injury and stability (**Fig. 34-1**). Stability indicates the energy of the injury, and the mechanism tells what associated structures might be damaged. For example, injuries that open the pelvis like a book not only disrupt the bony pelvis, but also tear the pelvic floor. Thus, the pelvic venous plexus is at risk. The more unstable the pelvis, the more likely these structures are to be damaged. Conversely, a lateral compression mechanism causes the pelvis to collapse so the floor is not ripped. With this mechanism, luminal injuries are more likely to be seen. Although these fractures can bleed, heavy blood loss can usually be attributed to a source other than the pelvis.

V. Evaluation

A. Pelvic Disruption

A pelvic disruption, especially in a young person, indicates a high-energy injury and mandates that the patient be evaluated as a multiple trauma victim using the standard advanced trauma life support (ATLS) protocol. A standard anteroposterior (AP) pelvic radiograph is an important part of the primary survey and helps with the overall patient evaluation. With the current generation of fast, high-quality computed tomography (CT) scans, a tendency is seen to skip the plain radiographs and move directly to CT. Unless three-dimensional reconstructions are immediately

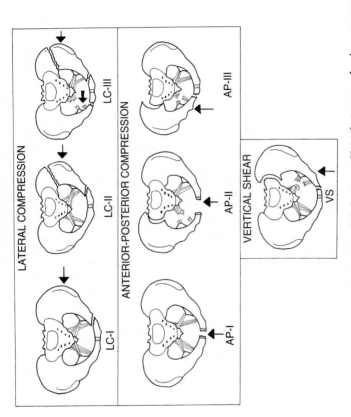

Figure 34-1. Young Burgess classification of pelvic fractures. Note that any mechanism can result in a stable or unstable pelvis. Vertical sheer fractures are completely unstable by definition.

available, more information is obtained from the plain films. Similarly, surgeons sometimes skip the AP pelvis radiograph because the pelvis does not "feel" unstable. In reality, it is extremely difficult to determine pelvic stability or mechanism of injury based on examination. Moreover, the AP pelvis radiograph is essential in the evaluation of patient with blunt trauma and should not be eliminated.

Even though a plain pelvic radiograph is essential for the initial management of the patient, it is not sufficient for the definitive pelvic management. It is difficult to determine the exact nature of the posterior injury from a plain radiograph. For this, a CT scan is essential. Because the pelvis is a ring, it rarely breaks in just one spot. A disruption in the anterior pelvis indicates that some injury has occurred in the back as well. This injury can be significant although it cannot be seen on plain films. Thus, a CT scan is mandatory in all young people where a disruption is noted in the anterior pelvis.

B. Evaluation of the Anteroposterior Pelvis
The primary survey AP pelvis should be viewed with an eye toward answering two questions:

1. What is the stability of the pelvic ring?
2. What was the mechanism of injury?

On the whole, these are easily answered by careful review of even a poor plain pelvic film. First, examine the overall symmetry of the pelvis. With the spine in the midline, the iliac wings and the obturator foramen should look similar on both sides. An open book type mechanism causes one or both ilia to rotate externally (open, like a book). A lateral compression mechanism causes the pelvis to collapse. When the pelvis opens like a book (open book mechanism), a displacement has to have occurred in the anterior pelvis. Most often, this is seen as a widening of the pubic symphysis or widening at fracture in the pubic rami. When the pelvis collapses from a lateral compression injury, the anterior rami usually fracture. Displacements of the anterior pelvis >2 cm indicate at least a partial instability. Complete disruptions of the posterior sacroiliac complex are indicated by translations at the sacroiliac joint.

VI. Initial Management
A. Airway, Breathing, and Circulation
Management priorities in a patient with a pelvic fracture are no different then those in a patient with a splenic injury: secure airway and breathing and then diagnose and manage shock. Any patient with a pelvic fracture will have lost some blood and the possibility exists of continued blood loss into the retroperitoneum. It is important to remember, however, that even if the patient is bleeding into the pelvis, bleeding may also be occurring somewhere else. When evaluating the patient, it is important to consider all potential sources of bleeding and not to be distracted by the possibility that the pelvis may be bleeding.

The most effective method for dealing with the bleeding pelvis is controversial. One school of thought suggests that it is most effective to provide tamponade by closing and stabilizing the pelvis using external fixation. Another school believes angiographic embolization is the most effective solution. Although several papers support both these approaches, the studies are small and poorly controlled. Nevertheless, it is worth reviewing this literature.

B.   Angiographic Embolization

Several studies have suggested that angiographic embolization is effective. Recently, Bassam et al. published a focused comparison of emergent orthopedic external fixation with angiographic embolization as first-line treatment for severe pelvic fractures. Hemodynamically unstable patients were managed either with external fixation or angiographic embolization. After intervention, both treatment groups required only an additional 2 units of blood. Nevertheless, the authors deemed external fixation to have failed in 50% of the patients. Generally, angiographic embolization was considered a success, although it is not clear how this determination was made. More importantly, three patients in the external fixation group developed significant buttocks and thigh hematomas and one of these patients died from sepsis secondary to breakdown of the buttocks followed by severe infection. None of the patients in the angiographic embolization group developed significant buttock hematomas. The hematomas likely developed from disrupted superior gluteal arteries. Thus, the study suggests that angiographic embolization is at least useful in controlling this artery.

C.   External Fixation

Several studies suggest that rapidly applied external fixators help to control blood loss and decrease all-cause mortality and shock. Riemer et al. compared mortality rates at a major trauma center before and after a protocol of external fixation for unstable pelvic fractures was introduced. Mortality rates in pelvic ring injury patients fell from 26% before the protocol was introduced to 6% once it was established. Because the study looks at patients over two successive time periods, however, it does not take into account many other things that might have changed in the management of the patients.

External fixation is believed to provide tamponade by decreasing the pelvic volume and, thereby, the space for blood loss. When the pelvis displaces, the volume of the true pelvis increases by the cube of the radius. Thus, reducing the pelvis necessarily decreases the volume. It is unlikely, however, that the true pelvis is the only space available for blood loss. Moss and Bircher evaluated volume changes in the true pelvis that occurred with progressive displacements in the pelvic ring using a cadaver model. On the whole, volume increases were less than previously assumed, and were far less than the usual replacement requirements for major fractures.

Similarly, Grimm et al. demonstrated that the space for blood loss with pelvic fractures is much greater than the true pelvis. Using nine unembalmed cadavers, they measured the intrapelvic pressure of fluid introduced through a catheterized femoral vein, both with and without simulated pelvic fractures. The intact pelves required 8 L of fluid to increase pressure to 50 mm Hg. Pressures in the disrupted pelvis did not reach this level even after 20 L of fluid had been introduced. Applying external fixators generated only a small increase in retroperitoneal pressures. Dissection revealed that fluid had not only filled the true pelvis, but also filled the abdominal retroperitoneum. Dissection also revealed that the pelvic floor had been disrupted, thus allowing fluid to escape into the perineum and the thighs.

Factors other than tamponade may explain the apparent clinical benefit of external fixation in some circumstances. It has been suggested that stabilizing the pelvis decreases the motion between bony fragments and allows bony surfaces to clot. Biomechanical evidence, however, clearly shows that external fixation does little to stabilize the posterior pelvis. Thus, although external fixation can provide useful stabilization for isolated anterior injuries, it probably does not prevent significant bony motion in cases of pelvic fractures that are unstable posteriorly. This has led to the development of clamps designed to stabilize the posterior pelvis (e.g., Ganz clamp). Little experience has been had with these clamps and reported complications are high. In recent years, the use of external fixators has declined in favor of simply wrapping with a sheet or other noninvasive binders, in part because of the time required to apply a fixator and in part because of complications associated with them (e.g., pin-site infection). If the goal is simply to close the pelvis, a sheet effectively achieves this. The sheet is wrapped around the patient at the level of the trochanters, pulled tight, and then fastened in place anteriorly with a towel clip.

D.   Management Protocols

In October of 2000, the Orthopaedic Trauma Association and the American Association for the Surgery of Trauma conducted a symposium in an attempt to reach some consensus on how a bleeding pelvis should be managed. Although no consensus was reached, the participants did generally agree on some currently accepted strategies. These are summarized in the algorithm in **Figure 34-2.**

VII.   Authors' Preferred Management

At the Massachusetts General Hospital, we follow general guidelines for the management of patients with pelvic fractures. Each patient is managed by standard ATLS protocols. A pelvic radiograph is taken as part of the primary survey and the management of shock is started immediately. We are particularly careful to control those factors that can contribute to a coagulopathy (e.g., hypothermia). If the pelvic radiograph demonstrates a pelvic fracture with significant displacement, a sheet is wrapped around the patient's pelvis for reduction and stabilization. The sheet is applied at the level of the patient's greater trochanters and clamped or tied once pulled tight around the patient. While the workup and search for other potential sources of blood loss continues, fluid and blood

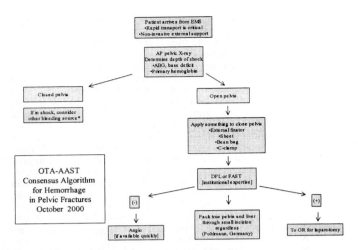

Figure 34-2. Flowchart for the management of pelvic fracture. (From meeting transcript, Orthopaedic Trauma Association–American Association for the Surgery of Trauma combined annual meeting, October 2000, San Antonio, Texas; available at http://www.hwbf.org/ota/s2k/panel/pfset.htm.) Accessed April 2003.

requirements are monitored to determine if the patient is continuing to bleed. Once we are confident the blood loss has stopped, we feel comfortable in removing the sheet. If blood loss continues and no source other than the pelvis is identified, the patient is taken to angiography for embolization. If the patient requires a laparotomy for any reason, the orthopedic surgeons proceed to the operating room with the general surgeons and stabilize the pelvis surgically. In instances wherein massive blood loss is occurring from the pelvis, the pelvis is stabilized and packed. The packs are left in place to be removed once the bleeding has stopped.

VIII. Definitive Management
Definitive management of pelvic injuries is beyond the scope of this chapter. An unstable pelvis, however, requires definitive stabilization. Although this is not an urgent procedure, we prefer to do it as early as possible, which allows early mobilization of the patient and can contribute to the patient's overall recovery.

IX. Summary
Patients with pelvic fractures should be managed by standard ATLS protocols, paying particular attention to the pelvis as a potential source of blood loss. Early on, determine the stability of the pelvis by pelvic radiograph. The degree of instability indicates the energy of the injury and helps in evaluating the risk of other injuries. The greater the instability, the higher the energy of the insult. Be particularly concerned if the pelvis is opened like a book or if one of the wings is displaced vertically. This situation suggests that the pelvic floor has been damaged and increases the likelihood that the pelvis is a major source of blood loss. Along with fluid resuscitation, the initial management of the unstable

pelvis should include some method of temporary pelvic stabilization. We prefer to use a sheet wrapped around the patient at the level of the greater trochanters. Further acute management can include external fixation, angiographic embolization, or both, depending on the resources of the particular institution. Most importantly, both the general surgeon and the orthopedic surgeon should be involved early on so that a combined treatment plan can be formulated.

SELECTED READING

Agolini SF, Shah K, Jaffe J, et al. Arterial embolization is a rapid and effective technique for controlling pelvic fracture hemorrhage. *J Trauma* 1997;43(3):395–399.

Barlow B, Rottenberg RW, Santulli TV. Angiographic diagnosis and treatment of bleeding by selective embolization following pelvic fracture in children. *J Pediatr Surg* 1975;10(6):939–942.

Bassam D, Cephas GA, Ferguson KA, et al. A protocol for the initial management of unstable pelvic fractures. *Am Surg* 1998;64(9): 862–867.

Burgess AR, et al. Pelvic ring disruptions: effective classification system and treatment protocols. *J Trauma* 1990;30(7):848–856.

Dalal SA, et al. Pelvic fracture in multiple trauma: classification by mechanism is key to pattern of organ injury, resuscitative requirements, and outcome. *J Trauma* 1989;29(7):981–1000.

Ganz R, Krushell RJ, Jakob RP, et al. Anterior versus posterior provisional fixation in the unstable pelvis. A biomechanical comparison. *Clin Orthop* 1995;(310):245–251.

Gordon RL, Fast A, Aner H, et al. Control of massive retroperitoneal bleeding associated with pelvic fractures by angiographic embolization. *Isr J Med Sci* 1983;19(2):185–188.

Grimm MR, Vrahas MS, Thomas KA. Pressure-volume characteristics of the intact and disrupted pelvic retroperitoneum. *J Trauma* 1998;44(3):454–459.

Moss MC, Bircher MD. Volume changes within the true pelvis during disruption of the pelvic ring—where does the haemorrhage go? *Injury* 1996;27(Suppl 1):A21–A23.

Palmer S, Fairbank AC, Bircher M. Surgical complications and implications of external fixation of pelvic fractures. *Injury* 1997;28(9–10): 649–653.

Panetta T, Sclafani SJA, Goldstein AS, et al. Percutaneous transcatheter embolization for massive bleeding from pelvic fractures. *J Trauma* 1985;25:1021–1029.

Pennal GF. Pelvic disruption: principles of management. *Clin Orthop* 1980;151:56–64.

Perez JV, Hughes TM, Bowers K. Angiographic embolization in pelvic fracture. *Injury* 1998;29(3):187–191.

Riemer BL, Butterfield SL, Diamond DL, et al. Acute mortality associated with injuries to the pelvic ring: the role of early patient mobilization and external fixation. *J Trauma* 1993;35(5):671–675; discussion 676–677.

Simonian PT, Routt ML Jr, Harrington RM, et al. The pelvic C-clamp for the emergency treatment of unstable pelvic ring injuries. A report on clinical experience of 30 cases. *Injury* 1996;27(Suppl 1): S-A38–A45.

Tile M, Pennal GF. Pelvic disruption: principles of management. *Clin Orthop* 1980;151:56–64.

Orthopedic Trauma 3: Extremity Fractures

David W. Lhowe, MD

I. Introduction

Although rarely life threatening, extremity injuries are potentially limb threatening and extremely common. The spectrum ranges from simple sprains and contusions to severe composite injuries of bone and soft tissues. Extremity injuries, a frequent component of multiple trauma, are sometimes neglected in the initial stages of evaluation and treatment, occasionally with detrimental consequences. Competent trauma care includes the initial assessment and stabilization of injured extremities, proceeding to definitive care, where appropriate, or working in conjunction with orthopedic, vascular, and plastic surgical specialists for more complicated injuries.

A. Examination Principles

A thorough examination of the injured extremity can be quickly accomplished. *Visual inspection* for deformity, swelling, discoloration, or skin break is accomplished simultaneously with *gentle palpation* to localize tenderness, soft tissue defects, or crepitus, and to assess pulses and skin temperature. The initial *neurologic examination,* which should emphasize light touch sensibility and the presence of active voluntary contraction, can be accomplished with minimal movement and discomfort. *Manipulation* can then proceed to test for joint instability, but it is guided by the prior findings. *Specific maneuvers* performed by the patient can then follow (e.g., voluntary straight-leg raising against gravity).

B. Diagnostic Testing

1. Plain Radiographs

Plain radiographs remain the most valuable initial diagnostic study when fracture or dislocation is suspected. They must be obtained in two orthogonal views. When the injury lies between two joints (thigh, lower leg, forearm), the films must include the joints above and below the site of injury. **Computed tomography (CT) scans** are a valuable adjunct to plain films for fractures involving certain joint surfaces, particularly the acetabulum, and can help clarify if a hip or shoulder joint is completely reduced when plain films are equivocal. **Magnetic resonance imaging (MRI) scans** are rarely used in the primary evaluation of extremity trauma. They are the most sensitive method, however, for detecting certain occult injuries such as femoral neck fracture in the setting of hip pain with normal x-ray study or an Achilles tendon rupture where examination is equivocal. MRI of an extremity is used most frequently to evaluate suspected meniscal or rotator cuff injuries. It is usually performed after an initial period of observation when symptoms persist. There may or may not be a history of antecedent trauma.

2. Compartment Pressure Measurement

Compartment pressure measurement using a hand-held device is valuable in assessing a swollen extremity where elevated compartment pressures are suspected.

3. Bacteriologic Cultures

Bacteriologic cultures are routinely obtained in the presence of an established septic process (abscess, draining sinus), but they have *not* proved useful in the setting of acute trauma (open fracture). Data obtained from swabbing the exposed bone in an open fracture does *not* predict the potential infecting organism nor help guide selection of antibiotic prophylaxis.

C. Treatment Principles

1. Severe Deformities

Severe deformities need to be realigned promptly. Vascular compromise and tenting of skin over prominent fracture fragments (or normal bony prominences) can rapidly produce ischemic injury to skin, muscle, or nerve. With a patient under adequate analgesia, a gentle axial pull on the deformed extremity will often improve alignment and promptly restore perfusion to the compromised areas. If unsuccessful, repeated manipulation should not be performed until x-ray films are reviewed and consultation with an orthopedic surgeon is obtained.

2. Antibiotic Prophylaxis

Antibiotic prophylaxis for all open fractures and severely contaminated soft tissue injuries should be given intravenously (1 g cefazolin). In cases of suspected agricultural contamination, four million units of aqueous penicillin G should be added as prophylaxis for Clostridial sepsis. Aminoglycoside coverage with gentamicin (80 to 100 mg) is often added in grade III open fractures, but the evidence supporting this practice is minimal. For injuries in need of emergent operative treatment (e.g., open fractures), the wound should be carefully documented at the initial examination and then covered with a damp gauze dressing that should not be removed until the patient is in the operating room.

3. Immobilize

Immobilize the injured extremity to provide comfort and prevent further injury. Circumferential wraps must not be too tight, and particular care is needed over bony prominences, which are frequent sites of blistering. Unyielding circumferential casts should be avoided in acute trauma and any immobilization used must not prevent periodic reexamination.

4. Elevate and Apply Ice
Elevate and apply ice to the affected area. A general rule is to apply the ice for 20 minutes at a time, with 10 minutes between applications. Excessive amounts of padding will hinder the effectiveness of the ice.

5. Reexamination
Periodic reexamination is performed as appropriate to the injury. Swelling and skin or neurovascular compromise can evolve rapidly despite adequate initial diagnosis and management.

D. Patients Being Discharged From the Emergency Room

1. Weightbearing
Weightbearing is usually restricted; in most cases, however, touchdown weightbearing is permissible and safer for the patient than absolute nonweightbearing because balance is improved and subsequent falls are less likely. If a patient cannot reliably maintain touchdown status, it is probably simpler and safer to keep to strict nonweightbearing.

2. Follow-up
Appropriate follow-up is arranged and the patient provided with an alternative in case the patient cannot obtain the recommended appointment.

3. Patient Instruction
Patient instruction is provided for care of the injury and symptoms and signs that indicate a possible complication.

II. Injury Description

A. Fractures
Fractures are described by localization within the bone (proximal, middle, distal), displacement, angulation, and comminution.

B. Dislocations
Dislocations are described in terms of the distal bone position. For example, an *anterior shoulder dislocation* indicates that the humeral head lies anterior to the glenoid, whereas a *posterior elbow dislocation* describes the articular surface of the ulna as being posterior to end of the humerus.

C. Open Fracture Grading
Open fracture grading is most commonly performed using the Gustilo-Andersen criteria. Although more detailed schemes exist, this classification is still universally understood. More important than the measured length of the soft tissue injury is its severity; crushing degloving injuries represent more significant injuries than long, relatively confined wounds resulting from the "inside-out" extrusion of a fracture fragment.

Grade I: Bone extrusion wound <1 cm
Grade II: Bone extrusion wound 1 to 10 cm
Grade IIIA: Bone extrusion wound >10 cm
Grade IIIB: Extensive exposed bone that will require surgical coverage

Grade IIIC: Any open fracture associated with an arterial disruption

D. Muscle Strength Assessment

Muscle strength assessment is based on the patient's ability to move a joint, using the following criteria:

0 of 5: No visible contraction
1 of 5: Contraction visible, but no movement of joint produced
2 of 5: Joint moves, but cannot overcome force of gravity
3 of 5: Joint moves, against gravity alone
4 of 5: Joint moves against gravity and some resistance from examiner
5 of 5: Full strength

III. Injury Mechanism

A. High-Energy Extremity Injury

High-energy extremity injury can occur with falls from heights, motor vehicle accidents, and when pedestrians are struck at any speed. The resulting fractures are typically more comminuted or open, and the associated soft tissue trauma is more severe. Associated injuries must be suspected and rapid evolution of swelling anticipated, secondary to bleeding from disrupted muscle and bone as well as transudation of edema fluid as a response to local injury. Although associated injuries of the head, chest, or abdomen will take precedence, evolving skin compromise or compartment syndrome must be treated simultaneously should they occur.

B. Crush Injury

Crush injury can present in a benign and misleading fashion. The skin may have no signs of injury and initially minimal pain and swelling can lead the examiner to underestimate the extent and severity of underlying muscle damage. Within hours, there may be elevated compartment pressures and impending compartment syndrome, as the muscle becomes ischemic. Alternatively, the skin that initially appeared normal goes on to a full-thickness necrosis as the result of an unrecognized "internal degloving" that occurred during the crush. Because crush severity is a factor of both time and force, suspect a crush injury when *either* factor is significant (e.g., transient "bumper injury" to a pedestrian leg or prolonged, low-intensity pressure on an extremity when an unconscious patient lies immobile for many hours).

C. Compartment Syndrome

Compartment syndrome is an evolving injury that is typically triggered by trauma to muscle or spontaneous bleeding within a confined space (e.g., lower leg compartments). As edema and bleeding increase, the pressure within the compartment rises, causing the arteriovenous pressure gradient to decrease. With sufficiently high compartment pressure, blood flow within the microcirculation supplying muscle and nerve tissues declines to a critical level, and these tissues become ischemic. Pain develops first, followed by hypesthesia, and motor weakness. To prevent progression to tissue necrosis, the compartment must be decompressed by fasciotomy that restores blood flow to the tissues that are still viable. The diagnosis of compartment syndrome is usually made on clinical grounds, but the serial measurement of compartment pressures is helpful in establishing the diagnosis and following the progression. The threshold above which the diagnosis is made remains controversial and no universally accepted pressure measurement defines the condition, although 30 mm absolute and two thirds of the patient's diastolic pressure are frequently used guidelines. Pressure measurements should be made whenever compartment syndrome is suggested by the appearance of the extremity. For patients who are obtunded or who have abnormal sensibility, the need for serial pressure measurements is much greater because an inability to follow symptoms or physical signs of neuromuscular dysfunction. Suspected compartment syndrome is treated by placing the extremity at the *level of the heart* (elevation <u>immediately</u> <u>decreases</u> the arterial pressure) and removing any constricting cast or dressing. Simultaneous correction of anemia, hypotension, and hypoxia will maximize oxygenation of the compromised tissues. Once the diagnosis is made, treatment is immediate fasciotomy, at the bedside, if necessary.

IV.   Patient Factors

A.   Unconscious Patients

Unconscious patients require more frequent monitoring and need more imaging studies because localization of fractures by pain and tenderness is impossible. Compartment pressure measurements must be made serially in cases of significant extremity swelling.

B.   Anticoagulated Patients

Anticoagulated patients are increasingly common. With even minor extremity injury, hemarthrosis and extensive hematomas can form, potentially precipitating a compartment syndrome. Although closed extremity injuries are theoretically limited to a certain absolute blood loss, elderly or anemic patients can become rapidly compromised. Immediate icing and gentle compressive dressings are particularly important in this group of patients, and correction of excessive anticoagulation should be done rapidly.

C.   Osteoporotic Patients

Osteoporotic patients tend to sustain typical fracture patterns, which localize to the areas of thinnest cortex—the metaphyses of the long bones. These periarticular fractures (proximal humerus, distal radius, proximal femur) predominate in the elderly in whom midshaft, diaphyseal fractures are less frequent. In addition, osteoporotic bone is more susceptible to stress or insufficiency fracture, particularly involving the pelvis and proximal femur (hip). MRI may be needed to help make the diagnosis.

V. Upper Extremity Injuries
A. Shoulder Girdle
1. **Sternoclavicular Dislocation**
   a. **Evaluation Keys.** Assess anterior versus posterior. Possible intrathoracic injury with posterior type, usually high energy with associated multiple trauma.
   b. **Imaging.** Chest x-ray study initially; CT scan in most cases.
   c. **Initial treatment.** Anterior: sling or analgesics. Posterior: immediate thoracic consult.
   d. **Follow-up.** Anterior: orthopedic follow-up in 3 to 5 days; often left unreduced. Posterior: admission, possible operative reduction.
2. **Clavicle Fracture**
   a. **Evaluation Keys.** Neurovascular deficits, skin breaks; rule out pneumothorax.
   b. **Imaging.** Anteroposterior chest x-ray study.
   c. **Initial Treatment.** Sling or figure-of-8 strap. Analgesics; consult orthopedics for neurovascular (NV) deficits, skin compromise, severe comminution.
   d. **Follow-up.** Orthopedic follow-up in 3 to 5 days.
3. **Acromioclavicular (AC) Separation**
   a. **Evaluation Keys.** Tenderness at AC joint with or without palpable step-off.
   b. **Imaging.** Anteroposterior shoulder (weight-bearing views *not* needed).
   c. **Initial Treatment.** Sling or analgesics.
   d. **Follow-up.** Orthopedic follow-up in 3 to 5 days. Most treated nonoperatively, with resulting visible deformity but good function.
4. **Shoulder Dislocation**
   a. **Evaluation Keys.** Differentiate common anterior from rarer posterior type. Look for axillary nerve dysfunction.
   b. **Imaging.** Anteroposterior shoulder with scapular "y" or axillary view.
   c. **Initial Treatment.** Anterior: reduce with appropriate analgesia or sedation, using progressive elevation of shoulder. Postreduction films in sling-and-swathe. Posterior or with associated fracture or nerve deficit: consult orthopedics before attempting reduction.
   d. **Follow-up.** Orthopedic follow-up in 3 to 5 days. Recurrent dislocations are treated surgically.
5. **Proximal Humerus Fracture**
   a. **Evaluation Keys.** Local swelling, tenderness; pain with any movement.
   b. **Imaging.** Shoulder films; transthoracic lateral helpful if unable to rotate shoulder.
   c. **Initial Treatment.** Sling-and-swathe. If fracture involves tuberosities or articular surface,

or shows severe angulation or displacement, consult orthopedics.

d.   Follow-up. Orthopedic follow-up within a week. Most are treated nonoperatively, with physical therapy. Severe displacement or tuberosity involvement may be treated surgically.

6.   **Scapula Fracture**

  a.   Evaluation Keys. Usually associated with high-energy injury. Assess for possible intrathoracic injury.

  b.   Imaging. Chest x-ray study, shoulder films; CT usually needed, if glenoid involved.

  c.   Initial Treatment. Sling-and-swathe. Admission, typically for associated injuries.

  d.   Follow-up. Most are treated nonoperatively, with surgery reserved for those fractures with significant glenoid displacement.

7.   **Humeral Shaft Fracture**

  a.   Evaluation Keys. Gross instability. Evaluate radial nerve function carefully, *before* any manipulation of fracture.

  b.   Imaging. Anteroposterior and lateral view of the humerus.

  c.   Initial Treatment. Coaptation splint and sling. Consult orthopedics if radial nerve is involved, especially if function is lost during a manipulation.

  d.   Follow-up. Orthopedic follow-up in 3 to 5 days. Treatment is usually with a brace, with surgery for delayed healing or persisting radial nerve palsy.

8.   **Biceps Tendon Rupture**

  a.   Evaluation Keys. Abnormal contour of biceps ("Popeye" deformity). Determine whether rupture is proximal or distal.

  b.   Imaging. Anteroposterior and lateral view of the humerus (include shoulder and elbow).

  c.   Initial Treatment. Sling. If distal rupture suspected, consult orthopedics.

  d.   Follow-up. Proximal ruptures are treated symptomatically. Distal ruptures may need surgical repair, and should be seen within 3 days for orthopedic evaluation.

9.   **Rotator Cuff Tear**

  a.   Evaluation Keys. Acute or acute-on-chronic pain. Inability to maintain shoulder abduction; inability to lift back of hand off buttock

  b.   Imaging. Shoulder films.

  c.   Initial Treatment. Sling.

  d.   Follow-up. Orthopedic follow-up in 3 to 5 days; MRI scan may be obtained at that time.

B.   **Elbow**

1.   **Distal Humerus Fracture**

  a.   Evaluation Keys. Usually unstable on examination. Assess NV status carefully. Reassess after any manipulation or splint application.

  b. Imaging. Anteroposterior and lateral view of elbow (comparison views of opposite side are helpful in children).

  c. Initial Treatment. Posterior splint, with immediate confirmation that distal pulse is not diminished, and neurologic examination seems intact. May need to decrease flexion of elbow. Consult orthopedics for all displaced or intraarticular fractures, NV compromise, or for *any* pediatric distal humerus fracture.

  d. Follow-up. Admission for operative repair or observation (all children and certain adults) or discharge in splint with follow-up in 2 to 3 days.

 2. Radial Head Fracture

  a. Evaluation Keys. Tenderness over radial head with restricted pronation or supination. Assess wrist carefully for associated sprain or fracture because fracture usually results from *indirect* force delivered through a fall onto the hand.

  b. Imaging. Anteroposterior and lateral view of entire forearm, *including* wrist and elbow.

  c. Initial Treatment. Posterior splint. Consult orthopedics for angulation >30 degrees or for displacement of joint surface.

  d. Follow-up. Orthopedic follow-up in 3 to 5 days to reassess and begin range of motion (ROM) exercises. Follow-up sooner or admit, if operative repair or radial head replacement required.

 3. Olecranon Fracture

  a. Evaluation Keys. Usually results from a *direct* blow to the olecranon.

  b. Imaging. Anteroposterior and lateral view of elbow.

  c. Initial Treatment. Posterior splint; consult orthopedics for probable repair.

  d. Follow-up. Admit for repair or discharge with orthopedic follow-up in 2 to 3 days.

 4. Elbow Dislocation

  a. Evaluation Keys. Prominent olecranon with more common posterior dislocation. Anterior dislocation: assess NV status carefully.

  b. Imaging. Anteroposterior and lateral view of the elbow.

  c. Initial Treatment. Closed reduction with posterior splint at 90 degrees for posterior dislocations and 20 degrees for anterior dislocations. Consult orthopedics for inability to reduce, postreduction instability, or NV deficits.

  d. Follow-up. Orthopedic follow-up in 3 to 5 days.

C. Forearm and Wrist

 1. Forearm Fractures

 Both bones/Monteggia/Galeazzi variants

  a. Evaluation Keys. Forearm swelling with possible elbow or wrist involvement. NV examination usually intact, but swelling can occasionally precipitate a compartment syndrome.

b. Imaging. Anteroposterior and lateral view of the *entire* forearm, including wrist and elbow.

c. Initial Treatment. Posterior splint. Admit for surgery or discharge with close orthopedic follow-up.

d. Follow-up. These fractures are almost always treated operatively.

2. **Distal Radius Fracture**

a. Evaluation Keys. Visible deformity of wrist. Assess for any median nerve dysfunction. Look for occult skin break.

b. Imaging. Anteroposterior and lateral view of wrist. Include elbow, if examination findings warrant.

c. Initial Treatment. Closed reduction under hematoma or intravenous regional (bier) block. Charnley splint. Consult orthopedics for all displaced fractures requiring reduction. Urgent reduction needed in presence of NV compromise.

d. Follow-up. Discharge in splint with observation for developing NV compromise. Follow-up in 2 to 3 days. Possible admission for operative repair, per orthopedic consult.

VI. Lower Extremity Injuries

  A. Hip and Proximal Femur

    1. Hip Fractures

    Intertrochanteric/Femoral Neck

a. Evaluation Keys. Inability to perform straight-leg raise. Groin pain with passive rotation.

b. Imaging. Anteroposterior and lateral of hip; an anteroposterior view with the hip joint <u>internally</u> <u>rotated</u> can be useful, if initial views are normal. MR scan, if diagnosis clinically suspected despite negative films.

c. Initial Treatment. Buck's traction (5 to 10 pounds) for comfort. Medical evaluation to clear for surgery. Young patients with displaced femoral neck fractures are candidates for *urgent* surgical repair to reduce risk of osteonecrosis.

d. Follow-up. Admit for operative repair when medically stable. Hemiarthroplasty is performed in most displaced femoral neck fractures. Young patients (who are poor candidates for hemiarthroplasty) are treated with prompt operative reduction and fixation.

    2. Greater Trochanter Fracture

a. Evaluation Keys. Tenderness over trochanter. Pain with attempted abduction.

b. Imaging. Anteroposterior and frog lateral of hip.

c. Initial Treatment. Assess for ability to mobilize weight bearing as tolerated. Consider facility admission for gait training and custodial care, if unable to ambulate.

d.   Follow-up. Usually treated nonoperatively. Orthopedic follow-up in 3 to 5 days not admitted.

3.   Hip Dislocation

a.   Evaluation Keys. Usually posterior and secondary to high-energy trauma. Anterior knee trauma sustained with flexed hip (e.g., dashboard injury) is a common mechanism. *Always assess ipsilateral hip in presence of anterior knee trauma.*

b.   Imaging. Anteroposterior and 45-degree oblique (Judet) views of hip. CT scan *after* hip is reduced.

c.   Initial Treatment. Consult orthopedics for prompt closed (or open) reduction.

d.   Follow-up. Operative repair of any associated acetabular fracture can be delayed several days, if hip joint is concentrically reduced and stable.

4.   Femur Fractures
Subtrochanteric/Shaft/Supracondylar

a.   Evaluation Keys. Usually from high-energy trauma in younger persons, with lesser forces seen in the presence of osteoporotic bone. Suspect pathologic fracture with known carcinoma or history of prior pain or when fracture has resulted from minimal trauma.

b.   Imaging. Anteroposterior and lateral view of femur, including hip and knee. Close scrutiny of femoral neck to rule out associated fracture.

c.   Initial Treatment. Consult orthopedics. Splint or place in Buck's traction for comfort prior to surgery. *Distal* femur fractures can be adequately stabilized in a knee immobilizer.

d.   Follow-up. Admit for operative repair.

B.   Knee

1.   Patella Fracture

a.   Evaluation Keys. Usually secondary to a direct blow to the anterior knee. Check ipsilateral hip for possible fracture or dislocation.

b.   Imaging. Anteroposterior and lateral view of knee. Anteroposterior pelvis film for any suspected hip injury.

c.   Initial Treatment. Knee immobilizer. Consult orthopedics for possible admission versus discharge TDWB until seen at follow-up.

d.   Follow-up. Orthopedic follow-up in 2 to 3 days if discharged. Surgical repair in most cases.

2.   Patellofemoral Dislocation

a.   Evaluation Keys. Patella lies displaced on lateral side of joint. Joint held rigidly by patient.

b.   Imaging. Anteroposterior and lateral view of knee.

c.   Initial Treatment. Intravenous sedation or analgesia, as appropriate. Closed reduction by extending knee and manually pushing patella medially over the lateral femoral condyle and into the trochlear groove. Knee immobilizer with lateral patellar pad to maintain reduction.

d.   Follow-up. Orthopedic follow-up in 2 to 3 days.

3.   Tibial Plateau Fracture

a.   Evaluation Keys. Secondary to simultaneous axial and valgus load. Vascular injury can be seen with severely displaced fractures.

b.   Imaging. Anteroposterior and lateral view of the knee. CT scan helpful to assess fracture in preparation for surgery.

c.   Initial Treatment. Knee immobilizer. Consult orthopedics for probable admission. Observe for possible compartment syndrome.

d.   Follow-up. Operative repair when soft tissues permit (1 to 10 days).

4.   Knee Dislocation

a.   Evaluation Keys. Usually high-energy injury, including athletics. Knee is grossly unstable. Distal NV examination needs careful assessment before and after reduction.

b.   Imaging. Anteroposterior and lateral view of the knee; MRI scan. Arteriogram indicated only for clinical evidence of vascular injury.

c.   Initial Treatment. Consult orthopedics. Knee must be promptly reduced, usually with distal traction. Knee immobilizer with serial vascular checks.

d.   Follow-up. Usually, admit for observation. Ligamentous repairs can be performed acutely or delayed for several weeks.

5.   Extensor Mechanism Disruptions
Quadriceps and Patellar Tendon Tears

a.   Evaluation Keys. Usually the result of a forceful quadriceps contraction against a flexing knee. Elderly and steroid-using patients may present with lesser trauma. Inability to perform or maintain a straight-leg raise. Palpable defect may be noted, if seen within 24 hours of injury.

b.   Imaging. Anteroposterior and lateral view of the knee looking for abnormal position of patella. MRI scan, if diagnosis is uncertain.

c.   Initial Treatment. Knee immobilizer. Assess ability to mobilize PWB. Consult orthopedics for admission versus discharge for office follow-up.

d.   Follow-up. Orthopedic follow-up in 2 to 3 days, if discharged. Surgery is usually required unless tear is incomplete and extensor mechanism remains in continuity.

C.   Leg and Ankle

1.   Tibial Shaft Fracture

a.   Evaluation Keys. Assess soft tissues carefully, especially in high-energy injury (motor vehicle collisions, falls, crush mechanisms). Look carefully for small breaks in skin that may represent protrusion of fracture ends, even if distant from position seen on the films. Be alert to any developing compartment syndrome.

b. Imaging. Anteroposterior and lateral view of the tibia, including knee and ankle.

c. Initial Treatment. Posterior splint. Consult orthopedics to plan for admission versus discharge TDWB on crutches.

d. Follow-up. Orthopedic follow-up in 2 to 3 days, if discharged. Most unstable tibia shaft fractures are repaired with an intramedullary nail.

2. Tibial Pilon Fracture

a. Evaluation Keys. Fracture extends to the distal articular surface of the tibia. Fibula can also be fractured. Soft tissue status takes precedence in planning treatment.

b. Imaging. Anteroposterior and lateral view of distal tibia and ankle. CT scan to assess fracture pattern in preparation for surgery.

c. Initial Treatment. Posterior splint. Consult orthopedics to plan treatment, with timing dependent on swelling and any associated soft tissue injury.

d. Follow-up. Operative repair when soft tissues permit (1 to 14 days).

3. Ankle Fractures

a. Evaluation Keys. If displaced, assess for skin compromise, especially over the malleoli. Palpate leg proximally over fibula to rule out an associated proximal fibula fracture.

b. Imaging. Ankle films (anteroposterior, lateral, and mortise). *Anteroposterior or lateral view of leg, if tender proximally.*

c. Initial Treatment. Closed reduction for displaced or severely angulated fractures. *Perform promptly in cases of any skin compromise from the deformity.* Consult orthopedics to plan for either admission for surgery or office follow-up.

d. Follow-up. Displaced or unstable fractures are repaired. Nondisplaced fractures are immobilized in cast.

4. Gastrocsoleus Tear

a. Evaluation Keys. Severe calf pain and tenderness proximally. Ecchymosis may be present. Injury is usually more medial than lateral. Differentiate from deep venous thrombosis (DVT) if no history of trauma, or if examination reveals distal edema.

b. Imaging. Anteroposterior and lateral view of leg. MRI scan if diagnosis cannot be made by examination. Vascular ultrasound if DVT is suggested.

    c. **Initial Treatment.** Brace or posterior splint with crutches. Weight bear as tolerated.

    d. **Follow-up.** Orthopedic follow-up in 3 to 5 days.

5. **Achilles Tendon Tear**

    a. **Evaluation Keys.** Pain and swelling near the Achilles tendon. If seen within 24 hours of injury, a defect can be palpable. Thompson Test establishes whether or not tendon is in continuity.

    b. **Imaging.** Anteroposterior and lateral view of ankle to r/o bony avulsion from calcaneus. MRI scan, if diagnosis cannot be made by examination.

    c. **Initial Treatment.** Posterior splint with ankle in slight plantar flexion. Consult orthopedics to plan either admission or discharge home in splint.

    d. **Follow-up.** Orthopedic follow-up in 2 to 3 days, if not admitted for surgery. Treatment can be either surgical or nonsurgical.

D. **Foot**

1. **Hindfoot fractures: Talus, Calcaneus**

    a. **Evaluation Keys.** Usual mechanism is either fall or floorboard injury in motor vehicle crash.

    b. **Imaging.** Ankle and foot films. CT scan usually obtained for calcaneus fractures.

    c. **Initial Treatment.** Posterior splint. Displaced talus fractures are often operated on urgently to reduce risk of osteonecrosis. Dislocated talonavicular or subtalar joints need prompt reduction. Consult orthopedics.

    d. **Follow-up.** Most displaced fractures will be surgically treated. Timing is dependent on soft tissue swelling, particularly for calcaneus fractures.

2. **Midfoot Fracture and Dislocations**

    a. **Evaluation Keys.** Present following severe torsional injury, but can occur with lesser trauma in persons with neuropathy. Look for tenderness, instability, or palpable step-off across midfoot joints.

    b. **Imaging.** Foot films. CT can help define more complex injuries.

    c. **Initial Treatment.** Posterior splint. Consult orthopedics to plan for probable operative repair.

    d. **Follow-up.** Orthopedic follow-up in 2 to 3 days, if discharged. Operative repair for displaced midfoot joints.

3. **Metatarsal Fractures**

    a. **Evaluation Keys.** Most common is an avulsion fracture of the proximal end of the fifth metatarsal. Typically, occurs as an inversion injury. Differentiate more severe crush injuries with multiple metatarsal fractures and potential skin compromise from the more common and benign isolated fractures.

    b. **Imaging.** Foot films.

    c. **Initial Treatment.** Posterior splint or post-operative shoe. Crutches with touchdown wight bearing gait for isolated fractures. Consult orthopedics for fractures resulting from high-energy or crush mechanism.

    d. **Follow-up.** Orthopedic follow-up in 3 to 5 days for isolated or minimally displaced fractures. Nonoperative treatment in nearly all cases. Severe foot trauma can require admission for observation and possible repair of multiple or displaced metatarsal fractures.

4. **Phalangeal Fractures**

    a. **Evaluation Keys.** Assess for visible mal-alignment or open fracture.

    b. **Imaging.** Foot films.

    c. **Initial Treatment.** Closed reduction of angulated fracture under appropriate anesthetic block. Stabilize by taping to adjacent toe. PWB with crutches or cane.

    d. **Follow-up.** Orthopedic follow-up in 3 to 5 days.

SELECTED READING

Browner BB, Jupiter JB, Levine AM, et al., eds. *Skeletal trauma,* 3rd ed. Philadelphia: WB Saunders, 2003.

Fu FH, Stone DA, ed. *Sports injuries,* 2nd ed. Philadelphia: Lippincott Williams & Wilkins, 2001.

Simon RR, Koenigsknecht SJ. *Emergency orthopedics—the extremities.* Hartford: Appleton & Lange, 1995.

36

Hand Injuries

J. Alejandro Conejero, MD, David A. Lickstein, MD, and Jonathan M. Winograd, MD

I. **Introduction**
  A. **Clinical Significance**
     1. Hand injuries account for 5% to 10% emergency visits.
     2. Seemingly minor injury can result in prolonged recovery, loss of employment, or disability.
     3. Besides skin and superficial tissues, the many muscles, ligaments, and tendons of the hand are vulnerable to injury, as are the nerves and blood vessels that supply those structures.
     4. Adequate treatment of hand injuries requires a considerable knowledge of the processes by which these different tissues heal. Understanding the time, course, and manner in which each tissue heals enables the surgeon to incorporate changes into the treatment plan.
  B. **Common Mechanisms of Injury**
     1. **Blunt Trauma (Crush Injury, Contusions, Abrasions)**
     2. **Lacerations and Penetrating Trauma**
     3. **Avulsion, Ring Avulsion**
     4. **Burns**

II. **Definitions**
The surface anatomy of the hand is shown in Figure 36-1.
  A. **Appropriate Anatomic Descriptions**
     1. **Dorsal**
     2. **Volar**
     3. **Radial**
     4. **Ulnar**
  B. **The Hand Has Five Digits: Four Fingers and a Thumb**
     1. **Thumb**
     2. **Index**
     3. **Middle or Long**
     4. **Ring**
     5. **Small**

III. **History**
  A. **General**
     1. **Age**
Children are often reluctant to cooperate for fear of further injury. Aged patients have slower wound healing, decreased breaking strength, and decreased collagen synthesis.
     2. **Handedness**
     3. **Profession**
The patient's occupation can dictate goals of treatment.
     4. **Hobbies and Other Activities Requiring Use of Hands**

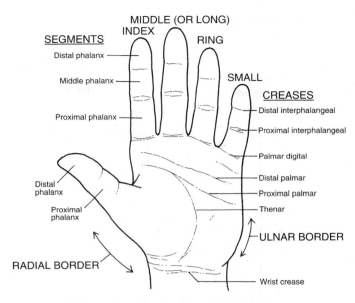

Figure 36-1. Surface anatomy of the hand.

5. **Medical History**
   a. **Prior Hand Injury or Trauma**
   b. **Prior Hand Surgery**
   c. **Diabetes Mellitus**
   d. **Collagen Vascular Disease**
   e. **Gout**
   f. **Rheumatologic Disease**
   g. **Congenital Deformity or Condition**

B. **Trauma**
   1. **Time of Injury**
   When significant time has elapsed since the injury or in the case of a heavily contaminated crush injury, it is best to delay closure.
   2. **Where Injured: Work or Home**
   3. **Equipment Involved**
   If work related, type of equipment involved, type of forces applied, and duration of exposure.
   4. **Mechanism of Injury**
   Reconstruct the exact mechanism of injury and position and action of hand at time of injury.
   5. **Contamination**
   Is wound clean, contaminated, or heavily contaminated? Assess for presence of foreign material.
   6. **Initial Treatment Before Evaluation**
   What treatment was administered before evaluation: irrigation, antiseptic solutions, immobilization, use of tourniquet.
   7. **Tetanus Status**

IV. **Surgical Anatomy**
   A. **Blood Supply**
      1. **Radial Artery**
         The radial artery enters the hand between the heads of the first and second metacarpal bones. It gives off a superficial branch that contributes to the superficial palmar arch, then continues to form the deep palmar arch.
      2. **Ulnar Artery**
         The ulnar artery enters the hand anterior to the flexor retinaculum, lateral to the ulnar nerve and the pisiform bone. It gives off a deep branch that contributes to the deep palmar arch, then continues to form the superficial palmar arch. Usually, it is the dominant blood supply to the hand.
      3. **Palmar Carpal Arch**
         The palmar carpal arch receives contributions from the interosseous, radial, and ulnar arteries. The deep palmar arch receives contributions from all four forearm vessels.
      4. **Common Palmar Digital Arteries**
         Formed by the anastomoses between the palmar metacarpal arteries from the deep palmar arch and the three palmar digital arteries from the superficial arch, the common palmar digital arteries travel to the webspace along the lumbricals, then divide into a pair of proper palmar digital arteries.
      5. **Proper Palmar Digital Arteries**
         The proper palmar digital arteries course with the digital nerves along radial and ulnar borders of each finger.
      6. **Dorsal Digital Arteries**
         The dorsal digital arteries extend distally to the proximal interphalangeal (PIP) joint level and receive same contributions as the dorsal carpal rete.
      7. **Princeps Pollicis Artery**
         A branch of the radial artery just distal to the snuffbox prior to radial artery diving deep into palm, the princeps pollicis artery bifurcates at the base of proximal phalanx of the thumb into common digital artery of the thumb and radialis indicis (supplies lateral side of index finger)
   B. **Muscles**
      1. **Intrinsic Muscles of the Hand**
         a. **Thenar Eminence**
            (1) **Abductor Pollicis Brevis**
            (2) **Flexor Pollicis Brevis**
            (3) **Opponens Pollicis**
         b. **Hypothenar Eminence**
            (1) **Abductor Digiti Minimi**
            (2) **Opponens Digiti Minimi**
            (3) **Flexor Digiti Minimi**
            (4) **Palmaris Brevis**

   c.   **Lumbrical Muscles**
     (1)   **Flex Digits at Metacarpophalangeal (MCP), Extend at the Interphalangeal (IP) Joints**
     (2)   **Radial Aspect of Flexor Tendon for Each Finger**
   d.   **Interossei**
     (1)   **3 Palmar: Adduction, IP Extension**
     (2)   **4 Dorsal: Abduction, IP Extension**
   e.   **Adductor Pollicis**
 2.   **Extrinsic Flexors of the Hand**
The extrinsic flexors of the hand arise from medial epicondyle as flexor or pronator mass.
   a.   **Digital Flexors**
     (1)   **Flexor Pollicis Longus (FPL)**
     (2)   **Flexor Digitorum Profundus (FDP)**
     (3)   **Flexor Digitorum Superficialis (FDS)**
   b.   **Wrist Flexors**
     (1)   **Palmaris Longus (PL)**
     (2)   **Flexor Carpi Radialis (FCR)**
     (3)   **Flexor Carpi Ulnaris (FCU)**
   c.   **Forearm Pronators**
     (1)   **Pronator Quadratus. Arises in distal forearm between the radius and ulna.**
     (2)   **Pronator Teres**
 3.   **Extrinsic Extensors**
The extrinsic extensors arise from the lateral epicondyle and ulna.
   a.   **Digital Extensors**
     (1)   **Abductor Pollicis Longus (APL)**
     (2)   **Extensor Pollicis Brevis (EPB)**
     (3)   **Extensor Pollicis Longus (EPL)**
     (4)   **Extensor Indicis Proprius (EIP)**
     (5)   **Extensor Digiti Minimi (EDM)**
     (6)   **Extensor Digitorum Communis (EDC)**
   b.   **Wrist Extensors**
     (1)   **Extensor Carpi Radialis Brevis**
     (2)   **Extensor Carpi Radialis Longus**
     (3)   **Extensor Carpi Ulnaris**
   c.   **Forearm Supinators**
     (1)   **Supinator**
     (2)   **Anconeus**
   d.   **Landmarks**
     (1)   Median nerve lies underneath the PL and radial to the FCR.
     (2)   The Ulnar nerve and artery travel deep to the FCU at the wrist level.
V.   Hand Examination
 A.   General
  1.   **Observe**
The first step should be a visual assessment of the patient's injuries.

a. **Posture of the Hand and Cascade.** Position at rest and abnormal angulation of bones and joints.

b. **Document Injuries and Areas of Questionable Viability.** Document and reevaluate diagrammatically.

c. **Sweating.** Provides information about the status of innervation of the hand. Normal skin is slightly moist. Loss of sympathetic tone results in drying of the skin.

d. **Muscle Wasting**

e. **Color Changes**

f. **Scars.** Previous trauma or surgery.

g. **Asymmetry.** Always compare both hands.

h. **Deformities.** Posttraumatic or congenital.

i. **Dimpling.** Over the thenar eminence. Dislocation of the MCP joint over the thumb.

2. **Palpate.** Before the administration of a local anesthetic, sedation or potent pain medication.

a. **Feel.** For areas of deformity, tenderness or instability.

b. **Palpate Pulses (see section IV.a.)**

c. **Allen Test.** Determines the patency of both the radial and ulnar arteries. Both arteries are compressed at the level of the wrist. The hand is exsanguinated by elevation, while the patient simultaneously flexes and extends the fingers. The radial artery is released. Prompt return of color and capillary refill indicate a patent radial artery and palmar arch. The entire test is then repeated for the ulnar artery. Normal filling time should be <5 seconds.

d. **Sensory Evaluation.** The simplest and most reliable way is the measurement of "two-point" discrimination. Tell the patient to keep the eyes closed during the examination. Start with 8 mm and decrease distance progressively. Small children and unconscious patients may need surgery to exclude diagnosis of injury. Normal value is <6 mm for static two-point discrimination.

e. **Motor Evaluation.** Active and passive movements and range of motion of all joints. Compare muscle strength with uninjured side. Correlate with sensory examination to determine level of nerve injury.

f. **Compartment Syndrome.** Always keep in mind the possibility of compartment syndrome, which can be indicated by palpably swollen compartments, pain on stretching of muscles, decreased strength, hypesthesia in the distribution of the nerve located in the involved compartment, and loss of distal pulses. For the pediatric or unconscious patient, measure intracompartmental pressures, if necessary.

g. **Bone and Ligaments.** A complete examination remains essential as a diagnostic tool and to direct radiographic examination. If sensation is normal, acute fractures and ligamentous injuries are always associated with pain over the site of injury.

h. Skin. Check for lacerations, nailbed injuries, burns, bites, infections.

B. **Innervation (Fig. 36-2)**
1. **Median Nerve**
   a. **Observe**
      (1) **Wasting of the Thenar Musculature**
      (2) **Sudomotor Changes in the Nerve Distribution**
   b. **Evaluation of Motor Function**
      (1) **Median Nerve at the Elbow**

      - Palpable tendon of FCR with resisted wrist flexion
      - Anterior interosseous nerve sign: inability to make an "O" sign: denervation of FDP to the index finger and FPL

      (2) **Pronation of the Forearm.** Elbow extended to neutralize biceps brachii.
      (3) **Motor Branch of Median Nerve**

      - Weak abduction of the thumb (APB)
      - Opposition to the little finger

   c. **Sensory Evaluation**
      (1) **Static and Moving Two-point Discrimination**
      (2) **Sharp or Blunt Sensation**
2. **Ulnar Nerve**
   a. **Observe**
      (1) **Interosseus Guttering and First Dorsal Interosseous Wasting**
      (2) **Hypothenar Wasting**
      (3) **Ulnar Claw Hand**
      (4) **Sudomotor Skin Changes**
   b. **Evaluation of Motor Function**
      (1) **Froment's Test.** Adductor pollicis.
      (2) **Resisted Abduction.** The index finger (first dorsal interosseous) and little finger—abductor digiti minimi (ADM).
      (3) **Flex.** The MCP joint of the little finger with the proximal interphalangeal straight—flexor digiti minimi (FDM).
      (4) **Absent Flexion.** At the distal IP joint of the ulnar two fingers.
   c. **Sensory Evaluation**
      (1) **Static and Moving Two-Point Discrimination**
      (2) **Sharp or Blunt Sensation**
3. **Radial**
   a. **Observe**
      (1) **Sudomotor Changes.** In the superficial branch of radial nerve distribution.

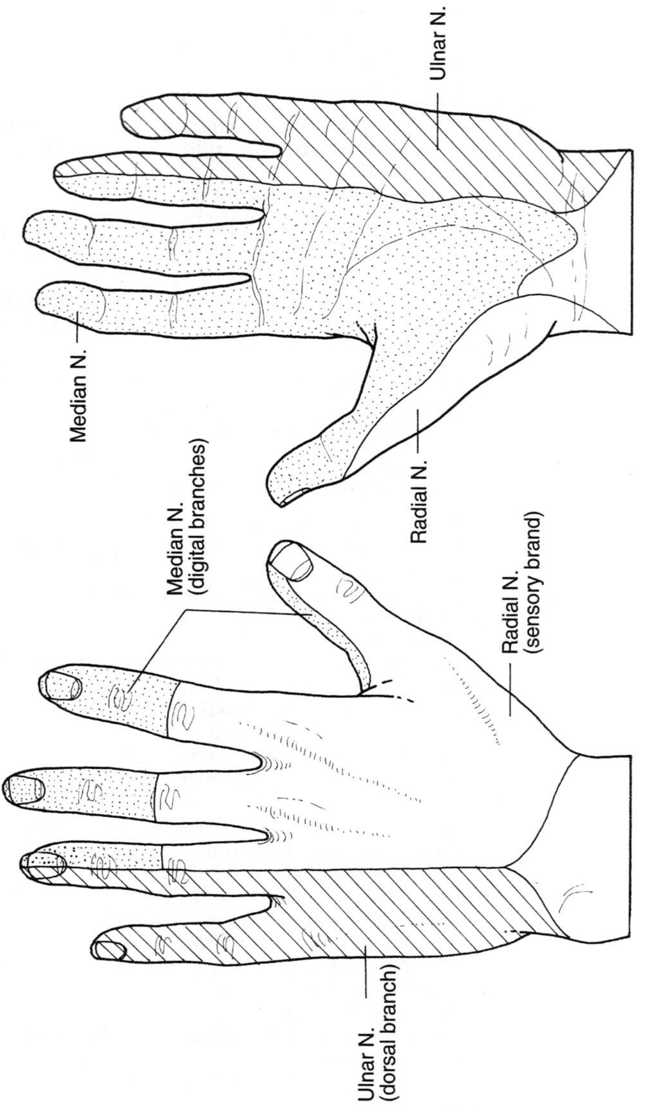

Figure 36-2.   Sensory innervation of the hand.

(2) **Wrist Drop**
(3) **Muscle Wasting**
b. **Evaluation of Motor Function**
(1) **Posterior Interosseous Nerve.** Supination with the elbow extended to neutralize biceps (supinator).
(2) **Thumb Extension with the Palm Flat (EPL)**
c. **Sensory Evaluation**
(1) **Static and Moving Two-Point Discrimination**
(2) **Sharp or Blunt Sensation**
C. **Circulation (see section IV.A.)**
1. **Assess Color, Temperature and Capillary Refill**
If refill after blanching is >2 seconds or incomplete, suspect arterial injury.
2. **Occlusion or Laceration**
Occlusion or laceration of the brachial artery proximal to its division usually results in distal extremity ischemia.
3. **Radial or Ulnar Injuries**
Radial or ulnar injuries can be difficult to determine because the remaining patent vessel can be providing adequate blood flow (**see Allen Test on section V.A.(2)**).
4. **Palmar Arches**
The radial artery makes a greater contribution to the deep palmar arch. The ulnar artery continues to form the superficial palmar arch. Fractures and penetrating injuries to the hand can cause injury to these arches.
5. **Distal Interphalangeal (DIP) Joint**
Distal to the DIP joint, the proper digital arteries divide into multiple branches.
6. **Doppler**
A Doppler probe may be helpful in vascular evaluation.
VI. **Diagnostic Methods**
A. **Radiographs**
Always consider clinical history and physical examination. Do not accept poor quality radiographs. Evaluate with an adequate number of proper projections.
1. **Routine Evaluation**
Posteroanterior, lateral, and oblique view are needed for routine evaluation.
2. **Stress Views**
For suspected ligament injury, stress views are needed.
3. **Anteroposterior Clenched Fist View**
For wrist instability and subtle fractures, an anteroposterior clenched fist view is needed.
4. **Comparison Views**
For pediatric and wrist injuries, comparison views are needed.

B. Doppler Flowmeter/Pulse Oximeter

In the assessment of perfusion of the hand or fingers, a Doppler flowmeter or pulse oximeter is useful.

C. Stryker Monitor

Use a Stryker monitor to measure compartment pressure.

D. Ultrasound

Ultrasound (US) is useful in examining structures during active motion. It provides detail of soft tissues. US can help in evaluating the internal character of tendons, as well as their functional and anatomic characteristics; the status of many ligaments, cartilage, and osseous surfaces; and soft tissue masses. It is rarely used since the advent of computed tomography (CT) and magnetic resonance imaging (MRI).

E. Computed Tomography

Spiral CT technique allows multiplanar reconstructions in any desired plane and high-quality three-dimensional reconstructions by a single examination. It is useful in the evaluation of carpal bone fractures not clearly visualized by plain radiography.

F. Magnetic Resonance Imaging

Examination using MRI has been shown to have a high sensitivity in detecting ruptured tendons, ligamentous injuries of the wrist, nondisplaced fractures, nonunion, and osteomyelitis.

VII. Emergency Department Care

    A. Injuries that Require Immediate Treatment

        1. Vascular Injury with Associated Hemorrhage or Ischemia

        2. Compartment Syndromes of the Hand and Arm

        3. Open Metacarpal or Wrist Fractures or Dislocations

        4. Amputations That are Candidates for Replantation

        5. Burns

        6. High-energy Injuries

    B. Treatment

        1. Initial Examination (see section V)

        2. Imaging Studies (see section VI)

        3. Local Anesthesia

        4. Wound Irrigation or Débridement

A physiologic irrigant dilutes the concentration of bacteria already present. An irrigant can also dislodge dirt fragments and, most importantly, facilitates identification of partially avulsed fat fragments and other devitalized tissue. Select a 30-mL syringe and a 25-gauge needle to assure optimal irrigation force.

        5. Repeat Hand Examination (see section V)

        6. Skin Closure, When Appropriate

            a. Skin. Use 4-0 monofilament, nonabsorbable suture. For the nailbed, use 6-0 plain gut or chromic suture.

            b. Suture Removal

Remove sutures in 7 days if not over a joint, 10 days if stressed over a joint.

c. **Single or Multiple Layers, as Appropriate**
d. **Simple or Horizontal Mattress Sutures**
7. **Antibiotic Prophylaxis**
   a. **Open Fractures**
   b. **Contaminated Wounds**
   c. **Bites.** Antibiotic prophylaxis is not mandatory for fresh, uninfected dog bites. Cat and human bites are usually treated prophylactically. The drug of choice for all of these bites is amoxicillin and clavulanic acid.

C. Anesthesia Techniques for Nerve Blocks (Fig. 36-3)

1. **Lidocaine (1% to 2%) or Bupivacaine (0.25% to 0.5%) without Epinephrine**
2. **Radial**
Radial, a superficial branch, is blocked three fingerbreadths proximal to the radial styloid. Injection is done around the dorsal radial aspect of the wrist.

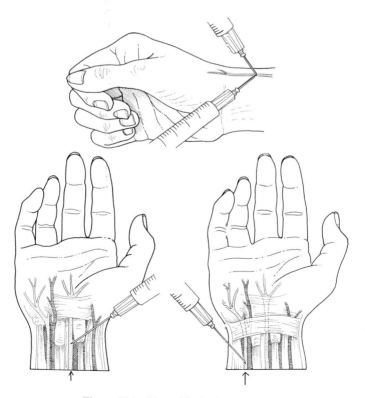

Figure 36-3. Nerve blocks for the hand.

3. Median
The median nerve is found at the proximal flexion crease of the wrist between palmaris longus and FCR tendon, angling underneath palmaris tendon.

4. Ulnar Nerve. The ulnar nerve lies under the FCU tendon proximal to the wrist crease. To avoid ulnar artery puncture, inject just proximal to the pisiform bone and direct dorsally underneath the FCU tendon.

5. Digital

  a. Palmar Injection. Palmar inject is over the A1 pulley and flexor sheath.

  b. Intermetacarpal Injection. Inject at the level of the metacarpal heads from dorsal aspect of web space and direct separately at each digital nerve.

  c. Distal ring. Local anesthetic is placed at the base of finger.

6. Hematoma Block at Site of Fracture

VIII. **Presentation, Diagnosis and Treatment of Specific Injuries**

  A. **Fingertip and Nailbed Injuries**

  1. Inspection
Inspect the nail plate in crush or lacerating injuries to the fingertip. Although such injuries are often managed with decompression, it can result in undertreatment of many nailbed injuries. We recommend removal of the nail plate and inspection of the nailbed when a hematoma encompasses >50% of the nailbed. In the presence of a fracture of the distal phalanx, a certain nailbed laceration exists that requires repair and antibiotic coverage.

  2. Hematoma Decompression
Subungual hematomas exert a painful pressure that distracts the nail plate away from the nailbed. It is necessary to perforate the nail plate and decompress the hematoma. A scalpel with a no. 11 blade, a 16-gauge needle, or a small electrocautery device that will burn through the nailbed to decompress the hematoma are excellent ways to decompress a hematoma.

  3. Repair
Ragged stellate nailbed lacerations result typically from crush injuries. Remove the nail plate to expose the area of the laceration, using small scissors and a hemostat to detach it from the nail fold. It is best to use loupe magnification and absorbable sutures (e.g., 6-0 chromic) to repair the nailbed. Injuries to the matrix decrease the adhesion of the nail plate to the nailbed, resulting in a nail that is elevated from the nailbed.

  4. Closure
Apply a protective surface over the repair. Either a large piece of nail that has been soaked in povidone-iodine or a piece of foil can be held in position with sterile strips or small mattress sutures.

B. Fingertip Amputations

Classify the amputation by location, obliquity of injury, and percentage of remaining matrix.

1. Type 1

Type 1 amputations are <1 cm in diameter, with no bone exposed. The injuries can be treated with wet to dry dressings and allowed to close secondarily. Healing in this manner results in a sensate fingertip. Free grafts or V-Y advancement flaps can also be used.

2. Type 2

In type 2 amputations >50% of the nail is lost or damaged. It is advisable to excise the remaining nailbed. It is important to remove the entire germinal matrix, including the portion of the dorsal nail matrix on the undersurface of the eponychial fold. Frequently, enough tissue remains to allow a primary closure. Removal can be deferred in the setting of limited soft tissue to achieve closure. If the fingertip is salvaged with <50% of the original nail, a hook nail deformity will result. Thenar or cross finger flaps may be necessary for coverage.

3. Type 3

Oblique injuries that spare >50% of the nail and often have open wounds at the tip that are >10 mm in diameter are classified type 3. Local flap coverage is recommended. In cases in which substantial cutaneous tissue is available on the fingertip, use full-thickness grafts or healing by secondary intention.

4. Type 4

In type 4, amputations are at the level of the DIP joint. In sharp amputations, replantation can be considered with excellent results. In severe crush injuries, revision amputation is the best treatment.

C. Replantation

1. Patient Selection

a. Considerations

(1) Age. Replantation in children is technically challenging. Elderly patients are less likely to have enough inflow to sustain replantation.

(2) Sex

(3) Occupation. Patient's occupational and recreational requirements for the injured extremity affect plans for reconstruction.

(4) Mechanism of Injury. Sharp amputations have better outcome than blunt injuries or avulsions.

(5) Level of Amputation. Zone II and proximal forearm amputations have fair prognosis.

(6) General Health of Patient. Replantation is less favorable in cases of diabetes, steroid use, and connective tissue disorder, or with a history of smoking.

(7) Duration of Ischemia. Best results if <24 hours of cold ischemia and <12 hours of warm ischemia.

(8) **Self-inflicted Injuries.** Consider psychiatric consultation.

b. Outcome. The likelihood of a successful outcome must exceed the potential morbidity of long anesthetic and potential need for anticoagulation.

c. Examination of Patient and Amputated part. Evaluate site of amputation and status of amputated part, including degree of contamination.

d. Proper Preservation of Amputated Part. Wrap hand or finger in moistened gauze, place in bag over ice.

2. **Indications**
   a. **Sharp Mechanism of Amputation Most Amenable**
   b. **Thumb**
   c. **Single Digit Distal to FDS Insertion**
   d. **Multiple Digits**
   e. **Partial Hand**
   f. **Wrist or Forearm**
   g. **Elbow or Upper Arm**
   h. **Pediatric Population**

3. **Contraindications**
   a. **Absolute**
      (1) **Associated Life-threatening Injuries**
      (2) **Systemic Illness or Condition that Prohibits Long Anesthesia**
   b. **Relative**
      (1) **Crush or Avulsion Mechanism**
      (2) **Multiple Level Injury**
      (3) **Amputation in Flexor zone 2**
      (4) **Systemic Disease**
      (5) **Smoking**
      (6) **Prolonged Warm Ischemia Time**
      (7) **Mentally Unstable Patient**
      (8) **Self-inflicted Injury**

4. **Complications**
   a. **Among Complications.** Loss of motion, chronic pain, cold intolerance, tendon adhesions, bony nonunion, painful neuroma formation, incomplete wound coverage.
   b. **Anticoagulation.** Patients may require anticoagulation, which carries a higher risk of bleeding and blood transfusions.

5. **Patient Expectations**
   a. **Commitment.** Replantation requires a strong commitment both from the patient and the surgeon. Evaluate benefits of replantation versus completion amputation.
   b. **Work.** Patient will be out of work between 6 and 12 weeks.
   c. **Additional Surgery.** Between 30% and 50% of patients will require further surgery.
   d. **Rehabilitation.** Patients are expected to participate in hand rehabilitation with an experienced hand therapist.

    e. **Recovery.** Best motion and sensation in a replanted part is not achieved until 12 to 18 months after surgery.

D. Fractures
  1. Closed
    a. **Carpus.** Attempts at closed reduction under local anesthesia should be made for fracture and dislocations.
      (1) Splint in Neutral Position
      (2) Associated Edema. Can cause median or ulnar nerve compression necessitating emergent decompression.
      (3) Require Operative Reduction and Fixation

- Irreducible or unstable fractures
- Comminuted fractures
- Intraarticular fractures
- Fractures with unacceptable angulation, rotation, shortening, or displacement (oblique or spiral pattern, segmental bone loss)

    b. **Metacarpal**
      (1) Closed Reduction. Attempts at closed reduction under local anesthesia should be made using the Jahss or another indicated maneuver.
      (2) Splint in Neutral Position
      (3) Require Operative Reduction and Fixation

- Irreducible or unstable fractures
- Comminuted fractures
- Intraarticular fractures
- Fractures with unacceptable angulation, rotation, shortening, or displacement (oblique or spiral pattern, segmental bone loss)
- Rolando, Bennett, or reverse Bennett (Teneb) fracture

    c. **Phalangeal**
      (1) Closed Reduction. Attempt closed reduction with the patient under local anesthesia.
      (2) Splint in Neutral Position
      (3) Similar Indications for Operative Reduction and Fixation as Metacarpal Fractures

  2. Open
    a. **Carpus or Metacarpal**
      (1) Urgent Operative Irrigation and Débridement of Wound
      (2) Operative Reduction and Fixation
      (3) Repair Associated Injuries

        (4) Appropriate Antibiotic Coverage

        (5) Tetanus Prophylaxis

    b. Phalangeal

        (1) Irrigation and Débridement. Irrigate and débride the wound in the emergency room with the patient under local anesthesia.

        (2) Tuft Fractures. These fractures rarely require operative reduction and fixation.

        (3) Consultation. Needs urgent operative reduction and fixation, and repair of associated injuries in consultation with hand surgeon.

E. Dislocations

    1. DIP. Stabilized by collateral ligaments and adjacent flexor and extensor tendons, making dislocations of this joint uncommon. If a dislocation does occur, it usually is directed dorsally and often is associated with an open wound. Treatment is similar to that for PIP dislocations.

    2. PIP. The ligaments of the PIP joints are those most commonly injured in the hand. Dorsal dislocations are the result of a blow to the extended digit, causing a combination of axial loading and dorsal deviation. They can be associated with a fracture. Volar dislocations are uncommon because the joint does not resist motion in this direction. Lateral dislocation is the result of a tangential load applied to the extended digit that ruptures a collateral ligament and disrupts the volar plate. Attempt reduction in the emergency department with the patient under local anesthesia. Once reduction is achieved, splint the digit splinted with the MCP joint flexed 70 to 90 degrees, and the PIP joint flexed 50 degrees. Irreducible dislocations require operative reduction.

    3. MCP. Dislocation of the MCP joint is uncommon, but when it occurs, deviation is usually dorsal. The common mechanism of injury is the application of a dorsal-directed force that is sufficient to rupture the volar plate. Dorsal dislocations that are in 60 to 90 degrees of hyperextension and are without intervening soft tissue are simple dislocations. Complex dislocations, which have the volar plate entrapped between the metacarpal and the proximal phalanx, require operative reduction.

    4. Thumb. The IP joint is very stable and seldom injured. Dislocations are often dorsal and open. The MCP of the thumb is one of the most frequently injured joints. Injury is commonly caused by hyperextension force sufficient to rupture the volar plate and cause dorsal dislocation. The complex dislocation is characterized by entrapment of the proximal phalanx between the tendons on the dorsum of the thumb.

F. Ligament Injuries

    1. Ligament injuries occur frequently and are often misdiagnosed. Sequelae range from chronically painful to unstable or chronically deformed joints.

2.   Ability to hold objects between the thumb and fingers depends on an intact ulnar collateral ligament (UCL).

3.   Gamekeeper's Thumb. A chronic injury to the UCL, caused by forceful abduction of the thumb. Any patient with pain in the distribution of the UCL or an inability to forcefully oppose the thumb should raise suspicion for an injury to the UCL.

4.   Rupture of the Radial Collateral ligament (RCL). A less common injury, resulting from forceful adduction of the thumb in any position.

G.   Tendon Injuries

1.   Superficial location predisposes tendons to injury from seemingly trivial lacerations as well as avulsions, crushes, and burns.

2.   Can be sustained as the result of forced hyperextension or forced flexion of an extended digit.

3.   Injuries include complete or partial transection, avulsion, or maceration.

4.   Tendons can remain functional despite a 50% to 90% laceration. A high index of suspicion and careful clinical examination are required when the mechanism and location of the injury are consistent with a possible tendon laceration or rupture.

5.   Zone of tendon injury should be described as with the fingers and thumb extended.

   a.   Verdan's Zones of Flexor Tendon Lacerations

     (1)   Finger

- **Zone 1:** Insertion of the FDP to the insertion of FDS
- **Zone 2:** Between the insertion of FDS and the A1 pulley (distal palmar crease). "No man's land" (Bunnell); critical zone (Boyes)
- **Zone 3:** From the A1 pulley to the distal border of the carpal tunnel.
- **Zone 4:** Carpal tunnel
- **Zone 5:** Carpal tunnel to musculotendinous junctions

     (2)   Thumb

- **Zone 1:** From the oblique pulley to the insertion of FPL
- **Zone 2:** A1 to oblique pulley
- **Zone 3:** A1 pulley to carpal tunnel; then as above

H.   Extensor Tendon Injuries

1.   Repair

The superficial location facilitates evaluation and permits repair in the emergency department.

2.   Partial Tendon Injuries

Injuries (<40% to 50% of the width) usually do not require repair. They should be splinted. Length of immobilization depends on degree of injury.

3.   Complete Extensor Tendon Injuries Repair
Use 3-0 or 4-0 nonabsorbable suture material. A running horizontal mattress or a modified Kessler suture technique is used, burying the knot on the palmar aspect of the tendon.

4.   Wound Closure
Failure to easily identify the lacerated ends of the tendon necessitates closure of the skin, splinting of the hand in 30 degrees of extension at the wrist with the MCP in neutral position, and referral for operative repair. Do not make multiple attempts to grasp the tendon beneath the proximal and distal skin flaps. Occupational therapy for range of motion is required following period of immobilization.

I.   Flexor Tendon Injuries
   1.   Lacerated tendons often retract beneath the skin and are sensitive to manipulation and susceptible to form adhesions. Primary repair should *never* be attempted in the emergency room.

   2.   Primary Tendon Repair
   Primary tendon repair in zones I and II has advantages: Tendon is returned to its normal length, period necessitated by wound healing and later grafting is reduced, joint stiffness is decreased, and results of secondary lysis, when necessary, should be better.

   3.   Perform a primary multistrand repair whenever possible. Modified Becker or Massachusetts General Hospital repair. Use nonabsorbable suture material.

   4.   Flexor tendons receive nutrition in two ways: small blood vessel networks called vincula and synovial diffusion. Avoid vincular injury during repair to preserve tendon blood supply.

   5.   Zone 1 injuries may require a reinsertion technique.

   6.   Up to 60% tendon division will have greater strength with an epitendinous stitch alone than if a core stitch is inserted. Protected motion of partial tendon lacerations is essential.

   7.   Failure of proximal interphalangeal joint flexion of the small finger:
       a.   Do not have FDS to little finger in 15% of cases
       b.   A nonfunctioning FDS to little finger in 15% of cases
       c.   Adhesions between FDS of ring finger and small finger can prevent independent motion
       d.   Referral to an occupational therapist for an early motion protocol is essential.

J.   Sequelae
   1.   Stiffness and Scar Contractures
       a.   The most common complication of any hand injury.
       b.   Prevention is more effective than attempts at correction.
   2.   Cosmetic Deformity
   3.   Hyperpigmentation

4. Complex Regional Pain
5. Reflex Sympathetic Dystrophy
6. Dysfunctional Motion
Protective mechanisms lead to maladaptive patterns of use after injury.
7. Compartment Syndrome
Compartment syndrome can develop after crush injury, reperfusion following fracture-related ischemia, intravenous injections, crush or blast injury, or prolonged pressure on the hand or arm. The late consequence is Volkmann's ischemic contracture, which involves muscle contracture and local ischemic neuropathy.
8. Cold Sensitivity
9. Nail Deformity

SELECTED READING

Agur AM. *Grant's atlas of anatomy.* Philadelphia: Lippincott Williams & Wilkins, 1999.

Eaton C. *The electronic textbook of hand surgery.* Available at: http://www.eatonhand.com; accessed March, 2003.

Green DP. *Operative hand surgery,* 4th ed. Philadelphia, PA: Churchill Livingstone, 1999.

Harrison BP, Hilliard MW. Emergency evaluation and treatment of hand injuries. *Emerg Med Clin North Am* 1999;17(4):793–822.

Ingari JV, Pederson WC. Update on tendon repair. *Clin Plast Surg* 1997;24(1):161–173.

Martin DS, Collins ED. *Manual of acute hand injuries.* St. Louis: Mosby, 1998.

Peimer CA. *Surgery of the hand and upper extremity.* New York: McGraw-Hill, 1996.

Rockwell WB, Butler PN, Byrne BA. Extensor tendon: anatomy, injury and reconstruction. *Plast Reconstr Surg* 2000;106(7):1592–1603.

Stern PJ. Management of fractures of the hand over the last 25 years. *J Hand Surg* 2000;25(5):817–823.

Stone C. *Plastic surgery: facts.* Greenwich: Medical Media, 2002.

Taras JS, Gray RM, Culp RW. Complications of flexor tendon injuries. *Hand Clin* 1994;10(1):93–109.

Wassermann RJ, Howard R, Markee B, et al. Optimization of the MGH repair using an algorithm for tenorrhaphy evaluation. *Plast Reconstr Surg* 1997;99(6):1688–1694.

Winograd J. *Plastic surgery. Advanced surgical recall.* Baltimore: Williams & Wilkins, 2000.

37

Techniques of Soft Tissue Reconstruction

Bohdan Pomahac, MD, and
Jonathan M. Winograd, MD

I. Introduction

Soft tissue reconstruction is an essential part of the management of a trauma patient. Open wounds serve as a port for bacterial invasion, which can cause disability or even death. The patient's proper functional and esthetic outcome is critically influenced by initial management.

II. Anatomic Principles

Based on embryologic development, the major arteries run close to the bones of the axial skeleton. Their branches enter the intermuscular septae, where they divide to supply the muscles, bones, tendons, nerves, and deep fat deposits. Cutaneous blood supply is derived from the cutaneous perforators, which usually arise from muscular or fasciocutaneous branches and enter the subcutaneous fat after piercing the deep fascia.

After emerging from the deep fascia, the cutaneous vessels follow the connective tissue framework around the fat lobules. Following multiple branching, they eventually reach the dermal level, where they create a subdermal plexus.

The three-dimensional territory of tissue supplied by a vessel is called an "angiosome." An angiosome is connected by anastomotic vessels. The anastomotic vessel can be of normal caliber or decreased caliber (e.g., the choke vessels serving as connectors between two angiosomes). These vessels play an important role in skin flap survival because of their inherent capacity to dilatate.

Complex wounds with exposed vital structures or wounds with significant functional and esthetic consequences usually require muscle or musculocutaneous flap. Based on vasculature, some muscle flaps are more suitable for reconstruction than others. As a basic rule, the ones with a defined blood supply (e.g., one dominant pedicle) are more predictable and, therefore, safer to use than those with multiple pedicles or segmental blood supply (sternocleidomastoid, sartorius muscles).

Based on the blood supply, the muscle flaps are divided into the following classes:

Type I: Single vascular pedicle (gastrocnemius muscle, tensor fascia lata muscle, vastus lateralis muscle)

Type II: Dominant vascular pedicle(s), and minor vascular pedicle(s) (gracilis muscle, trapezius muscle, biceps femoris)

Type III: Two dominant pedicles (rectus abdominis muscle, gluteus maximus muscle, serratus anterior muscle)

Type IV: Segmental vascular pedicles (sartorius muscle, extensor and flexor digitorum muscles)

Type V: Dominant vascular pedicle and secondary segmental vascular pedicles (latissimus muscle, pectoralis major muscle).

Muscle perforators supplying the overlying skin can be elevated with the muscle flap and transferred as musculocutaneous flap. Pay attention to where the vessels enter the overlying skin. Generally, the vessels radiate from fixed to mobile areas. If the skin over a muscle is mobile, the supply from the muscle can be tenuous. In suitable cases, the concomitant sensory nerve can be anastomosed in the recipient site, creating a sensate flap.

III. Important Physiology

Wound healing can be characterized as a process of wound contraction, extracellular matrix synthesis, angiogenesis, and epithelialization. Three types of wound healing are traditionally described. These are:

A. Healing

  1. Primary Healing
  Wound closure by direct approximation, pedicle flap, or skin graft.

  2. Healing by Secondary Intention
  Wound is left open to heal spontaneously.

  3. Tertiary Healing
  Delayed wound closure after several days. Sometimes, called "delayed primary healing," it is a technique used to treat contaminated wounds.

B. Factors that Influence Wound Healing

For simplicity, these factors can be divided into local, and systemic.

  1. Local Factors

   a. Tissue Trauma. Must be minimized

   b. Hematoma. Associated with higher infection rate.

   c. Blood Supply. Must be adequate and preserved.

   d. Infection

   e. Radiation

   f. Technique and Suture Material

  2. Systemic Factors
  Systemic factors influencing wound healing are nutrition, age, effects of steroids, chemotherapy, and chronic illness, to name just some. Physiology of wound healing has to be maintained by proper technique of wound care and dressings. As a general rule, wounds in wet environment heal faster than in moist environment, and these heal faster than dry wounds. The tissues, therefore, should not be left to desiccate; partial thickness wounds should be covered with occlusive or semi-occlusive dressings. Dirty wounds should be sharply débrided, irrigated, and left open for frequent débriding dressing changes (e.g., wet to dry). A new dressing modality is vacuum-assisted wound closure device (VAC). Proper studies comparing standard dressing changes with VAC are yet to be done.

IV. Evaluation of Reconstructive Requirements

The first step in patient's evaluation for reconstruction is a correct diagnosis. The extent and composition of the missing tissues dictates the reconstructive plan. The goal is to replace "like" with "like." Reconstructive ladder provides general guidance according to the level of complexity of the problem; however, in many cases it may not render a proper solution. For example, if the patient is missing half of a nose, neither skin graft nor free flap will solve the problem. The defect needs to be analyzed and tissues rearranged, possibly by using all levels of reconstructive ladder, to provide mucosal lining, cartilage or bony support, and properly matching skin coverage. In other occasions, the levels of the reconstructive ladder can be switched to provide superior esthetic or functional result.

As a general rule, plan an operation with a back-up plan. Sometimes, a minor change in the original plan saves a second option for later should the reconstruction fail. The reconstructive ladder involves the following:

A. **Healing by Secondary Intention**
B. **Skin Grafts**
C. **Random Flaps**
D. **Axial Flaps**
E. **Free Flaps**

1. Healing by Secondary Intention

Most of the wounds heal spontaneously with appropriate care. The esthetic and functional results are often acceptable or even superior to any other method. Certain types of finger pulp injuries, foot ulcers, or healing of forehead flap donor sites could serve as an example of wounds that successfully heal this way. Most acute wounds, however, should be closed primarily.

2. Skin Grafts

Skin grafts consist of epidermis and dermis of variable thickness. Based on thickness, the grafts are called "partial thickness" (thin, medium, thick), or "full thickness" (if the entire dermis is contained). As a rule, they do not carry their own blood supply. Their survival, therefore, depends on diffusion of nutrients from the recipient bed until the graft capillaries connect with the bed. The thinner the graft is, the more it contracts both primarily (after harvest) and secondarily (during healing in the recipient bed). Meshing can increase the skin graft surface area and pliability.

3. Random Flap

Random flap is a pedicle flap that does not carry a defined arteriovenous supply. As such, the distance of flap transposition is limited. Based on designed geometry, the flaps can arc around a pivot point or advance directly into the defect. Flaps moving about a pivot point can be further divided into rotation, transposition, and interpolation flaps. Advancement flaps are either a single or double pedicle, or a V-Y.

4. Axial Flap

Certain skin territories have well defined vascular pedicle. An area of skin that can be safely elevated based on known arteriovenous pedicle is called an "axial flap." An example of one of these territories is a forehead flap based on supraorbital artery and vein. Principally, all muscle or musculocutaneous flaps are also axial.

5. Free Flap

Free tissue transfer is the next logical step in flap translocation to distant areas. The tissue's dominant or major vascular pedicle can be elevated and divided at the donor site and reconnected to the vessels of the recipient site using microvascular techniques. The first successful free tissue transfer in a true sense of the word was the kidney transplant in 1954 by Dr. Murray. Microvascular transplantation is possible with any axial flap, including skin, subcutaneous tissue, fasciocutaneous muscle, myocutaneous, osteomyocutaneous, omental, and other intestinal flaps.

Free flaps are particularly important in areas where local flap options are limited (e.g., the head and neck region and the distal third of the lower extremity). Free flap options for reconstruction are wide, most commonly including muscle, myocutaneous, osteomyocutaneous, or osteomuscular flaps.

V. Common Scenarios
A. Head and Neck
1. Scalp Reconstruction

Scalp injuries are rarely life threatening, although ongoing blood loss from an unrepaired laceration in the scalp can be significant. Most such injuries are treated in the emergency room (ER) with minimal functional or esthetic sequelae. The most common are simple scalp lacerations. General principles of irrigation, débridement, and hemostasis apply, and healing is usually good. Complications are uncommon, but hematoma or abscess can develop. Spread of infection to the orbit and even intracranially via diploic veins is rare.

Defects up to 3 cm can be closed primarily with undermining of the surrounding scalp. Partial thickness loss of the scalp can be treated with defatting and grafting of avulsed skin, or split thickness skin grafting as long as pericranium remains intact. If the pericranium is not viable or is missing, exposed bone is in danger of desiccating and undergoing superficial necrosis and colonization. In such as case, the outer table of the skull can be removed and skin graft applied to the vascularized diploic bed after a suitable period to allow for granulation. Local advancement flaps are valuable for defects from 3 to 6 cm. Flaps are raised in the subgaleal plane with galeal scoring. Flap options include bipedicle or broad-based rotational flaps and skin grafting of the donor site. Large defects (>6 cm) of the scalp are managed with multiple flaps (three- or four-flap technique) or tissue expanders. Industrial injuries (e.g., scalp avulsion) sometimes can be suitable for microvascular replantation and avulsed parts must be preserved. There are three paired major arteries to the scalp, including the supratrochlear, superficial temporal, and the occipital arteries. Any one artery will often suffice for revascularization of the entire scalp. Stretch injury to the scalp vessels often makes replantation difficult because of the extensive longitudinal damage done to the vessels.

B. Upper Extremity

History and physical examination are crucial in upper extremity management. The patient's age, hand dominance, occupation, and history of prior upper extremity injuries should be obtained, as well as the mechanism of the current injury. The examination must include careful evaluation of circulation and sensibility. During examination of the wound, note any skin deficits or devitalized areas. Careful examination of deeper structures, which requires adequate anesthesia, may need to be performed in the operating room. Unless the patient is uncooperative or unresponsive, most diagnoses can be made with history and physical examination alone, without the need for a direct exploration in the ER. Clamping of bleeders in the hand or forearm is absolutely contraindicated in the ER setting, unless adequate lighting, magnification, and experience warrant such an approach. Many nerve injuries have been sustained in these situations because the major nerve of the upper extremity travels in close proximity to the major arteries.

Based on severity and urgency, the upper extremity injuries can be divided into:

1. Severe and requiring immediate treatment: massive hemorrhage, necrotizing infections, amputations
2. Severe and requiring early treatment: open fractures, flexor tendon lacerations, vascular injury without circulatory compromise, nerve injuries, joint injuries
3. Less severe injuries

Planning of surgical reconstructions begins with assessment of all injured structures by history, physical examination, and operative exploration. Once the defects are characterized, the treatment can begin with regard to the importance of the following:

1. Reconstructive Strategy

Normal hand structure and function will be restored, if possible. Unsalvageable parts will be altered to better restore function or removed. The complexity of the reconstructive plan will incorporate not simply what is surgically possible but what is the most efficient functional restoration for the particular patient.

2. Circulation

Decisions are based not simply on viability but also on functional demands. A digit can be perfused without digital artery continuity and a hand can be perfused through interosseous arteries alone. Cold intolerance in the digit or claudication in the hand musculature, however, would make the part useless or worse in terms of functional outcome.

3. Soft Tissue Coverage Options

The reconstructive ladder.

4. Skeletal Stability

Internal stabilization provides a more stable platform for early rehabilitation than either Kirschner wires or cast immobilization; however, it is more invasive and more likely to incur severe scarring.

5. Nerve Repair

Repair with or without grafting is essential to functional restoration. An insensate hand represents an extremely compromised part, often more difficult to use than one with less motion. Newer techniques use knowledge of internal neural architecture and the fact that motor and sensory fascicles usually have segregated distal to the elbow to perform separate motor and sensory nerve repairs. This has led to better return of sensory and motor function because of greater precision in directing regenerating fibers toward their proper targets distally.

6. Restore Active Motion

Tendon repair or reconstruction with grafting or transfers is essential in providing motor function to the injured limb. Passive range of motion of joints crossed by a tendon must be maximized before tendon reconstruction and at the earliest possible time after repair.

C. Torso

1. Chest Wall

The chest is unique in that it provides a protective shell for the intrathoracic organs as well as a mechanical support for reparation. Important concerns when considering reconstructive options are wall stability, thickness, reliability, and durability. Muscle or musculocutaneous flaps are usually required for major chest wall injuries. An important factor is the location of the defect. Several large muscles are most commonly used. The pectoralis major flap, based medially from the internal mammary perforators or superiorly from the thoracoacromial artery, has a versatile range for transposition. The latissimus dorsi is one of the most versatile muscles or musculocutaneous flaps, with excellent reach to both anterior and posterior chest wall defects. The function of the transposed latissimus is well substituted by surrounding musculature and presents little functional deficit. The trapezius muscle is most useful for midline defects of the posterior chest and cervical or thoracic spine. Other options involve the abdominal donor area. The rectus abdominis, with or without overlying skin paddle, or omentum are useful flaps for chest wall reconstruction. Omentum and latissimus dorsi muscles are good flaps for intrathoracic reconstruction because of their bulk.

It is generally accepted that skeletal stabilization is necessary if more than four ribs are resected or the full-thickness defect measures >5 cm. Restoration of skeletal stability includes the following options:

a. Autogenous

(1) Rib Grafts

(2) Fascia

(3) Muscle Flaps with Vascularized Bone Grafts from Rib

b.   Synthetic
Synthetic materials are often used for their strength and the absence of a donor defect. They are covered with transposed muscle for stabile coverage.
> **(1)   Teflon, Acrylic, Polypropylene Mesh, Gore-Tex**
> **(2)   Composite Mesh**
> **(3)   Marlex and Marlex-methyl Methacrylate Sandwich**

2.   Abdominal Wall
Before starting reconstruction, it is helpful to understand the function of the parts to be constructed. The main features of abdominal wall function are as follows:
> **a.   Protection of the Internal Organs**
> **b.   Barrier Preventing Herniation**
> **c.   Torso and Body Contour**

3.   Reconstruction
Abdominal wall reconstructions usually deal with large areas of extensive soft tissue loss, often the result of direct destruction by trauma or from chronic fistulae or extensive herniation. In the setting of acute trauma or chronic fistulae, the abdominal wound is contaminated with enteric contents or frank stool. Although exposed viscera can be directly skin grafted, such coverage is temporary and often accepts a large abdominal hernia as its outcome. If sufficient soft tissue coverage in the form of skin and subcutaneous tissue or local flaps exists, the treatment of choice in this setting is fascial reconstruction with synthetic mesh or tensor fascia lata free grafts or flaps.

Tensor fascia lata grafts and flaps will tolerate a small amount of contamination. The synthetic meshes can become exposed if placed in the setting of contamination. Gore-Tex mesh usually mandates removal after exposure, whereas polypropylene mesh does not. A new Gore-Tex mesh impregnated with chlorhexidine and silver may show promise in resisting contamination. Component separation can be used for smaller midline, vertically oriented defects with preservation of the rectus abdominus muscle and fascial sheaths. The fascia is released at the external oblique insertion on the lateral rectus sheath and the posterior sheath is released from its attachment to the linea alba. Estimated gains in closure are up to 20 cm in the midline at the level of the umbilicus, based on cadaveric studies.

D.   Lower Extremity
Common scenarios for lower extremity trauma include motor vehicle accidents, sports injuries, and falls. Plastic surgeons get involved in cases of extensive soft tissue loss. Several points should be considered before the reconstructive plan is formulated.

1.   Mechanism of Injury
Low, medium, or high-energy injuries will all likely have different levels of bony and soft tissue involve-

ment. An open tibial fracture caused by a fall from a sitting or even standing position will have a less extensive *zone of injury* compared with a pedestrian struck by a rapidly moving car. Planning for reconstruction needs to take into account the zone of injury to avoid using injured tissues for muscle flap donation or as a vascular pedicle for free flap reconstruction. Angiograms are necessary for free flap reconstruction and deep venous thromboses need to be ruled out to ensure adequate outflow for free tissue transfer.

2. Extent of Bone and Muscle Injury: Blood Supply and Sensation of the Lower Extremity Although most of the bony injuries can be treated from the orthopedic standpoint, it is important to consider final functional outcome of the leg in determining the best option for reconstruction and in considering whether to undertake lower extremity salvage. A foot without sensation is susceptible to recurrent ulcers, which can add to the morbidity over time, and a foot without functional muscles, at best, is comparable to a prosthesis in terms of function if not appearance.

VI. **General Rules for Lower Extremity Amputation**
   A. **Severe Combined Injury to Bone, Skin, Joint, Nerves, and Vessels**
   B. **Absence of Sciatic or Posterior Tibial Nerve Function**
   C. **Severe Infection or Contamination, Especially with Systemic Sepsis**
   D. **Multilevel Severe Injury**
   E. **Classification**

Classification of open tibial fractures with relation to fracture pattern and soft tissue injury is useful in describing injuries and prognosis. The most commonly quoted classification for open fractures is that of Gustilo, first outlined in 1976 and then modified in 1983 (**Table 37-1**).

Most of the injured limbs can be salvaged using current techniques. The chosen procedure depends on the size and location of the wound.

Table 37-1. Gustilo classification of open fractures of the tibia

Type	Description
I	Open fracture with a wound <1 cm
II	Open fracture with a wound >1 cm without extensive soft tissue damage
III	Open fracture with extensive soft tissue damage
IIIA	With adequate soft tissue coverage
IIIB	With soft tissue loss with periosteal stripping and bone exposure
IIIC	With arterial injury requiring repair

1. Location of Wound: Thigh, Lower Leg; Proximal, Middle, Distal Third, and Foot

Location and extent of the wound is key for the choice of soft tissue coverage. Skin grafts can be used if underlying muscle, paratenon, or periosteum is healthy. Local fasciocutaneous or muscle flaps are useful to cover small to moderate defects of bone or to cover exposed vessels or tendons. Bulky muscles surround a thigh and, consequently, thigh wounds are rarely a challenge for closure. More difficult is soft tissue coverage of lower leg wounds. As a general rule, even a small defect will often require a large local skin and subcutaneous flap to be rotated or advanced over the wound. Skin grafting of donor sites is not unusual. Take care not to exceed length-to-width ratios of these flaps. Local flaps (e.g., gastrocnemius or soleus muscles) can cover defects of the proximal or middle third of the leg. A hemisoleus muscle can be taken with preservation of function of the opposite half of the soleus muscle. Smaller defects can also be covered by the tibialis anterior muscle or other muscles of the anterior or lateral compartments, although these do not advance over great distances and often are within the zone of injury. These muscles generally have a less reliable blood supply, which limits their size and versatility. If the local muscle flaps are in the zone of injury, microvascular free tissue transfer is the only choice.

Defects of the lower third of the leg are difficult to reach with any local muscle flaps, and usually require free flap coverage. The most common choice for these defects is use of muscle flaps because of their ability to conform to the surfaces of deeper defects and bone gaps. Other choices include fascial flaps, which do have the advantage of being thin in a thin patient, in comparison with muscle. They do not require skin grafting. Vascularized bone can be included with many flaps or added as a second flap in tandem to provide the best chance of healing an extensive bone gap.

High-energy lower extremity injuries with extensive soft tissue damage or exposure of vessels and nerves have been historically a vexing problem, resulting most commonly in amputation. With the development of microvascular techniques, free tissue transfer and salvage of complex lower extremity injuries has become more feasible. The basic principles of adequate débridement apply and it appears that the adequacy of the débridement, rather than the rapidity, is the more important factor in achieving successful wound closure. In experienced hands, the success rate should be 80% to 90%.

VII.   Postoperative Care of Wounds

Dressings serve multiple purposes. They mechanically protect the wound, facilitate healing, and prevent infection. Dry dressings to open wounds cause desiccation, delayed wound healing, and pain. Moist and, ideally, wet wounds heal faster than dry, both experimentally and clinically. Open contaminated wounds should be treated by débridement, either with wet to dry saline gauze dressings or with surgery. A VAC seems to be a promising tool to adequately débride wounds, even for conservative management of exposed hardware or tendons. It works best when plentiful soft tissue can be recruited from the adjacent areas (e.g., abdomen, thigh, hips, back).

Postoperative care following microsurgery requires intensive monitoring by experienced practitioners. Free flaps are at highest risk in the first 72 hours following surgery. Patients should be kept in a warm room (80°F) and should be well hydrated, with adequate pain control and an anxiolytic, when necessary. Venous thrombosis is by far the most common cause of flap failure, which will be followed in short succession by arterial thrombosis and flap demise. Salvage rates of up to 70% after thrombosis and successful operative revision are only possible when flap failures are recognized early in their course. Another cause of early flap failure is severe, intractable arterial spasm that does not respond to the conservative measures of patient warming, adequate analgesia, anxiolytics, and even local sympathectomy. Eventually, this leads to thrombosis. For this reason, flaps must be monitored every hour for the first 72 hours and institutional support must available for emergent return to the operating room for recognized problems.

Commercially available resorbable Doppler cuffs can be wrapped around the outflow vein and continuously followed for signals. Alternatively, the best site of Doppler signal reception should be marked on the flap in the operating room. Hourly checks of the flap should be performed for Doppler signal, color, warmth, and turgor. Venous thrombosis will result in a tense, cyanotic, often warm flap with a preserved arterial signal. Venous augmentation, a Doppler signal obtained by pushing a pulse wave manually in the flap, is a sign of venous patency, which will be lost within a short time after the onset of venous thrombosis. Arterial thrombosis results in a pale, cool, deflated flap with no Doppler signal. No reflow, a state of widespread microthrombosis within the flap, usually following prolonged flap ischemia or a hypercoagulable state, prevents further efforts at flap perfusion. Early reversal of the no reflow state can be attempted with thrombolytics, but only if flap perfusion is still possible through the vascular pedicle.

VIII.   Rehabilitation and Delayed Complications

Rehabilitation of the reconstructed areas is guided by several basic rules. Motion is permitted as early as possible but should not jeopardize stable soft tissue coverage required for healing. Dangling of lower extremity skin grafts and flaps is allowed after the skin graft has reepithelialized its interstices and is done with compression of the graft or flap. This is performed to condition the patient to the pain that often accompanies the return to the dependent position for a wound or fracture. A commonly asked question of many patients is when can a scar be revised. Most surgeons wait for at least 6 months, if not a year, to allow for scar maturation and softening. Steroid injections of hypertrophic scars can aid in improving the appearance or symptoms of the scar, which include pain and pruritus. Silicone oil applied topically or silicone sheeting is also effective in treating the appearance and symptoms of hypertrophic scars.

SELECTED READING

Arnold PG, Pairolero PC. Chest-wall reconstruction: an account of 500 consecutive patients. *Plast Reconstr Surg* 1996;98(5):804–810.

Clark AF. *The molecular and cellular biology of wound repair,* 2nd ed. New York: Plenum, 1996.

Cohen M. Reconstruction of the chest wall. In: Cohen M, ed. *Mastery of plastic and reconstructive surgery.* Boston: Little, Brown, 1994: 1248–1267.

Fix RJ, Vasconez LO. Fasciocutaneous flaps in reconstruction of the lower extremity. *Clin Plast Surg* 1991;18(3):571–582.

Godina M. Early microsurgical reconstruction of complex trauma of extremities. *Plast Reconstr Surg* 1986;78:285.

Gustilo RB, Mendoza RM, Williams DN. Problems in the management of type III (severe) open fractures: a new classification of type III open fractures. *J Trauma* 1987;24:742–746.

Hui K, Lineweaver W. Abdominal wall reconstruction. *Adv Plast Reconstr Surg* 1997;14:213–244.

Livingston DH, Sharma PK, Glantz AI. Tissue expander for abdominal wall reconstruction following severe trauma: technical note and case reports. *J Trauma* 1992;32:82–86.

Manson PN. Maxillofacial injuries. In: Siegel J, ed. *Management of trauma.* New York: Churchill-Livingstone, 1986.

May JW Jr, Rohrich RJ. Foot reconstruction using free microvascular muscle flaps with skin grafts. *Clin Plast Surg* 1986;13(4):681–689.

Meara JG, Guo L, Smith JD, et al. Vacuum-assisted closure in the treatment of degloving injuries. *Ann Plast Surg* 1999;42(6):589–594.

Pomahac B, Svensjo T, Yao F, et al. Tissue engineering of skin (review). *Crit Rev Oral Biol Med* 1998;9(3):333–344.

IV

Special Considerations

38

Pediatric Trauma 1: Resuscitation and Initial Evaluation

Rashini Dasgupta, MD, and Daniel P. Ryan, MD

I. Introduction

Pediatric trauma became an entity unto its own when Peter Kottmeier established the first pediatric trauma unit in 1962 in Brooklyn, New York. The American College of Surgeons standardized pediatric trauma protocols by publishing, *Resources for Optimal Care of the Injured Patient,* which established guidelines for pediatric trauma centers in 1976.

Each year, 22 million injuries occur to children. It is the leading cause of death in children, exceeding all other causes of death combined. In the age group from 1 to 14 years, more than half of the mortality is related to trauma. Approximately 15,000 children die from trauma each year and 100,000 children are permanently disabled. The estimated cost of pediatric trauma is in excess of $15 billion each year.

II. Type of Injuries

A predominance of blunt versus penetrating trauma injuries is seen in the pediatric population. Falls are the leading cause of injuries, most common among the toddler age group. The next major mechanism is motor vehicle crashes with children either as occupants or as pedestrians who have been struck. Of injuries, 10% involve bicycles. Penetrating traumas, including gunshot wounds and stabbing, comprise another 5% of injuries.

III. Prevention Programs

The American Trauma Society has a "Play Safe" campaign that includes board games and educational videos to teach school-aged children about safe behaviors.

Bicycle injuries are common among the pediatric age group; only 1% of children admitted for bicycle trauma had been wearing a helmet. Studies suggest that a bicycle helmet law can significantly increase helmet use among children. Currently, however, fewer than 20 states have a statewide helmet use law. These laws vary by age affected, penalty, and type of enforcement

IV. Important Differences in Anatomy and Physiology

The primary survey must involve evaluation of the child's airway, breathing, and circulation. Airway control is the first priority.

    A. **Airway**
        1. **Shorter Neck**
        2. **Smaller and More Anterior Larynx**
        3. **Short Trachea**
        4. **Intubation**
           In-line cervical spine immobilization.

Airway size = (16 + age in years) ÷ 4 = internal tube diameter in millimeters
Reasonable estimate is size of fifth phalanx at the base

5. **Floppy Epiglottis**
6. **Large Tongue**
7. **Narrow Subglottic Trachea**
   Use of uncuffed tubes in children ≤8 years of age to minimize tracheal trauma. If unable to orally intubate, use needle or open cricothyroidotomy because of decreased incidence of secondary subglottic stenosis.

B. **Breathing**
   1. **Infants and Children are Diaphragmatic Breathers**
   2. **Abdominal or Diaphragmatic Trauma Compromises Ventilation**

C. **Circulation**
   Children have significant cardiovascular reserve and signs of shock may not present until >30% of blood volume lost

D. **Normal Vital Signs Based on Age (Table 38-1)**

E. **Vascular Access**
   1. **Percutaneous**
      Percutaneous intravenous catheter access is first choice, avoiding the external jugular vein until the cervical spine is cleared.
   2. **Catheter**
      Place at least a 20-gauge intravenous catheter in the bilateral upper extremities.
   3. **Intraosseous Access**
      If peripheral access cannot be obtained quickly or in three attempts, attempt an intraosseous access. Intraosseous infusion allows rapid fluid administration can be safely used in children <6 years.
      a. **Technique (Fig. 38-1)**

      - Prepare the skin using povidone-iodine disinfectant, drape off the area, usually 1 to 2 cm inferior to the midpoint of a line drawn from tibial tuberosity to the medial aspect of tibia.
      - Using a commercially available needle, or a 16- or 18-gauge spinal needle, advance the needle perpendicular to the tibia in a screwing motion until "a give" occurs when the needle penetrates the cortex—usually no deeper than 1 cm.
      - Remove trocar and confirm position by aspiration of marrow and blood.

Table 38-1.   Normal vital signs based on age

Age	Pulse	Systoloic Blood Pressure (mm Hg)	Respirations (breaths/min)
Newborn	95–145	60–90	30–60
Infant	125–170	75–100	30–60
Toddler	100–160	80–110	24–40
Preschool	70–110	80–110	22–34
School age	70–110	85–120	18–30

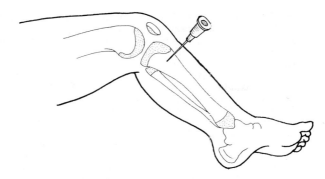

Figure 38-1. Intraosseous infusion.

- A secure needle and can accept volume infusions of 10 mL/min, bolus will require pressure assistance.

F. Complications
  1. Extravasation and Infection
Remove the intraosseous line as soon as a vein can be cannulated.
  a. In older children, a cutdown of the saphenous vein at the ankle or antecubital vein of the arm is often a rapid way of gaining vascular access. If the patient is known to have poor access (was a premature infant or had long hospitalizations in the past), consider saphenous vein or femoral cutdown in the groin.
  b. Percutaneous placement of lines in groin, or elsewhere, using Seldinger technique should be left after the resuscitation is well under way and the patient is in the operating room of pediatric intensive care unit (PICU).

G. Fluid Resuscitation
  1. Initial boluses of 10 to 20 mL/kg of warmed lactated Ringer's solution, depending on vital signs; if the patient continues to be hemodynamically unstable, repeat. If no response to >40 mL/kg of crystalloid solution, consider adding blood products.
  2. Maintenance fluids should be warmed and adjusted to maintain a urine output of 1 to 2 mL/kg/hour.

V. Imaging Studies
  A. Initial Trauma Series and Cervical Spine Clearance
These studies should be as are done with adult patients.
  B. Other Imaging
Mechanism, history, and physical examination determine other appropriate studies.
  C. Computed Tomography in Our Emergency Ward is Mode of Choice
Head, neck, chest, abdomen, and pelvis imaging, as indicated.

D. Diagnostic Peritoneal Lavage and Focused Abdominal Sonogram for Trauma

These procedures have limited roles because the presence of fluid does not dictate a need for surgery.

E. Angiography

In rare cases of pelvic fractures, angiography may be helpful to control bleeding.

VI. Specific Injuries by System

A. Central Nervous System Trauma

Central nervous system injuries are the most common cause of death and disability. Children can have significant trauma without skull fracture with a greater incidence of epidural hematomas. They tend to have diffuse injuries and early imaging may show little evidence of injury. In children aged ≤2 years, abuse is the most common cause of head injury. Shaken baby syndrome is characterized with little evidence of external trauma, subdural, subarachnoid hemorrhage, and retinal hemorrhage.

1. Glasgow Coma Scale (Pediatric modification for nonverbal children) Scoring

  a. Eye Opening
- **(1)** Spontaneous: 4
- **(2)** To speech: 3
- **(3)** To pain: 2
- **(4)** No response: 1

  b. Best Verbal Response
- **(1)** Oriented (infant coos or babbles): 5
- **(2)** Confused (infant irritable or cries): 4
- **(3)** Inappropriate words (infant cries to pain): 3
- **(4)** Incomprehensible sounds (infant moans to pain): 2
- **(5)** No response: 1

  c. Best Motor Response
- **(1)** Obeys (infant moves spontaneously and purposefully): 6
- **(2)** Localizes (infant withdraws to touch): 5
- **(3)** Withdraws to pain: 4
- **(4)** Abnormal flexion to pain (decorticate): 3
- **(5)** Extensor response to pain (decerebrate): 2
- **(6)** No response: 1

2. Degree of Traumatic Brain Injury Based on Glasgow Coma Scale Score

  a. Glasgow Coma Scale
- **(1)** Mild: 13 to 15
- **(2)** Moderate: 9 to 12
- **(3)** Severe: 3 to 8

3. Treatment

  a. Dependent. Oxygenation, ventilation, and blood pressure are factors that help determine treatment.

  b. Preventive Measures. It is important to prevent hypoxia, hypoventilation, fluid overload, and hypoperfusion to avoid secondary injury.

      c. Intracranial Pressure (ICP) Monitors. ICP monitors should be used early in severe and in some moderate injuries.

      d. Adjuncts. Diuretics and hyperventilation are also good temporary adjuncts in selected patients.

  4. Spinal Cord Injury

      a. Uncommon in Pediatric Population. Most commonly involves C1-C2.

      b. Spinal Cord Injury Without Radiologic Abnormalities (SCIWORA)

      c. Accounts for Most Cervical Spine Injuries in Children. Occurs in children <8 years of age because of the elasticity of the cervical spine, which can allow severe cord injury without radiologic findings.

      d. Diagnosis of Exclusion

      e. Treatment. Spine immobilization.

B. Thoracic Trauma

- Thoracic trauma is the second leading cause of death, 25% of all deaths related to trauma
- Approximately 90% are caused by blunt injury in motor vehicle accidents
- Greater compliance of the chest wall and the increased mobility of structures within the mediastinum in children means that children can have serious intrathoracic injuries without rib fractures

  1. Common Injuries

- Airway laceration
- Tension pneumothorax
- Cardiovascular injuries and tamponade
- Massive hemothorax
- Flail chest
- Diaphragmatic rupture
- Esophageal injuries

  2. Indications for Operative Intervention (Table 38-2)

C. Abdominal Trauma

- Far more blunt abdominal injuries occur in children than in the adult population, accounting for 10% of trauma deaths
- In children, the abdomen begins at the level of the nipples. The spleen, liver, and kidneys are especially vulnerable to injury

  1. Splenic Injury Grading System (Table 38-3)
  2. Liver Injury Grading System (Table 38-4)
  Grades seen on CT scan are *not* well correlated with need for operative intervention

  3. Guidelines for the Clinical Management of *Isolated* Blunt Hepatic or Splenic Injuries

  As with any guideline, the clinical judgment of the surgeon is the ultimate gold standard of care. We

Table 38-2. Indications for operative intervention

Immediate Thoracotomy
–Massive continuing pneumothorax
–Cardiac tamponade
–Open pneumothorax with extensive soft tissue injury
–Esophageal injury
–Massive air leak from tracheobronchial injury
–Aortic or other vascular injury
–Acute diaphragmatic rupture
Delayed Thoracotomy
–Chronic rupture of diaphragm
–Persistent hemothorax
–Persistent chylothorax
–Chronic atelectasis from traumatic bronchial stenosis

Table 38-3. Splenic injury grading system

Grade	Description of Injury
I	Capsular tear, parenchymal injury <1 cm depth
II	Capsular tear, parenchymal injury 1–3 cm depth, no involvement of trabecular vessel
III	Laceration, >3 cm parenchymal depth involving trabecular vessels; ruptured subcapsular or parenchymal hematoma; intraparenchymal hematoma >5 cm or expanding
IV	Lacerations involving segmental or hilar vessels, producing major devascularization, >25% of spleen
V	Shattered spleen, or hilar vascular injury that devascularizes spleen

Table 38-4. Liver injury grading system

Grade	Description of Injury
I	Capsular tear >1 cm in depth
II	Capsular tear 1–3 cm in depth <10 cm in length
III	Capsular tear >3 cm in depth
IV	Parenchymal disruption 25% to 75% of hepatic lobe
V	Parenchymal disruption >75% of hepatic lobe; injury to retrohepatic vena cava

hope that the guidelines will provide appropriate levels of care and resource utilization, without any compromise of the clinical outcome.

Severity of injury will be categorized as minimal, moderate, and severe, using a combination of clinical findings, laboratory tests, and radiographic imaging. The decision to operate is based on the clinical judgment of the attending surgeon, along with the patient's wishes.

4.   Discharge Criteria for All Levels of Injury (Table 38-5)

- Stable or increasing hematocrit
- Resolution of abdominal tenderness
- Tolerating regular diet
- Absence of symptoms ambulating in hospital (e.g., orthostasis)

To take this a level further, we should also *standardize* the observation protocol for the residents. We would suggest the following:

a.   Minimal

1. Admit to floor
2. Serial hematocrit every 6 hours until nadir is reached or passed
3. No nasogastric tube unless persistent emesis
4. Start oral feeding when tenderness resolved and hematocrit is stable
5. Complete blood count on day of discharge

b.   Moderate

1. Admit to monitored bed, either on floor or in ICU
2. Serial hematocrit every 6 hours until nadir is reached or passed

Table 38-5.   Discharge criteria for all levels of injury

Criteria	Minimal	Moderate	Severe
Hemodynamic instability	—	± minimal	± prolonged
Transfusion	—	–	±
Minimal hematocrit	>30	>25	<25
Computed tomography grade	I–II	III	IV–V
Free fluid by ultrasound or computed tomography	–/minimal	± definite	mod-large
Abdominal tenderness	±	±	+
Suggested intensive care unit stay	—	±	+
Time in hospital (days)	2–3	3–5	5–10

3. No nasogastric tube unless persistent emesis
4. Start oral feeding when tenderness resolved and hematocrit is stable
5. Complete blood count on day of discharge

c. Severe

1. Admit to ICU
2. Serial hematocrit every 4 hours until hemodynamically stable, then every 8 hours until nadir reached
3. Transfer to floor when stable examination, hematocrit, hemodynamics
4. Foley catheter for urine output monitoring
5. Nasogastric tube, if clinically indicated
6. Start oral feeding when tenderness resolved and hematocrit is stable
7. Complete blood count on day of discharge

d. Principles of Nonoperative Management

1. Close observation, serial physical examinations, serial hematocrits.
2. Floor observation reasonable for many isolated liver or spleen injuries
3. Length of observation related to degree of injury

e. Indications for operative intervention

1. Hemodynamic instability
2. Continued hemorrhage
3. Presence of other injuries requiring operative intervention

5. Special Injuries to Consider
Seatbelt sign as an indicator of small bowel perforation, pancreatic injury or transection with traumatic pancreatitis are special considerations.

    a. Operative Intervention. Operative intervention to repair the duct can be indicated. Late appearance of a pseudocyst is also possible.

    b. Duodenal Hematoma. A duodenal hematoma can be caused by blunt force to the upper abdomen, as from a bicycle handlebar. Can be seen on CT and often presents with gastric outlet obstruction symptoms. Conservative management takes a long time; operative drainage is a better option in most cases.

D. Musculoskeletal Trauma

    1. Determining Treatment and Outcome
Status of bone development and injuries involving the growth plate are essential in determining outcome and treatment.

    2. Salter-Harris Classification of Epiphyseal Fractures

        a. Type I: Pure physeal separation

        b. Type II: Metaphyseal fracture and physeal separation

        c. Type III: Epiphyseal fracture and physeal separation

        d. Type IV: Fracture through epiphysis and metaphysis

        e. Type V: Crush injury of physis

   3. Treatment

        a. Type I and II: Closed Reduction

        b. Type III and IV: Open Reduction and Internal Fixation

        c. Type V: Open reduction and Internal Fixation, Associated with Growth Failure

   4. Greenstick Fractures

Because of the pliability of pediatric bone, angulation of a long bone causes the bone to break only on the convex side, leaving the concave periosteum and cortex intact.

   5. Fracture Complications

        a. Limb Growth Disturbances

        b. Avascular necrosis of Epiphyses

        c. Joint Instability

V. Child Abuse

   A. Suspect in the Following Cases

      1. History

The history is inconsistent with the physical examination findings.

      2. Discrepancy

Accounts of injury vary and stories change.

      3. Multiple Injuries in Various Stages of Healing

      4. Reaction

Pay special attention to the reaction of parents (babysitter or others) to the situation.

      5. Report all *suspected* cases of abuse.

SELECTED READING

American Trauma Society. *National guidelines for pediatric trauma care,* 2002.

Dodson, TB Kaban LB. Special considerations for the pediatric emergency patient. *Emerg Med Clinic North Am* 2000;18(3):539–548.

Kapklein M, Schunk J. Pediatric trauma. *Mt Sinai J Med* 1997; 64(4–5):302–310.

National Pediatric Trauma Registry Fact Sheets.

Pediatric Trauma 2: Definitive Care

Akemi L. Kawaguchi, MD, David Lawlor, MD, and Jay J. Schnitzer, MD

I. Introduction

Accidents account for 65% of all injury related deaths in patients <19 years of age. As discussed in the previous chapter, all trauma patients should first be evaluated and resuscitated using advanced trauma life support (ATLS) and pediatric advanced life support (PALS) guidelines.

II. Unique Pediatric Considerations in Transport and Destination

A. Criteria for Transfer

Similar to adults, any pediatric patient with needs that exceed the available resources of the initial hospital should be transferred to a trauma center. The patient's condition should be optimized before transfer, including establishment of two intravenous (i.v.) access lines with fluid resuscitation, control of external hemorrhage, and airway management with endotracheal intubation or a surgical airway, if indicated. Children with a significant possibility of airway obstruction, airway edema, or decreased mental status should be intubated before transfer. Critically ill children should be transported by a team familiar with the care of children. Pediatric equipment (e.g., endotracheal tubes, Ambu bags oral airways, laryngoscopes, i.v. supplies, and other items should be available. Proper weight-adjusted dosages for emergency medications should accompany the patient in transfer.

B. Securing the Pediatric Airway

Use extra precautions when securing the airway of a child. A small airway can be extremely difficult to regain if lost during patient transfer or if the patient is accidentally extubated. We routinely secure an endotracheal tube in place with umbilical or tracheal tape rather than adhesive tape.

III. Unique Pediatric Considerations in Neurologic Injury

A. Background

Head injuries alone or those associated with other injuries comprise most fatal traumatic injuries in children. Brain injury is also the leading cause of long-term disability in children and young adults. The Glasgow Coma Scale (GCS) for children can be used as a guide to injury severity, and the score directly correlates with outcome. A GCS score of 13 to 15 is considered mild, 9 to 12 moderate, 5 to 8 severe, and 3 to 4 very severe. Mild injuries tend to have good outcomes. Children with moderate and severe head injuries are at high risk for cognitive and behavioral problems.

Children with very severe head injuries who survive usually have a prolonged comatose state with posttraumatic amnesia, and cognitive, behavioral, and physical disabilities. It is essential to involve a pediatric neurosurgeon early in the care of a pediatric patient with a neurologic injury.

B. Management

Once a neurologic injury has occurred, little can be done to lessen the primary damage. The goal is to minimize secondary damage that can occur from bleeding, edema, hypoxia, and ischemia. Cerebral perfusion pressure, which is defined as mean arterial pressure (MAP) minus the intracranial pressure (ICP), must be maintained to prevent further injury. Adequate blood pressure must be maintained, sometimes requiring the use of pressors. ICP should be monitored in children with head injuries with GCS score ≤7, patients who cannot have a neurologic examination, patients who require prolonged anesthesia for surgical procedures, and patients who require paralysis for ventilatory control.

1. Methods for Decreasing Intracranial Pressure

a. Cerebrospinal Fluid Removal. Remove cerebrospinal fluid (CSF) via ventriculostomy.

b. Osmotic Therapy. We use mannitol 0.5 to 1.0 g/kg loading dose, followed by 0.25 g/kg every 2 to 4 hours, titrated to achieve a maximal serum osmolality of 315 to 320 mOsm/L.

c. Hyperventilation (Judicious). Titrate to a goal $PaCO_2$ of 30 to 40 mm Hg.

d. Barbiturate Coma. Phenobarbital loading dose 3 to 5 mg/kg, followed by maintenance dose of 0.5 to 1.0 mg/kg/h.

2. Corticosteroids

Current studies do not support the use of corticosteroids for the treatment of acute head trauma.

C. Epidural and Subdural Hematomas

Manage epidural and subdural hematomas in children as in adults. Children tend to have a better prognosis than do adults with the same injury pattern. A neurosurgical consultation should be obtained for all patients with an intracranial hemorrhage.

D. Admission Criteria

For children who have an isolated head injury but are alert and awake at the time of consideration, admission criteria include one or more of the following:

1. Loss of consciousness
2. Abnormal behavior (e.g., persistent vomiting, irritability, sleepiness)
3. Seizures
4. Evidence of a CSF leak
5. Inability for caregivers to provide a safe home

E. Cervical Spine Injuries

Children under 8 years of age are particularly susceptible to spinal cord injury without radiographic abnormality

(SCIWORA) and may be more difficult to assess secondary to communication difficulties or inability of the patient to cooperate with an examination secondary to fear. The immature and relatively lax cervical ligaments, incomplete bone ossification, and horizontally oriented articular surfaces of the vertebral bodies in children put them at higher risk for subluxation and spinal cord injury. In addition, children have relatively larger heads with immature neck musculature, leading to a fulcrum effect in the C2-C3 area. Younger children, therefore, more often suffer a higher cervical spine injury than do adolescents and adults.

An algorithm we developed for the evaluation of cervical spine injuries in children is shown in **Figure 39-1.** Patients are first evaluated for the presence of midline neck pain or tenderness, decreased level of consciousness, physical signs of neck trauma (i.e., ecchymosis, crepitus), distracting injuries (i.e., painful fracture or laceration), or an abnormal neurologic examination. An in-collar lateral cervical spine plain film should be performed immediately. Transient neurologic symptoms or unexplainable hypotension can indicate SCIWORA. If the answer is "no" to all of these questions, then an out-of-collar lateral cervical spine plain film is done. If this is negative, the immobilization collar can be removed. If the answer to any of these questions is positive or the examiner is unable to assess the patient, then three-view plain films, including the anteroposterior (AP), lateral, and odontoid views can be done. If these cannot be completed and the patient has neurologic symptoms or is already scheduled for a head or abdominal computed tomography (CT) scan, then a helical CT scan of the neck with three-dimensional reconstructions of the cervical spine is performed. Steroid therapy is given in the standard dosage of methylprednisolone (30 mg/kg i.v.) push for one dose, followed by 5.4 mg/kg/h for 24 hours if spinal cord injury is strongly suspected because clinical examination findings or if it has been diagnosed by radiographic study.

F.   Child Abuse

Physical abuse is the leading cause of head injury in infants. Child abuse should be considered any time when the injury pattern is not consistent with the mechanism of injury, the caregivers are evasive regarding mechanism, or if other signs are seen of neglect or intentional injuries. These children can come to the hospital as a trauma patient after a "fall" or other mechanical event.

Shaken baby syndrome is a clearly definable and potentially life-threatening form of child abuse. Although this injury pattern has been documented in children 5 years of age, it most often occurs in infants and children <2 years of age because of the size disparity between the caregiver and victim. Shaken baby syndrome results from violent shaking of the child, which causes acceleration and deceleration of cranial contents. This results in retinal hemorrhages, subdural or subarachnoid hemorrhages, all with little evidence of other trauma. Mild symptoms can include poor feeding, lethargy, and irritability. More severe cases

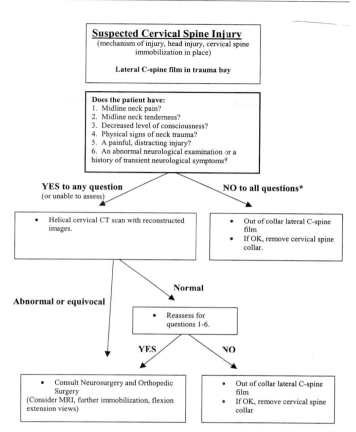

Figure 39-1.   Algorithm for the evaluation of pediatric spine trauma.
*A negative clinical exam (NCE) can only be performed if the patient
is awake, alert, old enough to respond to questions, and without significant distracting injuries. It requires that the alert patient deny
significant neck pain, that physical examination reveal no significant
tenderness of the cervical spine, and that the patient is able to
move the neck through a full voluntary range of motion without
significant pain.

can result in mental status changes, loss of consciousness,
bradycardia, apnea, and death. The workup includes CT
scan for immediate assessment for subdural and subarachnoid hemorrhage, mass effect from edema, and other
trauma. In addition, magnetic resonance imaging (MRI)
can be performed 2 to 3 days later, which may show evidence of diffuse axonal injury, edema, and hemorrhage. A
pediatric ophthalmologist and neurologist or neurosurgeon
should see these patients. The proper authorities should
also be notified.

IV. Unique Pediatric Considerations in Chest Injury

A. Radiographic Evaluation

All patients with a suspected thoracic injury should have a plain chest radiograph early in the initial evaluation. Most life-threatening injuries can be diagnosed with plain film. Chest CT scan with intravenous contrast material, which can be used to evaluate other injuries, has recently been found to be a highly sensitive test for great vessel injury. Aortography, however, remains the gold standard for evaluation of traumatic aortic injury. Occasionally, echocardiography and bronchoscopy can be useful in the evaluation of thoracic injuries.

B. Traumatic Asphyxia

Traumatic asphyxia is an injury seen almost exclusively in children. This occurs with sudden compression of the abdomen or chest against a closed glottis. A rapid rise in intrathoracic pressure occurs that is transmitted to all of the veins draining into the valveless superior vena cava. Capillary extravasation occurs in the upper half of the body, the sclerae, and sometimes the brain. Signs and symptoms include hyperemic sclera, seizures, disorientation, petechiae on the upper half of the body, and respiratory failure. Traumatic asphyxia is clinically diagnosed and has a good prognosis. Treatment is supportive care. Associated injuries can include pulmonary contusions, central nervous system injuries, and intraabdominal injuries.

C. Rib Fractures

Because of the increased compliance of children's ribs, fractures are much less common than in adults and require a greater force of injury. When rib fractures are present, it is a likely indicator of more severe underlying injury, so maintain a low threshold for further testing. With child abuse, the typical site of fracture is at the neck of the rib, near the articulation of the rib and transverse process. These are often undetectable in infants because the head of the rib is cartilaginous. Other signs include cystic lesions in the posterior portion of the ribs and multiple rib fractures at various stages of healing. Treatment of rib fractures involves pain control and rest, with most rib fractures healing within 6 weeks.

D. Pneumothorax and Hemothorax

Management of pneumothorax and hemothorax is similar in adults and children. In general, chest tube placement at the level of the nipple (approximately fourth or fifth intercostal space) in the anterior axillary line is appropriate. Recommended chest tube sizes include (1) newborns 12F to 16F, (2) infants 16F to 18F, (3) younger children 18F to 24F, and (4) adolescents 28F to 32F. Chest tubes are placed to closed suction drainage and monitored closely for air leak and drainage. In most patients, chest tube thoracostomy is sufficient. Indications for thoracotomy with bronchoscopy include large, persistent air leak (which can indicate tracheobronchial injury), initial drainage of >20% of estimated blood volume, continued bleeding at a rate >1 to 2 mL/kg/h, increased rate of bleeding, and inability to drain the pleural space of blood and clots.

E. Pulmonary Contusion

Pulmonary contusion is one of the most common injuries in blunt thoracic trauma in the pediatric population. Children with severe contusions should be admitted to an intensive care unit (ICU) with continuous oxygen saturation monitoring and administration of supplemental oxygen, as needed. Patients should have fluid intake restricted and be provided with adequate analgesia and aggressive chest physical therapy. Intubation is not often indicated and most contusions clear within 2 weeks.

V. Unique Pediatric Considerations in Abdominal Injury

A. Background

Children are more susceptible to abdominal injuries than are adults because their rib cages are smaller and more pliable, therefore offering less protection. Children's organs are also relatively larger in relation to the abdomen, making them more vulnerable to injury. Moreover, the thin abdominal wall musculature provides less protection from both blunt and penetrating trauma. Serial examinations are essential because young children are often not able to provide a full history or cooperate with the initial examination.

B. Radiologic Evaluation

In the hemodynamically stable patient with a suspected abdominal injury based on the history, mechanism of injury, physical examination, abnormal laboratory values, or other concerns, an abdominal or pelvic CT scan should be performed. CT scan has been demonstrated to be sensitive for solid organ and retroperitoneal injury. It lacks sensitivity, however, for hollow viscous injury. Diagnostic peritoneal lavage (DPL) is largely reserved for patients with coexisting extraabdominal injuries that need urgent operative intervention, without the opportunity for CT scan. Warm isotonic fluid (10 to 15 mL/kg) should be used for the lavage. Focused abdominal sonography for trauma (FAST) has not been shown to be an accurate method of detecting solid organ injury in children at our institution and it is not generally used for our pediatric patients.

C. Splenic Injuries

The spleen is the most commonly injured abdominal organ in children. Previously, splenectomy was the treatment of choice for even a minor splenic injury. More recently, it has been clearly demonstrated that most splenic injuries can be managed nonoperatively. Nonoperative management is particularly important to children because they are at high risk for postsplenectomy bacterial sepsis. This syndrome is most commonly seen in children <5 years of age. Following splenectomy, all patients should be vaccinated against encapsulated organisms: *Haemophilus influenza, Streptococcus pneumoniae,* and *Neisseria meningitides.*

When a splenic injury is diagnosed, management includes placement of large-bore i.v. lines and nasogastric tube, serial hematocrit measurements, bedrest, and close monitoring, preferably in an ICU setting. Patients should have frequent serial abdominal assessments by a consistent, experienced examiner. Operative indications include persistent hemodynamic instability, continuing hemorrhage with need for transfusion of more than half of blood volume, diffuse peritoneal irritation with abdominal distension and hypovolemia, and signs of significant injury to other intraabdominal organs. Splenectomy is reserved for only those patients who have irreparable damage to the organ, uncontrollable hemorrhage, or a multitude of life-threatening injuries that place the patient at risk for coagulopathy, hypothermia, and vascular collapse. Many operative techniques exist for splenorrhaphy, including pledgeted sutures, vertical mattress sutures, simple sutures, and absorbable mesh wraps. These can be reinforced with omental buttressing. Devascularized segments of the spleen should be resected.

Children who are managed nonoperatively are allowed out of bed after their abdominal tenderness resolves. They can return to light activity at home and school in 1 week. For children who participate in contact sports, they are allowed to resume full activity in 2 to 6 months, largely depending on the severity of injury. Imaging should be repeated in patients with any recurrent or persistent local symptoms.

D.   Hepatic Injuries
The liver is the second most commonly injured organ in the child's abdomen. Much like management of splenic trauma, most liver injuries can be managed nonoperatively with careful monitoring. Operative indications are similar to those of patients with splenic injuries: hemodynamic instability, ongoing transfusion requirements, and other associated injuries.

E.   Trauma to Hollow Abdominal Organs
Stomach rupture is rare, but can occur following an abrupt blunt force to the abdomen following a full meal. This has been seen in falls, motor vehicle collisions, and as the result of child abuse. Intramural duodenal hematoma is the most common small bowel injury in children. It occurs as the duodenum is forced posteriorly against the vertebral body. Symptoms include postprandial epigastric and right upper quadrant pain occurring immediately to 7 days following the initial injury. Persistent bilious emesis is common. Most patients will respond to nasogastric tube decompression and nonoperative management. Patients with complete obstruction may require total parenteral nutrition (TPN) until the hematoma reabsorbs.

VI.   Unique Pediatric Considerations in Orthopedic Injury
A.   Background
The major differences between bone in adult and children include the presence of the physis or "growth plate," more rapid remodeling, and decreased bone density. Children have a much greater ability to quickly remodel injured

bone. In fact, fractures set with <30% of angulation in a prepubescent child will provide adequate healing. Children often have accelerated growth at the area of long bone fractures, which can lead to a discrepancy in bone length as the bone heals. Allowing the fracture to heal in anatomic alignment, with a 1-cm overlap, often reduces this inequality. Varus, valgus, angulation, and rotation will not be compensated with remodeling. It is essential to provide proper traction and splinting to prevent further soft tissue damage and minimize unnecessary pain for the patient before further lengthy trauma evaluation. The length of immobilization depends on the age of the child and the forces specific to the bone involved.

B. Orthopedic Injuries Particular to Children (Fig. 39-2)

1. Plastic Deformity
Excessively bowed bone without radiographic evidence of cortical disruption is referred to as "plastic deformity."

2. Torus Fracture
Torus fracture, or "buckle" fracture at the junction between the epiphysis and metaphysis results from compressive forces.

3. Greenstick Fracture
A greenstick fracture occurs at the opposite side of the force of impact.

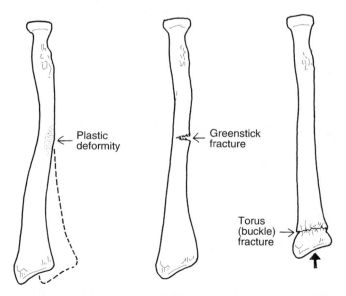

Figure 39-2. Unique pediatric fracture patterns. Left: Plastic deformity. Right: Torus (buckle) fracture. Middle: Greenstick fracture.

4. Fractures Involving the Physis

Up to 18% of pediatric fractures are those that involve the physis or "growth plate." The cartilaginous composition of the physis makes it softer and more vulnerable to injuries. This is particularly true during times of rapid growth. In 1963, Robert Salter and Robert Harris classified growth plate injuries into groups with associated clinical treatment as well as prognosis. In general, the higher the number, the more serious the injury. The Salter-Harris classification of epiphyseal plate injuries is as follows **(Fig. 39-3)**:

a.   Type 1. Fracture is through the physis only. With minimal or no displacement, this type of fracture may not be evident on plain radiographs. If a patient has tenderness over the area of the physis, treat with immobilization, as if a fracture were present. Prognosis is excellent.

b.   Type 2. Fracture is through the physis and metaphysis with a fragment of metaphysis remaining attached to the epiphysis. Treat with immobilization. Prognosis is excellent.

c.   Type 3. Fracture begins intraarticularly and travels through the epiphysis into the physis. This requires precise reduction with anatomic alignment to prevent arthritis and growth abnormalities. Prognosis is good with proper alignment.

d.   Type 4. An intraarticular fracture that extends through the epiphysis, physis, and metaphysis. These require precise reduction, often accomplished operatively.

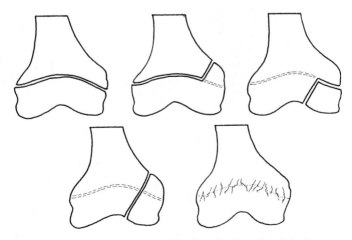

Figure 39-3.   Salter-Harris classification of epiphysial plate fractures. Top Left: Type 1. Top Middle: Type 2. Top Right: Type 3. Bottom Left: Type 4. Bottom Right: Type 5.

e. **Type 5.** The physis is crushed without any other injury to the bone. This injury is often not appreciated on the initial radiographs. It carries a poor prognosis with premature growth cessation at the physis.

5. **Supracondylar Fractures**

A supracondylar fracture is considered an orthopedic emergency. It is the most common elbow fracture in pediatric patients and usually results from a fall onto an outstretched arm. The patient will usually hold the arm pronated and resist elbow flexion secondary to pain. A careful neurovascular examination is warranted because damage can have occurred to the radial nerve, ulnar nerve, median nerve, anterior interosseus nerve, and brachial artery. The patient should have an immediate evaluation by an orthopedic surgeon.

6. **Femur Fractures**

In the pediatric population, children with femur fractures are treated differently at varying ages. In children <1 year of age, most are treated nonoperatively with a spica cast, traction and casting, or Pavlik harness. As children get older, femur fractures are increasingly likely to be repaired operatively with intramedullary rodding.

C. **Child Abuse**

Documentation of skeletal injuries is essential for any child who may have suffered from abuse. A skeletal survey consists of AP and lateral chest and skull films and a complete skeletal survey, including the long bones, hands, and feet. A CT scan may be necessary. Children who have been abused can have several injuries in various states of healing. Radiographic findings include evidence of callus formation from older fractures, epiphyseal septations, periosteal hemorrhage, periosteal shearing, and shearing of the metaphysis.

VII. **Unique Pediatric Considerations in Critical Care**

A. **Temperature Regulation**

In comparison with adult patients, young children have a higher body surface area-to-mass ratio. They are more susceptible to heat loss by radiation, convection, and evaporation. It is critical to maintain the patient's body temperature in the field, the trauma resuscitation area, the operating room, and at the bedside. This should be accomplished by increasing the ambient room temperature, and using warmed fluids, warmed blood products, warming lights, warm air blankets, and incubators (for infants).

B. **Fluid and Electrolytes**

Young children have a remarkable cardiovascular reserve; consequently, hypovolemia can be underestimated. Children will not show signs of decreased urine output and hypotension until 30% of their blood volume has been lost. Immature kidneys of infants have difficulty both excreting high salt loads and concentrating the urine relative to adults. Hourly maintenance fluids for children by weight can be calculated with the "4, 2, 1 rule," with 4 mL/kg/h for the first 10 kg, 2 mL/kg/h for the next 10 kg, and 1 mL/kg/h for each kilogram above 20 kg. For example a 25-kg child would require 65 mL/h intravenous fluid for maintenance. Insensible losses from the skin, respiratory tract, and gastrointestinal tract must also be considered.

C. Nutrition and Metabolism

We routinely start our patients on enteral nutrition as soon as possible. The type of nutrition depends on the patient's age and ability to safely tolerate oral intake. If possible, we use enteral tube feedings and avoid parenteral nutrition because it is associated with central line placement complications, bacteremia, fungemia, and liver failure. The incidence of TPN-induced hepatic failure is higher in children than in adults.

D. Pain Management

Acetaminophen is the most commonly used nonopioid analgesic at our institution. If needed, opioids (e.g., morphine or fentanyl) can be used for pain control. We transition our patients to oral medications as soon as they are able to tolerate enteral intake. For children with severe pain who are unable to tolerate oral medications, continuous i.v. infusions can be used. Children on opiates require frequent assessment of respiratory rate, oxygen saturation, and level of arousal. Children who are >7 years of age may also benefit from a patient-controlled anesthesia (PCA), which allows the patient to self-administer small intermittent dosages of i.v. narcotic medications. This can be advantageous for older children because PCA can give them a sense of control over their pain management.

E. Rehabilitation Issues

Children on our trauma service are regularly followed by our PRIME (Pediatric rehabilitation, Injury Management, and Evaluation) team, which consists of social services, speech and language therapists, physical therapists, occupational therapists, rehabilitation medicine clinicians, case managers, and the pediatric trauma nurse coordinator. Together, this team coordinates patient care and involves the family members. This multidisciplinary approach is essential for optimizing patient care and allowing our pediatric patients to achieve an optimal functional recovery as efficiently as possible.

VIII. Common Pitfalls in the Care of the Pediatric Trauma Patient

A. Relying primarily on the blood pressure as the sign of hypovolemia.

B. Failure to obtain prompt vascular access for resuscitation.

C. Failure to recognize the magnitude of possible blood loss from isolated injuries, particularly intracranial bleeding in infants with open sutures that allow the skull to expand, femur fractures, and pelvic fractures.

D. Failure to recognize inadequate resuscitation and the child's ability to compensate and create an illusion of hemodynamic normalcy.

E. Failure to use appropriate-sized equipment and supplies for the individual patient. This includes the laryngoscope, endotracheal tube, nasogastric tube, oral and nasal airways, oxygen masks, cervical spine collar, urinary catheters, splints, i.v. catheters, and other equipment.

F. Failure to identify physical or sexual abuse and to document a detailed history of the episode, including who was with the child, medical history of neglect or abuse, complete details of examination, photographs of injuries, genital examination, and a statement of compatibility of injuries and their explanation.

G. Failure to listen to parents who note abnormal behavior in their child or their child's refusal to use an injured limb.

SELECTED READING

American Academy of Pediatrics Committee on Child Abuse and Neglect, 2000–2001. Shaken baby syndrome: rotational cranial injuries—technical report. *Pediatrics* 2001;108(1):206–210.

Bond S, Eichelberger M, Gotschall C, et al. Nonoperative management of blunt hepatic and splenic injury in children. *Ann Surg* 1996;223(3):286–289.

Sanchez J, Paidas C. Trauma care in the new millennium: childhood trauma, now and in the new millennium. *Surg Clin North Am* 1999;79(6):1503–1535.

Vicellio P, Simon H, Pressman B, et al. A prospective multicenter study of cervical spine injury in children. *Pediatrics* 2001;108(2):E20.

40

Considerations in the Pregnant Woman

Larry Rand, MD, and
Kevin C. Dennehy, MB, BCh, FFARCSI

I. **Introduction**
   A. **Statistics and Epidemiology: Maternal**
      1. **Physical Trauma**
      Physical trauma is estimated to complicate 1 of every 12 pregnancies in the United States. Trauma is a leading cause of death in women of reproductive age.
      2. **Motor Vehicle Accidents**
      The most significant contributor to fetal death from trauma is a motor vehicle accident. In industrialized nations, two thirds of all trauma results from automobile crashes. Female drivers are more likely to be involved in car accidents than male drivers according to the National Safety Council.
      3. **Other Causes of Trauma**
      Other common causes of trauma during pregnancy are falls and direct assaults to the abdomen. Blunt trauma is the far more likely scenario than sharp.
   B. **Statistics and Epidemiology: Fetal**
      1. **Fetal Loss**
      Accurate statistics on the number of fetal losses caused by trauma are not yet available. Estimates, however, indicate that between 1300 and 3900 pregnancies are lost each year in the United States as a result of trauma.
      2. **Effect of Maternal Trauma**
      A fetal loss rate of 40% to 50% is associated with life-threatening maternal trauma, such as shock, head injury and coma, and maternal emergency laparotomy. A pregnancy loss rate of 1% to 5% resulted from minor or non life-threatening injuries.
      3. **Effect of Minor Injuries**
      Because minor injuries are much more common, most losses result from these. Several case series studies indicate that >50% of fetal losses occur in association with minor or seemingly insignificant trauma. Abruption complicates 40% to 50% of pregnancies sustaining severe trauma, whereas it only has an incidence of 1% to 5% in non life-threatening trauma.
      4. **Injury Severity Score**
      The standardized Injury Severity Score (ISS) has been shown to be a poor predictor of adverse fetal outcome, presumably because of so many losses occurring with more minor maternal trauma.

C. Abuse in Maternal Trauma

1. Assault

Two million women per year are reported to have been assaulted by their male partners. The prevalence of violence against pregnant women ranges from 1% to 20%. In an inner-city setting, domestic violence can occur in 1 of every 12 pregnancies. Of victims, 60% report two or more episodes of physical assault during pregnancy.

2. Risk Factors

Pregnant women are at particularly high risk for violence for multiple reasons. Partners may react negatively toward the pregnancy; they may view the fetus as stealing the mother's attention; and they may take advantage of the pregnancy as something of value to the mother. Thus, the unborn fetus and pregnant abdomen are a common target for trauma by abusers.

II. Primary Survey

A. Guiding Principle

The guiding principle in trauma to a pregnant patient is ensuring that the woman is medically stable before evaluating the fetus. Thus, the parturient is examined first and the fetus is assessed at the start of the secondary survey.

B. Airway Management

Airway management involves assessing for the effects of trauma on the pregnant airway while taking into account the anatomic and physiologic changes of pregnancy. Optimal patient positioning (**Fig. 40-1**) may not be possible if spinal injury precautions are being maintained. In this setting, it is important to have an airway management algorithm that considers the difficulties presented by the effects of trauma on the airway and, especially that of the parturient.

1. Physiologic Changes

Among the physiologic changes to consider is engorgement of the capillaries and mucosa of the nasal, oropharyngeal, and laryngeal structures, thus nasal intubation is not recommended. The average weight gain during pregnancy is approximately 26 pounds. This weight gain is made up of increases in protein, fat, and fluid throughout the body. Breast enlargement can make laryngoscope insertion into the mouth difficult (**Fig. 40-1**). Lower esophageal sphincter tone is reduced during pregnancy. If intubation attempts are not immediately successful, these patients are at high risk of aspiration. Oxygen consumption increases 30% to 60% during pregnancy and functional residual capacity is reduced by 20% at term. These factors combine to cause rapid desaturation if the patient is rendered apneic.

2. Comorbid Disease

Hypertensive disorders of pregnancy can lead to a loss of consciousness (e.g., eclampsia) followed by traumatic injury. Elevated blood pressure is thought to make interstitial edema worse and can make laryngoscopy difficult.

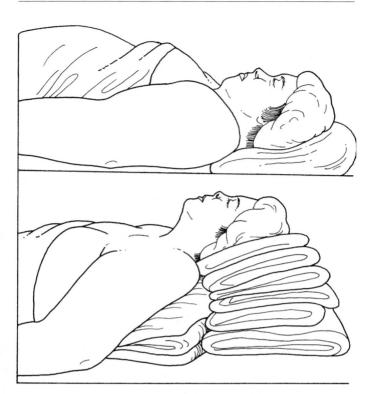

Figure 40-1.   Positioning of the patient with blankets under the back, shoulders and head improves the distance between the chin and the chest wall and allows better alignment of the airway axis. This positioning is possible if no concern is seen regarding injury to the spine. (From Cohen SE. Anesthesia for the morbidly obese pregnant patient. In: Shnider SM, Levinson G, eds. *Anesthesia for obstetrics,* 3rd ed. Philadelphia: Williams & Wilkins, 1993:581–595, with permission.)

3.   Airway Evaluation

Assess the patient's head, face, neck, and mouth attributes to evaluate the airway. Mouth opening and visualization of oropharyngeal structures (**Fig. 40-2**) can predict difficulty associated with intubation. Other factors that have been associated with a difficult intubation in the obstetric patient include a short neck, receding mandible, and protruding upper incisors. The relative risk of these factors making intubation difficult, compared with a class I airway, is listed in **Table 40-1.**

4.   Airway Management

The patient's current clinical condition and how that is expected to evolve, including investigations and

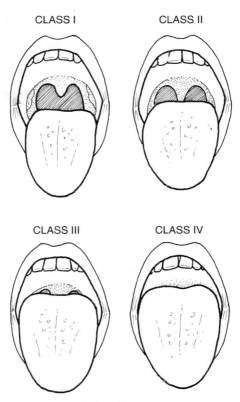

Figure 40-2. Visualization of the oropharyngeal structures is the basis of the Samsoon and Young airway classification system. (From Samsoon GLT, Young JRB. Difficult tracheal intubation: a retrospective study. *Anaesthesia* 1987;42:487–490, with permission.)

subsequent treatment, determine airway management. If a head injury is apparent with the Glasgow Coma Scale (GCS) score <8, intubation should be performed. If the GCS score is >8, but the mental status is altered and multiple investigations are planned for operative intervention, then intubation should be strongly considered. Once the decision to intubate is made, the method of intubation must be chosen. This can be by awake, fiberoptic intubation with or without sedation, and local anesthetic applied to the airway versus general anesthesia in the form of a rapid sequence induction with cricoid pressure and manual in-line stabilization of the cervical spine. Alternatively, a surgical airway may be indicated based on the presence of trauma to the face and airway.

Table 40-1.   The relative risk of factors that make intubation difficult in the parturient as compared with Samsoon and Young airway class I

Risk Factor	Relative Risk
Samsoon and Young Classification	
Class I	1
Class II	3.2
Class III	7.6
Class IV	11.3
Short neck	5.0
Receding mandible	9.7
Protruding upper incisors	8.0

(From: Rocke DA, Murray WB, Rout CC, et al. Relative risk analysis of factors associated with difficult intubation in obstetric anesthesia. *Anesthesiology* 1992;77:67–73, with permission.)

C.   Breathing

The breathing pattern is slightly altered during pregnancy. Tidal volume increases by 45% and respiratory rate remains unchanged. Alveolar ventilation is increased, which results in a compensated respiratory alkalosis, as indicated in **Table 40-2.**

D.   Circulation

Circulation is also altered during pregnancy.

1.   Cardiac Output

Cardiac output increases by 30% to 50% during pregnancy and by 100% to 150% during labor and immediately postpartum. This occurs through an increase in both stroke volume and heart rate. Systemic vascular resistance decreases by 20%. The resultant effect on blood pressure is that systolic pressure decreases by 6% to 8% and diastolic pressure decreases by 20% to 25%. Increased skin perfusion results in increased skin temperature, with resultant increased heat loss in the trauma setting. The use of vasopressors to restore maternal blood pressure should be

Table 40-2.   Arterial blood gases during pregnancy

Blood Gas	Nonpregnant	Pregnant
$Paco_2$ (mm Hg)	40	30
Pao_2 (mm Hg)	100	105
pH	7.4	7.44
Hco_3^- (mEq/L)	25	20

(From Conklin SE. Anesthesia for the morbidly obese pregnant patient. In: Shnider SM, Levinson G, eds. *Anesthesia for obstetrics,* 3rd ed. Philadelphia: Williams & Wilkins, 1993:581–595, with permission.)

avoided until appropriate volume resuscitation has been administered. They should not be withheld if they become necessary, despite their likelihood of reducing uterine blood flow.

2. Blood Volume

During pregnancy, blood volume changes. Plasma volume increases by 50% to 55% and red cell volume increases by 30% steadily during pregnancy, which results in 10%, 30%, and 45% increases in blood volume during the first, second, and third trimesters, respectively.

3. Coagulation

Coagulation changes during pregnancy because the concentration of most coagulation factors increases. The results of thromboelastography and sonoclot analysis in the parturient are consistent with a hypercoagulable state. These changes, in association with immobility, predispose to the development of venous thromboses and prophylaxis against this should be provided.

E. Disability and Obstetric Evaluation

  1. Integrated Efforts Required

  Optimal management of the seriously injured gravida requires the integrated effort of multiple specialties.

  2. Obstetricians

  Obstetricians play a central role in the management of injured pregnant women. A focused effort to emergently consult an obstetrician or gynecologist for co-management of the patient is emphasized.

  3. Critical Management Issues

  For the obstetrician, critical management issues include the effects of various drugs on uterine blood flow; potential teratogenic and mutagenic effects of diagnostic radiation and medications; the effect of surgery on pregnancy; assessment of gestational age; and detection and management of any superimposed complications of pregnancy (e.g., placenta previa, placental abruption, or preeclampsia).

  4. Transfer to Obstetrics

  Consider transfer of primary care to obstetrics once the trauma issues are treated and stabilized. Moreover, the labor and delivery unit may be the most appropriate place for patient and fetal monitoring once postoperative recovery is complete, depending on gestational age.

F. Exposure (Positioning of the Mother)

  1. Following midpregnancy (fundus palpable at or near the umbilicus), displacement of the uterus off the inferior vena cava (IVC) and the abdominal aorta should be affected.

  2. This can be done by having the patient lie in the lateral decubitus position. If the patient must remain supine (in cases of suspected spinal injury or cardiopulmonary resuscitation [CPR]), manual displacement of the uterus laterally with a hand or placement of a wedge under the backboard or stretcher mattress will accomplish the same goal.

G. **Immediate Therapy for Life-Threatening Situations**

1. **Cardiopulmonary Resuscitation of the Pregnant Patient**

a. **Cardiac Arrest.** In the pregnant patient, cardiac arrest is rare, estimated to occur in 1 of 30,000 deliveries. Trauma, although not one of the leading causes of maternal mortality, is a recognized cause and efforts should be made to determine the exact cause of the cardiorespiratory collapse while instituting resuscitative measures.

b. **Venous Access.** Place venous access above the diaphragm. The enlarged uterus and its contents cause obstruction of venous return to the heart via the inferior vena cava (IVC). Drugs or fluids administered through an intravenous (i.v.) access in the femoral or saphenous veins can take excessively long to reach the central circulation. The extent of the trauma will determine what sites are readily accessible for i.v. access. Cephalad displacement of the lung by the enlarged uterus can increase the risk of pneumothorax if the subclavian route is chosen.

c. **Left Uterine Displacement.** Providing 30 degrees of left lateral tilt to the abdomen will reduce the obstructive effect of the gravid uterus on the IVC.

d. **Closed Cardiac Massage.** Institute closed cardiac massage immediately. The compressive force that can be generated on the sternum with the abdomen tilted at 30 degrees is reduced to 80% of the force generated in the supine position.

e. **Intubation.** If not already accomplished, perform intubation of the airway.

f. **Open Cardiac Massage.** If no response occurs during closed cardiac massage, open cardiac massage is recommended.

g. **Cesarean Delivery.** If CPR is not successful within the first 4 to 5 minutes, cesarean delivery of the fetus is recommended. Anecdotal reports have described maternal survival after CPR and cesarean delivery of the near term fetus. Neonatal survival has been quoted to be between 50% and 70% with good neurologic outcome, provided delivery occurs within 5 minutes of maternal arrest.

h. **Perimortem Cesarean Delivery of Fetus**

(1) The uterus can be evacuated (even of a demised fetus) when a patient is unresponsive to attempts at resuscitation during cardiopulmonary arrest. The term "postmortem" cesarean delivery is replaced with "peri-

mortem" in an attempt to aid the resuscitative effort.

(2) Fetal survival is unlikely if more than 15 to 20 minutes have transpired since the loss of maternal vital signs.

(3) Based on isolated case reports, cesarean delivery should be considered for both maternal and fetal benefit 4 minutes after a woman has experienced cardiopulmonary arrest in the third trimester.

(4) Perform a perimortem abdominal delivery by making a vertical incision from the umbilicus to the pubic symphysis, using deep force. It should take no more than three passes with the scalpel to get to the fetus. A vertical incision is the fastest and most hemostatic incision for abdominal delivery.

III. Secondary Survey

A. Assessment of Uterine Size (Gestational Age)

1. Gestational age assessment is valuable both to determine the need for fetal assessment as well as maternal trauma management. Once the mother is stabilized, gestational age should be assessed as soon as feasible.

2. Gestational age can be estimated by pushing firmly on the abdomen to feel the location of the uterine fundus (the top of the uterus). Landmarks for gestational age include 12 weeks at the level of the pubic symphysis, 20 weeks at the umbilicus (considered to be 20 cm from the pubic symphysis), and then by adding 1 week per centimeter to the 20 cm for each centimeter above the umbilicus. If the mother is stabilized and a reasonably experienced operator is available to perform a bedside ultrasound (US), a more exact estimation of gestational age can be made radiologically. Even US dating is limited after the first trimester, however. Second trimester (12 to 28 weeks) dating can be off by ±2 weeks, and third trimester (28 weeks to term) dating can be off by up to ±3 weeks. Ultrasound dating is obtained by measuring the fetal biparietal diameter (BPD), abdominal circumference (AC), and femur length (FL).

3. Fetal viability in the extrauterine environment begins after 24 weeks gestation in a tertiary care center with an available neonatal ICU. Determination of gestational age >24 weeks can thus significantly change management decisions with evidence of fetal compromise.

4. Uterine size after 18 weeks gestation will compress both the aorta and IVC in the supine position, increasing the likelihood of both maternal hypotension and decreased uterine perfusion (and fetal distress).

5. Based on gestational age, the type of trauma can affect the fetus differently. For example, abdominal trauma before 12 to 13 weeks' gestation is unlikely to affect the fetus, because the uterus is still protected by the bony pelvis. Trauma in the first trimester generally does not cause pregnancy loss, unless it is associated with profound hypotension and uterine hypoperfusion.

B. Documentation of Fetal Heartbeat

1. Given the heightened medicolegal environment of pregnancy, it is highly advisable to document clearly the visualization or assessment of the fetal status on secondary survey once the mother is stable enough for the providers to do so.

2. A bedside US can be used to find the fetal heartbeat if a relatively experienced operator is available. This is the quickest way to document fetal status while attempting to get through the secondary survey.

3. A fetal Doppler-tone monitor can be placed on the abdomen to assess the fetal heart rate. The advantage to using a fetal heart rate monitor is that it can be left strapped to the abdomen or held in place for a period of time to obtain a recorded fetal heart tracing on paper, which can be informative.

4. If a fetal heartbeat cannot be found with a Doppler monitor, US should be used to visualize the fetal heart. Intrauterine death must be diagnosed on US with an adequate view of the cardiac chambers and absence of cardiac activity.

5. Although US visualization of the fetal heart rate allows fast acknowledgment of the living status of the fetus, it can be challenging to tell if the heart rate is displaying signs of fetal distress, such as late decelerations (usually caused by placental insufficiency, abruption, or uterine rupture). A monitor allows the providers to visualize the heart rate pattern over a few minutes to assess whether a stable baseline is present or the heart rate, in fact, is a terminal bradycardia, tachycardia, or displaying repetitive decelerations.

C. Pulmonary

1. Maternal Respiratory Rate

Maternal respiratory rate is normally minimally elevated above baseline but the tidal volume is increased by 45%. A higher incidence is seen of venous thromboembolism during pregnancy and the immediate postpartum period, thus examine for a pleural rub and monitor with pulse oximetry. If pulmonary embolism is suspected, evaluation should proceed as for any other patient with computed tomography (CT) angiography preferred to a V/Q scan.

2. Amniotic Fluid Embolism

Rarely, amniotic fluid embolism can occur with the mother presenting with respiratory distress. Chest radiographic findings range from minimal findings to diffuse, bilateral infiltrates.

D. Cardiac

1. Often, a grade 1 to 2 SEM is heard, consistent with the increased plasma volume of pregnancy. With any suspicion for an abnormal or overly loud murmur, perform an echocardiographic examination. In cases of preexisting valvular heart disease or prosthetic parts, provide prophylaxis with ampicillin/gentamicin (or clindamycin/gentamicin for penicillin allergy) for any procedures. Mitral valve prolapse by itself does not require prophylaxis, whereas mitral regurgitation does.

E. Abdomen

1. The abdomen is of particular importance because a substantial percentage of serious injuries will involve the uterus, intraperitoneal structures, and the retroperitoneum.

2. Palpate the uterus and examine for evidence of gross deformity, tenderness, or the presence of contractions.

    a. The onset of a regular pattern of contractions as a result of trauma is highly suggestive of the presence of placental abruption.

    b. Open peritoneal lavage is advocated over a blind needle insertion to lessen the likelihood of needle injury to the uterus or other displaced intraperitoneal organs. Open lavage can be effective in the diagnosis of intraperitoneal hemorrhage in pregnancy. Perform open lavage with sharp dissection and opening of the anterior abdominal peritoneum under direct vision, usually periumbilically.

F. Genitourinary

1. Pregnancy predisposes patients to asymptomatic urinary tract infections. Urinalysis should be performed and culture and sensitivity, if warranted. Macrobid can be started as a baseline antibiotic until sensitivities are available.

G. Hematologic

1. If the mother has experienced abdominal trauma and is determined to have an $Rh^{(-)}$ blood type, consider administering Rh_oD immune globulin (RhoGAM, Ortho Diagnostic Systems, Raritan, NJ) to protect from D alloimmunization.

2. The mean estimated blood volume of fetal cells injected into the maternal circulation during trauma is usually <15 mL, and >90% of these fetal-maternal hemorrhages are <30 mL. One ampoule (300 µg) of RhoGAM protects against 30-mL fetal-maternal hemorrhage and, thus, would protect nearly all $Rh^{(-)}$ trauma victims.

3. A Kleihauer-Betke assay will quantitate the amount of fetal-maternal hemorrhage and identify those few unsensitized $Rh^{(-)}$ women who are found to have a hemorrhage >30 mL and, thus, would need an additional ampoule of RhoGAM.

4. Before 12 weeks gestation, given the small fetal blood volume, maternal trauma rarely requires more than the "mini-RhoGAM" dose (50 µg). Because no adverse effect occurs in administering excess RhoGAM to Rh$^{(-)}$ patients, standard practice allows for safe administration of the 300 µg dose anytime in pregnancy, when indicated.

5. Rarely, amniotic fluid embolism will present in association with trauma. A coagulopathy (disseminated intravascular coagulation [DIC]) develops rapidly and can be refractory to treatment.

H. Extremities

1. Of parturients, 70% will develop worsening peripheral edema as pregnancy advances. This is not pathognomonic for preeclampsia.

IV. Perioperative Management for Nonobstetric Surgery

A. Fetal Monitoring Issues

1. Intraoperative fetal monitoring should be considered if the fetus is viable (>24 weeks gestation). This is a variable recommendation, and if the fetus has demonstrated reassuring testing and monitoring and the mother remains stable, pre- and postoperative monitoring may be sufficient. This decision is usually left to the obstetric provider.

2. For intraoperative monitoring of a viable fetus, a Doppler device or US transducer wrapped in a sterile plastic bag can be used, either on the abdominal skin or on the uterus if it is exposed during surgery.

3. For a nonviable fetus, a fetal heart check by Doppler needs to be done only at the start of the procedure and at the end. No heroic efforts or change in management would be undertaken for a previable fetus intraoperatively.

4. The need for exploratory laparotomy, by itself, is not an indication to proceed with cesarean delivery.

5. If the uterus has been penetrated and delivery must proceed, a neonatologist and pediatric surgeon should be in attendance, if possible.

B. Positioning (Fig. 40-1)

1. Maternal positioning in the operating room is done just as for a cesarean section. The patient can lie supine and a large roll (which may be fashioned from a rolled or folded-over blanket) is placed underneath the right flank to achieve a leftward tilt and displacement of the uterus off the great vessels.

2. Pneumoboots are not routinely used for cesarean delivery, but no contraindication is seen to their use and they should be placed, if indicated.

C. Postoperative Recovery

1. The patient should be brought to the recovery room for routine postoperative care indicated for the procedure performed. The uterus should remain displaced with a leftward tilt while the patient lies supine.

2. Supplemental oxygen should be given by nasal cannula or mask during the recovery period. Pay attention to maintaining adequate intravascular volume because any transient dehydration, especially in the postoperative setting, can trigger uterine contractions.

3. Fetal monitoring can be continued via a fetal heart rate monitor in the recovery room. Once a reassuring pattern is established, the obstetric team may opt for intermittent monitoring. If the pregnancy is previable (<24 weeks), only a fetal heart check is required to document the living status of the fetus.

4. Fetal monitoring is ideally coordinated by contacting the obstetrics team or obstetric nursing. They can bring the appropriate equipment and possess excellent knowledge of fetal heart pattern recognition.

5. If the patient is stable and medically suitable, she should be transferred from the recovery room to the labor and delivery unit for continuous fetal and uterine monitoring for at least 4 and up to 24 hours. If the mother's condition requires her to go to an intensive care unit (ICU) setting, this should preclude fetal monitoring issues, and obstetric comanagement can be coordinated in the ICU.

6. Uterine contractions are a common occurrence postoperatively in the recovery room. They are usually transient in nature and respond well to intravenous fluid (IVF) boluses. Terbutaline is not recommended as a first-line agent because it causes tachycardia, which is far from ideal for the postoperative patient. The obstetric team may recommend placement of an indomethacin (Indocin; Merck & Company, West Point, PA) suppository (50 to 100 mg) to help achieve tocolysis. Indocin is usually not recommended >34 weeks gestation if delivery is imminent because of its effect on the patent ductus arteriosus (PDA). If uterine contractions take on a regular pattern, increase in frequency or strengthen in character, intravenous magnesium sulfate may become necessary for tocolysis. This is usually administered as a 6-g bolus, followed by 2 g/hour continuous infusion. Magnesium levels can be checked every 6 hours to avoid toxicity, but are not necessary as toxicity is easily seen clinically on examination. As magnesium levels rise, deep tendon reflexes become decreased, and rales may be auscultated at the lung bases. The infusion can be turned down to 1 g/hour for symptomatic toxicity, or turned up to 3 g/h for a continued pattern of contractions not responding to the attempted tocolysis.

7. In cases of a reasonable chance of preterm delivery for the fetus, intramuscular steroids should be given at any gestation between 24 and 34 weeks. Steroids will help the fetus with lung maturation and help protect the neonate from intraventricular hemorrhage and necrotizing enterocolitis, the most common difficulties encountered with preterm births. Two doses need to be given 24 hours apart. The maximal effect occurs after 48 hours from the time of the first dose.

V. Penetrating Trauma

A. Cause

Most commonly, penetration is by gunshot or stab wounds.

B. Prognosis

Prognosis is significantly disparate for the mother and fetus. Maternal outcome is usually more favorable because the uterus and its contents, absorbing much of the projectile energy, shield the maternal viscera. Fetal loss usually occurs as a result of direct injury (or to the cord or placenta) of the penetration.

C. Bowel Injury

Bowel injury secondary to stab wounds is somewhat different in location in the gravid patient. Because the uterus displaces the bowel into the upper abdomen, a stab wound that might not normally be associated with bowel injury can be more complex in a pregnant patient.

D. Exit Wounds

Expected exit wounds of projectiles can be altered and unpredictable in pregnancy because of the uterus and shift of abdominal contents. If an exit wound cannot be seen on examination, radiographs of the area in multiple projections can be helpful.

VI. Abdominal Blunt Trauma

A. Key Obstetric Issues

Key obstetric issues to address are gestational age at time of injury, extent and severity of maternal injury, and mechanism of injury.

B. Blunt Abdominal Trauma

Placenta abruption or partial separation, uterine rupture, maternal shock, or some combination thereof can occur from blunt abdominal trauma. More than 50% of fetal losses, however, are the result of placental abruption. Placental abruption occurs because of the difference in tissue properties between the elastic myometrium and the relatively inelastic placenta. Any force to the uterus can cause the translation of a shear force to this tissue interface with resultant separation. Because the amniotic fluid translates this force, the risk of abruption is independent of the area of the uterus impacted or placental location.

C. Uterine Rupture

Uterine rupture is infrequent but life threatening. It occurs in only 0.6% of trauma in pregnancy, and usually only in cases of substantial direct abdominal force. Findings range from subtle (uterine tenderness, fetal heart patterns of distress) to rapid onset of maternal hypovolemic shock. Signs of peritoneal irritation (rebound, guarding, rigidity) are frequently detected on examination, but are less pronounced in pregnancy.

VII. Seatbelt Injury

A. Incidence and Severity

The appropriate use of automobile safety restraints has been shown to decrease the incidence and severity of injuries. Therefore, properly counseled pregnant patients are advised to use and be reassured of the safety of these devices during pregnancy.

B. Proper Use

Many women do not wear seatbelts properly. Current recommendations indicate that throughout pregnancy, they should be used with both the lap belt and shoulder harness in place. The lap belt, however, should be placed under the pregnant abdomen, over both anterior superior iliac spines and the pubic symphysis. The shoulder harness should be positioned between the breasts. Both belts should be applied as snugly as comfort will allow, without excessive slack.

Placement of the lap belt over the uterine fundus transmits significant uterine pressure on impact, and is associated with increased uterine and fetal injury.

C. Airbags

Based on the limited existing literature, no significant maternal or fetal risk of injury appears to occur from airbag deployment.

VIII. Pharmacology

A. Pain Management

The pregnant trauma patient can receive any indicated anesthetic or narcotic agent that would be used for a woman who is not pregnant. Non-steroidal anti-inflammatory drugs remain among the few pain medications that are contraindicated in pregnancy. Intravenous ketorolac, therefore, should be avoided.

B. Antimicrobials

Broad-spectrum antibiotics are safe in pregnancy. Among the only antibiotics not approved in pregnancy are the fluoroquinolones (levofloxacin, ciprofloxacin) based on animal studies and bone defects. Generalized broad-spectrum coverage can usually be achieved with intravenous ampicillin, gentamicin, and clindamycin or metronidazole. Vancomycin can be used in place of ampicillin in case of penicillin allergy. Cephalosporins of any generation are safe in pregnancy as well.

C. Other Medications

Most perioperative medications used for all patients are safe in pregnancy. This includes anxiolytics and benzodiazepines. For sleep, diphenhydramine or oxazepam is commonly used. Sudafed (Warner Wellcome, Morris Plains, NJ) and Robitussin (A. H. Robins, Richmond, VA) are safe for congestion and cough. Seizures can be treated with intravenous magnesium, midazolam, lorazepam, or diazepam. It should be noted that intravenous magnesium sulfate has been shown to be far superior to other epileptic drugs to treat and prevent seizures in pregnancy.

D. Tetanus

Indications for tetanus do not change in pregnancy, and appropriate candidates should be vaccinated.

IX. Radiation Exposure and Studies

A. It is absolutely imperative that no indicated radiologic procedure be denied to the patient or put in question because of the pregnancy. If the imaging is required and would be done for any other patient in the same circumstance, it should be performed.

1. Flat plate plain films such as chest x-ray study or kidney, ureter, bladder (KUB) are on the order of 0.5 rad.

2. CT scan of the abdomen and pelvis range in the order of 2 to 3.5 rad, depending on the proximity to the fetus. The further away the imaging is from the fetus, the fewer the rads. Thus, a chest CT and head CT are more on the order of 1 rad.

3. Fetal exposure >20 rad in early pregnancy and 50 rad in the third trimester can be sufficient to induce adverse effects, but these data are somewhat unclear and the rads clearly far in excess of what would be required for diagnostics in a trauma patient.

SELECTED READING

American College of Obstetricians and Gynecologists. *Obstetric aspects of trauma management.* Educational Technical Bulletin number 251, September 1998.

Awwad JT, Azar GB, Seoud MA, et al. High-velocity penetrating wounds of the gravid uterus: review of 16 years of civil war. *Obstet Gynecol* 1994;83:259–264.

Catanese CA, Gilmore K. Fetal gunshot wound characteristics. *J Forensic Sci* 2002;47:1067–1069.

Cohen SE. Anesthesia for the morbidly obese pregnant patient. In: Shnider SM, Levinson G, eds. *Anesthesia for obstetrics,* 3rd ed. Philadelphia: Williams & Wilkins, 1993:581–595.

Conklin KA. Physiologic changes of pregnancy. In: Chestnut DH, ed. *Obstetric anesthesia: principles and practice.* St. Louis: Mosby, 1994:17–42.

Dahmus MA, Sibai BM. Blunt abdominal trauma: are there any predictive factors for abruptio placentae or maternal-fetal distress? *Am J Obstet Gynecol* 1993;169:1054–1059.

Dannenberg AL, Carter DM, Lawson HW, et al. Homicide and other injuries as causes of maternal death in New York City, 1987 through 1991. *Am J Obstet Gynecol* 1995;172:1557–1564.

Fries MH, Hankins GD. Motor vehicle accident associated with minimal maternal trauma but subsequent fetal demise. *Ann Emerg Med* 1989;18:301–304.

Katz VL, Dotters DJ, Droegemueller W. Perimortem cesarean delivery. *Obstet Gynecol* 1986;68:571–576.

Leggon RE, Wood GC, Indeck MC. Pelvic fractures in pregnancy: factors influencing maternal and fetal outcomes. *J Trauma* 2002;53:796–804.

Pearlman MD, Tintinalli JE, Lorenz RP. A prospective controlled study of outcome after trauma during pregnancy. *Am J Obstet Gyncecol* 1990;162:1502–1510.

Pearlman MD, Phillips ME. Safety belt use during pregnancy. *Obstet Gynecol* 1996;88:1026–1029.

Pearlman MD, Tintinalli JE, Lorenz RP. Blunt trauma during pregnancy. *N Engl J Med* 1990;323:1609–1613.

Rocke DA, Murray WB, Rout CC, et al. Relative risk analysis of factors associated with difficult intubation in obstetric anesthesia. *Anesthesiology* 1992;77:67–73.

Samsoon GLT, Young JRB. Difficult tracheal intubation: a retrospective study. *Anaesthesia* 1987;42:487–490.

Schiff MA, Holt VL, Daling JR. Maternal and infant outcomes after injury during pregnancy in Washington State from 1989 to 1997. *J Trauma* 2002;53:939–945.

Schiff MA, Holt VL. The injury severity score in pregnant trauma patients: predicting placental abruption and fetal death. *J Trauma* 2002;53:946–949.

Williams JK, McClain L, Rosemurgy AS, et al. Evaluation of blunt abdominal trauma in the third trimester of pregnancy: maternal and fetal considerations. *Obstet Gynecol* 1990;75:33–37.

Geriatric Trauma

Kari Rosenkrantz, MD,
and Robert L. Sheridan, MD

I. Introduction

The elderly, defined as persons 65 years of age or older, currently comprise 12% of the total population of the United States, yet account for >28% of the trauma admissions and consume nearly 33% of the total healthcare dollars spent annually on traumatic injuries. The elderly represent a fragile population with significantly depleted physiologic reserves and often potentially confounding comorbidity. The care of this population, therefore, requires a delicate attention to detail and a careful evaluation of subtle signs and symptoms. As the population of the United States continues to age, trauma in the elderly is poised to become a more lethal and more costly phenomenon.

A. Population Changes

1. Increase in Population Size

Census figures project a 55% increase in the elderly population over the next 50 years. This rate of increase is greater than twice that of the population under 65. Most significantly, the greatest rate of increase in the elderly population is in the very old, a group 85 years of age or older.

2. Defining the Old and Very Old

Because of the increasing size of the elderly population and the distinctions in the predictability of outcomes, several authors have begun to differentiate between the *old,* patients 65 to 84 years of age, and the *very old,* patients 85 years of age and older. Of patients within the *old* group, 10% will die following a trauma, whereas 50% of the *very old* will die after trauma.

3. Changes in Health and Activity

With the recent advances in scientific understanding and technology, the health and functional status of the elderly population continue to improve and life expectancy continues to increase. As a group, the elderly are more mobile and more active than in previous generations. These more active lifestyles expose the elderly to greater potential trauma.

B. Costs of Geriatric Trauma

1. Physical

Physically, the impact of trauma on the elderly population far exceeds that in the younger population. The literature attests to a significantly increased risk of death following trauma in the elderly patient. Of trauma patients >65 years of age, 15% to 30% will die as a result of their injuries versus 4% to 8% of younger patients. These rates have been adjusted for injury severity. For the elderly surviving injury, reports of long-term outcomes vary in the literature. Although 89% of survivors return home upon recovery, 33% to 47% never regain functional independence.

2. Financial

The number of elderly trauma patients represents a small percentage of total patients; hospital costs for the injured elderly, however, particularly the very old, are disproportionately elevated. Sixty-one billion dollars in direct and indirect costs are spent annually on care of the injured in the United States. Elderly trauma patients consume >$20 billion of these costs. Elderly trauma patients experience more post-traumatic complications than the younger population, resulting in increased morbidity and mortality, longer hospitalizations, and higher hospital costs. Geriatric trauma patients are also more likely to require significant care after discharge from the hospital. This contributes significantly to the financial burden associated with the elderly trauma patient.

II. Epidemiology

A. Population Growth in the Elderly

The population of the United States has more than tripled in the last century. Although every age group continues to increase in absolute number, the rate of increase among the elderly is twice as rapid as the remainder of the population. Within the elderly population, the very old has increased its representation from 4% of the elderly to 10% of the elderly population. Currently, >32 million are elderly Americans. As this group continues to increase in size, longevity, and activity level, the emotional, physical and financial costs of healthcare will continue to grow.

B. Trauma

Injury is currently the fifth leading cause of death in the elderly. Of elderly Americans, 25% will die as a result of injury. The elderly represent approximately 12% of the population of the United States, yet account for 28% of trauma admissions. The rate of trauma admission in the elderly is nearly twice that of the younger population. The rate of death in the elderly following injury is more than six times that of the younger population.

III. Mechanisms of Injury

A. The Old

Mechanism of injury varies with age between both the elderly and the youthful populations, and within the elderly population. Overall, falls, motor vehicle accidents, and thermal injuries account for >75% of all injury in persons over 65 years of age. Motor vehicle collisions represent the most common mechanism of injury in the *old* population and the second most common mechanism of injury in the elderly population as a whole.

B. The Very Old

Falls, which dominate the *very old* population as the most common mechanism of trauma, remain the leading cause of accidental death in the elderly. The elderly are ten times more likely to fall than younger patients. Given the fragility

of this population, >10% of all fall victims suffer significant injury. The causes of falls are many, but up to 25%
are thought to result from cardiac dysrhythmias. Motor
vehicle crashes and struck pedestrians represent the
second and third most common mechanisms of injury in
this population. More than 50% of all pedestrians struck
by vehicles are elderly.

IV. Changes in the Elderly

As persons age, individual organ systems deteriorate in function
and lose capacity to react adequately to stress. Anatomic changes
predispose the elderly to injury. Thus, seemingly low-energy mechanisms or minor appearing injuries, in fact, can severely disrupt
the equilibrium of the elderly patient and lead to catastrophic
outcomes.

A. Neurologic

1. Decreased Reserves

Elderly trauma patients often suffer from preexisting
neurologic deficit or cognitive dysfunction, including
dementia and cerebrovascular disease. This presents
a challenge to clinicians attempting to discern acute
from chronic signs following a traumatic event.

2. Anatomic Changes

Further complicating the ability to diagnose potentially life-threatening neurologic conditions is an increased intracranial space present in many elderly
patients. As persons age, the brain atrophies loga-
rithmically (an average of 10% between the ages of 30
and 70), thereby expanding the intracranial space.
This allows for greater stretch in bridging veins and,
therefore, a predisposition to subdural bleeding. The
increased intracranial space also permits significant
accumulation of blood before the onset of neurologic
symptoms. The elderly are three times as likely to
suffer a subdural hematoma, but much less likely to
exhibit early symptomatology. Thus, heightened clinical suspicion is a necessity in evaluating head trauma
in the elderly.

B. Cardiac Decreased Reserves

As humans age, the myocardium stiffens, leading to decreased stroke volume and poor diastolic relaxation. When
challenged by the stress of injury or hypotension, the
elderly heart is often unable to compensate satisfactorily.
Given increasing incidence of atherosclerosis of the coronary vessels, attempts at an appropriate stress response
predispose elderly patients to ischemia and infarction. As
persons age, coronary blood flow is often reduced even in
the absence of atherosclerotic disease. The ability of the
conducting system within the heart to respond to catecholamines also deteriorates over time, which further jeop-
ardizes the stress response.

C. Pulmonary

1. Decreased Reserves

Loss of elasticity in the lungs and chest wall lead to
decreased pulmonary compliance in the elderly. Simultaneously, the number of alveoli diminishes. Mucosal

atrophy and changes in oral flora predispose the elderly to pulmonary infection. These physiologic changes, alone and in combination, decrease the pulmonary reserve and increase the work of breathing for the elderly patient.

2. Anatomic Changes

A propensity for rib fractures, a result of decreased bone density, and an increased incidence of traumatic hemopneumothorax further contribute to the increased work of breathing and potential infectious complications.

D. Renal Decreased Reserves

Renal reserves deteriorate over time, as glomeruli are lost. It is difficult, however, to closely monitor the effect of injury on the kidney in the elderly patient. As muscle mass diminishes with age, the accuracy of serum creatinine as a measure of renal function loses its accuracy. Creatinine clearance, rather than serum creatinine, provides a more reliable index of renal function.

E. Orthopedic Anatomic Changes

Incidence of arthritis and osteoporosis increase steadily with age. These conditions predispose the elderly trauma patient to bony injury, but also can mask or confuse radiographic findings. Careful physical examination and judicious use of radiographs are warranted.

V. Evaluation and Management of the Injured Elderly Patient

A. Routine Trauma Care

1. Airway, Breathing, and Circulation

The injured elderly patient is first and foremost a trauma patient. Thus, the priorities outlined in the advanced trauma life support (ATLS) algorithms remain steadfast. Pay careful attention to the airway, breathing and circulation (ABCs) of the patient.

2. Immobilization

Proper immobilization of the spine is a necessity in any trauma patient. Given the increased incidence of osteoporosis and arthritis, the elderly are at higher risk for spinal injury. Heightened attention to immobilization is mandatory because seemingly low-impact trauma can injure the brittle bones of the elderly.

3. Primary and Secondary Surveys

The primary survey adheres to ATLS protocol in the injured elderly. Following evaluation and necessary management of the ABCs, a concise evaluation is done to assess potential thoracic, abdominal, and pelvic injury. Aggressively monitor vital signs, including temperature, as well as efficiency of oxygen delivery. Make corrections rapidly in the face of any abnormalities. Once this is complete, perform a more thorough and methodic secondary survey. In the stable patient, complete a full physical examination, including neurologic, orthopedic, and a more detailed thoracic and abdominal assessment.

4. Studies
Recommendations for initial diagnostic studies in the elderly mirror those outlined by ATLS. Cervical spine series, and chest and pelvic x-ray studies are standard. Further examinations including additional plain films, computed tomography (CT) scans, and angiography are dictated by findings from the initial evaluation.

B. Special Attention in the Elderly
1. Underlying Pathology
As mentioned, in comparison to a younger population, the elderly are physiologically more depleted and harbor significantly more comorbidity. Of all patients >75 years of age, 65% will have at least one comorbid condition. These factors must be taken into account in the evaluation and management of the injured elderly. Injuries can present subtly in the elderly and clinical suspicion is mandatory in evaluating these patients. Subdural bleeding and other intracranial processes can present slowly and liberal CT scanning of the head is indicated. Similarly, the elderly often do not exhibit early signs of peritonitis or intraperitoneal injury. Again, judicious CT scanning of the abdomen and pelvis are suggested. Clinicians must, however, remain cognizant of the baseline renal deterioration and risks of CT contrast material use in the elderly. In the unstable patient diagnostic peritoneal lavage (DPL) is a reasonable alternative diagnostic modality. Given deficiencies in cardiac conduction as well as potential medication effects, tachycardia can be absent as an early indicator of shock. Thoughtful and frequent evaluation of the circulation is required.

2. Risk of Fracture
As discussed, the elderly are at greater risk of fracture than their youthful counterparts. At least 5% of elderly patients seen in emergency departments after falls are discharged with undiagnosed fractures. Index of suspicion must remain high.

3. Medical History
A detailed medical history, to the extent permitted in a trauma situation, can greatly facilitate the diagnosis and management of the injured elderly patient. Preexisting conditions can increase susceptibility to injury (e.g., osteoporosis), limit the patient's ability to respond to the stress of injury (coronary artery disease), and predispose the patient to a prolonged recovery and potential complications (lung disease, renal insufficiency). An awareness of these underlying pathologies should direct trauma evaluation and management strategy.

4. Medication History
Geriatric patients are more likely than younger patients to be taking one or more medications. A careful medication history can provide insight into an underlying cause of trauma and into the patient's physiologic response to trauma. Common medications, including

beta-blockers and diuretics, alter the manifestations of shock and confound volume status and resuscitation requirements.

C. **Triage and Disposition—Decisions in the Field**
1. **Rapid Assessment**
Given the depleted physiologic reserves of the elderly, the main goal of transport is rapidity. Studies have documented that prolonged transport times predict worse outcomes in this population. After a rapid assessment and management of the ABCs, the elderly must be swiftly transported to an emergency facility.

2. **Destination**
Studies have hypothesized that age should dictate transport decisions. Currently, data suggest that seriously injured elderly patients warrant direct transport to a level I trauma center. Patients exhibiting hemodynamic stability and without evidence of head or spinal injury or an immediate surgical problem, however, can be safely transported to the closest emergency facility for complete trauma evaluation.

3. **Hospital Triage**
The injured elderly often present to the emergency room with misleading stability. Head injuries, peritoneal injuries, and vascular injuries can present in delayed fashion. The geriatric trauma patient, however, is fragile with a poor ability to recover from hypotensive and hypoxemic episodes. Thus, cautious monitoring is wise in this population. In any elderly patient with significant mechanism and injury score, observation in the intensive care unit (ICU) is advised.

D. **Monitoring—ICU and Aggressive Care**
Elderly trauma patients require close observation because altered physiology, medication use, and comorbidity can mask underlying injuries. Studies have documented that early invasive monitoring successfully dictates management and improves outcomes. The early implementation of a pulmonary artery catheter helps determine volume status during resuscitation and provides a more accurate index of cardiac function and oxygenation. Both over and under resuscitation are serious risks in the physiologically depleted elderly patient. The catheter also offers early evidence of clinical decompensation and enables the ICU team to avert disaster. Although clinicians may be reluctant to initiate such aggressive measures, studies have shown that it is extremely difficult to discern an injury for which the patient will not survive in the initial phases of resuscitation. Thus, the elderly merit full treatment in the early period after trauma.

E. **Surgical Disease**
1. **Preoperative Consultation**
In the unstable trauma patient for whom time is not a luxury, surgical intervention must proceed on an emergent basis. Little, if any, preoperative assessment is feasible. In less urgent cases, however, take care to assess the elderly patient before operation.

The clinical team must elicit a thorough medical history. Specialists with respect to any comorbid conditions should provide consultation to maximize organ function preoperatively. Again, aggressive interventions, including Swann-Ganz catheterization, can aid in the optimization of cardiac function and organ perfusion. Feeding can be initiated to enhance nutritional status and facilitate postoperative healing. Monitor glucose closely.

2. Timing of Surgery

Trauma in the elderly strains an already delicate physiologic system. The overwhelming stress response following injury increases metabolic demands, thereby burdening the heart and placing other end organs at risk of hypoperfusion. When feasible, the overall health of a patient should be optimized before surgery. Delaying surgery until the acute stress response abates can improve outcome for the patient. The delay of nonemergent procedures, particularly orthopedic fixation, compromises neither the short-term care nor the long-term functional outcome of these patients.

F.   Nonoperative Management

Nonoperative therapy for solid organ injury can be successful in the elderly, although there is some data suggesting a lower success rate with nonoperative management of splenic trauma. Nonoperative management should be considered on a case-by-case basis dictated by the dynamic clinical scenario.

VI.   Comorbid Conditions

A.   Prevalence

As persons age, the number of comorbid conditions steadily increases. In the fourth decade of life, premorbid disease affects 17% of the general population. By the eighth decade, this percentage increases to 69%.

B.   Secondary Effects

1.   Medications

A history of premorbid disease and medicinal treatments thereof can alter the clinical picture of a trauma patient.

a.   Cardiac Medications. Several cardiac medications, including ace inhibitors, calcium channel blockers, beta blockers, and diuretics, can significantly affect the stress response and confuse the clinical picture and management of a trauma patient. In particular, beta blockade can blunt the tachycardic response to hypovolemia. This can result in significant hypoxemia because the body's adaptive responses are muted. The absence of tachycardia can also lure a clinical team into complacency. The presence of calcium channel blockers and ace inhibitors confound accurate assessment of preload and afterload. Diuretics decrease circulating volume and can increase the demands for volume resuscitation. Again, invasive monitoring with a pul-

monary arterial catheter can clarify the clinical
picture.

b. Anticoagulants. Anticoagulation use is increasing in the older population. Well anticoagulated patients are at greater risk of serious
hemorrhage. Clinicians must maintain a low
threshold of suspicion for injuries, including
subdural hematoma in the anticoagulated
patient.

C. Management of Comorbid Conditions

Time pressure and medical emergency take precedence
over the evaluation of preexisting conditions. As time
permits, however, consult a specialist to optimize the
functioning of individual body systems. In the event of
management conflicts, the trauma team must negotiate
the disunity in the best interest of the patient.

D. Effect on Outcomes

Although difficult to quantify, it is clear that comorbid
conditions manifest a significant negative impact on all
trauma patients. Increased length and cost of hospitalization and mortality are all positively correlated with
preexistent medical conditions. Preexisting renal disease, hepatic disease, and malignancy prognosticate the
worst outcomes. Cardiac, pulmonary, and endocrine disease, however, represent the most common comorbid
conditions.

VII. Long-term Concerns

A. Mortality

Geriatric trauma patients are at least twice as likely to
die from equivalent injuries as are younger patients.
The likelihood of dying following trauma increases 6.8%
per year after 65 years of age. Multiple organ failure is
generally the cause of death in the elderly. The
increased risk of death is attributable to age, preexisting medical conditions, and higher complication rates.
Often, death in the elderly is delayed as the patient sur-
vives the initial insult, but lacks the reserves to fend off
complications. Despite the increased incidence of death
in elderly trauma patients, no algorithm has been developed to satisfactorily select the patients at highest risk
for death at the time of admission. Head injury, spinal
injury, and hypotension on admission are poor prognostic signs.

B. Complications

Complications in elderly patients are prevalent and
lethal. A sound knowledge of potential complications can
help prevent them. Sepsis and cardiac failure represent
the most common complications that lead to death in the
elderly population. Respiratory failure resulting from
chemical pneumonitis, infection, or chest wall trauma
also poses significant issues for the critically ill geriatric
patient. Finally, renal failure resulting from ischemic
insult or nephrotoxic injury can trigger the death of a
patient.

C. Preventing Complications

A cognizance of potential complications and an awareness of early signs and symptom can decrease the morbidity and the mortality of the elderly trauma patient. Specific measures have been shown to decrease the incidence of life-threatening complications.

1. Prophylatic Procedures

a. Early Tracheostomy. Early tracheostomy in a patient requiring long-term ventilatory support decreases risk of aspiration pneumonia and aspiration pneumonitis.

b. Early Venal Caval Filter. Given the decreased physiologic reserve of elderly lungs, the insult of a small pulmonary embolism can lead to death in older patients. With the high incidence of head trauma and often the inability to use anticoagulants, filters can significantly decrease the risk of death from an embolism.

c. Invasive Monitoring. As mentioned, elderly patients often manifest symptoms late in the course of disease. Their fragile physiologic balance cannot withstand such insults. Invasive monitoring allows clinicians to monitor subtle and potentially correctable physiologic change.

2. Nutrition

The elderly are often nutritionally depleted before a traumatic event. Traumatic injury significantly increases metabolic demand. Without proper nutrition, elderly patients are predisposed to poor wound healing, prolonged ventilation, and infectious complications. Clinicians must supplement the elderly trauma patient with enteral feeding as rapidly as is tolerated. Be cautious in the use of enteral feeding, however, as aspiration is the most common preventable complication leading to death in these patients. Parenteral nutrition should be used until enteral feeding is satisfactorily accomplished. A regular calculation of nitrogen balance and implementation of the metabolic cart may be required to assess nutritional status.

3. Pain Management

Pain management is an essential component of care of all trauma patients. Comfort is a priority. In the elderly, pain management takes on heightened significance as pain can lead to hyperventilation, anxiety, and tachycardia. The ability of the older heart to meet oxygen demands is limited at baseline. Pain can exacerbate these demands and stress an overburdened system.

D. Rehabilitation

1. Physical Rehabilitation

Early rehabilitation predicts improves discharge functioning. Physical therapy for the patient maintains muscle strength and flexibility.

2. Placement Issues at Discharge

Given the inability of physicians to predict survival early in the clinical course, discharge planning should begin for all patients at the time of discharge. Education of, and interaction with, family members in this regard increases the likelihood that a discharge plans will satisfy both the patient and family.

E. Quality of Life

1. Controversies

Given the increasing numbers of elderly, the rising incidence of geriatric trauma, and the escalating cost of trauma care, clinicians and ethicists continue to review the posttraumatic quality of life of these patients.

Whereas one study reports that 72% of trauma patients remain in nursing homes 1 year following injury, another suggests that 87% of the injured elderly will return home following discharge. Of this group, 57% achieve prehospitalization levels of functioning.

2. Goals and Recommendations

Currently, most elderly trauma patients appear to enjoy an acceptable quality of life. Thus, until predictors of nonsurvival improve significantly in accuracy, ethicists insist that all elderly trauma patients receive the full support of the trauma system in the initial phases of illness. Close communication with the family is essential. Advance directives should be reviewed and care must be taken to adhere to the wishes of the patient and the family in managing this fragile population.

VIII. Conclusions

A. Elderly Trauma Patients are Unique

1. Pitfalls

As people age, physiologic reserves decline and fragility increases. Elderly trauma patients, therefore, are more likely to experience significant injury, but lack the homeostatic mechanisms to compensate. Moreover, given changes in anatomy and neurologic function, symptoms can manifest in unusual and subtle ways. Missed symptoms and missed injuries as well as later complications are of increased danger in this brittle population. Recovery from hypotensive and hypoxemic insults is difficult in the face of minimal physiologic reserve.

a. Vigilant Imaging and Surveillance. Given the conditions noted above, maintain a high index of suspicion for occult injuries in the elderly. The threshold for imaging studies and invasive interventions must be significantly lowered not to overlook injury.

b. Comorbidity. An awareness of the likelihood of comorbid conditions in this population is mandatory. Medications can mask or exacerbate signs and symptoms of injury. Decreased functioning of an organ system because of preexisting conditions can have a significant impact on the care and outcome of an individual patient. The trauma team should invoke the skills of specialists liberally.

SELECTED READING

Cocanour C, Moore F, Ware D, et al. Age should not be a consideration for nonoperative management of blunt splenic injury. *J Trauma* 2000;48:4:606–612.

DeMaria E. Evaluation and treatment of the elderly trauma victim. *Clin Geriatr Med* 1993;9:2:461–471.

Furner S, Brody J, Jankowski L. Epidemiology and aging. In: *Geriatric medicine.* New York: Springer-Verlag, 1997.

Grossman M, Miller D, Scaff D, et al. When is an elder old? Effect of preexisting conditions on mortality in geriatric trauma. *J Trauma* 2002;52:2 242–246.

Mandavia D, Newton K. Geriatric trauma. *Emerg Med Clin North Am* 1998;16(1):257–274.

McMahon D, Shapiro B, Kauder D. Comorbidity and the elderly trauma patient. *World J Surg* 1996;20(8):1113–1119.

McMahon D, Shapiro B, Kauder D. The injured elderly in the trauma intensive care unit. *Surg Clin North Am* 2000;80(3):1005–1019.

Perdue P, Watts D, Kaufmann C, et al. Differences in mortality between elderly and younger adult trauma patients: geriatric status increases risk of delayed death. *J Trauma* 1998;45(4):805–810.

Wardle T. Co-morbid factors in trauma patients. *Br Med Bull* 1999; 55(4):744–756.

Trauma Radiology

Thomas Ptak MD, PhD, MPH,
and Andrew Hines-Peralta, MD

I. **Overview**
   A. Imaging has assumed a great role in trauma care in recent years. Imaging protocols in acute blunt trauma vary widely, from plain film techniques to complex cross-sectional imaging. This section introduces guidelines for imaging with suggested protocols. We will also point out common life-threatening injuries and criteria for radiographic diagnosis.
   B. A quick initial plain film series is commonly incorporated into the primary trauma evaluation. Portable anteroposterior (AP) views of the chest and pelvis and a single portable lateral view of the cervical spine can be useful in providing initial details of severe injury. These films can often be acquired during the primary or secondary assessment.

II. **Craniocerebral Trauma**
   A. **Imaging Technique**
      1. **Computed Tomography Imaging**
      Computed tomography (CT) is currently preferred for the initial evaluation.
      2. **Slice Thickness**
         a. **Supratentorial:** 5 to 7 mm
         b. **Posterior Fossa:** thinner, typically 2 to 3 mm (optional)
         c. **Facial Bones and Orbits:** 2 to 3 mm
         d. **Temporal Bones:** 2 to 3 mm
            (1) Can usually be reconstructed from existing posterior fossa images.
      3. **Reconstruction Algorithm**
         a. **Brain:** low spatial frequency soft tissue detail
         b. **Facial and Temporal Bones and Orbits:** high spatial frequency bone detail
      4. **Window (W) and Level (L) Settings**
         a. **Brain:** W120 to 140/L30 to 40
         b. **Posterior Fossa:** W70 to 80/L30 to 40
         c. **Blood:** W50 to 70/L20 to 30
         d. **Bone:** W2200 to 2500/L250 to 500
      5. **Reformations**
      Coronal and sagittal
         a. **Orbit and Facial Bones:** 2.5 mm thick with 20% overlap
         b. **Temporal Bones:** 1.25 mm thick with 20% overlap
      6. **Magnetic Resonance Imaging—Advanced**
         a. **T1:** sagittal sequence
         b. **T2 fast spin echo (FSE):** axial sequence

      c. Fluid Attenuated Inversion Recovery (FLAIR): axial sequence

      d. Magnetic susceptibility sequence: axial sequence

      e. All sequences: 4 to 6 mm thick

      f. Add magnetic resonance angiography (MRA) in cases of question of a skull base fracture passing through the vascular channel or if dissection suspected.

         (1) May need to add fat-saturated T1WI or neck to rule out vascular dissection.

B. Brain and Coverings

   1. Use windows designed specifically for each compartment: supratentorial, infratentorial, and extraaxial blood windows.

   2. Brain Parenchymal Injury

      a. Contusion. A contusion can be hemorrhagic or bland.

         (1) A bland injury can involve microhemorrhage, glial, or avascular injury to the neuropil. Can be evident as only cytotoxic or vasogenic edema with low density, loss of gray and white interface, or local sulcal effacement.

         (2) Hemorrhagic injury can range from microhemorrhagic injury to frank sublobar or lobar parenchymal laceration.

         (3) Commonly occurs at the crests of gyri from direct impact—*coup injury.*

         (4) Can occur from a direct impact to the brain opposite the side of impact as a result of elastic recoil forces—*contra coup* injury.

      b. Diffuse Axonal Injury or Shear Injury. Ranges from stretch of axons with dysfunction, but limited permanent injury, to complete tear of axons and surrounding blood vessels. CT may show microhemorrhage and punctate edema in the white matter.

         (1) Common at gray and white interface, and in corpus callosum, especially the splenium

         (2) Severe injury can occur in the posterolateral brainstem.

   3. Extraaxial Hemorrhage

      a. Any of these can be isodense to brain.

      b. Epidural

         (1) Lens-shaped or biconvex

         (2) Does not cross sutures

         (3) Hyperdense (>50 to 60 Hounsfield units [HU])

      c. Subdural

         (1) Crescent shaped

         (2) Follows the inner table of the skull, even across sutures. Will track into the falx cerebri and tentorium cerebelli.

         (3) Usually hyperdense, although can vary, depending on phase of blood products. If chronic, can have near cerebrospinal fluid (CSF) density.

  d. Subarachnoid
    (1) Follows sulci, fissures, and cisterns.
    (2) Can be hyper- or isodense to adjacent brain. Reports indicate 5% of "missed" subarachnoid hemorrhage (SAH) are actually isodense and limited in area. A lumbar puncture is needed SAH is suspected. Middle cerebral artery (MCA) and other arteries can appear hyperdense if surrounded by adjacent isodense blood *hyperdense artery sign*. Look for *missing* anatomy (e.g., missing Sylvian fissure, basal cistern, and convexity sulci).

4. Calvaria and Skull Base
  a. Axial CT views are most useful.
  b. Temporal bone fractures
  c. Longitudinal and transverse types
  d. Ossicular dislocation
  e. Can disrupt seventh (transverse) or eighth (longitudinal) nerves.

5. Facial Bones and Orbits
  a. Coronal reformats are helpful in delineating sloping orbital floor and complex facial buttresses.
  b. Blowout fractures (inferior) are more obvious on coronals. Medial blowout are more obvious on axial view.

6. Common Traps and Decision Dilemmas
1. Posterior fossa and brain stem are severely compromised because of surrounding bony anatomy. If injury is suggested here, magnetic resonance imaging (MRI) is needed.
2. Extraaxial blood products may be very difficult to detect depending on the stage of organization. Isointense hemorrhage may be missed. Look for symmetric CSF cisterns. Be sure they have the proper configuration and CSF density.

III. Cervical Trauma
A. Imaging Technique
  1. Slice Thickness
    a. Bone: 1 to 3 mm
    b. Soft Tissue: 3 to 5 mm
  2. Reconstruction Algorithm
    a. Bone: high spatial frequency bone detail
    b. Soft Tissue: low spatial frequency detail
  3. Windows
    a. Bone: W2200 to 2500/L250 to 500
    b. Soft Tissue: W120 to 140/L60 to 80
  4. Reformations
    a. From thin soft tissue algorithm images
    b. Coronal and sagittal
    c. 2.5 mm thick with 20% overlap
    d. Useful for examining craniocervical junction

B.   Craniocervical Junction: Upper Cervical Segment

1.   Jefferson Fracture

Burst fracture of C1: Common after direct vertex axial load. Direct indications include cortical disruption, especially notable in the anterior arch on AP view. Secondary indicators of C1 ring injury include the following:

    a.   Lateral atlantodens interval on AP open-mouth view should be symmetric within ±2 mm.

    b.   Anterior atlantodens interval on lateral view should be ≤3 mm in adults; ≤5 mm in children <8.

    c.   Joint spaces of atlantooccipital joints on AP open-mouth projection should be symmetric and 1 to 2 mm in height.

    d.   Joint spaces of atlantoaxial joints on AP open-mouth view should be symmetric and 2 to 3 mm in height.

2.   Hangman Fracture

Classically, an avulsion fracture at the pars interarticularis of the C2 vertebral body

    a.   Direct indicators include clear disruption in the cortex on lateral view with a break in the ventral cortex or posterior axial line.

    b.   Disruption of hyperdense ring on lateral projection ("ring sign") indicates fracture extending through the body of C2.

    c.   Dens may appear posterior angulated on lateral view. Rarely, anterior angulated (<5%). Look for evidence of fracture.

    d.   Displacement of C2 lamina from the spinal-laminar line can indicate disruption of the C2 ring.

3.   Atlantoaxial Dissociation

    a.   Ligamentus injury involving the transverse, vertical (i.e., cruciate), alar, or axial ligaments. Look for indirect evidence of misalignment of the joint.

    b.   Lateral View. Distances to check.

        (1)   Atlantodens Interval (ADI). As in Jefferson fracture (see **1.b. above**)

        (2)   Dens Basion Interval (DBI). Distance from basion to dens tip should be <12 mm.

        (3)   Posterior axis-basion line (PABL). Line drawn from base of C2 along the posterior cortex of C2 to the level of the basion. Basion should be <12 mm anterior to PABL (**Fig. 42-1**). In <15% of normal individuals, PABL can lie up to 4 mm anterior to the basion tip.

    c.   Cervical Spine: Lower Cervical Segment

        (1)   MUST IDENTIFY VERTEBRAE C3 TO T1. Mobility of the cervical spine occurs above the cervicothoracic junction and is more fixed below the thoracic inlet. This junction between mobile cervical elements and fixed

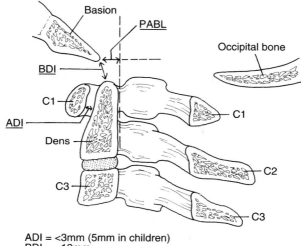

ADI = <3mm (5mm in children)
BDI = <12mm
PABL = <12mm

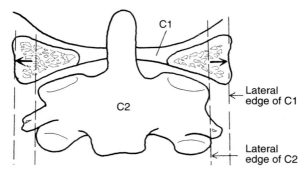

Figure 42-1. Anatomic relationships at the craniocervical junction.

thoracic elements renders this inflection point more vulnerable to injury.

(2) This region is often difficult to visualize because of the thickness of the shoulders. It may be necessary to proceed to CT with sagittal reformation.

(3) Fracture and misalignment in C3 to C7 are assessed using the following criteria from the lateral view.

(4) Normally has smooth lordotic curve (**Fig. 42-2**).

(5) Can be straightened because of positioning, spasm, or injury.

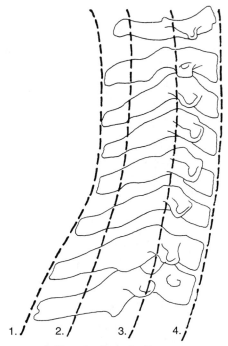

1. Tips of spinous bodies
2. Spinolaminar line
3. Post. vertebral body line
4. Ant. vertebral body line

Figure 42-2.   Lines used to inspect cervical alignment.

- Anterior spinal line
- Posterior spinal line
- Spinal lamina line
- Spinous process line or orientation: the spinous processes normally converge on a point posterior to the midcervical segment.
- Lateral mass integrity and alignment: should appear as a parallelogram with overlapping "shingled" appearance.

d.   Soft Tissues
(1)   Muscles and Ligaments. Best evaluated by MRI. FSE-T2WI with fat saturation makes edema or hemorrhage apparent.
(2) T2 hyperintense ligaments do not always indicate mechanical instability.

(3) Hyperintensity crossing hypointense fibrous ligament suggests tear.

(4) Larynx and Pharynx. MRI better than CT. Need thin (≤3 mm) section.

(5) MRI signal indicates edema or hemorrhage in cartilage and muscle.

(6) Alteration in signal or density of paraglottic fat pad can indicate injury.

(7) Look for architectural alterations in thyroid and cricoid cartilage and hyoid bone.

   e. Vessels. Difficult to evaluate on noncontrast CT examination. CT angiogram is better. Noncontrast MRI axial T1 or proton-density imaging most sensitive. T2WI low sensitivity.

   (1) Flow voids are sensitive for identifying moving blood on noncontrast and non-MRA images.

   f. Common Traps and Decision Dilemmas

1. Must see all vertebral elements from occipital junction to upper thoracic region. Points of attachment are vulnerable to injury. May need CT with reformation to fully evaluate the craniocervical junction and thoracocervical attachment.

2. Evaluation of cervicospinal ligaments using MRI is helpful. Bear in mind that currently *no conclusive literature* indicates that an abnormal signal in the ligaments directly correlates with mechanical instability or loss of load-bearing structural integrity. Abnormal ligaments found on MRI, at least for now, necessitate mechanical assessment of structural integrity and stability (i.e., flexion-extension views).

3. To avoid injury to the cord by herniated disk, spinal stenosis or extradural hematoma, MRI should be performed on high suspicion cases *before* flexion-extension series.

IV. Chest Trauma

   A. Chest trauma is associated with 16% morbidity and 36% mortality.

   B. Start with plain film in trauma bay.

   1. Portable chest x-ray (CXR) is often insensitive because of supine portable technique, but can give early indication of serious injury or pending disaster (e.g., tension pneumothorax or aortic injury).

   C. Computed Tomography Imaging Technique

   1. 5 mm thick CT sections are common.

   2. Arms positioned over the head, when possible.

   3. Contraindicated in fractured limb or shoulder.

   4. Contrast enhanced for visualization of great vessels and mediastinum.

   a. A twenty-five second pre scan delay is typical.

5. Image from C6-C7 to midrenal level to ensure coverage of the entire intrathoracic pulmonary parenchyma and thoracic cage.

6. Image During Quiet Breathing

Often cannot be controlled in trauma patient.

7. Reconstruct to 2- to 3-mm thick sections, small field of view (for spine) for reformation of axial images to sagittal and coronal planes.

D. Thoracic Spine

1. Thoracic spine is best evaluated using thin section CT axial reconstructions with coronal and sagittal reformations for assessment of anteroposterior and transverse alignment.

 a. Axial CT imaging alone diminishes sensitivity because it does not allow evaluation of alignment or intervertebral relationships.

 b. In the absence of complex helical CT imaging, AP and lateral inspiration technique plain films specific to the thoracic spine provide full spatial evaluation of the thoracic spine. Plain film techniques become insensitive because of thoracic summation shadows obscuring evaluation of fine detail.

 c. Carefully and methodically evaluate alignment, vertebral architecture, and relationship of vertebral bodies and disks as described in the cervical spine section.

 d. Fracture and Subluxation. Apparent through disrupted vertebra, disk space, and malalignment. Can involve only posterior elements and posterior ligamentous complex with intact vertebral body.

  (1) Chance Fracture. A specific shear or distraction force injury, with the fracture plane extending horizontally through the vertebral body, pedicles, articulating facets, and into the lamina and spinous process. Think of this type of injury in lap belt mechanism.

  (2) MRI is necessary to evaluate thoracic cord and conus. Dural compromise caused by bone fragments, disk herniation, or intracanalicular hematoma should also be assessed using MRI.

E. Chest Wall

1. CT imaging is best for evaluation of bony thorax. Pay attention to rib and sternum. Ribs are easily evaluated on axial images, but sternum can be viewed only fully with sagittal and, to a lesser degree, coronal reformations.

2. Fractures of the first through third ribs indicate sufficient force deposited to the thoracic cage to significantly injure intrathoracic and, specifically, mediastinal structures.

3. Also consider injury to brachial plexus and subclavian vessels.

4. Three or more adjacent ribs containing two or more fractures result in a free-floating chest wall segment, resulting in a significant loss of structural rigidity. The region of floating thoracic cage is referred to as a *flail segment* (i.e., flail chest). Paradoxic or absent lung motion in the region of the flail segment can contribute to respiratory compromise.

5. Chest wall hematoma can be seen on CT with limited sensitivity.

    a. Muscular tear can be recognized by subpleural or extrathoracic hemorrhage. Tear of intercostal artery or vein contributes to hematoma and hemothorax.

    b. MRI provides increased sensitivity for injury to the muscular chest wall. MRI can be hampered in the acutely injured patient because of tachypnea or inability of the patient to cooperate with the breath-holding required during imaging sequence.

6. **Scapular Injury**

    a. Protected by muscular covering. Fractures here are infrequent.

    b. If scapula fracture, suggests significant force.

    c. If scapula is fractured, at risk for the following:

        (1) Pulmonary contusion, hemo- or pneumothorax in 40%

        (2) Closed head injury in 25%

        (3) Spinal fracture in 18%

    d. **Scapulothoracic Dissociation**

        (1) A "closed amputation" or avulsion type injury where the scapula is torn from chest wall connections.

        (2) Associated with neurovascular injury

        (3) Bony injuries include sternoclavicular and acromioclavicular separation and distracted clavicle fracture.

F. Diaphragm

    1. Difficult to image because of anatomic, spatial, and contrast limitations.

    2. MRI is best, but logistically difficult.

        a. Good for a detailed, noncritical assessment

        b. Motion sensitive. Tachypnea reduces image quality.

    3. CT with sagittal and coronal reformation is most sensitive and specific.

    4. Plain film CXR is next in sensitivity.

    5. Imaging sensitivity to detect diaphragmatic injury falls for all modalities in intubated patients on positive pressure breathing.

    6. Increased intrathoracic pressure opposes visceral excursion into the chest: displacement of viscera is the key to making the diagnosis.

G. Lung and Pleura

    1. Pulmonary Contusion

        a. Direct impact transferred to lung parenchyma

      b. Appear as patchy areas of air space disease that defy lobar boundaries

      c. **Phases**

          (1) Interstitial hemorrhage

          (2) Edema follows 1 to 2 hours later.

          (3) Alveolar hemorrhage and protein by 24 hours

      d. Contusion may not show on initial films. Is most radiographically evident on CXR within 6 hours of injury.

      e. **CT more sensitive than plain film**

          (1) CT shows more contusions and defines area involved better than CXR.

      f. **Associated Lung Malfunction**

          (1) V/Q mismatch

          (2) Diminished pulmonary compliance

      g. All typically resolve in 3 to 5 days

          (1) If >25% of lung parenchyma involved, patient would benefit from mechanical ventilation.

  2. **Pulmonary Laceration**

      a. CT is most sensitive for defining character and extent of pulmonary laceration.

          (1) Laceration will show an ovoid cavity surrounded by pseudomembrane on CT.

          (2) Can have blood-air level.

          (3) Clotted blood can give a crescent or meniscoid appearance. Blood clots can be seen as a resolving nodule on plain film CXR.

          (4) Uncomplicated laceration will resolve on its own over several weeks. Complicated lesions can have bronchial tears or air leaks, which may require surgical intervention.

  3. **Pleural Injury**

      a. **Pneumothorax**

          (1) Air goes to most nondependent space. In the supine patient, look in the anteromedial and subpulmonic regions. Air in these areas result in the *deep sulcus and double diaphragm* signs, respectively. In the upright position, look at apex and superolateral boarders.

      b. **Tension Pneumothorax**

          (1) Occurs from a one-way flap valve effect of a pleural tear

          (2) Predominantly, a clinical diagnosis

          (3) A simple pneumothorax seen in blunt trauma can convert to a tension pneumothorax.

          (4) Can persist despite thoracostomy tube.

          (5) Look for a shift of mediastinum away from the side involved or inversion of the ipsilateral hemidiaphragm.

          (6) Communicate diagnosis immediately! Can result in circulatory and respiratory collapse.

c. **Hemothorax**
   (1) Can originate from various venous or
   arterial sources. Venous = self-limited. Arterial hemothorax can accumulate rapidly and
   require a thoracostomy tube or open thoracostomy.
   (2) Fluid in the pleural space on CXR: nonspecific
   (3) CT is more sensitive. Helps discrimi-
   nate between blood (~>45 to 50 HU), chyle, or
   serous fluid (~<30 HU).

H. **Mediastinum**
   1. Start with plain film, then consider CT to evaluate mediastinum.
      a. **Pneumomediastinum**
      b. Most commonly occurs from alveolar rupture
      into the interstitium, with tracking back to the
      hilum and mediastinum.
      c. Air between the heart and mediastinal pleura
      d. Air can track along the esophagus and aorta
      beyond the mediastinal reflection.
      e. Air under the heart: *continuous diaphragm*
      sign
      f. Pneumomediastinum can convert to pneu-
      mothorax by rupturing through the mediastinal
      pleura.
      g. Air can track through diaphragmatic hiatus
      and present as air in the retroperitoneal space,
      which can then rupture through the peritoneum
      and present as pneumoperitoneum.
   2. **Vascular Injury**
      a. **Aorta**
         (1) Plain film signs include the following:

         • "Widened mediastinum" >8 cm at vascular
           infundibulum: NOT SENSITIVE ALONE
         • Loss or enlargement of aortic arch contour
         • Loss of AP window
         • Loss of left pulmonary artery shadow
         • *Apical cap:* free pleural fluid tracking
           superomedially into the medial left apex

         (2) **Computed Tomographic Signs**

         • Hemorrhage adjacent to aorta
         • Most common at junction of proximal de-
           scending segment and arch
         • Hemorrhage NOT immediately in contact
           with the aorta is unlikely due to aortic
           injury, but can be atelectasis, consolida-
           tion, or pleural fluid.
         • Irregular aortic lumen suggests intimal
           derangement and possibly breech.
         • Flap in lumen or circumferential narrow-
           ing suggests aortic dissection. Dissections
           can be posttraumatic or previously exist-
           ing. Not easily distinguishable.

b. Brachiocephalic Vessels
(1) Computed Tomographic Signs

- Hemorrhage adjacent to origin of great vessels extends to superior mediastinum
- Nonfilling of great vessels or a flap seen in lumen, which can indicate dissection

3. Cardiac Injury
a. High-density (>=45 HU) fluid in the pericardial sac

b. Consider myocardial injury.

> **(1)** Myocardial laceration or rupture
>
> **(2)** Posttraumatic cardiac aneurysm
>
> **(3)** Aortic root injury, especially at the coronary artery origins. Tends to bleed below attachment of pericardial reflection and into the sac, giving a pericardial effusion.

c. Can result in *cardiac tamponade* and circulatory collapse.

d. Pneumopericardium can be confused for pneumomediastinum or pneumothorax.

> **(1)** Can be seen in blunt trauma.
>
> **(2)** Can develop into *tension pneumopericardium.*

4. Airway Injury
a. Accounts for 1% to 2% of mortality.

> **(1)** Most mortalities of this type are prehospital.
>
> **(2)** Survival is inversely proportional to size of tear.

b. Full evaluation of airway can require thin section (1 to 3 mm) CT examination with coronal and sagittal reformations.

> **(1)** Thinner sections are imperative to detect minimally displaced tears.

c. Tracheal Injury

> **(1)** More common in penetrating neck trauma
>
> **(2)** Diagnostic signs are largely secondary: rightward deviation of the endotracheal tube tip; extension of the endotracheal tube cuff beyond the tracheal walls on CXR. Clinically, a persistent pneumothorax or "air leak" seen.

d. Bronchial Injury

> **(1)** 80% occur within 2.5 cm of the carina.
>
> **(2)** Bronchoscopy is test of choice.
>
> **(3)** Right bronchus is more likely injured than is the left.
>
> **(4)** "Fallen lung" sign is a pathognomonic but rare finding. The lung falls posterior and laterally on supine film. Normally, it pulls toward hilum. The lung falls inferiorly when upright. Normally, it is held up by hilum.
>
> **(5)** Acute angulation or change in caliber of bronchus

(6) Blood clot displacing hilar contents suggests concomitant hilar vessel injury.

I. **Common Traps and Decision Dilemmas**

1. Respiratory motion can severely compromise image quality.
2. Coronal and sagittal CT reformations can give false indication of extravasation or fracture.
3. Intubated patients on ventilator can suspend respirations during acquisition. Positive pressure limits sensitivity for detecting diaphragmatic injury.
4. Tachypnea severely limits MRI quality.
5. Know positioning (e.g., upright vs. supine) on plain films! Do not look for an apical pneumothorax on a supine film.
6. Be aware of easy to miss diagnoses (e.g., diaphragmatic or tracheobronchial injuries). Findings are often subtle and secondary in nature.

V. **Abdominal Trauma**
   A. **Introduction**
      1. CT of the abdomen is the primary imaging modality for the trauma patient.
      2. Multidetector CT scanners now allow scanning of patients who previously were deemed too unstable.
      3. Sonography plays an important role in detecting blood within the abdomen in the unstable patient.
      4. The principal goal of imaging is to first assess for injuries necessitating emergent operative intervention. Afterward, evaluation can proceed to accurately characterize the spectrum of intraabdominal injuries.
   B. **Focused Abdominal Sonography for Trauma (FAST)**
      1. **Technique**
         a. 3.5-MHz transducer
         b. Abdominal presets
         c. Window depth to visualize the crus of the diaphragm
         d. Time Gain Compensation (TGC) optimized to area of interest
      2. Primary goal of the FAST is to assess for hemoperitoneum in unstable patients.
         a. Physical examination is negative in ~20% of patients with hemoperitoneum.
         b. Sonography is 85% to 99% sensitive for hemoperitoneum.
         c. ~400 mL of blood is necessary before sonography becomes reliable.
      3. **Probe Placement**
         a. Subxiphoid space for visualization of pericardial fluid
         b. Right midaxillary line for the right subphrenic space, Morison's pouch, and right paracolic gutter
         c. Posterior left axillary line for the left subphrenic, perisplenic space, and left paracolic gutter

      d. Abdominal midline two to three finger-breadths above the pubic symphysis for fluid in the pelvic cul-de-sac

4. Appearance of Blood on Ultrasound

      a. Unclotted blood: low echogenicity. Appears black.

      b. Clotted blood: more echogenic. Can be hard to distinguish from spleen or liver. Failure to identify the spleen or liver raises the concern of adjacent clot.

5. Abdominal Organ Injuries

      a. False-negative findings are common.

      b. Organ injuries without hemoperitoneum are missed in one third of patients.

      c. CT is always necessary once patients become stabilized.

C. Computed Tomography

    1. Primary imaging modality for all hemodynamically stable patients

    2. High sensitivity and specificity for detecting all types of abdominal trauma

    3. Characterizes progression of injury, enabling nonoperative management for traumatic conditions that need close supervision.

      a. Assess first for signs of life-threatening injury: active arterial contrast extravasation, hemoperitoneum, pneumothorax, pneumoperitoneum, and signs of the hemodynamic status.

      b. Assessment then proceeds with orderly review of the abdominal organs, muscles, and bones.

    4. Technique

      a. 5-mm slices at a pitch of 1.5 with oral and intravenous contrast

      b. Oral contrast: ~600 mL of Gastrografin (meglumine diatrizoate)

      c. Intravenous contrast: 120 to 150 mL of 60% contrast material at 2 to 3 mL/sec.

      d. Rectal contrast (up to 1 L) can be administered for sufficient enhancement of the entire colon in suspected intestinal injuries.

      e. Oral contrast only typically reaches the stomach and proximal small bowel. Injuries to unenhanced portions of the small bowel can be difficult to identify.

      f. Foley catheter is clamped to maximize bladder filling (to detect bladder tears).

      g. Scanning begins 70 to 90 seconds after administration of the intravenous contrast to balance arterial and portal vein enhancement.

      h. Motion artifacts can greatly restrict the diagnostic capacities of CT.

      i. Uncooperative patients should be sedated, if possible.

D. Intraabdominal Hemorrhage and Air

    1. Single most important sign in trauma. Usually necessitates emergent surgery or embolization.

2. CT is very sensitive. Contrast-enhanced blood is easily visualized escaping from an injured vessel.

 a. Attenuation of contrast-enhanced blood is hyperdense, usually ~100 HU.

3. Active bleeding has same attenuation as contrast-enhanced aorta.

 a. May not bleed freely into the abdomen.

 b. Known as pseudoaneurysm or arteriovenous fistula.

  (1) Well-circumscribed area of contrast attenuation

  (2) Freely extravasating blood has no distinct margin.

 c. Some pseudoaneurysms and arteriovenous fistulas resolve spontaneously, whereas others require intervention.

 d. Active extravasation can be present in up to 18% of cases.

4. Splenic and Hepatic Bleeding

 a. Spleen more than liver is most common site for active arterial extravasation.

 b. Of cases, ~70% with active hemorrhage go to surgery or embolization.

 c. Coil embolization is very effective in treating active bleeding from spleen and liver.

 d. Hepatic Venous Bleeding

  (1) Extravasation from major hepatic or portal veins must be evaluated during the portal venous phase of the contrast flow.

  (2) Angiography is often necessary to identify patients for surgical intervention.

5. Mesenteric Bleeding

 a. Angiography is performed before embolization to better visualize the injured artery and to direct placement of the coil.

 b. Never use arterial embolization for active bleeding from mesenteric arteries because of the high risk of infarcting the bowel.

 c. Active bleeding from mesenteric arteries is hard to distinguish from bowel perforation.

  (1) Both are visualized as extravasation of contrast material.

  (2) Both mesenteric artery hemorrhage and bowel perforation need surgical intervention.

6. Peritoneal Fluid

 a. Fluid seen in the abdomen can represent blood, urine, bile, bowel contents, or some combination.

 b. Trace amount of simple fluid not uncommon in the posttraumatic patient.

  (1) Not necessarily indicative of organ injury

 c. A trace amount of fluid in the pelvis is normal in menstruating women.

  (1) More than a trace is often associated with visceral organ injury.

d. Even if no other sign of solid organ injury exists, almost half of patients with more than trace free fluid will have organ injuries requiring exploratory surgery.

(1) Most from bowel or mesentery

7. Fluid Attenuation

a. Urine and bile near-water attenuation: ±10 HU

b. Unclotted blood: ~25 to 40 HU

c. Contrast-enhanced arterial blood: >100 HU

d. Fluid combinations attenuate at the average of the components.

e. Clotted blood: 45 to 65 HU

(1) Will not mix with other fluid.

(2) Shows a distinct attenuation, even in the presence of other fluid.

(3) Clots form near sites of injury, which are called *sentinel* clot sign.

8. Pneumoperitoneum

a. Upright chest radiograph and CT are very sensitive for free abdominal air.

b. Air in the abdomen can be caused by air tracking from a pneumothorax.

c. Use lung windows when looking for free extraluminal air on CT.

(1) Often disguised next to bowel gas.

(2) If detected, seek other signs of bowel injury.

d. Pneumoperitoneum is a possible sign of bowel rupture requiring exploratory surgery.

(1) Perforations can be detected on reimaging after oral and rectal contrast.

(2) Chest CT needed to exclude pneumothorax.

9. Hemodynamic Status

a. Radiographic signs of insufficient intravascular volume depletion are visible before shock.

(1) Flattened vena cava

(2) Flattened renal veins

(3) Small, hypoattenuated spleen

(4) Small or contracted aorta (especially in children)

E. Spleen

1. Of all abdominal organ injuries, 35% are identified by CT.

2. Most common cause of preventable death in trauma patients

3. Often accompanies other left-sided injuries.

a. Left-sided rib fractures should heighten suspicion of splenic injury.

4. Clot Formation

a. Clot adjacent to the spleen indicates splenic injury = *sentinel* clot sign.

5. Splenic Injury Types

a. Contusion (see Parenchymal hematoma)

b. Hematoma

> **(1)** Parenchymal hematoma: round area of low attenuation expanding the parenchyma
> **(2)** Subcapsular hematoma: peripheral curved shape that can compress the splenic parenchyma

c.   Laceration
> **(1)** Low attenuation lines within the splenic parenchyma
> **(2)** Hemoperitoneum, if laceration extends through capsule.

d.   Fracture (see Laceration).

e.   Hilar Injuries
> **(1)** Can cause hypoperfusion to the spleen.
> **(2)** Low attenuation because of lack of contrast enhancement. Note: the upper pole can remain normal from collateral vasculature.
> **(3)** Small spleen can result from hypoperfusion because of shock. May or may not show low attenuation.
> **(4)** Active arterial bleeding can be helpful in identifying patients not conducive to conservative management.
> **(5)** Active splenic bleeding can be successfully treated with embolization.
> **(6)** Most splenic injuries are managed nonoperatively with embolization and careful observation.

F.   Liver
1.   The liver is the second most injured abdominal organ in blunt trauma.
2.   Injuries are much more common in the right lobe than the left.
> **a.**   Likely result from compressive force against the spine.

3.   Radiographic appearance of these injuries is similar to that of the spleen.
4.   Liver injuries are described in terms similar to splenic injury:
> **a.   Contusion**
> **b.   Laceration**
> > **(1)** Lacerations are linear hypoattenuation in the liver parenchyma.
> > **(2)** Hemoperitoneum results from liver injury when lacerations extend through Glisson's capsule.
> **c.   Fracture**
> > **(1)** Lacerations extending through the liver fracture it into distinct fragments.
> **d.   Hematoma**
> > **(1) Parenchymal:** round, low attenuation within the liver parenchyma
> > **(2) Subcapsular:** crescent-shaped at liver margin
> **e.   Peritoneal Bleeding**
> > **(1)** Occurs with injury to the bare area of the liver, where there is no peritoneal reflection.

(2)   Extra peritoneal blood from bare area injury collects in the right pararenal space. This is not specific for hepatic injury because organ injuries (e.g., to the duodenum) can bleed into the same area.

f.   Hepatic injuries can be staged just as those to the spleen. Grade V hepatic injuries usually require surgery and carry a high morality rate (70% to 80%).

g.   Of blunt hepatic injuries, 80% are treated nonoperatively, in part, because of coil embolization and improved monitoring with CT.

h.   Infarction after coil embolization is rare because of the dual blood supply of the liver.

5. **Further Imaging**

   a.   For suspected portal or hepatic bleeding, imaging during the maximal venous phase is necessary.

   b.   Current three-dimensional reformations of CT angiograms and CT venograms will provide as much information as invasive standard angiography.

G. **Gallbladder**

1. **Gallbladder Injury is Rare**

   a.   Occurs if distended during traumatic compression.

   b.   Lacerations and contusions to the gallbladder appear as a distorted gallbladder border, blood in the gallbladder, or both.

   c.   Pericholecystic fluid is a nonspecific finding often seen in trauma patients with no injury to the gallbladder.

   d.   Avulsion of the gallbladder shows the gallbladder displaced from its usual location in the gallbladder fossa.

H. **Bowel**

1.   Sensitivity of helical CT for bowel and mesentery injury is >90%.

2.   Bowel injuries are especially important to detect because signs of perforation or perfusion injury indicate emergent exploratory surgery.

3.   Injury can be missed if subtle signs are not appreciated.

   a.   **Intraperitoneal Free Air**

      (1)   Intraperitoneal free air is the most widely known sign of perforation.

      (2)   Specific (98%) but not sensitive (76%) for full-thickness bowel injury. Sensitivity and specificity are reduced because free air can also result from other injuries (e.g., pneumothorax).

      (3)   Often, just a few small air bubbles are seen in the mesentery.

   b.   **Extraperitoneal Free Air**

      (1)   Can result from injury to the duodenum or large bowel.

(**2**) Air usually tracks to the right pararenal space.

c. Extravasation of Contrast-enhanced Intestinal Contents

(**1**) Diagnostic for perforation

(**2**) Short delay to scan in emergent trauma elicit caution because oral contrast will only reach stomach, duodenum, and proximal jejunum, resulting in an inability to fully evaluate distal jejunum, ileum, colon, or rectum unless delayed scans performed.

4. The most common site of injury from blunt trauma occurs near the ligament of Treitz.

    a. Tethering site during deceleration

5. Mesenteric Vessel Injury

    a. Missed mesenteric vessel injuries are likely to result in bowel infarction, perforation, and sepsis.

    b. Signs of mesenteric vessel injury include hematoma within the mesentery, active bleeding, and poor bowel perfusion.

    c. May be the only sign of mesenteric vessel injury.

    d. Seen as hypoattenuation of the bowel wall on CT.

    e. Active mesenteric bleeding requires surgical intervention. Coil embolization is generally not performed given the high risk of bowl infarction.

5. Other nonspecific signs of bowel injury include the following:

1. Bowel wall thickening
2. Adjacent fat stranding
3. Fluid between bowel loops
4. Mesenteric vessel injury

6. Further Imaging

    a. In suspected large bowel injuries, abdominal CT with rectal contrast is helpful.

    b. Delayed imaging for bowel extravasation in distal small bowel

    c. Endoscopy and coloroscopy may be necessary to confirm suspected tears.

I. Kidneys and Adrenals

1. Renal injury occurs in 1% to 5% of all trauma cases.

    a. Usually secondary to blunt injury.

    b. Suspected in patients with the following:

1. Gross hematuria
2. Microscopic hematuria with shock
3. Hematuria with hemoperitoneum

    c. Most injuries to the kidney are treated conservatively.

    d. Delayed diagnosis can lead to the loss of a kidney.

  e. Most renal vascular injuries result in loss of renal function.

  f. Parenchymal renal injuries include the following:

    (1) Contusion: suggested by patchy areas of parenchymal hypoattenuation.

    (2) Laceration: shows as a linear parenchymal hypoattenuation, which can be associated with perirenal hemorrhage.

    (3) Hematoma: subcapsular hematoma presents as a crescent of hypoattenuation constrained by an intact renal capsule.

    (4) Urinary collecting system injuries: lacerations result in extravasation of urine if they involve the collecting system.

  g. **Renovascular Injury**

    (1) Vascular Avulsion

    (2) Renal Artery Dissection

    (3) **Thrombosis of the Renal Artery or Vein**

    (4) CT Signs of Vascular Injury

    - Inadequate arterial or venous flow with poor parenchymal contrast enhancement
    - Parenchyma can enhance in complete renal artery occlusion if capsular collaterals are present.
    - A small branch occlusion can result in segmental infarction.
    - Persistent renal enhancement on delayed scanning can indicate renal vein thrombosis

 2. **Adrenal Injuries**

  a. Adrenal injuries are uncommon.

  b. They almost never require surgical intervention.

  c. Hemorrhage can appear as a round mass within the adrenal or may be poorly circumscribed.

  d. Hemorrhage can be difficult to differentiate from the parenchyma and, thus, injury often appears as a swollen or enlarged gland with surrounding fat stranding.

 3. **Further Imaging**

  a. Delayed images should be taken at 2 to 10 minutes to allow contrast to enhance excreted urine.

  b. MRI can be helpful in select cases.

    (1) Can characterize the age of hematoma using the difference between T1 and T2 signals.

    (2) Can help elucidate ambiguous CT findings.

J. **Pancreas**

 1. The pancreas is the most difficult organ to assess in trauma.

  a. Incidence of pancreatic injury is only 1% to 2% in patients with blunt or penetrating trauma.

b. Injuries are occasionally missed, especially if imaged in the initial phases of injury.

c. Other midline organs (e.g., duodenum and left lobe of liver) are also injured.

d. Injuries include

(1) Laceration: indicated by lines of hypo-attenuation on contrast-enhanced CT with disruption of pancreatic parenchyma.

(2) Hematoma: a focal or regional area of hypoattenuation. Can appear as an isodense expansion of parenchyma or a pancreatic mass. Any irregularity in attenuation or contour of the pancreas should raise the suspicion of a hematoma or contusion. Fluid surrounding the pancreas suggests pancreatic injury. Look for fluid especially in the lesser sac, around the superior mesenteric artery, and between the pancreas and splenic vein.

(3) Pancreatic duct injuries: require surgical repair. Mortality and morbidity from pancreatic trauma directly relates to involvement of the main pancreatic duct. More than half of patients with pancreatic trauma will have involvement of either the main pancreatic duct or major branches.

(4) Early endoscopic retrograde pancreatography should be performed in patients with suspected ductal injury, as delays lead to increased morbidity.

2. Further Imaging

a. Patients with pancreatic injury visualized on CT should be imaged with endoscopic retrograde cholangiopancreatography (ERCP) to assess for ductal involvement.

K. Common Traps and Decision Dilemmas

1. Motion artifacts: can greatly restrict the diagnostic capacities of CT. Uncooperative patients should be sedated, if possible.

2. Active bleeding: active venous bleeding can be more easily visualized if scans are taken during the maximal venous phase.

3. Pneumoperitoneum: extraluminal air can be missed if lung windows are not specifically used for visualization.

4. Pneumoperitoneum: look for pneumothorax as a possible cause of air in the abdomen.

5. Liver: blood in the right pararenal space can be caused by injury to the bare area of the liver or extraperitoneal organs.

6. Gallbladder: pericholecystic fluid is a nonspecific finding often seen in trauma patients with no injury to the gallbladder.

7. Spleen: splenic fragment can be mistaken for active bleeding if the attenuation of the fragment is not carefully noted.

8. Kidney: extravasating urine can look like active arterial bleeding. Active arterial bleeding is seen within 1 to 2 minutes from the injection of contrast. Urine extravasates after 2 to 10 minutes.

9. Pancreas: the pancreas is the most difficult organ to assess with CT. False-negative findings are rare, but possible.

VI. Pelvic Imaging

A. Introduction

1. Plain radiographs and CT are best for initial imaging of the pelvis. Imaging options are outlined in.

2. Portable pelvis, chest, and lateral cervical spine are performed as a screening procedure for patients with multiple trauma.

3. Pelvic CT is far superior to pelvic radiography as the primary pelvic imaging modality in the stable patient. Forgo plain pelvic imaging if the patient will also be examined by CT.

B. Pelvic Radiography

1. A portable AP view should be taken of the pelvis in severely injured patients.

2. Pelvic fractures are a potential source of major blood loss. Portable radiography, therefore, can lead to expedient pelvic angiography and embolization and, thus, improved survival.

3. Portable imaging enables quick visualization of significant fractures and major bleeding, but poor soft tissue contrast characteristics hamper visualization of further injuries.

4. Routine trauma plain film views include inlet, outlet, and bilateral oblique (Judet).

C. Computed Tomography

1. CT is sensitive and specific for pelvic injuries and has mostly replaced plain radiography in the trauma setting.

   a. Provides excellent detail for complex fractures and intraarticular disruptions.

   b. Up to one third of pelvic fractures detected on CT are missed on routine radiographs.

   (1) Of acetabular fractures, 40% are missed. Sections 1 to 2 mm thick may be necessary to characterize the fracture adequately.

   (2) Up to 50% of femoral head fractures are missed.

2. **Reformations**

   a. Useful for surgical planning in determining approach and screw placement

   b. Fractures usually appear more severe on multiplanar and three-dimensional reformations.

   c. Can change patient management in 30% of cases.

   (1) Immediate operative management may be indicated for what was originally thought to be nonemergent.

(2) Treatment can be delayed for later definitive arthrodesis or arthroplasty.

D. Further Imaging

1. Pelvic angiography is the gold standard. It is both diagnostic and therapeutic for life-threatening arterial bleeding.

2. Contrast-enhanced CT is 85% sensitive and 98% specific, and is the first line of diagnosis in the emergency department setting.

3. CT cystography can be used for suspected bladder injuries.

4. Retrograde urethrography is needed to detect anterior and posterior urethral injuries.

E. Assessment of Anteroposterior Plain Radiography

1. AP projection will pick up most injuries, but the other pelvic views enable detection of more subtle injuries.

2. Evaluate pelvis by assessing injuries in the center of the pelvis, progressing concentrically outward.

F. Classification of Injuries

1. Disruptions in the pelvic ring can often be predicted from knowledge of the offending force.

    a. Classified based on a system developed by Tile and modified by Young and Burgess (see chapter 34, *Pelvic Fractures*).

    b. Injuries are organized according to the impact (e.g., anterior or lateral blows, vertical shear injuries).

2. Iliac Fractures

    a. First Type: peripheral iliac fracture confined to the iliac crest. The sacroiliac joint is not involved

    b. Second Type: extends from the iliac crest into the greater sciatic notch with sparing of the sacroiliac joint. Gluteal vascular injuries are sometimes associated.

    c. Third Type: extends from the iliac crest into the anterior sacroiliac joint (crescent fracture-dislocation).

        (1) In this type of fracture, the stable portion is the posterior iliac fracture component, which remains attached to the dorsal sacrum.

3. Acetabular Fractures

    a. Anatomy

        (1) Four sections: anterior column, posterior column, anterior wall, posterior wall ("wall" is also referred to as "rim")

        (2) Columns are marked by the iliopectineal line (anterior column) and ilioischial line (posterior column). These lines join above the acetabulum and continue upward to the sciatic notch. The end product looks like an inverted Y. The bottom third (upside down Y portion) contains the articular surface, which is divided into the anterior half (anterior wall) and posterior half (posterior wall).

b.   Fractures

(1)   About 15% of patients with pelvic ring injuries will also have an acetabular fracture.

(2)   Posterior column fractures are more common than anterior column fractures.

(3)   Transverse fractures across both columns are common. The most common type of acetabular fracture is a Y-shaped fracture in which the acetabulum is broken into three or more fragments.

(4)   Some fractures are limited to the rim of the articular surface. Posterior wall (or posterior rim) fractures are more common than anterior wall (or anterior rim) fractures.

(5)   A *central hip dislocation* is when direct impact on the hip actually displaces the femoral head through the acetabulum.

c.   Visualization

(1)   The posterior wall of the acetabulum should be visualized on the AP pelvis film.

(2)   The anterior wall is more difficult to see on a plain AP projection.

(3)   The AP pelvic radiograph will reveal many acetabular fractures, but minimally displaced fractures can be hard to detect.

(4)   Normal appearance of the central acetabulum is made up of the quadrilateral plate, which can be seen on the AP view as a "teardrop." This may only be slightly distorted in fractures.

(5)   The most difficult fractures to identify on plain radiographs are acetabular rim fractures because of the overlap with the femoral heads.

(6)   Judet views can better demonstrate acetabular fractures.

(7)   CT, which will identify up to 30% of fractures missed on plain radiography, can detect intraarticular bone fragments that cannot be visualized on plain film. CT better defines the extent of the injury and can be invaluable in the surgical planning.

4.   Fractures Outside Pelvic Ring

a.   Fractures of a single pubic ramus is the most common type of pelvic fracture.

b.   Isolated fractures of iliac wing can occur from lateral impact to the ilium.

c.   Avulsion fractures can occur after sudden muscular movements in teenagers with immature bones.

d.   Sacrum fractures or coccyx fractures can occur from isolated impact.

(1)   Sacrum fractures are hard to detect except on CT.

(2) Coccyx fractures, which are hard to detect radiographically, are usually found by clinical diagnosis.

G. Pelvic Vascular Injuries

1. Hemorrhage is leading cause of death after pelvic fractures, accounting for a mortality rate of 10% to 15%.

2. Of individuals with high-energy pelvic trauma, 10% to 20% will have hemodynamic instability related to blood loss from the pelvic injury.

3. Routine use of intravenous contrast in pelvic CT allows a vascular map of the iliac and femoral vessels to be created.

4. CT is sensitive (84%) and specific (85% to 98%) for detection of active pelvic bleeding when compared with the angiographic gold standard.

5. Arterial bleeding typically occurs from the following:

a. Internal iliac (hypogastric) artery and its branches (most common)

b. Internal pudendal arteries

c. Superior gluteal arteries

6. Pelvic fractures that result in an increased intra-pelvic volume (e.g., anterior posterior compression [open book] injuries) can result in massive blood loss into the extraperitoneal dead space before tamponade.

a. A 2-cm symphyseal diastasis can increase pelvic volume from 1.5 L to 5 L.

7. Fractures into the sciatic notch, sacral crush injuries, and vertical shear injuries are also associated with more severe hemorrhage.

8. Fracture stabilization with volume reduction often stops venous bleeding, but arterial bleeding results in continued hemodynamic instability.

a. Angiography with therapeutic coil embolization is indicated for active arterial bleeding.

H. Bladder Injuries

1. Bladder injuries include contusion, hematoma, extraperitoneal rupture, and intraperitoneal rupture.

2. CT cystography and conventional cystograms are very sensitive and specific for bladder tears.

3. Detection of bladder rupture is contingent on a full bladder.

a. Extravasation of urine from the bladder is diagnostic for rupture.

b. The Foley catheter should be clamped while the patient is in the trauma bay.

c. If imaged with an incompletely distended bladder, spiral CT has been quoted to have an accuracy rate as low as 40% to 60%.

4. If patients with suspected bladder injuries are evaluated with CT cystography in conjunction with a routine CT, conventional cystography can be precluded.

       a. CT cystography is as effective in detecting rupture as conventional cystography.

I. Extraperitoneal Versus Intraperitoneal Rupture

    1. Extraperitoneal tears are much more common than intraperitoneal tears. Large extraperitoneal tears can be treated conservatively, whereas even small intraperitoneal tears require surgical intervention. Given the disparity in management, radiographic differentiation between the two types of tears is essential. Intraperitoneal and extraperitoneal tears will both be present in up to 10% of patients with bladder tears.

    2. Extraperitoneal Bladder Rupture

       a. Extraperitoneal bladder rupture usually arises from sheering forces.

       b. Pelvic fractures from these same sheering forces are common, and in fact, bladder tears can occur from direct puncture of broken pelvic fragments.

       c. The most sensitive sign in diagnosing bladder rupture is the presence of extravasated urine, which appears water-dense on CT.

       d. In extraperitoneal rupture, urine will extravasate into the soft tissues surrounding the bladder and can also track through inferior soft tissues down into the scrotum, thigh, or perirectal area.

    3. Intraperitoneal Bladder Rupture

       a. Classic history: restrained, intoxicated passenger involved in front-end automobile accident.

       b. A full bladder (as in heavily drinking alcohol) is more likely to rupture from compression between a seatbelt and spine.

       c. Most intraperitoneal tears occur on the dome of the bladder.

       d. Extravasated urine will be visualized in the peritoneal cavity down in the pelvis. Typically, the fluid will appear slightly denser than water because some blood commonly mixes with the urine.

       e. Water-dense fluid, however, is nonspecific for bladder injury and can be seen in a variety of injuries.

J. Further Imaging

If the bladder is not full when imaged, CT can miss small tears. CT cystography or conventional cystography should be performed in patients with suspected injury.

K. Urethral Injuries

    1. Urologic injuries occur in 10% to 20% of major trauma patients and can be the result of either blunt or penetrating trauma.

    2. Lower genitourinary tract trauma results from localized trauma, whereas injuries to the upper urinary tract (kidney and ureters) usually occur from high-energy blunt trauma.

3. Urethral injury must be assessed in a male patient with pelvic ring disruption.

4. Retrograde urethrography is used to visualize both anterior and posterior urethral injuries

    a. Extravasation of contrast material confirms the presence of urethral tearing.

    b. Injury is partial if bladder filling occurs. Complete tears will have no communication with the bladder.

    c. A negative retrograde urethrogram permits the safe placement of urinary catheters.

5. Urethral injuries in female patients are uncommon and more difficult to identify. Often, they are only identified at the time of surgical repair of a pelvic fracture.

L. Obstetric Injuries

1. Trauma is the primary nonobstetric cause of maternal death during pregnancy.

2. The leading cause of trauma during pregnancy is injury sustained during a motor vehicle crash.

    a. Domestic abuse is another common source of trauma to the pregnant mother.

3. Ultrasonography is useful in the pregnant patient to establish gestational age, assess fetal activity and heart rate, and estimate amniotic fluid volume.

    a. Also reveals any intraperitoneal fluid and blood.

4. Traumatic abruptio placentae can also be visualized with sonography, but the sensitivity is not high enough to exclude the diagnosis, and electronic fetal monitoring is also necessary.

5. Penetrating Trauma

    a. Radiography may be necessary to localize a bullet that has not exited the patient.

    b. Multiple gunshot wounds are not uncommon.

    c. The gravid uterus slows the progression of a bullet such that very few bullets that enter the uterus will have enough velocity to exit.

    d. The diagnostic benefit of CT in this instance outweighs the risk of radiation to the fetus.

M. Common Traps and Decision Dilemmas

1. The grooves of nutrient arteries of the iliac wing or acetabular dome can look like fracture lines.

2. The pubic symphysis can appear to be abnormally widened in the adolescent child.

3. Growth plates in children can mimic fractures.

4. Plain radiographs can miss up to a third of pelvic fractures.

5. Check human chorionic gonadotropin (hCG) in menstruating women.

6. **Bladder:** routine CT can miss bladder tears if the bladder is not fully distended. The Foley catheter should be clamped in the trauma bay for all patients,

and patients with suspected bladder injuries should be evaluated with CT cystography or conventional cystography.

VII. Extremity Imaging
A. Introduction
1. Imaging of extremity trauma is a voluminous and complex topic that has a varied impact on the patient with multiple trauma. Here, we present common radiographic features of key life-threatening injuries. Most distal extremity injuries, although sometimes incapacitating, are not often life threatening on their own. For this reason, a detailed description of distal extremity posttraumatic injury is not within the scope of this text.

2. Proximal extremity attachments, which lie at the junction between the axial and appendicular skeleton, are often associated with major vascular and neurologic bundles. Injury to these junctions and their associated neurovascular conduits can result in severe hemorrhage or threatened limb. A limited discussion of upper and lower proximal joint and extremity injury is presented in the following sections.

B. Technique
1. Plain radiography is the primary modality for assessing fracture in the extremities, except the shoulder and pelvis.

2. CT is used in musculoskeletal trauma for the shoulder and pelvis. CT is also used to detect or exclude a fracture that was equivocal on plain radiographs or to better characterize the true extent of a known fracture. Although CT is more expensive, CT offers significant savings in patient time, which can be important in the trauma setting.

3. MRI has emerged as an important modality in assessing the vast diversity of soft tissue injuries in trauma patients.

4. Because various modalities and views are used to assess for extremity injury, clinical suspicion must direct the imaging protocol or various injuries can be overlooked.

C. Computed Tomography
1. CT parameters for small areas (e.g., the wrist, sternoclavicular joints) are usually 2- to 3-mm slices, 2- to 3-mm table speed, reconstruction at 1 to 2 mm, and pitch 1 to 1.5 mm.

2. CT parameters for larger anatomic areas (e.g., the shoulder or pelvic), use thicker slices (3 mm) and faster table speeds (3 to 6 mm) to obtain adequate coverage in a spiral of 32 to 40 seconds. Thinner slices can be easily achieved with multidetector CT, if available. Pitch is typically 1 to 2 mm and reconstruction at 2- to 3-mm interval.

    a. Intravenous contrast is not necessary for CT of skeletal trauma, although it is often concomitantly used to evaluate visceral organs.

3. Multiplanar reformations in skeletal trauma are very helpful. Two-dimensional reformation images provide excellent anatomic detail.

4. Three-dimensional images are preferred by surgeons for surgical planning.

    a. Volume rendering algorithm is superior to shaded surface rendering for three-dimensional musculoskeletal imaging.

D. Shoulder

1. CT is the first-line modality for viewing shoulder trauma.

2. Three-dimensional reconstructed views of the shoulder in trauma are very useful for surgical planning.

E. Proximal Humerus Fractures

1. CT is superior to radiographs in identifying humeral fractures, fragment displacement, fragment rotation, and the status of the humeral head and articular surface.

2. The Neer classification system can be used at some centers (based on fragment displacement and rotation).

3. In elderly patients, fractures of the surgical neck are most common. They are often associated with avulsion fractures of the greater tuberosity.

4. All types of fractures occur in the shaft of the humerus.

5. Pseudodislocation

    a. Comminuted fractures of the humeral head and neck result in large hemarthroses.

    b. With a large joint effusion, the head is displaced inferiorly and laterally.

        (1) Widened joint space and obvious incongruity of the joint surfaces. The joint appears to be dislocated, but is not a true dislocation (= pseudodislocation).

F. Clavicle

1. Fractures usually occur in the middle third.

2. Cephalic angulation in the AP projection is often necessary to free the clavicle from the underlying scapula.

3. Fractures adjacent to the sternoclavicular joint are best seen by CT.

4. In younger patients, fractures of the clavicle, acromioclavicular joint separation, and dislocations of the glenohumeral joint are frequent.

G. Scapula

1. Scapular injuries are subtle on plain film and commonly missed.

2. Easily detected on CT.

3. Usually secondary to severe trauma.

H. Anterior and Posterior Shoulder Dislocations

1. Of shoulder dislocations, ~20% have an associated fracture.

2. The axillary view is the most sensitive plain film radiograph for dislocation.

3. CT is an excellent method to detect shoulder dislocations.

    a. CT shows associated fractures of the anterior glenoid rim and the greater tuberosity after anterior dislocations, as well as fractures of the less tuberosity and the posterior glenoid rim after posterior dislocations.

4. CT and MRI are excellent means of assessing associated compression fractures of the humeral head.

5. Anterior Dislocation

    a. Far more common than posterior, accounting for 95% of all shoulder dislocations

        (1) Most common dislocation of any human joint

    b. Can be associated with *Hill-Sachs lesion,* compression fracture of the posterolateral humeral head.

    c. Less commonly associated with *Bankart lesions,* anterior rim fracture of the glenoid fossa

        (1) Bankart lesions are often cartilaginous rather than bony. They can be impossible to identify on plain radiographs. They are better visualized on CT, but best on MRI.

6. Posterior Dislocation

    a. Comprises 5% of all shoulder dislocations.

    b. Result of epileptic convulsive seizures in 50% of cases.

    c. Produced by direct blow to the anterior aspect of the shoulder in 50% of cases.

    d. Diagnosis is difficult and such dislocations are overlooked in as many as 50% to 60% of cases.

    e. CT is superior to plain radiographs for determining the presence, size, and position of bony fragment in these fractures.

        (1) Findings are usually very subtle.

    f. Avulsion of the lesser tuberosity is common in posterior dislocations.

7. Anterior Oblique or "Y" View is Helpful

    a. Normally, oval glenoid is overlaid by circular humeral head.

    b. In posterior dislocation, the glenoid head faces posteriorly below the acromion.

8. Signs of Posterior Dislocation

    a. The head of the humerus is locked in internal rotation with the articular surface facing posteriorly.

    b. Second most common sign of posterior dislocation is the "trough line," an impaction fracture of the medical joint surface, seen as a line of cortical bone paralleling the medial cortex of the humerus.

    c. Third sign is the widening of the joint ("a positive rim sign").

        (1) Space between the anterior glenoid rim and medial aspect of the humeral head ≤6 mm.

I. Acromioclavicular Joint Separation
1. **Common Injury**
2. Caused by a fall on the shoulder.
3. Incomplete: termed a *subluxation*
4. In complete separation, the clavicle is displaced upward on the acromion and the ligaments attaching the clavicle to the coracoid process are ruptured.
5. Stress films often necessary to visualize separation.
   a. Upright AP views are obtained with patient holding 15- to 20-pound weights in each hand.
6. Two principal considerations in assessing acromioclavicular joint separation are:
   a. Width of acromioclavicular joint. Comparison with the opposite shoulder can be helpful. Normal = 3 to 5 mm.
   b. Length of coracoclavicular ligament between coracoid process of the scapula and the inferior, outer margin of the clavicle. Normal = <1.2 cm.

J. Sternoclavicular Joint
1. Dislocations result from closed chest injury.
2. Plain film cannot easily detect dislocation.
3. CT is sensitive and specific. Three-dimensional study is helpful for evaluating the orientation of posterior sternoclavicular joint dislocations.
4. **Anterior Dislocation**
   a. Readily detected on clinical examination.
5. **Posterior Dislocation**
   a. Difficult to detect on clinical examination.
   b. Associated with injury to the aorta and great vessels. Perform CT chest with intravenous contrast material to exclude vascular injury.
   c. Symptoms include cough, dyspnea, dysphagia, voice change, and vascular compromise.

K. Hip
1. Accounts for 30% of all fractures requiring hospitalization.
2. Plain radiography remains the initial imaging examination in the evaluation of trauma to the hip.
3. Standard hip radiographic series include an AP view of the pelvis, coned-down AP, and lateral views of the affected hip.
4. AP view of the pelvis allows evaluation of the contralateral hip for concomitant disease and can exclude osseous or articular abnormalities of the pelvis.
5. Judet views can be helpful in establishing fracture patterns of the acetabulum.
6. CT of the hip is used primarily in trauma. CT also helpful in predicting hip instability in posterior hip dislocations with associated posterior wall fractures.
7. MRI has had an increasing role in the evaluation of hip trauma in the elderly. Nondisplaced femoral neck or intertrochanteric fractures in elderly patients can be radiographically occult or difficult to diagnose.

a. MRI has proved to be the imaging modality of choice to exclude an occult hip fracture in the elderly.

(1) Radionuclide bone scan can be normal in the first 48 hours after a fracture in the elderly and is less sensitive than MRI in detecting occult hip fractures.

8. MR arthrography has largely replaced conventional arthrography, except for diagnostic hip aspirations and therapeutic injections.

9. MR arthrography is sensitive in the detection of intraarticular abnormalities (e.g., injuries of the acetabular labrum).

10. "If they can't walk, they can't go home" look for occult fracture.

11. Hip fractures are divided into intracapsular and extracapsular.

a. Intracapsular fractures characterized as fractures of the femoral head or femoral neck. Femoral neck fractures include subcapital, midcervical, or basicervical.

b. Extracapsular fractures are characterized as intertrochanteric or subtrochanteric.

12. Hip fracture is also usually classified according to cause: acute trauma, stress, or pathologic condition.

13. Intracapsular Fractures

a. Femoral Head Fractures

b. Usually associated with hip dislocations.

(1) Anterior dislocations are seen 22% to 77% of the time.

(2) Posterior dislocations occur 10% to 16% of the time.

c. Femoral head fractures are usually best seen on radiographs obtained following the reduction of the dislocation.

d. Femoral head fractures include depression, flattening, or transchondral fractures.

14. Femoral Neck

a. Unusual in healthy young persons and require high-energy forces.

b. Common in elderly.

c. Leg is shortened and externally rotated if the fracture is impacted.

d. Risk exists for avascular necrosis because of poor blood supply to femoral neck.

e. Nondisplaced or impacted fractures can be difficult to see on plain films. If femoral neck fracture is suspected, MRI or other studies are indicated.

f. When searching for a fracture of the femoral neck, carefully examine both the medial and lateral cortical margins of the femoral head and neck for the normal S and reverse S curve.

(1) Fracture will produce a tangential or sharp angle indicative of a disruption of the normal anatomic relationship.

15. **Subcapital Fractures**
   a. Occur at the junction of the femoral head and neck.
   b. Most common femoral neck fracture.
   c. Displacement is obvious on AP, but non-displaced may be occult.
   d. Most commonly missed fracture about the hip.
   e. Advanced studies (e.g., CT or MRI) are important in diagnosis of occult fractures.
   f. Radiographic signs of nondisplaced subcapital fracture include the following:
      (1) Disruption of the normally smooth line of the cortex
      (2) Superimposition of the base of the femoral head on the cortex of the femoral neck
      (3) Disruption of the normal trabecular architecture
      (4) Foreshortening of the femoral neck
      (5) Abnormal angle between the femoral neck and femoral head: normally, 120 to 135 degrees
      (6) Transverse band of increased density across femoral neck indicated impacted fracture

16. **Transcervical Fractures**
   a. Cross the mid portion of the femoral neck
   b. Uncommon
   c. Readily diagnosed on AP view.

17. **Basicervical Fractures**
   a. Involve the junction of the base of the neck and the trochanter.
   b. Uncommon
   c. Readily diagnosed on AP view.

18. **Extracapsular Fractures**
   a. **Intertrochanteric Fracture**
      (1) Most common extracapsular fracture
      (2) Results from falls in elderly
      (3) Leg is shortened and externally rotated to a much greater extent than with femoral neck fractures.
      (4) Rich blood supply allows potential for rapid healing with little risk of avascular necrosis.
      (5) Classified by the number of fragments:

      - In a two-part fracture, the fracture line extends between the greater and lesser trochanters.
      - A three-part fracture has an additional fracture line separating the greater or lesser trochanter as a free fragment.
      - A four-part fracture has both the greater and lesser trochanters separated as free fragments.

  b. **Greater Trochanter Fracture**
   (1) Greater trochanter fractures occur in adolescent athletes as avulsion injury and in elderly patient who land on their greater trochanter.
   (2) Patients with this type of injury are able to walk but have tenderness over greater trochanter.
   (3) Can be difficult to see radiographically because injury may not be suspected because of unimpressive clinical findings and the greater trochanter is usually overexposed when imaging the entire hip.
  c. **Lesser Trochanter Fracture**
   (1) Occurs in young athletes.
   (2) Caused by forceful contraction of the iliopsoas muscle.
  d. **Subtrochanteric Fracture**
   (1) Occurs up to 5 cm below the inferior margin of the lesser trochanter.
   (2) Caused by major trauma and occur in younger age group.
   (3) Proximal fracture fragment is flexed, abducted, and externally rotated, producing an outward protrusion of the greater trochanter.
   (4) Is easily diagnosed radiographically.
   (5) Because of high energy needed to cause injury, other associated injuries (e.g., acetabular fractures and hip dislocations) are common.
L. **Hip Dislocations**
 1. Occur in adults after high-energy force (e.g., motor vehicle accidents).
 2. Young children are more likely to dislocate their hips than to sustain a fracture of the femoral neck.
 3. Incidence of avascular necrosis increases with delayed reduction of the dislocation.
 4. **Posterior Dislocation**
  a. More common than anterior dislocations.
  b. Usually caused during motor vehicle accident when flexed knee strikes dashboard.
  c. Associated with fractures of acetabulum, patella, tibia, and femoral head, neck, and shaft.
  d. Affected leg is shortened, flexed, adducted, and internally rotated.
  e. On AP film dislocated femoral head is usually located superior to the acetabulum. Can also lie posterior to the acetabulum.
 5. **Anterior Dislocation**
  a. Less common than posterior dislocation, only 10% to 15% of all hip dislocations.
  b. Results from forced abduction and external rotation of the leg.
  c. Associated with femoral head fractures.

> **d.** Affected leg is abducted and externally rotated.
>
> **e.** On AP film, femoral head is usually located medial to the acetabulum.
>
> **f.** Lesser trochanter is prominent because the proximal femur is in external rotation.
>
> **g.** Affected femoral head appears larger because of magnification that results from its being farther away from the film cassette.
>
> **h.** Confirmed on cross-table lateral view.

6. Central Dislocation

> **a.** If thigh is abducted during front impact such as in a motor vehicle accident, the forces direct the femoral head through the acetabulum.

M. Common Traps and Decision Dilemmas

1. Shoulder

> **a.** Nondisplaced fractures of the lateral third of the clavicle can be missed on plain film.
>
>> **(1)** Region is usually over penetrated. Use of the "bright light" can help.
>>
>> **(2)** CT easily identifies all clavicular fractures.
>
> **b.** Nondisplaced fractures of the acromion and coracoid process can be overlooked. CT easily identifies all acromion and coracoid process fractures.

2. Hip

> **a.** The soft tissue linear lucency superolateral and in inferomedial to the femoral head and neck do not represent the hip capsule.
>
>> **(1)** Represents the fat within the fascial plane covering the gluteus minimus and then tendon of the iliopsoas muscle inferiorly. Do not use comparison of these lines on the symptomatic side with those of the unaffected side to determine if an effusion of the hip is present.
>
> **b.** Nondisplaced fractures of the femoral neck are often overlooked.
>
>> **(1)** Look for the smooth line of cortical bone. Any disruption in this line or in the trabecular pattern should heighten suspicion of fracture. Using MRI can be cost-saving because of quicker diagnosis.
>
> **c.** Avulsion fractures are often misdiagnosed as "muscle pulls."
>
> **d.** Gluteal skin fold can mimic a fracture line and can also overlie a fracture line.

SELECTED READING

Cerva DS Jr, Mirvis SE, Shanmuganathan K, et al. Detection of bleeding in patients with major pelvic fractures: value of contrast-enhanced CT. *AJR Am J Roentgenol* 1996;166:131.

Chiu SC, Cushing BM, Rodriguez A, et al. Abdominal injuries without hemoperitoneum: a potential limitation of focused abdominal sonography for trauma (FAST). *J Trauma* 1997;42:617–625.

Harley JD, Mack LA, Winquist RA. CT of acetabular fractures: comparison with conventional radiography. *AJR Am J Roentgenol* 1982;138:413–417.

Hunter JC, Brandser EA, Tran KA. Pelvic and acetabular trauma. *Radiol Clin North Am* 1997;35:559–590.

Mason MB. Some observations on fractures of the head of the radius with a review of one hundred cases. *Br J Surg* 1954:42:123.

Pao DM, Ellis JH, Cohan RH, et al. Utility of routine trauma CT in the detection of bladder ruptures. *Acad Radiol* 2000;7:317–324.

Peng MY, Parishky YR, Cornwell EE III et al. CT cystography versus conventional cystography in evaluation of bladder injury. *AJR Am J Roentgenol* 1999;173:1269–1272.

Pitt MJ, Ruth JT, Benjanmin JB. Trauma to the pelvic ring and acetabulum. *Semin Roentgenol* 1992;27:299.

Pretorius ES, Fishman EK. Spiral CT and three-dimensional CT of musculoskeletal pathology. *Radiol Clin North Am* 1999;37(5):953–974.

Stewart BG, Rhea JT, Sheridan RL, et al. Is the screening portable pelvis film clinically useful in multiple trauma patients who will be examined by abdominopelvic CT? Experience with 397 patients. *Emergency Radiology* (in press).

Yao DC, Jeffrey RB, et al. Using contrast-enhanced helical CT to visualize arterial extravasation after blunt trauma: incidence and organ distribution. *AJR Am J Roentgenol* 2002;178:17–20.

43

Organ and Tissue Procurement in Trauma

Andrew M. Cameron, MD, PhD,
and Francis L. Delmonico, MD

I. **Introduction**
   A. Currently, 80,000 people in the United States with end-stage organ failure are listed for transplantation. Most cadaveric donors come from or pass through the trauma or emergency room setting. This represents an important opportunity for healthcare providers involved in trauma to contribute to a group of patients in dire need. In fact, it is an obligation, both ethical, and medicolegally.
   B. A clear pathway can be described to convert potential to actual donors and strategies to maximize recovery rates have been demonstrated to work. Even so, they are not widely practiced. This chapter describes the organizations involved with organ donation in the United States, the steps by which appropriate donors are identified and managed, and the role of the trauma healthcare provider in facilitating this lifesaving act of generosity.
   C. Identifying potential donors involves understanding the criteria for declaration of brain death as well as contraindications to donation. Understanding the structure of organ procurement organizations (OPO) facilitates making referrals to them. Attempts to obtain consent for donation are required by law and can be done in a manner that has been shown to improve success rates. Support of the brain-dead potential solid-organ donor can be complicated and time consuming, but is facilitated by understanding the pathophysiology involved and is crucial to maximizing organ recovery and graft function in the recipient (**Table 43-1**).
II. **Identification of Potential Donors**
   A. **Indications: Brain Death**
      1. **Criteria for the Determining Brain Death in the United States**
      The criteria for the determination of brain death in the United States is based on the findings in the *Report of the Medical Consultants on the Diagnosis of Death to the President's Commission on the Study of Ethical Problems in Medicine and Biomedical and Behavioral Research of 1981*. Specifically, 36 states have defined brain death legislatively, whereas the other 14 states have opted for judicial determination of brain death on a case-by-case basis.
      2. **Conceptual Definition**
      The President's Commission specified brain death as the irreversible loss of cortical and brainstem function.

Table 43-1.   Four steps in the organ donation pathway

1. Identify all potential donors
2. Early referral to local organ procurement organization/determine brain death in a reliable and rapid manner
3. Approach all potential donor families for consent after brain death has been declared
4. Aggressively manage medical issues of all potential donors

Conceptually, therefore, trauma providers can think of brain death as *"the **irreversible cessation** of brain function in the **absence of complicating conditions**."*

3. **Clinical Evaluations**
   a. **Cessation**
      (1) **Of Cerebral Functioning.** Unresponsiveness, (i.e. Glasgow Coma Scale (GSC) score < 3, no verbal or meaningful motor responses to any stimuli indicates any cessation of cerebral functioning. Spinal cord reflexes can persist after death.
      (2) **Of Brainstem Functioning.** Papillary light reflex, corneal, oculocephalic (doll's eyes), oculovestibular (calorics), oropharyngeal (gag or cough), and respiratory reflexes are used to test brainstem functioning. Apnea test is accomplished by hyperoxygenating the patient and demonstrating absence of respiratory effort with P_{CO_2} >60 mm Hg.
   b. **Irreversibility**
      (1) **Cause of Coma.** The cause of coma is established and sufficient to account for loss of brain function (i.e., head computed tomography [CT] scan with evidence of overwhelming traumatic injury or bleed).
      (2) **Absence of Brain Function.** Absence of brain function persisting over an appropriate observation period confirmed by an electroencephalogram (EEG), complete cessation of circulation to brain for >10 minutes, or serial clinical examinations separated by at least 6 hours are all consistent with an irreversible injury.
   c. **Complication Conditions.** All complications must be carefully excluded and including the following:
      (1) Drug intoxication, metabolic coma
      (2) Hypothermia (temperature >35.5°C)
      (3) Shock
4. **Ancillary Tests**
No ancillary tests are required because the diagnosis of brain death is made clinically as described above. Furthermore, none are specified in any set of guide-

lines; however, they can be of confirmatory benefit in difficult or unclear cases Specifically, EEG has long been recognized to be of value and is minimally invasive, but may not be readily available. A four-vessel cerebral angiogram is the gold standard, but it involves both a dye load and a trip to the angiography suite. Nuclear medicine brain flow scans and transcranial Doppler blood flow studies are accurate and inexpensive alternatives (**Table 43-2**).

B. Contraindications

Following is a partial list of the most common and important exclusions to donation. Their presumed presence does not obviate the duty of the trauma provider to offer donation to relatives or to inform the OPO of a potential donor. Decisions about the ultimate appropriateness for donation of any or all tissues or organs will be made by the OPO and surgical team responsible for the potential recipient.

1. Extracerebral Malignancy

Except local skin cancers and carcinoma in situ (CIS) of the cervix

2. Uncontrolled Sepsis

3. Active Viral Infections

Hepatitis A, hepatitis B, cytomegalovirus, herpes simplex virus, human immunodeficiency virus (in some cases a hepatitis C positive donor can be used for a hepatitis C positive recipient. Again, the OPO and recipient surgical team make all such decisions.

III. Systems of Organ Procurement

A. United Network for Organ Sharing

The rapid expansion of transplantation in the early 1980s ushered in by cyclosporine usage resulted in public demand for a national system of organ procurement and allocation. In October of 1984, the United States Congress passed the National Organ and Transplant Act (NOTA), which established a new National Organ Procurement and Transplantation Network (OPTN) for this purpose. The Department of Health and Human Services awarded the contract for development and implementation of this network to the United Network for Organ Sharing (UNOS) on September 30, 1986. This network went into effect on October 1, 1987 and has been the operational guide for all

Table 43-2. Making the diagnosis of brain death

1. *Cessation*–Cortical function absent—no verbal or meaningful motor movement, GCS = 3
   - Brainstem function absent: Pupillary light, corneal, oculocephalic, oculovestibular, oropharyngeal, respiratory reflexes absent
2. Irreversibility: Cause is easily established, accounts for loss of brain function and is obviously irreversible
   - Cessation persists for appropriate observation period (serial clinical examinations)

GCS, Glasgow Coma Scale.

transplant centers, organ procurement organizations, and tissue typing laboratories ever since.

B.   Organ Procurement Organizations

Organ procurement had preceded this governmental formalization. Organ procurement organizations (OPO) initially developed from the newly conceived clinical transplant programs and were staffed by the surgeons and nurses who were performing the transplantations. The first OPO was the New England Organ Bank founded by Paul S. Russell, Joseph Murray, Francis Moore, and others in 1968. The Uniform Anatomical Gift Act was enacted in 1968 to provide statutory authorization for the recovery and transplantation being carried out by OPO and this was later further formalized by NOTA as described above. Currently, 59 OPO are operating in the United States.

C.   Healthcare Provider Responsibilities

In 1986, the Omnibus Reconciliation Act, section 1138 required that all hospitals participating in Medicare and Medicaid programs refer all deaths and imminent deaths to their local OPO for possible donor evaluation and that families of all potential organ donors be aware of their options to donate. This obligation is supplemented by state law in more than 40 states, which requires that hospitals ask families of all deceased patients to consider organ donation.

IV.   Support of the Brain-Dead Potential Solid-Organ Donor

A.   Overview

Severe physiologic complications are common in brain-dead potential donors. Awareness and understanding of these issues allows for attempts to maximize the stability of the donor and preserves organ viability, quality, and subsequent function in the recipient. These management principles represent a paradigm shift that takes place after the declaration of brain death in which treatment goals change from saving a patient's life to preserving organ viability in a potential donor.

B.   Autonomic Instability and Hypotension

Autonomic instability and hypotension occur in 80% of brain-dead donors. Cause is multifactorial: (1) a "catecholamine storm" refers to the massive release of vasoactive hormones that accompanies brain death; (2) potential hypovolemia from blood loss, from osmotic agents given for intracranial pressure (ICP) or from diabetes insipidus secondary to cerebral injury; (3) hypertension from Cushing's response as the body attempts to maintain cerebral perfusion pressure (CPP); and (4) hypotension from eventual compromise of ischemic catecholamine secreting autonomic nerves and adrenal medulla or from cardiac failure.

1.   Management

a.   Aggressive resuscitation with normal saline or lactate Ringer's solution until filling pressures are adequate to prevent hypotension. Monitor success by keeping mean arterial pressure (MAP)

>60, central venous pressure (CVP) >8, and urine output >30 mL/hour.

b. Once filling pressures are adequate, vaso-active agents are used to maintain MAP. Dopamine (1 to 20 μg/kg/min) is most commonly used, phenylephrine is avoided.

C. Neuroendocrine Failure

1. Diabetes insipidus with massive diuresis and resultant hypernatremia is by far the most common endocrine disorder (70%). Other endocrine disorders associated with brain dead donors include low thyroid hormone and cortisol levels, as well as temperature dysregulation.

2. Management

Treat hypernatremia with intravenous D5W, or with triiodothyronine, hydrocortisone, and vasopressin (0.1 to 2 units/hour).

D. Pulmonary Disability

1. Pulmonary Complications

Common pulmonary complications seen in brain dead potential donors include aspiration pneumonitis, pulmonary contusion, and neurogenic pulmonary edema. In fact, only 1 of 20 donors has lungs that are suitable for donation.

2. Management

a. Avoid Overhydration

b. Ventilation

The ventilatory modality of choice is continuous mandatory ventilation. Donor's airway pressure will dictate whether pressure control or volume control is used. Pressure control is preferred to reduce barotrauma.

E. Coagulation Abnormalities

1. Brain-dead donors often show a consumptive coagulopathy with high prothrombin time (PT) and low platelets because of a release of rich substrates of thromboplastic, fibrinolytic, and plasminogen from necrotic brain.

2. Management: fresh frozen plasma and platelets, as needed.

IV. Nonbeating Heart Donation

Nonbeating heart donation is defined as the surgical recovery of organs after the pronouncement of death based on cessation of cardiopulmonary function. Although this method of recovering cadaveric organs accounted for only 1% of cadaveric donors during the time period of 1994 1996, it is now becoming increasingly recognized as a potential option for expanding the donor pool. In this scenario, the family provides consent for donation before the removal of life support when irrefutable evidence shows devastating injury with no chance of a meaningful recovery. In cases of nonbeating heart donation, life support is usually withdrawn in the intensive care unit setting and the donor is then transported to the operating room for organ procurement. Alternatively, the entire process can be carried out in the operating room. The situation of nonbeating heart donation is less relevant to the trauma provider in an emergency room situation but is a reality and an option of which it is helpful to be aware.

V. **Family Counseling and Consent**

    A. **Counseling**

    Besides being a legal obligation of the healthcare provider to inform families of their right to donate as described above, providing family counseling is a humane and essential component of the provision of trauma care in times of tragedy. Providing support to assist families in understanding information and serving as a grief outlet is associated with improved donation rates. This counseling and the request for donation consent are best done in concert with representatives and guidance from the OPO.

    B. **Specific Measures**

    Specifically, not coupling the death notification with a request for consent, combined efforts in which both hospital staff and members of the OPO participate, as well as use of a private setting for the request have been shown to increase consent rates for organ donation to 75%. The best predictor of donation is a favorable initial response by the family to the request. The strongest negative predictor is a family perception that that the patient would decide against donation (**Table 43-3**).

VI. **Common Traps and Decision Dilemmas**

    A. Incomplete understanding of criteria for brain death can lead to a delay in contacting OPO, obtaining consent, and aggressively medically managing the donor.

    B. Anxiety over approaching a grieving family. Overcome by the knowledge of legal responsibilities, early involvement and support of OPO, and not coupling death notification and request for consent.

    C. Time demand required to coordinate donation efforts in a busy emergency room setting with other "salvageable" patients in need of attention. Aided by support from OPO and understanding of organ shortage crisis and many other patients in need waiting on list.

Table 43-3. Appropriate practice in obtaining consent from families of donors

---

1. Decouple the notification of death with request for organ donation consent: Frequent communication with family regarding patient before time of request; allow time for family to accept death

2. Request is made by hospital personnel and members of organ procurement organization such that requesters have experience with issues: Knowledge of the criteria for brain death, time to work with families, knowledge of organ and tissue donation process

3. Request is made in appropriate setting: A comfortable and stress-reducing environment allows unhurried approach and complete explanation of process

---

D. Meaning of a driver's license consent: The Uniform Anatomical Gift Act (see above) requires *explicit* consent rather than *implied* consent for organ donation. This can be granted by premortem exercises such as a driver's license. The law, however, also allows for individual donors or families to revoke that decision and, thus, driver's license consents and organ donor cards are rightly considered a means of public education rather a means by which to procure organs.

E. Brain-dead heart is denervated and, therefore, is atropine resistant. Arrhythmias can be difficult to treat.

F. Protective management of some donor organ systems can compete (e.g., aggressive hydration for renal protection can cause pulmonary edema).

SELECTED READING

Ehrle RN, Shafer TJ, Nelson KR. Referral, request, and consent for organ donation: best practice—a blueprint for success. *Crit Care Nurse* 1999;2(19):21–33.

Mone T. The business of organ procurement. *Current Opinion in Organ Transplantation* 2002;1(7):60–64.

Ramos HC, Lopez R. Critical care management of the brain-dead organ donor. *Current Opinion in Organ Transplantation* 2002;1(7):70–75.

Razek T, Olthoff K, Reilly P. Issues in potential organ donor management. *Surg Clin North Am* 2000;80(3):1021–1031.

UNOS website: http://www.unos.org. Last accessed October, 2003.

44

Psychiatric Issues in Trauma

John K. Findley, MD, and Lawrence Park, MD

I. Introduction

It is estimated that >50% of all trauma patients in the hospital setting have preexisting psychiatric disorders; patients with penetrating wounds have psychiatric comorbidity approaching 90%. Substance abuse and intoxicated states are also highly correlated with trauma. Studies demonstrate that 25% to 50% of acute trauma patients present intoxicated with alcohol or under the influence of other substances of abuse.

Despite the high prevalence of psychiatric disorders in trauma patients, preexisting psychopathology often goes unrecognized by the trauma service, and can be a significant factor in postoperative management and recidivism. For patients who survive trauma, the estimated rate of recidivism is 40%, with a 5-year mortality rate of 20%.

Agitation, bizarre behavior, and psychological distress complicate the management of many patients. Consultation psychiatrists are trained to recognize and treat alterations in mental state caused by organic dysfunction (delirium and dementia). Any trauma, including acute and chronic sequelae of brain injury, can also result in untoward psychological reactions; psychiatrists are trained to recognize, treat, and provide support for these patients. Substance abuse is another important area where psychiatrists can assist in optimizing patient management. Psychiatrists are also skilled in evaluating competency to assess whether patients possess the mental capacity to refuse (or accept) medical treatment.

II. Consciousness

Any psychiatric evaluation begins with an assessment of consciousness. Consciousness is composed of two components, *level of arousal* and *psychic content.*

A. Levels of Arousal

Plum and Posner characterize four different levels of arousal discussed below.

1. Alert: attentive, responsive, and interactive

2. Obtundation: mild-moderate reduction in arousal, attention, and responsiveness

3. Stupor: arousal maintained only by vigorous and continuous stimulation

4. Coma: unable to arouse, unresponsiveness

B. Psychic Content

Validated instruments can be used to objectively assess level of consciousness. One common instrument is the Glasgow Coma Scale (GCS) (see Chapter 8, *Secondary Survey of the Trauma Patient*). GCS score should take into account any conditions that can prevent appropriate response (e.g., intubation, paralysis, baseline level of verbal ability). Any GCS score <15 represents a significant alteration of consciousness. Suspicion for an underlying organic cause should be high and organic workup should be initiated. If GCS = 15, consciousness is largely intact.

III. **Mental State**
   A. **Mental Status Examination**
   Generally, the mental status examination (MSE) encompasses the emotional, cognitive, and behavioral condition of the individual. A comprehensive MSE when done by a psychiatrist consists of many components. These components are listed below.
   1. **Mental Status Examination**
      a. **Observation and Behavior**
      b. **State of Consciousness**
      c. **Manner of Dress and Hygiene**
      d. **Demeanor**
      e. **Attitude:** toward others and the situation
      f. **Eye contact**
      g. **Speech:** fluency, pressured, dysarthria, dysphasia
      h. **Motor activity:** retardation, hyperactivity, tremor, tics
   2. **Emotional state**
   Depressed, happy, euphoric, irritable, angry, anxious
      a. **Mood:** refers to patient's report of own internal state
      b. **Affect:** refers to outward appearance of emotional state; affect can be described as congruent or incongruent with mood, appropriate or inappropriate to situation, labile or restricted in variability
      c. **Suicidal, Homicidal, or Violent Ideation**
   3. **Thought State**
      a. **Content:** ruminations, obsessions, delusions, paranoia
      b. **Process:** linear, coherent, goal-directed, tangential, disorganized, incoherent
      c. **Cognitive:** logical, abstraction, calculation, organization or construction
      d. **Memory:** deficits in immediate recall, short-term, long-term memory
      e. **Perceptions:** hallucinations, illusions
      f. **Insight and Judgment**
   B. **General**
   Although it may not be practical for those on a busy surgical service to conduct a comprehensive mental status examination if not a psychiatrist, general impressions of a patient's mental state are useful. Roughly speaking, the MSE can be broken down into three main areas: emotion, behavior, and thought. For any psychiatric evaluation, it is important to have some basic assessment of each of these areas.
   As a mnemonic, remember the **Psychiatric ABCs:**

   1. Affect: emotional state
   2. Behavior: activity
   3. Cognition: thought state

C.   Changes in Mental States

One of the most confusing aspects of determining a patient's mental state is that no good rule of thumb exists for distinguishing between organic and psychiatric conditions solely on the basis of clinical presentation. A change in mental state secondary to an organic cause (delirium), therefore, can present in an identical way as someone in a depressed, manic, or psychotic episode. Some estimates have found that up to one third of patients in the surgical intensive care unit (ICU) have been in delirious states. Therefore, any change in mental state, as with any alteration in consciousness, is highly suggestive of delirium and necessitates a workup for an underlying organic cause. Primary psychiatric disorders should be considered diagnoses of exclusion, to be considered once a complete organic workup is negative (**Table 44-1**).

D.   Delirium Versus Dementia

If mental status changes are organic in nature, they typically follow one of two patterns: delirium or dementia. Delirium refers to acute changes in mental status that are the "direct physiological consequences of a general medical condition" [from DSM-IV]. Delirium is also known by other names: confusion, agitation, acute confusional state, encephalopathy, ICU psychosis, acute organic brain syndrome, or acute brain failure.

The hallmarks of delirium are:

1. Disturbance in consciousness
2. Change in cognition
3. Acute onset (over hours to days)
4. Fluctuating course

Typically, the delirious patient will present in a confused and agitated state. The patient will have difficulty focusing attention, may be disoriented, and may have problems with paranoia or delusions (false beliefs). Cognition, memory, language, and perception can also be affected. Perceptual disturbances are often represented by hallucinations or illusions. Visual and auditory hallucinations are most common, but other modalities of hallucinations (tactile, olfactory, gustatory) are highly suggestive of an organic cause. Symptoms of delirium are said to "wax and wane." This means that the mental status examination can vary unpredictably over time; at one moment a patient can appear calm and coherent, and the next moment, can become severely confused and agitated. Delirious states are almost always reversible, with the patient returning to baseline functioning. Risk factors for developing delirium include being elderly, history of brain damage or burn, drug dependency, acquired immunodeficiency syndrome (AIDS), and history of cardiac surgery.

Dementia, in contrast, represents a chronic, progressive process whereby a person's cognitive and memory functioning slowly declines. Dementia is typically associated with a chronic degenerative brain process and does not usually require immediate intervention.

Table 44-1.   Common medical causes of delirium

Causes	Evaluation
Withdrawal syndrome (alcohol, barbiturate or benzodiazepine)	Serum or urine toxicology, monitoring of vital signs, withdrawal symptoms
Wernicke's encephalopathy	Physical examination: change in mental status, ataxia, ophthalmoplegia
Hypoxia	Oxygen saturation, arterial blood gas
Hypoperfusion	Vascular studies, magnetic resonance imaging
Hypertensive crisis	Blood pressure
Hypoglycemia	Serum glucose
Electrolyte imbalances	Serum electrolytes
Intracranial hemorrhage	Computed tomography scan, magnetic resonance imaging
Central nervous system infection: meningitis, encephalitis	Lumbar puncture
Poisoning (including toxic environmental agents, drugs of abuse, medications)	Serum toxicology (see list of medications that can cause delirium below).
Pulmonary embolus	V/Q scan, pulmonary arteriography
Status epilepticus	Electroencephalogram
Other infections: pneumonia, urinary tract infections, subacute bacterial endocarditis	Infection workup: complete blood count, urinalysis, cultures, chest x-ray, echocardiography
Sepsis	Blood cultures
Renal failure	Renal function tests
Hepatic failure	Liver function tests
Hyperammonemia	Serum ammonia
Thyrotoxicosis or myxedema	Thyroid function tests

E.   Evaluation of Mental State

Presented below are two bedside instruments that provide a quick clinical measure of mental state. The **Folstein Mini Mental Exam** (MMSE) (**Table 44-2**) is a commonly used scale that provides a numeric score to gauge mental state. Possible scores range from 0 to 30 with 28 to 30 considered to be normal. Additionally, one can also use the quick and practical bedside test of **Frank Jones.** Regardless of which technique is used some objective means of assessing mental state is critical to document delirious states, which can fluctuate greatly over time.

Table 44-2.   Folstein mini mental state examination (MMSE)

Test Item	Score
1. What is the year, season, date, month, day?	5
2. Where are we? What state, country, town, hospital, floor?	5
3. Name three objects (e.g., paper, flower, penny)	3
4. Serial 7s (100-7, 93-7, 86-7, 79-7, 72-7); alternatively, spell "world" backward	5
5. Recall of three objects	3
6. Name a pencil, a watch	2
7. Repeat "no ifs ands or buts"	1
8. Follow three-step command, "take a paper in your right hand, fold it in half, and put it on the floor"	3
9. Read and obey the following: "close your eyes"	1
10. Write a sentence.	1
11. Copy a design (interlocking pentagons).	1
TOTAL	30

Adapted from Folstein MF, et al., 1975.

1.   Frank Jones

A quick bedside probe of mental functioning is the so-called "Frank Jones" story [adapted from Murray, 1997]. Response to this story is a rough indication of mental status when delirium is suspected. At the bedside, ask the patient what he or she thinks of the following story (tell story without emotional cues or facial expressions):

"I have a friend, Frank Jones, whose feet are so big he has to put his pants on over his head." After saying this, wait a few moments, allowing the patient to display an initial reaction, then ask, "can he do it?"

Possible Responses:

Type I: Mentation Intact. The patient knows it is a joke and smiles or laughs. Furthermore, when asked, "Can he do it?" the patient will respond in a way that indicates he or she knows that it is impossible (indicating that intellectual insight is preserved).

Type II: Suspect Delirium. The patient knows it is a joke and smiles, but is unable to explain why it cannot be done; he or she does not "get it." In this case, brain neocortical functioning is impaired, while limbic (subcortical) functioning is preserved.

Type III: Suspect Dementia. The patient does not know it is a joke and does not know it cannot be done. This demonstrates neocortical and limbic confusion and can represent underlying dementia.

The theory behind "Frank Jones" is that the initial emotional response tests the deep brain structures related to affect (the limbic system). The limbic system generally remains intact when a patient is delirious (type II). With many types of advanced dementia (type III), however, the patient is impaired both cognitively and emotionally. This indicates impairment of both neocortical and limbic structures.

IV. Causes of Delirium

A. Common Medical Causes of Delirium

Multiple medical conditions can be responsible for delirium. Below is a list of common medical causes of delirium and the typical workup that is indicated (see **Table 44-1**).

B. Head Trauma and Anoxic Injury

Head trauma and anoxic brain injury are frequent sequelae of trauma. Closed head injury is more common than open (or penetrating) head injury; in both cases, mental state can be significantly altered. Anoxic injury of the brain can also occur in trauma patients and lesions may not be immediately visible with head scanning (particularly, computed tomography [CT] of the head). All three of these conditions can result in major changes in psychiatric and neurologic function. Changes in function are typically correlated with the location and extent of injured brain tissue. Psychiatric changes include cognitive difficulties (problems with attention, focus, organization, memory, and planning), personality changes (impulsivity, irritability), and mood changes (depression, anxiety, increased mood lability). Postconcussive syndrome is a controversial syndrome that typically presents 1 to 3 months after a minor head injury. Common symptoms include headache, dizziness, and fatigue. Associated changes in mental state (e.g., irritability, anxiety, depression, memory, attention problems) can also be present.

C. Medications Commonly Associated with Delirium

Table 44-3 lists medications commonly associated with delirium. Other agents include the following:

- Anticholinergic agents: atropine, scopolamine, trihexyphenidyl, diphenhydramine, benztropine
- Tricyclic antidepressants: amitriptyline, clomipramine, desipramine, imipramine, nortriptyline, protriptyline, trimipramine
- Monoamine oxidase inhibitors (phenelzine, tranylcypromine)
- Barbiturates
- Benzodiazepines
- Nonsteroidal anti-inflammatory drugs (NSAID): ibuprofen, indomethacin, naproxen, sulindac
- Beta blockers
- Digitalis preparations
- Steroids

V. Symptomatic Treatment of Delirium

Delirious patients are at high risk for adverse outcomes. Being confused and agitated, they are at risk of pulling at tubes and lines, interfering with the function of supportive equipment, and otherwise jeopardizing their recovery secondary to behavioral dyscontrol. Delirious patients require increased attention and support

Table 44-3. Medications commonly associated with delirium

Acyclovir	Disulfiram	Phenytoin
ACTH	Ephedrine	Procarbazine
Amantadine	Ergotamine	Procainamide
Aminoglycoside	Ganciclovir	Quinidine
Aminophylline	Gentamicin	Ranitidine
Amphetamine	Interferon	Reserpine
Amphotericin	Isoniazid	Rifampin
Azacitidine	l-asparaginase	Sulfonamides
Baclofen	Levodopa	Tamoxifen
Bromocriptine	Lidocaine	Tetracycline
Captopril	Lithium	Theophylline
Cephalosporins	Meperidine	Thioridazine
Chloramphenicol	Methyldopa	Ticarcillin
Cimetidine	Methotrexate	Vancomycin
Clonidine	Pentazocine	Vinblastine
Cocaine	Phenylephrine	Vincristine
Cytosine arabinoside	Phenylpropanolamine	5-fluorouracil

from medical staff. They may require mechanical restraint (e.g., a posey jacket or wrist or leg restraints) and constant observation ("sitter"). Complications throughout the hospital course are also more likely (e.g., aspiration pneumonia, decubitus ulcers, falls). Moreover, every delirious state is caused by an underlying, and perhaps life-threatening, medical condition. Psychiatric consultation can provide aid in the medical workup as well as the behavioral and pharmacologic management of acute delirium.

The most important and definitive treatment for delirium is to discover and adequately treat the underlying organic derangement. Without proper treatment of the underlying pathology, symptoms of delirium will not remit and the patient will remain medically at risk.

In addition, symptomatic treatment is often necessary to treat affective, behavioral, and cognitive manifestations of delirium. Generally, first-line agents for delirium include neuroleptic (antipsychotic) medications. Neurochemically, these agents work by blocking dopamine receptors in the brain. Two classes of neuroleptic medications are available: typical and atypical agents. The typical agents, represented by haloperidol, perphenazine, and chlorpromazine, are available via oral (p.o.) and parenteral route of administration and have a long track record of effectively treating delirium. Concerns regarding their use most commonly stem from side effects of dystonia and prolongation of QT interval. Atypical agents, represented by risperidone, olanzapine, quetiapine, and ziprasidone, have also proved useful for delirium and are not associated with dystonic symptoms. Parenteral formulations of olanzapine and ziprasidone have been developed, but experience using them for delirium is limited at this time.

In addition to neuroleptic medications, other classes of medications can prove useful in the management of delirium and agitation. Benzodiazepines (e.g., lorazepam, diazepam, midazolam) can aid in symptomatically treating agitation, anxiety, and alcohol withdrawal states. Their sedative and anxiolytic properties are often useful for the delirious patient. Although respiratory depression is a possible complication of benzodiazepine use, many patients on a surgical trauma service are intubated, have a tracheostomy, or have their respiratory status closely monitored.

Opiate (narcotic) agents can also be helpful in the management of delirium. Often, trauma patients have experienced painful injury and opiate medication can be used both for analgesia and sedation.

Other less commonly used agents for delirium include barbiturates, propofol, mood stabilizers, or anticonvulsants. Mood stabilizers (valproic acid, carbamazepine, gabapentin) can be particularly useful for cases of head injury, anoxic brain injury, and other central nervous system lesions. For severe and refractory cases of delirium that have failed other interventions, general anesthesia and muscle paralysis (e.g., intravenous [i.v.] propofol and nondepolarizing muscle blocker) remain a final treatment option.

First and foremost, evaluate and treat potentially life-threatening causes of delirium. Then treat symptomatically. Neuroleptics are used to treat severe agitation states, disorganization, hallucinations, and other psychotic symptoms. Benzodiazepines are particularly useful to treat anxiety and agitation, and for sedation. Opiates are most useful for sedation and pain control. Concurrent use of pharmacologic agents often proves to be most successful in treating agitation and confusion.

A. Neuroleptics

The mechanism of action of neuroleptics is dopamine receptor blockade. These agents theoretically work by acting on the underlying mechanism of delirium. Neuroleptic agents are separated into two categories: typical and atypical. Typical neuroleptics (e.g., haloperidol, droperidol, perphenazine, chlorpromazine) are available via a parenteral route of administration. Although none have been approved for intravenous administration by the US Food and Drug Administration (FDA), haloperidol has a long and safe history of intravenous administration (n.b. in solution, haloperidol precipitates out when mixed with heparin or phenytoin). In addition, intravenous administration of typical neuroleptics can have less associated extrapyramidal symptomatology than oral or intramuscular (i.m.) routes of administration. Droperidol, until recently, had been a popular and effective intravenous agent for agitation. A recent black box warning issued by the FDA for QT prolongation has effectively ended its use. Atypical neuroleptics (e.g., risperidone, olanzapine, quetiapine, ziprasidone) are demonstrating good efficacy for delirium via the oral route of administration (aripiprazole, a new agent, may also prove efficacious for delirium). They have less associated extrapyramidal side effects. Parental formulations for ziprasidone and olanzapine have been FDA approved, but their safety and efficacy for use in delirium have not yet been established.

Neuroleptic agents can result in QT interval prolongation. Although the risk is low, prolonged QT predisposing to heart block or torsades de pointes (an unstable polymorphic ventricular tachycardia) has been reported. QT effects are most pronounced with intravenous use and, therefore, before administration, an electrocardiogram (ECG) is advised to assess QTc (especially in those with history of coronary artery disease, cardiac arrhythmia, structural cardiac disease, or age >50 years). When administering intravenous neuroleptics, follow QTc at least daily. If QTc is >450 msec, consider alternative medications. Electrolyte abnormalities can increase the risk of arrhythmia: check potassium (K) and magnesium (Mg). Aggressively replete K = 4, hyper-replete Mg >2.

To calculate QTc:

$$QTc = \frac{QT_{measured}}{r\text{-}r^{'1/2}}$$

1. **Haloperidol Administration for Agitation**
   a.   Check ECG, if QTc <450 msec
   b.   See below for starting doses (lower doses for children and the elderly)
      (1)   Mild agitation: 0.5 to 2 mg
      (2)   Moderate agitation: 5 to 10 mg
      (3)   Severe agitation: >10 mg
   c.   Administer first dose and monitor over 30 minutes.
   d.   If patient remains agitated, administer double the initial dose.
   e.   Monitor over 30 minutes and continue to double the dose until calm is achieved.
   f.   Dose that establishes calm will then equal total daily dose (administer over 24 hours in four to six divided doses)

2. **Atypical Neuroleptic Dosing for Agitation**
   a.   Risperidone: 0.5 to 6 mg p.o. (elixir also available)
   b.   Olanzapine: 2.5 to 20 mg p.o. (dissolvable wafer also available)
   c.   Quetiapine: 25 to 600 mg p.o.
   d.   Ziprasidone: 10 to 40 mg p.o., 10 to 20 mg i.m.

3. **Tapering and Side Effects**
Once the patient is calm and is tolerating tube feeds or is on oral feeding, neuroleptics can be tapered 10% to 25% per day.

All typical neuroleptics can cause extrapyramidal side effects such as dystonia or akathisia (feeling of restlessness). Treat dystonia with anticholinergic agents (benztropine 1 to 2 mg i.v. or diphenhydramine 50 to 100 mg i.v.) and remove the offending agent. Treat akathisia with beta blocker (propranolol 10 to 20 mg p.o. or i.v.) or benzodiazepine (lorazepam 1 to 2 mg p.o., i.m., or i.v.) and reduction or removal of offending agent.

4. **Treatment of Dystonia**
   a. **Stop Neuroleptic**
   b. Benztropine: 1 to 2 mg i.v. or i.m.
   c. Diphenhydramine: 50 to 100 mg i.v. or p.o.
5. **Treatment of Akathisia**
   a. **Stop Neuroleptic**
   b. Propranolol: 10 to 20 mg p.o. or i.v.
   c. Lorazepam: 1 to 2 mg p.o., i.m., or i.v.

B. Benzodiazepines

Benzodiazepines work as γ-aminobutyric acid (GABA) receptor agonists. As a result, they are extremely effective for anxiety and agitation states. In addition, they are cross-reactive with alcohol, which also has GABA effects, and therefore are used to treat alcohol withdrawal states. In some patients, particularly the elderly, paradoxic disinhibition can be seen with benzodiazepine use. Agents, which can be selected on the basis of pharmacokinetics, are listed below.

1. **Lorazepam**
   a. Starting dose: 0.5 to 2 mg
   b. Available routes of administration: p.o., i.m., i.v.
   c. Onset of action: fast to moderate
   d. Duration of action: short
2. **Diazepam**
   a. Starting dose: 5 to 20 mg
   b. Routes of administration: p.o., i.m., i.v. (by rectum available for status epilepticus)
   c. Onset of action: fast
   d. Duration of action: long (active metabolites)
3. **Midazolam**
   a. Starting dose: 0.5 to 2 mg
   b. Routes of administration: i.v. (p.o. syrup available)
   c. Onset of action: fast
   d. Duration of action: short
   e. Tolerance can quickly result, which requires increasing doses for the same effect.
      *Conversion of midazolam i.v. drip to diazepam p.o.: midazolam 1 mg/hour→diazepam 2 mg every 6 hours.

C. Opiates (Narcotics)

Trauma patients often require significant opiate medications (e.g., **morphine** or **hydromorphone**) for pain and sedation. Three types of opiate receptors are found in the brain. The *mu* and *delta* receptors are thought to mediate analgesia and mood and reinforce behavior. They are also thought to influence blood pressure, respiration, and gastrointestinal and endocrine function. The *kappa* receptors are thought to be responsible for dysphoria and analgesia. The positive reinforcing effects of opiates are mediated by the ventral tegmental area (VTA). In the VTA, opiate use is associated with firing of dopamine neurons that project to the nucleus accumbens, the so-called "pleasure center." This reinforcement pathway leads to a potent physical dependence syndrome. Although opiates are typically sedating medications, paradoxic agitation can develop (likely mediated by opiate stimulation of VTA dopamine release). If agitation to one opiate develops, switching to a different opiate medication is recommended. **Meperidine** and its metabolites (normeperidine) can lower seizure threshold and increase the likelihood of seizures. The use of meperidine, therefore, should be avoided in patients with an increased risk or history of seizures. **Methadone** is very sedating, with relatively fewer dopaminergic (euphoric) effects. It has a slow onset of action and long duration of action. Therefore, it is a good agent to use for agitation and may be used to wean or switch from intravenous to enteral (p.o., nasogastric [NG], or feeding tube) administration.

Opiate administration will quickly induce physical tolerance and dependence. Once tolerance develops, either as a result of treating the trauma or preexisting to hospitalization, slow tapers must be established to avoid physiologic withdrawal. Taper opiate dose by approximately 10% per day.

In addition, during the course of treatment for many trauma patients, medications need to be switched from intravenous to enteral administration (p.o., NG, or feeding tube). This needs to be done carefully with opiate medications because the risk for oversedation or relative withdrawal is high. We recommend the following conversion when switching from intravenous to enteral agents.

1. **Intravenous Morphine, Intravenous Hydromorphone, Oral Methadone Conversion**
   a. Morphine 1mg i.v.→morphine 1mg p.o.
   b. Morphine 1mg i.v.→hydromorphone 1mg i.v.
   c. Morphine 1mg i.v.→methadone 1.5mg p.o. (chronic), 1mg p.o. (acute).
   d. Hydromorphone 1mg →methadone 6mg p.o.
2. **Protocol for Intravenous to Oral Switchover**
   a. Administer one third of the total daily dose of opiate enterally (p.o., NG, or feeding tube).
   b. Decrease intravenous drip by 50%.
   c. Monitor level of sedation, respiratory status, other vital signs, and pupillary diameter.
   d. Adjust dose as needed.
   e. All conversions are estimates and doses should be based on duration of infusions, history of drug abuse, degree of absorption, and individual differences among patients.
   f. Conversion to methadone should only be done once the patient is medically stabilized and fully tolerating tube feeds or oral intake.

VI.   Substance Abuse

Alcohol and other substance abuse are of major concern on the trauma service. Concurrent substance abuse in trauma is now the rule rather than the exception. As a result, initial workup of trauma patients should always include both serum and urine toxicology. Check with the laboratory that runs the screens for a list of screened-for agents. Multiple agents can be used concurrently. Agents include marijuana, phencyclidine hydrochloride (PCP), hallucinogens, opiates, cocaine, stimulants, ecstasy, and γ hydroxybutyrate (GHB). Withdrawal states can also be encountered at presentation or during the hospital course. Of all withdrawal states, alcohol withdrawal is the most common and most pernicious. Psychiatric consultation can assist with the evaluation and management of substance intoxication and withdrawal states.

A. **Alcohol**
1. **Screening**
If patients are conversant and coherent on presentation, the CAGE questionnaire is an effective means of alcohol screening:

C Have you ever felt the need to **cut down?**

A Have people **annoyed** you by criticizing your drinking?

G Have you ever felt **guilty** about your drinking?

E Have you ever had an **eye-opener** to steady your nerves?

Affirmative response to two or more of these questions is considered clinically suspicious for alcohol abuse or dependence.

Given alcohol's rapid clearance from blood and urine (a matter of hours), a patient can have alcohol problems even if both urine and serum toxicology screens are negative. When alcohol is discontinued in a patient with physical dependence, withdrawal can occur anywhere from hours to up to 10 days after the patient's last drink (typically, begins within 1 to 2 days). Alcohol withdrawal is a **life-threatening** condition and requires immediate intervention. Benzodiazepines are the first-line treatment for alcohol withdrawal and are used to avert a withdrawal syndrome. Liver function will affect the metabolism of most of these agents and, therefore, it influences withdrawal management. In addition, folate, thiamine, and multivitamins should be administered to any patient thought to have alcohol abuse or dependence. Depending on the individual, benzodiazepines are not cross-reactive with alcohol and, in rare cases, may not be treat withdrawal symptoms. Lack of cross-reactivity should be suspected if withdrawal symptoms continue despite the administration of high doses of benzodiazepine. Should this occur, switch the patient to another benzodiazepine, barbiturate, neuroleptic, or propofol. In rare cases, when none of these agents are cross-reactive with alcohol; withdrawal can be treated with alcohol itself. Oral or intravenous alcohol can be administered to alleviate withdrawal symptoms and then tapered once the patient has stabilized.

2. **Treatment of Withdrawal (Table 44-4)**
a. Monitor vital signs at least every 4 hours while patient is awake.

Table 44-4. Treatment of withdrawal

Normal LFT	Elevated LFT
Intravenous: Diazepam 5–10 mg	Lorazepam 1–2 mg
Oral: Chlordiazepoxide 25–50 mg	Oxazepam 15–30 mg

    b. Administer benzodiazepine for any signs or symptoms of alcohol withdrawal: systolic blood pressure (SBP) >150, diastolic blood pressure (DBP) >100, heart rate (HR) >100, tremor, diaphoresis, nausea and vomiting, anxiety, confusion.
    c. Use benzodiazepines as frequently as needed to alleviate signs and symptoms of withdrawal (as frequently as every hour, if necessary).
    d. Establish a standing dose for active withdrawal: Twice daily (b.i.d.) dosing for diazepam and chlordiazepoxide, four times (q.i.d.) daily dosing for lorazepam and oxazepam
    e. Titrate benzodiazepine dose to alleviate signs and symptoms of withdrawal.
    f. Start thiamine (100 mg), (folate 1 mg), multivitamin (i.v. daily for 3 days; switch to p.o. route of administration if gastrointestinal absorption is intact).

3. Delirium Tremens
Delirium tremens, which represents a state of severe alcohol withdrawal, was initially described by Raymond Adams as the prototypical hyperdopaminergic state of delirium. Symptom onset is generally between 8 and 9 hours after the last drink, though cases have presented as far as 10 days out. Patients with alcohol dependence, who chronically maintain high blood alcohol levels, can begin to show signs of withdrawal even with a detectable blood alcohol level. Early symptoms include flushing, diaphoresis, disorientation, hallucinations or seizures. Late symptoms, which can occur 48 to 96 hours after the last drink, include tremor, profound disorientation, autonomic instability, and visual hallucinations. Seizures generally do not occur. Delirium tremens is a life-threatening condition with mortality rate of 5% to 10%, even when appropriately treated.

4. Alcohol Withdrawal Seizures
Seizures occur roughly 24 to 48 hours after last drink. Seizures are usually of the generalized tonic-clonic variety. They are often isolated events; however, they can recur 3 to 6 hours after the initial seizure. Management includes aggressive treatment of withdrawal (per above) and seizure prophylaxis in the acute setting. Check glucose, electrolytes, and ammonia level because these are often abnormal.

B. Opiates

Opiates are associated with pronounced dependence and withdrawal syndromes. Although withdrawal from opiates is uncomfortable (and patients are vocal about their discomfort), it is **not** generally a life-threatening condition. Psychiatry consultation can be useful in determining actual withdrawal states from medication-seeking behavior.

1. Treatment of Opiate Withdrawal

Signs and symptoms of opiate withdrawal can include combinations of the following: pupillary dilatation, diffuse myalgias, diarrhea, fever, insomnia, diaphoresis, piloerection, rhinorrhea, dysphoric mood, and autonomic instability. The best indication of opiate intoxication is pupillary contraction (pinpoint pupils). The best indication of opiate withdrawal is pupillary dilatation. Particularly in the ICU, opiate withdrawal states often mimic *Clostridium difficile* infection (to distinguish between the two, monitor pupil examination). If a patient is currently using opiates and tolerance is established (e.g., patient prescribed opiates for pain management), tapering the opiate agent at 10% per day will minimize withdrawal discomfort.

   a. Clonidine, an alpha-$_2$-adrenergic agonist, can reduce some of the physical discomfort of withdrawal at a dose of 0.1 mg p.o. q.i.d.; hold for SBP <90, HR <60.

   b. Dicyclomine: 10 mg p.o. q.i.d, prescribed for abdominal cramps

   c. Quinine: 325 mg p.o. b.i.d., as needed for leg cramps

   d. Phenergan: 25 to 50 mg p.o. q.i.d., as needed for nausea and vomiting

2. Treatment of Opiate Intoxication

If patients are over-sedated, respiratory status is at risk. Opiate intoxication can be reversed with naltrexone (0.4 mg i.v.); repeat as needed.

C. Cocaine

Cocaine can be used orally, intranasally, smoked, or injected intravenously. Abusers often prefer alkaloid forms of cocaine (free base and crack) because of their extremely rapid onset of action (<10 seconds). Cocaine use blocks the reuptake of dopamine, serotonin, and norepinephrine by the presynaptic neuron. As with opiates, the euphoric effects of cocaine are thought to be mediated by dopamine effects in the nucleus accumbens. Cocaine is very fast acting and has a short duration of action. This lends to its addiction potential. Cocaine is only transiently detectable in serum (during acute intoxication; hours) and urine (4 to 6 hours). Although cocaine has a high addiction potential, no associated physical withdrawal syndrome occurs with its use. Cocaine, however, is associated with multiple medical comorbidity, including hypertension, cardiac ischemia, cardiac arrhythmias, and coronary and cerebral vasospasm.

VII. Anxiety Disorders

Anxiety is a normal and transient response to stress. Any patient who has experienced a traumatic injury should be expected to have some type of anxiety symptoms. Anxiety disorders include generalized anxiety disorder, panic with or without agoraphobia, phobias, obsessive-compulsive disorder, and pathologic reactions to stress. Anxiety symptoms can be mental in nature (nervous, restless, poor attention irritable, panic, worry or fear) or physical in nature (palpitations, diaphoresis, trembling, shortness of breath, chest pain, nausea, dizziness). If anxiety symptoms are distressing to the patient, they should be treated. Anxiety is not only common during the hospital course for patients sustaining traumatic injury, but is often the chief complaint when presenting to the out-patient clinic. Patients should be routinely asked if they have **anxiety,** problems with **sleep,** or **nightmares.**

In terms of treatment, one helpful rule of thumb is to determine if the primary psychic state is **anxiety** or **fear.** Determination of the primary psychic state can guide pharmacotherapy. Benzodiazepines, with a GABA agonist mechanism of action, have well-established efficacy for anxiety. Alternatively, some theories of fear link the emotional state to an amygdala substrate (involving dopaminergic neurons). This underlying dopamine pathway is not affected by benzodiazepines, but can be modulated with neuroleptics. Neuroleptics often reduce anxiety when patients appear to be resistant to benzodiazepines (even in high doses). Clinically, anxiety and fear can be difficult to distinguish. Anxiety, however, tends to be less directed toward a single object and more generalized over time. Fear tends to be episodic, situational, and directed toward specific concerns.

Consider psychiatric consultation for any anxiety symptoms that are refractory to initial treatment with benzodiazepines or neuroleptics. Psychiatrists can also help in the diagnosis and supportive care of patients with acute stress disorder or posttraumatic stress disorder.

A. Acute Stress Disorder

Acute stress disorder (ASD) and posttraumatic stress disorder (PTSD) are particular pathologic reactions to trauma. In both cases, symptoms include reexperiencing the traumatic event (through flashbacks and nightmares), increased sensitivity to stimulation, and dissociative symptoms (e.g., feeling numb, detached, out of one's body or "zoned out"). Temporal characteristics distinguish these two disorders with acute stress disorder occurring within 4 weeks of the traumatic event and lasting no longer than 4 weeks. If symptoms last longer than 4 weeks, by definition the diagnosis is PTSD.

B. Posttraumatic Stress Disorder

Posttraumatic stress disorder is a psychiatric reaction to being the victim of severe, life-threatening trauma (or being witness to such trauma). The prevalence of PTSD in the general population exposed to trauma is 3.5% to 15%. Symptoms can occur as early as the first month after the traumatic event, or they may not appear for years after the initial event. Often, these patients present to the surgical outpatient clinic with complaints of decreased sleep, nightmares, flashbacks, and difficulty with work or personal relationships. Commonly, they will avoid thoughts or activities associated with the trauma. Symptoms can also include increased arousal characterized by sleep disturbance, irritability and anger; difficulty concentrating; hypervigilance, and an increased startle response.

Treatment includes acute management of anxiety, sleep, and other symptoms with antianxiety agents (e.g. benzodiazepines), long-term pharmacologic treatment with agents (e.g., selective serotonin reuptake inhibitors [SSRI], and supportive psychotherapy.

VIII. Mood Disorders

Along with anxiety disorders, disturbances in mood are the most common psychiatric complications in trauma patients. Mood disturbance can range from normal variation in emotion to severe depression, irritability, or mania. Whereas major mood disorders can exist before experiencing a traumatic event, it is more likely that anxiety, sadness, grief, or depression can be a reaction to trauma. If this reaction is relatively mild and lasts <3 months, it is classified as an **adjustment disorder.** If depression is severe and longer lasting, the diagnosis may be **major depressive disorder. Manic** episodes can be precipitated by trauma, although it is more likely the case that manic episodes (in the context of long-term bipolar illness) result in erratic behavior and are the cause of many traumatic events.

A. Depression

1. Diagnosis

The prevalence of depression on the trauma service is high, both as a preexisting condition and as a result of the physical trauma. Although substance abuse is the most common preexisting psychiatric disorder seen on a trauma service, many of these patients present with a substance abuse disorder in conjunction with a comorbid mood disorder (dual diagnosis). Depression is not typically a normal reaction to stressful events, but rather is defined as a clinical syndrome that requires the persistence of the following symptoms for **2 weeks** associated with a **dysphoric mood** or anhedonia (loss of pleasure in usual activities).

2. Clinical Features (Associated Symptoms of Depression)

The acronym **SIGECAPS describes the clinical features of associated symptoms of depression:** decreased **sleep,** loss of **interest,** feelings of **guilt,** poor **concentration,** lack of **energy,** decreased **appetite, psychomotor** retardation or agitation, **suicidal** ideation, or recurrent thoughts of death. At least five of the symptoms must be present during the same 2-week period to make the diagnosis.

3. Suicidal Ideation

Commonly, suicidal ideation is a symptom of major depression, but can also be associated with bipolar illness, schizophrenia, and substance abuse. Traumatic injury can be the result of suicide attempts. Physicians have a legal obligation to prevent people from committing suicide, if aware of any intent. With any question of suicidal intent, the trauma team should secure the patient (either by constant observation, locked door seclusion, or mechanical restraint) and prevent him or her from leaving the hospital. Psychiatry should then be consulted. Prompt psychiatric evaluation is essential to the timely evaluation and proper management of the suicidal patient.

4. Treatment

Selective serotonin reuptake inhibitors are the most common antidepressant medications because they are well tolerated and have few drug interactions. These medications, however, can take 6 to 8 weeks to demonstrate effect. Dextroamphetamine (a psychostimulant) can often provide mood elevation and improve associated symptoms of depression within 48 hours. When used at **low dose** (5 to 10 mg p.o. every morning), dextroamphetamine stimulates mood, appetite, and motivation. It should be used cautiously in patients with a history of substance abuse because of its abuse potential as well as in patients with cardiac pathology or problems with insomnia.

B. Mania and Mixed States

1. Diagnosis

Patients with persistently expanded or elevated (euphoric) moods can be described as manic. This mood state is the characteristic state of bipolar illness, which is a disorder that is marked by manic and depressed episodes. When patients are manic or depressed, they can have such severe symptomatology that associated psychotic symptoms (delusions, hallucinations) are also present.

Mixed state is characterized as a state of elevated or agitated mood that meets criteria for both a manic or hypomanic state and a depressed state.

2. Clinical Features (Associated Symptoms of a Mania)

The acronym **DIGFAST** describes the clinical features of associated symptoms of mania: easily **distractible,** increased **indiscretions, grandiosity, flight of ideas,** increased goal directed **activity,** decreased need for **sleep,** and **talkative** with pressured speech. Mania is distinguished from hypomania in that it is more severe and associated with significant social or occupational dysfunction. Many types of substance intoxication can mimic a manic or hypomanic presentation.

3. Treatment

Mania is commonly treated with mood stabilizers: lithium, valproic acid, or carbamazepine. If the patient is critically ill, requiring significant fluid resuscitation, however, these agents are difficult to manage (given their narrow therapeutic windows). In the setting of rapid changes in fluid status, ineffective or toxic levels can result. Therapeutic ranges are as follows:

    a. Lithium: 0.6 to 1.0 mmol/L
    b. Valproic acid: 50 to 100 µg/mL
    c. Carbamazepine: 6 to 10 µg/mL
    d. Acute manic symptoms can also be managed with neuroleptic agents. Psychiatric consultation should be promptly obtained for aid in managing manic and mixed states.

C. Psychosis

Psychosis is a gross impairment of reality testing that can result from a variety of psychiatric and medical problems. Characterized by hallucinations, delusions, or as a formal thought disorder, this disruption in the organization of thinking can be preexisting or as the result of the trauma or its treatment. An evaluation of the patient's mental status is required to differentiate these symptoms as secondary to delirium or to a preexisting disorder (e.g., schizophrenia). Consultation can aid in the evaluation and management of psychotic states.

IX. Legal Issues

Issues regarding informed consent and emergency treatment frequently arise on the trauma service. In the course of treating trauma patients, one may have to deal with a patients ability to consent for or refuse medical care. Laws dealing with consent vary on a state-to-state basis, and psychiatric consultation may often be useful in negotiating these complicated situation.

A. Informed Consent

Informed consent refers to the right of the patient to make personal decisions about medical care. For any medical test or intervention, the patient must give permission to the physician for treatment to proceed. Informed consent must be voluntary and cannot be attained through coercive means. The patient has the right to waive consent ("Doctor, do what you need to do."). Informed consent can be implied if the patient puts himself or herself in a situation in order to receive care (e.g., the patient voluntarily presents to the emergency room for treatment).

The patient must be provided with sufficient information to make an informed decision:

    1. Nature of the medical condition
    2. Risks and benefits of the treatment
    3. Likelihood of the risks and benefits, including the inability to absolutely predict the outcome of treatment
    4. Irreversibility of the treatment, if applicable
    5. Availability of alternative treatments

B. Patient's Competency and Capacity

The patient must be competent to give informed consent. That is, the person must have the mental capacity to make such a decision.

    1. Competency is a legal determination arrived at in the courts.

    2. Capacity is a clinical determination made by any physician that a patient has the mental ability to assent to or refuse treatment.

    3. Capacity is not an absolute concept. The threshold for capacity is dependent on the nature of the medical condition, being low for procedures with minimal risk and high for more risky procedures (i.e., the threshold for consent or refusal of exploratory laparotomy is higher than that of a blood test).

C. Substituted Judgment (for the Commonwealth of Massachusetts)

If a patient is found to be incompetent or lacking in capacity to make medical decisions, then some form of substituted judgment must be instituted. **Substituted judgment** refers to the assignment of a substitute decision-maker who has the power to make healthcare decisions for the patient. Substituted judgment must be accompanied by written documentation that clearly defines the substitute decision-maker and what specific decisions that person can make. In emergency situations, if informed consent has not been obtained (or cannot be obtained) and when failure to act would result in a serious and imminent deterioration in the patient's condition, the physician can serve as the agent of substituted judgment (make treatment decisions for the patient).

D. Treatment Refusal

All competent individuals have the right to refuse treatment that others believe is in their best interest. Treatment of a patient without consent can be the basis of medical malpractice and, in legal terms, can constitute battery. Regarding treatment refusal, patients are presumed competent unless determined otherwise. Likewise, patients who are mentally ill are presumed competent unless their mental illness interferes with their decision-making capacity. Patients who are deemed incompetent or are unable to express a preference may have consistently and specifically expressed their preferences at some earlier time when they were competent. If this can be discovered, then medical management should proceed according to their wishes. The laws regarding treatment refusal vary state by state, and physicians should check the laws in their own state. Psychiatry consultation can assist in determining capacity and interfacing with patient and family when a question of treatment refusal presents. In addition, psychiatry and the legal office of the hospital are valuable resources for clarifying state law.

SELECTED READING

Cassem NH et al: Psychopharmacology in the ICU. In: Chernow B, ed. *The pharmacologic approach to the critically ill patient.* Baltimore: Williams & Wilkins, 1995.

Cottrol C, Frances R. Substance abuse, comorbid psychiatric disorder, and repeated traumatic injuries. *Hospital and Community Psychiatry* 1993;44:715–716.

Diagnostic and statistical manual of mental disorders, 4th ed. Washington, DC: American Psychiatric Association Press, 1994.

Folstein MF, Folstein SE, McHugh PR. "Mini-mental state," a practical method for grading the cognitive state of patients for the clinician. *J Psychiatr Res* 1975;12:189–198.

Heckers S. Delirium. In: Stern TA, Herman JB, eds. *Psychiatry update and board preparation.* New York: McGraw-Hill, 2000:41–46.

Jennett B, Teasdale G. Aspects of coma after severe head injury. *Lancet* 1977;1:878.

Mayfield D, McLeod G, Hall P. The CAGE questionnaire: validation of a new alcoholism instrument. *Am J Psychiatry* 1974;131:1121–1123

Murray GB. Limbic Music. In: Cassem EH, ed. *Massachusetts General Hospital handbook of general hospital psychiatry.* St. Louis: Mosby, 1997:11–23.

Plum F, Posner J. *The diagnosis of stupor and coma.* Philadelphia: FA Davis, 1982.

Whetsell LA, Patterson MC, Young DH, et al. Preinjury psychopathology in trauma patients. *J Trauma* 1989;29(8):1158–1162.

Rehabilitation of the Trauma Patient

Ricardo Knight, MD, and Robert L. Sheridan, MD

I. **Disability Following Trauma**
   A. Injury is the leading cause of both death and functional limitation in adults <45 years of age, with post-trauma disability rates ranging from 19% to 80%.
   B. Good functional planning is perched on a foundation of good functional assessments. Prognosticating about functional recovery is based on a through understanding of the functional consequences of the injury or knowledge of its natural history, and awareness of the available range of medical and therapeutic interventions

II. **Overview of the Rehabilitation Process**
   A. The **initial phase** of rehabilitation begins with a comprehensive assessment of the patient's primary impairment. In this first phase, medical and therapeutic interventions are put in place to prevent or limit any secondary impairment that can lead to functional compromise. These secondary impairments include joint contractures, muscle weakness, peripheral nerve injury, heterotopic ossification (HO), and deconditioning. Bracing, range of motion (ROM), functional positioning, early mobility, and muscle and nerve blocks might prevent secondary impairment.

   The **second phase** of rehabilitation, which focuses on getting the patient ready for discharge to the most appropriate subacute setting, occurs simultaneously with medical and surgical efforts to stabilize the patient. Activities during this active second phase include functional mobility training, strengthening, training with assistive devices, and trails of function-enhancing medications.

   The **third phase** is the postacute phase, which can take place in a number of settings including acute rehabilitation hospital, subacute centers, skilled nursing facilities, or home. The discharge disposition and the rehabilitation activities depend on the medical, cognitive, and functional status of the patient. The postacute transition occurs as soon as the medical or surgical team feels the patient no longer requires the medical intensity of the acute care hospital. The goal of rehabilitation during this phase is attainment of functional independence and unsupervised medically stability.

   In the **final phase,** the rehabilitation process involves environmental acclimation and maintenance, which usually takes take place at home with appropriate rehabilitation follow-up.
   B. **Trauma Rehabilitation Team**
      1. **Physiatrist**
         This is a physician with expert knowledge about the adverse functional consequences of traumatic disor-

ders, who advises the trauma team on medical and therapeutic interventions aimed at limiting impairment, preventing disability, and restoring function. As a member of the trauma team, the physiatrist provides long-term prospective to the team, patients, and the families. Other PM&R personnel make functional prognoses and advise about appropriate discharge dispositions.

2. Physical Therapist

The physical therapist (PT) is licensed professional whose responsibilities include providing therapeutic exercise, functional training, therapeutic bracing, and protective bracing. A PT is involved in the care at the earliest possible moment, and works to prevent the negative effects of immobility.

3. Occupational Therapist

The occupational therapist (OT) is also involved with therapeutic activities and bracing that promote functional recovery. The OT is particularly interested in the necessary activities of daily living (ADL), such dressing, grooming, bathing, and toileting.

4. Speech-Language Pathologist

The domain of speech-language pathologist (SLP) includes the evaluation of treatment of disorders of verbal and writing communication, swallowing, and cognitive dysfunction after a traumatic injury.

5. Psychologist

Rehabilitation psychologists play a crucial role in the comprehensives assessment of cognition, emotional state, and behavior. Neuropsychological assessments are used to tailor cognitive interventions and behavioral plans. The psychologist provides counseling in areas of adjustment to disability and management of posttraumatic stress.

III. Rehabilitation Following Orthopedic Trauma

    A. Cervical Spinal Injuries

        1. Cervical spine injuries are common following certain kinds of trauma, particularly involving motor vehicle accidents. Cervical spine injuries include soft tissue injuries, vertebral artery, ligamentous, and spinal cord injuries. The first priority in the management of cervical traumatic injuries is to rule out major vascular, bony, or neurologic compromise. All injuries should be stabilized and cleared before any mobility-related activities begin.

        2. Cervical strains, commonly referred to as "whiplash injuries," are associated with a large constellation of symptoms. Neck pain and stiffness is the most common complaint, but dizziness, headache, tingling sensations in the neck and shoulders, blurred vision, vertigo, balance problems, hoarseness, and cognitive dysfunction are also described. Radiographic findings usually absent except for the loss of cervical lordosis, which indicates spasm. Initial treatment usually consists of relative rest with a soft cervical collar, ice, nonsteroidal anti-inflammatory drugs (NSAIDS), narcotics, and muscle relaxants for the first 2 weeks.

After the first 2 weeks, rehabilitation efforts focus of restoring normal ROM, relieving spasms, and managing pain. Physical therapy can be helpful in the postacute period, using heat modalities (e.g., ultrasound), moist heat in conjunction with soft mobilization, muscle energy, passive cervical ROM, and massage. Spray and stretch, electrical stimulation, biofeedback, and acupuncture are often helpful adjuncts to therapy. If tingling, burning, or paraesthesias comprise prominent symptoms drugs (e.g., gabapentin, lamotrigine, and tricyclics antidepressants) can be adjuncts to the medication regiment.

In recalcitrant cases, pain and spasms might persist or worsen for >6 weeks. If such recalcitrant cases are associated with finding of prominent trigger points, then trigger point injections may be indicated. The points could be injected with a dry needle, a local anesthetic alone or in a combination of corticosteroids and local anesthetic. Severe, painful spasms or dystonias can be treated with selected botulinum toxin muscle blocks. Pain in the occipital area caused by occipital neuritis can be ameliorated with occipital nerve blocks. When painful spasm has subsided and ROM is restored, strengthening activities should commence, with emphasis on strengthening muscle that stabilize the cervical spine.

Return to work and normal activities are encouraged. A work hardening program can make for a smother transition back to work, particularly for physically demanding jobs. Most people improve within the first 2 months, but 42% can have persistent symptoms for >1 year, and 33% for >2 years.

3. Cervical radiculopathy describes a condition characterized by signs and symptoms along a predictable cervical nerve root distribution (**Table 45-1**), which are generally caused by compression of a nerve root, usually by a prolapsed intervertebral disk (**Table 45-2**). Focus of treatment, which can be done by several means, is on eliminating the noxious stimuli that can be affecting the nerve root and causing symptoms. NSAIDS and steroids given orally, or by epidural injection, can act against the pain causing inflammatory mediators at the site of encroachment. Traction produces mechanical distraction that can relieve pressure directly on a nerve root or prolapsed disc, as well as provide a prolonged stretch to spastic guarding muscles.

Symptomatic relief from pain and spasms, also a primary objective of initial treatment, can be achieved by using a number of symptom-directed medications. If the predominant symptom is paraesthesias or radiating electrical pain, a drug (e.g., gabapentin or a tricyclic antidepressant drug) can be efficacious. If the

Table 45-1. Localization of cervical level

Disc Level	Findings	Reflex Deficit
C4–C5	Radiation to lateral elbow; weakness of deltoid, biceps, and rotator cuff; impaired sensation in lateral shoulder	Biceps
C5–C6	Radiation to lateral arm to thumb and lateral scapula, weakness in biceps and wrist extensors (ECRL&B), impaired sensation in dorsolateral aspect of thumb and index finger	Brachio-radialis
C6–C7	Radiation to medial scapula, lateral arm to middle finger, weakness in triceps and pronator, finger extension, wrist flexion, sensory changes in index and middle fingers and dorsum of hand	Triceps, pronator
C7–C8	Radiation along medial arm to digits 4 and 5; weakness in intrinsic muscles, ulnar deviation of wrist	None

predominant symptom is spasms, a muscle relaxant can be a helpful addition. For sharp, stabbing, or severe constant pain, the limited use of narcotics may be necessary to break up the pain cycle. Physical modalities (e.g., heat, ice, and electric stimulation) could reduce pain and spasms and be good adjunctive therapies. Acupuncture, biofeedback, and massage can also aid in symptomatic relief of pain and spasms. Chiropractic manipulation is contraindicated in the presence of neurologic findings.

Table 45-2. Definitions of disk pathology

Bulging disk	The annulus is displaced concentrically beyond the body endplate
Herniated disk (*prolapsed disk*)	Focal displacement of the nucleus pulposus through a defect in the annulus with the nuclear material remains connected to the parent nucleus. Herniations can be located central, posterolateral (paracentral), or lateral (foraminal)
Extruded disk	Extrusion of disk material such that the fragment is not connected to the parent disk
Sequestered disk	The herniated nuclear material is not contiguous with the remaining intraannular nucleus within the intervertebral disk space

B. Thoracic and Lumbar Injuries

1. Thoracic spine injuries should be classified as stable or unstable before any rehabilitation is considered. Early mobilization after spine trauma is important to the promotion of good pulmonary toilet and the prevention of thromboembolism, pressure ulcers, and deconditioning. When the spine is unstable, mobilization is allowed after it is stabilized through protective bracing or surgery. Physical activity is allowed within the parameters set by the surgeon, with allowances made for pain. In the acute and immediate postacute period, aggressive pain management, using a combination of short- and long-acting narcotics, facilitates efforts to mobilize the patient.

2. Spinal trauma can result in an acute radiculopathy, usually as intervertebral disk rupture, and cause nerve root encroachment. Acute rehabilitation intervention in the acute and immediate postacute period is generally targeted toward alleviation of symptoms, and maintenance of functional mobility and strength. Rest is discouraged for >3 days. A short course of corticosteroids or NSAIDS is often indicated. For symptoms of radicular pain, drugs (e.g., gabapentin, lamotrigine, or tricyclic antidepressants) can be helpful. In cases of accompanying muscle spasms, relaxants can be very useful. Physical therapy modalities (e.g., moist heat, ice, electrical stimulation, massage, and soft tissue mobilization) help to decrease pain and promote function.

In the subacute period, rehabilitation emphasis is switched to restoration of preinjury strength and mobility. Physical therapy is very important in this phase, with more emphasis placed on strength and flexibility exercises. Some patients might require structured work-hardening programs, where task-specific training and back injury prevention education is emphasized. In some patients, selective spinal injections can alleviate symptoms and restore function.

C. Upper Extremity Injuries

1. Fracture

Trauma to the upper extremities could be functionally devastating, especially with joint involvement or peripheral nerve injury. Active or passive joint ROM is often contraindicated with interarticular injures, which rapidly lead joint capsule restrictions, which can progress to adhesive capsulitis, a painful debilitating condition.

2. Injuries involving the shoulder girdle can lead to rotator cuff tears and brachial plexus injuries. Suspect rotator cuff tears if the patient has difficulty initiating or maintaining shoulder adduction, or has weak external or internal rotation. Weakness following scapula fractures can injure the suprascapular or infrascapular nerve, leading to weakness that can be misinterpreted as a rotator cuff tear. Humeral neck

fracture and shoulder dislocation can be associated with axillary nerve injury, which can cause persistent shoulder adduction weakness and affect the ability to do overhead activities.

3.   Midhumeral shaft fractures can be associated with radial nerve injury, which can lead to weakness in wrist and finger extensors. With radial nerve injuries, wrist and finger flexors muscles have unopposed flexion which predispose to wristdrop and MCP contractures. Grip power is also diminished with radial nerve injury because of lack of the tenodesis effect, wherein the wrist and MCP are stabilized by the wrist extensors allowing optimal finger flexion. Wrist bracing will be required to prevent wristdrop, maintain web space, and assist with wrist and thumb extension. A forearm or volar-based wrist extension splint with dynamic extension outriggers for the fingers and thumb will enhance hand function.

4.   Elbow injury, including fractures and dislocations, can cause loss in elbow mobility and injury to the ulnar and median nerve. When immobile, the elbow joint rapidly develops joint capsule restrictions that can limit functionally important elbow flexion and supination. Early movement is pivotal to the maintenance of elbow function, but should be guided by the orthopedic surgeon. When possible, dynamic bracing should be applied and active movement encouraged within the safe joint range.

Medial epicondyle fracture could be associated with ulnar nerve injury, leading to impairment in hand function and creating an intrinsic negative or claw hand. Ulnar nerve injury can lead to a loss of full hand opening, making it difficult to grasp large objects. The thumb also loses its ability to oppose and generate a strong pinch.

A splint that blocks the MCP joints from fully extending will prevent claw hand formation. The splint can be dynamic or static and can be an opponens type orthosis with a fourth and fifth MCP extension stop set at 30 degrees of flexion.

Because the flexor digitorum profundus (FDP) is weakened by ulnar nerve injury at the elbow, the claw hand deformity is not as prominent as distal nerve injuries, making splinting less important. The median nerve could also be involved in an elbow injury, which could have a grave effect on hand function.

Patients with median nerve injury at the elbow will present with weakness in elbow pronation, wrist flexion, second and third MCP flexion, and thumb opposition, flexion, and adduction. The goals of functional splinting in patients with proximal median nerve injury is to maintain the (1) thumb web space, (2) thumb in opposition, and (3) assist with finger flexion. To restore proper hand function, tendon transfer may be necessary, in which case, a functional hand splint is appropriate to maintain the hand in wrist extension, thumb opposition, and MCP flexion (**Fig. 45-1**).

5. Fractures involving the forearm can also cause functionally consequential radial, median, and ulnar nerve injury. Posterior interosseous nerve injury (radial nerve) will cause weakness in the extensor digitorum and in thumb extension. The brace needed with more distal radial nerve injuries is the same as used with proximal injuries. Distal median nerve injuries can lead to unopposed action of the adductor pollicis, which can then lead to contractures. A splint is necessary to maintain the thumb web space; a soft

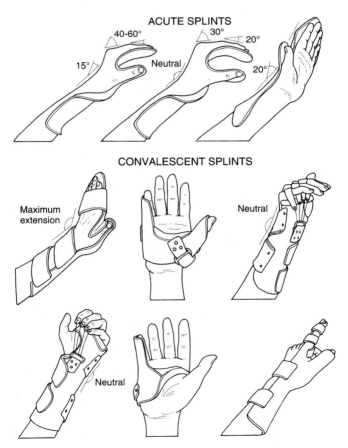

Figure 45-1. Selected splints useful for hand rehabilitation.

dynamic thumb splint, a thumb spica splint, or a C-bar could accomplish this. A distal ulnar injury can cause loss of intrinsic muscle function in the fourth and fifth digit, leading to a partial claw hand or a "Benedictine sign." The bracing requirements for a distal ulnar injury are the same as for proximal injures.

D. Lower Extremity Injuries

1. The goal of rehabilitation after lower extremity fractures is to return the patient quickly back to independent functioning. The rehabilitation team works closely with the orthopedic surgeon, keeping within weightbearing and mobility restrictions (**Table 45-3**). Mobility restrictions need to be fre-

Table 45-3. Rehabilitative precautions after hip fracture and dislocation

Injury Type	Precautions
DISLOCATIONS WITHOUT FRACTURE	
Anterior	After stabilization, weightbearing, as tolerated, with limited extension and abduction
Posterior	After stabilization, weightbearing, as tolerated, with limited flexion, adduction, and internal rotation
Dislocations with fracture	Same as above; additional limitations based on fracture type
Femoral neck fracture	
Nondisplaced	Weightbearing, as tolerated, by second postoperative day
Displaced	If internal fixation is used, weight-bearing is variable, but usually foot-flat to partial for 4 to 6 weeks. If cemented endoprosthesis is used, weightbearing, as tolerated immediately. No hip flexion, adduction, or internal rotation if endoprosthesis is used.
INTER OR SUBTROCHANTERIC FRACTURE	
Stable	If internal fixation is used, weight-bearing is variable, but usually as tolerated by the second post-operative day. No range of motion limits. If internal fixation is used, weightbearing is variable.
Unstable	Usually foot-flat to partial for 4 to 6 weeks No range of motion limits.

quently reassessed and updated not to delay in the rehabilitation process.

2. The rehabilitation period following lower extremity injuries has many challenges, including pain, deep venous thrombosis (DVT) prophylaxis, infections, wound care, and management of comorbidity. Mobility is better facilitated when acute and subacute pain is treated using a short-acting narcotic given 30 minutes before activity. Long-acting narcotics can be required if the patient needs short-acting drugs more than every 4 hours.

Many complications can occur during the rehabilitation. Complications directly related to the trauma of surgery are wound infection, heterotopic ossification, venous thromboembolism (VTE), prosthetic loosening, periprosthetic fracture, decubiti, wound dehiscence, and nerve injuries. VTE is common after a fractured hip and always requires prophylaxis. Full anticoagulation with heparin or warfarin (international normalized ration [INR] >2) is the most effective form of prophylaxis, but carries the highest risk of bleeding complications. To prevent DVT in this population, low-dose warfarin (INR 1.8 to 2) or low molecular weight heparin is more affective than low-dose unfractionated heparin.

3. Hip fractures account for approximately half of all inpatient days for fracture care and billions of dollars in healthcare cost. Most patients will require some form of rehabilitation service following a hip fracture. Rehabilitation care following a hip fracture begins typically on postoperative day 1, with bed and chair transfer mobility training, and exercises in the chair (**Table 45-4**). On postoperative day 2, the patient can start progressive gait training with a protective device or in the parallel bars, as well as ADL training, including dressing, bathing, and grooming. By postoperative day 3 to 4, patients can be discharged home and receive home rehabilitation services if they are medically stable and have mastered all the functional skills needed to return to their living environment with the supports they have. Acute inpatient rehabilitation is needed if further medical management of the hip fracture, complications, or comorbidity is needed. During this phase of rehabilitation, further functional mobility training takes place, including gait training on level surfaces and elevations, tub and car transfers, and kitchen mobility. This second phase, which can range from 7 to 14 days, usually is limited by the medical stability of the patient. Patients who are stable from a medical point of view but do not have skills to function in their environment with the assistance that they have or are unable to participate in a full inpatient rehabilitation, might need a skilled nursing facility or subacute rehabilitation unit for the second phase. The goal, by end of the second phase, is to make the patient independent in household level

Table 45-4.   Rehabilitation after hip fracture

Stage	Number of Postoperative Days	Program
ACUTE	1	Comprehensive evaluation. Bed-level strengthening, range of motion and conditioning exercises. Out of bed to chair, chair-level exercises. Review extremity weightbearing and ROM limits
	2–4	Basic transfer skills, wheelchair skills, pregait activities, ambulation training, bath-room mobility, basic ADL. Transfer to rehabilitation facility if slow to progress (see "Rehabilitation," below).
	4–7	Advanced transfer skills, stair climbing, advanced ADL. Equipment procurement. Return home if possible.
	5–40	Home or outpatient physical therapy for household mobility, community mobility, endurance training. Return to work and driving by 6 to 8 weeks postoperatively.
REHABILITATION		
	5–25	Advanced transfer skills, stair climbing, advanced ADL, community mobility, and household mobility with home evaluation. Equipment procurement. Return home. Return to work and driving by 6 to 3 weeks postoperatively.

ROM, range of motion; ADL, activities of daily living.

mobility, and in performing all ADL in their desired environment with the assistance that they have.

The third phase of rehabilitation, typically done on an outpatient basis, concentrates on returning the patient as close as possible to the prefracture state. Emphasis here is placed on strengthening, condition-ing, and higher-level instrumental ADL (e.g., shopping, doing laundry, housekeeping or employment-related activities).

4.   Pelvis fractures are classified as stable or unstable, the distinction usually determines weightbearing sta-

tus. Fractures that involve the pelvic ring in two or more sites, open book fractures, vertical dislocations, or those involving the posterior sacroiliac ligament are inherently unstable and required long periods of weightbearing restrictions. Functionally significant neurologic injury involves the sacral plexus or sciatic nerve injury. Patients with pelvic fractures are at a high risk for heterotopic bone formation.

5.   Posterior dislocations are associated with a number of complications that can be divided into acute and chronic. Acute complications can include infection, rent in posterior hip capsule, glenoid lip avulsion, avascular necrosis of the femoral head, soft tissue or bony fragment joint interposition, and sciatic nerve injury. Chronic complications of hip dislocation include malunion, posttraumatic degenerative joint disease, and recurrent dislocations. Avascular necrosis can occur as late as 2 years after injury. Sciatic nerve injury is present in 10% to 20% of patients with posterior hip dislocation. Sciatic nerve injury is usually neuropraxic, but can leave permanent sequelae in approximately 20% of cases.

6.   Peripheral nerve injury, which can occur as a complication of lower extremity fractures (**Table 45-5**), can have negative functional consequences. Sciatic

Table 45-5.   Lower extremity peripheral nerve injury

Nerve	Injury Site	Physical Findings
Sciatic	Posterior to hip	Hamstring weakness, weak DF and PF
Common peroneal	Piriformis syndrome	Foot drop, toe extension weakness, foot inversion and eversion
	Fibula neck	Sensory deficits over the lower anterolateral leg and dorsum of the foot
Lateral femoral cutaneous	Deep to the inguinal ligament at the anterior superior iliac spine	Pain over the lateral thigh
Tibial	Under the arch of the soleus	Weak deep leg and plantar foot muscles. Sensory deficits over the plantar foot
Tarsal tunnel	Behind the tibial malleolus	Weak plantar muscles and sensory deficits involving the entire plantar skin

DF, dorsiflexion; PF, plantarflexion.

nerve injury can occur with posterior hip dislocation, affecting mostly the peroneal branch. Patients with tibial branch injury can present with weak knee flexion, weak plantar flexion, or dropfoot, if the peroneal branch is injured. The femoral nerve can be involved in pelvic fractures or anterior hip dislocations, causing hip flexion weakness during swing, and knee buckling during the stance phase of gait. The common peroneal nerve could also be injured with fibula neck fractures, resulting in dropfoot. The tibial nerve can be injured with posterior dislocations, resulting in plantar flexion weakness and problems with knee stability and push-off during ambulation.

7. Electrodiagnostics (electromyogram [EMG]) can be used to diagnose injury, predict chances of recovery, and track recovery. Nerve injures can be classified as neurapraxia, axonotmesis, and neurotmesis. Neurapraxia injuries usually result from compression forces causing local myelin injury. EMG might show a conduction block across the compressed segment, but 100% recovery is expected in weeks to months. In axonotmesis, the nerve axon is physically disrupted with preservation of the endoneurium. These nerve injures are caused by pressure or traction and undergo wallerian degeneration. Because the endoneurium remains intact, the nerve will grow back along its original route and an excellent prognosis for recovery is seen. Neurotmesis carries a poor prognosis because the entire nerve and all the connecting tissues are severed, leaving surgical reconnection the only hope of regaining neurologic function.

In the acute period after a nerve injury, the EMG may remain normal (**Table 45-6**). After an injury, degeneration progresses at a rate of 2 mm/hour during the first 3 days after nerve injury. The most proximal muscle might show evidence of denervation (fibrillations) in 3 days, but it might take 4 weeks to see any evidence in distal muscles. EMG is most useful 4 to 5 weeks after injury, unless the goal is to rule out preexisting disease.

IV. Rehabilitation Following Spinal Cord Injury

A. Spinal cord injuries (SCI) can have devastating functional consequences and an impact on multiple organ systems. After SCI, impairment can be seen in the central nervous system (CNS), peripheral nervous system (PNS), skin, respiratory system, bowel, bladder, and musculoskeletal and cardiovascular systems. Early involvement of the rehabilitation team is important to maximize functional outcome. The most important predictors of long-term functional outcome are the level and completeness of injury.

B. The American Spinal Injury Association (ASIA) (see Chapter 15, *Nervous System 2*) neurologic classification system is the most widely used system to classify SCI by

Table 45-6. **Electromyographic time line**

Weeks	Spontaneous Activity	Recruitment	CMAP	NCV	H reflex/ F-wave
1	Normal	Decreased	Normal	Normal	Prolonged or absent
1–4	Increased in paraspinal and proximal muscles with large fibrillation potentials	Decreased >12% poly-phasic large MUP	Low	Slight reduc-tion Normal SNAP	Prolonged or absent
4–12	Proximal and distal show increase insertional activity, fibrillations, and positive sharp waves	Decreased Increase dura-tion and amplitude of MUP and polyphasics	Low	Slightly reduced Normal SNAP	Prolonged or absent
>3 months	Fibrillations with small (<25 mV), complex repetitive discharges Spontaneous activity and PSW may disappear	Increase dura-tion and amplitude of MUP and polyphasics	May re-main low	NCV may remain slightly reduced; SNAP is normal	Prolonged or absent

CMAP, compound muscle action potential; NCV, nerve conduction velocity; MUP, motor unit potential; SNAP, sensory nerve potential; PSW, positive sharp waves.

rehabilitation professional. ASIA classification system is based on motor examination of key muscles and sensory examination. The ASIA score also indicates the level and completeness of injury. A complete injury is one in which is seen an absence of rectal sensation of voluntary rectal motor function.

C. The functional outcome after spinal cord injury depends on the level and completeness of the injury. For complete injuries, or ASIA injuries, prognosis for of function below the level of injury is poor. Prognosis for recovery of motor strength is better when injuries are incomplete, with one study showing 85% of muscles that were manual muscle tested (MMT) at one fifth to two fifths improved to three fifths at 1 year. More than a third of patients with incomplete tetraplegia will be able to ambulate in 1 year.

Most motor recovery occurs in the first 3 months, and generally plateaus after 1 year.

The functional potential is closely linked to the level of injury (**Table 45-7**). Patients with injury level between C3 and C6 can potentially achieve independent mobility in a power wheel chair, but invariably require assistance with transfers and some ADL. Patients with C6 injury can use wrist-driven orthoses to facilitate grip function. The highest level of injury that allows independent living, with the assistance of a manual wheel chair and adaptive equipment, is one at C7. Independent ambulation is possible in highly motivated patients with injuries at T9. These high paraplegics use walkers and knee-ankle-foot orthosis (KAFO), and use their abdominal muscle to achieve lower extremity swing through. Driving is possible in specially adapted vans for patients with C5 injuries. Patients with C7 injuries can independently drive a car with hand controls and are able to put away their own wheel chairs.

D. Neurogenic bowel, which can occur with a CNS injury between the rostral pons and the sacral spinal cord, is characterized by an inability to voluntarily evacuate the bowel or to perceive when the bowel is evacuated. During spinal shock most patients experience diarrhea, but as spinal reflexes and normal rectal tone returns, inability to evacuate becomes apparent. Neurogenic bowel occurs as a result of reduced expulsive force or from anorectal dyssynergia, which is increase in external anal sphincter tone as rectal volume increases. The initial goals of bowel management are to achieve continence and avoid bowel overdistension. Dietary maneuvers to gaining bowel control include maintaining a high-fiber diet and adequate hydration. Medications play an important role in bowel management, along with taking advantage of the gastrocolic reflex. Rectal suppositories containing bisacodyl, polyethylene glycol-based, or sodium bicarbonate preparations given 30 minutes after a meal should achieve colonic emptying within an hour. If evacuation is not achieved, deep digital stimulation can attain desired effect. Oral medications that increase water content of the stool (e.g., docusate sodium) should be used on a twice daily regiment, in combination with at least one daily promotility agent, given 6 to 12 hours before the desired effect. The bowel should be evacuated at least every 48 hours.

E. Neurogenic bladder is seen in patients with traumatic spinal cord injury who are still in spinal shock and have detrusor areflexia, where the bladder has no contractions. The SCI patient soon develops detrusor hyperreflexia, where the bladder contacts with small volume and detrusor sphincter dyssynergia where the detrusor and the external sphincter contract at the same time. To attain continence, intermittent catheterization (ISC) is preferred to indwelling catheter because of the lower risk of infections, kidney stones, and carcinoma. ISC should be done every 4 to 6 hours to maintain volumes <500 mL.

Table 45-7. Functional potential after injury by level

Injury Level	Bed Mobility	Grooming	Feeding	Dressing	Bowel and Bladder Management	Bathing	Wheelchair Transfers	Wheelchair Propulsion	Ambulation
C3–C4	Total dependence	Total dependence	Set up with a BFO and universal cuff with adapters and a long straw	Total dependence	Total dependence	Total dependence	Total dependence	Independent with power chair using mouth or head controls	Non-ambulatory
C5	Minimal assistance	Independent with adapted equipment and set up	Independent with adapted equipment and set up	Assistance for upper body, dependent for lower	Total dependence	Total dependence	Assistance of one person	Independent with power chair on any surface, and indoors surfaces with an adapted manual chair short distances	Non-ambulatory
C6	Independent with equipment	Independent with adapted equipment	Independent	Independent with upper body, dependent with lower	Independent with bowel, assistance with bladder	Assistance for upper and lower body with equipment	Independent using sliding board	Independent with manual chair on level surface using plastic-coated rims. Assistance outdoors and on uneven surfaces	Non-ambulatory

C7	Independent	Independent	Independent	Independent with adaptive equipment	Independent	Independence with equipment	Independent except with floor transfers	Independent with standard manual chair on level surfaces, some assistance with elevation	Non-ambulatory
C8–T8	Independent	Independent	Independent	Independent	Independent	Independent	Independent	Independent	
T9–T12	Independent	Independent	Independent	Independent	Independent	Independent	Independent	Independent	Independent with bilateral KAFO and a walker on level surfaces
T12–L3	Independent	Independent	Independent	Independent	Independent	Independent	Independent	Independent	Independent with bilateral KAFO with lofstands on all surfaces
L4–L5	Independent	Independent	Independent	Independent	Independent	Independent	Independent	Independent	Independent with bilateral AFO, crutches or canes on all surfaces

BFO, Balance forearm orthosis; KAFO, knee ankle foot orthosis; AFO, ankle foot orthosis.

F.   Pulmonary problems haunt SCI patients in all phases of recovery. Atelectasis, pneumonia, and respiratory failure, the most common pulmonary problems after acute SCI, are the leading causes of death in these patients. Rehabilitation interventions consist of aggressive chest PT, postural drainage, and assisted cough (quad cough), in combination with the administration of bronchodilators and mucolytic agents. In most cases, early and frequent upright positioning can help with chest and lung expansion. Supine positioning in quadriplegics, however, allows the abdominal viscera to push up on the diaphragm improving the vital capacity.

G.   Autonomic dysreflexia results from an interruption in the autonomic nervous system below T6 because of loss of modulation sympathetic discharges. Symptoms of autonomic dysreflexia consist of systolic hypertension, bradycardia, pounding headaches, pallor and sweating above the injury level, and complains of nasal congestion, and anxiety. Autonomic dysreflexia can be triggered by any noxious stimulation (e.g., bladder or bowel distension, gallstone), or pain from any source. The definitive treatment for autonomic dysreflexia is to eliminate the irritating source. Immediate measures consist of placing the patient in an upright position and lowering the blood pressure using agents (e.g., transdermal nitroglycerin ointment and intravenous hydralazine).

H.   Immobilization hypercalcemia can occur after an SCI, especially in young men. Symptoms of hypercalcemia include lethargy and abdominal pain. Treatment of immobilization hypercalcemia include mobilization, loop diuretics, saline infusion, and, occasionally, calcitonin.

I.   Orthostatic hypotension results from the failure of normal hemodynamic responses to upright positioning leading to a fall in blood pressure, an increase in heart rate, and feelings of dizziness or lightheadedness. Spinal cord patients are particularly susceptible to this phenomenon because of lost sympathic tone. Treatment includes measures to decrease dependent vascular pooling (e.g., lower extremity ace wrapping and abdominal binding) in combination with slow progression to full upright positioning. A tilting wheelchair allows quicker acclimation to upright position because it allows the patient to be out of bed without being completely upright. Medical maneuvers to treat orthostatic hypotension include liberal salt and water intake, and the use of ephedrine and fludrocortisone.

J.   Heterotopic ossification (HO), extraskeletal deposition of new bone, occurs in both spastic and flaccid paralysis. HO causes pain, limits joint mobility, and can interfere with functional recovery. Symptoms include warmth, swelling, pain with ROM, and loss of joint mobility. It is often mistaken for DVT. Early HO plain x-ray study often misses the new bone growth, but pooling in the third phase of a triple phase bone scan is highly correlative. Elevated alkaline phosphatase can be a metabolic marker of active bone formation in HO. Treatment includes ROM to maintain joint mobility and the early use of bisphosphonates. Disodium etidronate has been shown to be effective at slowing down HO. Surgery, once the HO is mature, can improve joint mobility and enhance function.

K. Central pain is a phenomenon seen in SCI patients. It is usually described as a burning pain below the level of injury, of which the cause is not clear. Drugs that can be effective against central pain include tricyclic antidepressants, carbamazepine, gabapentin, intrathecal morphine (with or without clonidine), and baclofen. Shoulder pain is a common complaint among tetraplegics and, at times, is related to adhesive capsulitis or calcific tendonitis, both of which can be relived by an intraarticular steroid injection and ROM.

L. Spasticity, defined as a velocity-dependent increase in muscle tone, is a consequence of upper motor neuron (UMN) injury, and it can have a significant functional impact. To manage this condition, a clear distinction should be made between other disorders exemplified by resistance to passive movement. A muscle contracture, an anatomic shortening of a muscle, occurs commonly in SCI patients with spasticity, but the resistance to passive stretch is irrespective of the velocity of which the body segment is moved. Unlike spasticity, dystonia, which is often confused for spasticity, occurs with the conspicuous absence of other UMN signs (e.g., hyperreflexia and Babinski response). The hypertonicity seen with Parkinson's disease is characterized by catch and release or "clasp-knife" type phenomenon. Spasticity can cause pain, lead to muscle and joint contractures; interfere with positioning, transfers, and hygiene; and predispose patients to skin breakdown.

The goal of rehabilitation is to control the spasticity and to prevent and restore functional muscle length and joint positioning. In SCI patients, spasticity emerges as spinal shock dissipates. Physical measures that can be used to inhibit spasticity or its effects include prolonged heat, sustained muscle stretch, prolonged ice, and slow, rhythmic activities. The aggressive use of early splinting in functional joint positions is recommended, using low temperature thermoplastic custom splints, and plaster or fiberglass cast. With a few exceptions, medications to treat spasticity are usually targeted toward the γ-aminobutyric acid (GABA) receptors (**Table 45-8**). Baclofen is the usual first-line treatment. The dose should be increased every 3 days until the desired effect is reached, untoward side effects occur, or the maximal dose is reached. In patients where sedation is a problem, dantrolene may be the first therapeutic choice, but the effect of muscle weakness above the level of injury must be considered.

M. Therapeutic procedures used in the treatment of spasticity are either targeted toward the muscle's peripheral motor nerve or the spastic muscle. Selected nerve,

Table 45-8. Commonly used oral antispasticity medications

Medication	Target Receptor	Common Effects	Relative Contra-indications
Baclofen	GABA-B	Sedation, hepatoxicity, lower seizure threshold	Cognitive impairment
Diazepam	GABA-A	Sedation, confusion	History of benzodiazepine abuse
Tizanidine	Alpha-adreno receptors	Sedation, dry mouth, hepatoxicity	Cognitive impairment
Clondine	Alpha-adreno receptors	Sedation, dry mouth, orthostatic hypotension, dysrythmias	Liver disease
Dantrolene	Calcium influx into the sarcoplasmic reticulum	Weakness, hepatoxicity, occasional weakness, hypotension, diarrhea	Liver disease

GABA-A/B, γ-aminobutyric acid; tid, three times daily; bid, twice daily; qid, four times daily.

stimulator-guided, perineural phenol injections directed toward the motor branch of the nerve can be effective in eliminating spasticity. Phenol works by denuding the nerve, which can be permanent. The most common side effect of the procedure, particularly if a mixed nerve or sensory branch is injected, is segmental pain and dysesthesia. Injected botulinum toxin, with or without electromyographic guidance, is taken up in the presynaptic motor neuron and permanently prevents the release of acetylcholine, making the muscle incapable of contracting. Botulinum toxin, type A is often required to get the desired effect. The clinical effects are usually evident in 3 days, peak in 3 weeks, and last for 3 months. The combination of medications, therapeutic injections, and aggressive physical therapy is the best strategy to prevent muscle and joint contractures and restore functional joint positioning. Intrathecal baclofen, delivered by a surgically place programmable pump, can effectively control lower extremity spasticity in recalcitrant cases. Neurosurgical procedures (e.g., myelotomy and dorsal rhizotomy) are also used in selected cases.

N. Venous thromboembolism is extremely prevalent in SCI, occurring in 47% to 60% of patients in the first 2 weeks following the injury. Prophylaxis with external pneumatic compression devices, graduated compression stockings, and low-dose heparin is recommended, unless otherwise contraindicated. Lower molecular weight has been found to be more effective than unfractionated heparin in the prevention of VTE in the SCI population. If heparin is initially contraindicated because of bleeding risk, an intravenous filter may prevent pulmonary embolus, but heparin should be started when the bleeding risk has dissipated because it is still desirable to prevent VTE. VTE prophylaxis is recommend for 3 months in SCI patients.

O. Decubitus ulcers cause tremendous problems for patients with SCI and require fastidious attention to prevent. Tissue ischemia occurs in SCI patients when sustained pressure is applied to insensate skin, particularly over bony prominences. Ulceration can occur in as few as 2 hours if pressure is left unrelieved. Factors that contribute to the formation of ulcers are shear forces, friction forces, moisture, spasticity, poor nutrition, and old age. The most common sites of breakdown in SCI patients are the ischium, sacrum, heels, greater trochanters, and occiput. Rehabilitation efforts to prevent breakdown include frequent position changes and lower extremity splits with relief for the heel. Ideally, lower extremity splints should have a derotation bar that is laterally placed to prevent hip external rotation, avoiding pressure over the greater trochanter. Wheel chairs should be tilt-in-space chairs rather that just reclining to minimize shear forces in the sacral area. Footplates should be set up at a height that does not transfer weight to the ischium but allows this weight to be borne by the thighs. Wheelchairs should always be well fitted and have the appropriate pressure relief cushion. During transfers, patients should be lifted rather than slid to avoid friction forces.

VI. Traumatic Brain Injury

A. Impairments that occur as a result of traumatic brain injury (TBI) can be broadly categorized as physical, cognitive, and neurobehavioral. TBI often occurs in a setting of other multiple traumas, any of which can significantly impair physical functioning. One of the first roles of the rehabilitation team is to understand all the impairments and therapeutically intervene, on the premise of, the sooner a therapeutic plan is in place, the sooner the resolution of the problems. The list of physical and cognitive impairments that can affect function is exhaustive (**Table 45-9**) and may not be evident for some time after the acute hospitalization. Every member of the trauma team should be constantly upgrading the impairment list based on their

Table 45-9. Neurologic impairments

PHYSICAL IMPAIRMENTS

Spasticity	Rigidity	Paresis-pelegia	Ataxia
Tremor	Autonomic dysfunction	Causalgia	Entrapment Neuropathy
Field cuts	Diplopia	Dysphagia	Hearing loss

COGNITIVE IMPAIRMENTS

Arousal	Orientation	Apraxia	Aphasia
Attention	Memory	Agnosia	Abstraction

NEUROBEHAVIORAL DEFICITS

Apathy	Aggressiveness	Emotional lability	Impulsivity
Anxiety	Lack of initiative	Depression	Restlessness
Irritability			

examination of the patient. The physiatric physical examination is a combination of thorough neurologic, musculoskeletal, and mental status findings needed to predict functional recovery and make a comprehensive rehabilitation plan, including the determining the appropriate rehabilitation setting.

B. Making functional prognosis after TBI is important to rehabilitation planning and to helping the patient and family put this catastrophic injury in some contextual framework. Age is inversely related to functional outcome even after the severity of injury is controlled. Other poor prognostic indicators are Glasgow Coma Scale (GCS) score in the first 24 hours of <7 and prolonged comma. The duration of posttraumatic amnesia is inversely related to good functional outcome, with less than one third of patients with >4 weeks of posttraumatic amnesia achieving good recovery. Injury characteristics that portend poor functional outcome are homodynamic instability, absence of cranial nerve responses, decorticate or decerebrate posturing, intracerebral pressure >20 mm, and subdural hematoma with shift. Computed tomography indicators of poor prognosis are temporal lobe lesions with >4 mm of shift and diffuse edema. Magnetic resonance imaging findings correlate poorly with functional outcomes. Normal evoked potentials imply a good functional prognosis, whereas patients with TBI and profoundly abnormal evoked potentials have a 0% probability of good recovery at 1 year.

C. The Coma Patient

The Rancho Los Amigos Scale (RLA) (**Table 45-10**), a description of neurobehavioral recovery based on observation, helps clinicians describe general patterns of behaviors. Patients can pass through these levels slowly, rapidly, or become arrested at one level for a protected period. Coma

**Table 45-10. Rancho Los Amigos levels
of cognitive function**

I	No response	Unresponsive to all stimuli
II	Generalized response	Inconsistent, nonpurposeful
II	Localized response	Inconsistent localized response related to the type of stimuli
IV	Confused-agitated	Disorientated, inappropriate, agitated behavior
V	Confused-inappropriate	Nonagitated, alert, nonpurposeful, responds to simple commands
VI	Confused-appropriate	Goal directed, responds appropriately to task but incorrect
VII	Automatic-appropriate	Robotlike, poor insight and judgment
VIII	Purposeful-appropriate	Carries over new learning, some abstract reasoning difficulties

is defined as a state with lack of awareness or arousal without a sleep wake cycle, and is considered ended when the patient demonstrates some ability to follow commands. **D.** Patients in vegetative states are similar to those in coma states, but these patients have sleep-wake cycles. The so-called "minimally responsive patients" are those who are more responsive than vegetative patients; they might inconsistently follow command, visually tract, and demonstrate goal-directed purposeful movements. Patients who remain in coma or minimally responsive states for a long time require rehabilitation attention for stimulation to prevent some of the secondary effects of immobilization. **E.** The outcome after a prolonged vegetative state is better than might be thought, with one study showing that almost half of the patients were independent in ADL, and another 20% were only partially dependent after being vegetative for 1 month. In fact, 11% were able to resume working in the open job market, whereas 48.6% were engaged in sheltered workshops. Of the study's patients, 70% were considered socially integrated, enabling them to enjoy a reasonable quality of life. Most patients in a prolonged vegetative state who progress beyond that state do so in the first 3 months. **F.** The rehabilitation priority for vegetative patients is to get them to the stage where they can benefit from a full physical, cognitive, and neurobehavioral rehabilitation program. To get them ready for rehabilitation, emphasis is placed on activities that stimulate recovery, prevent contractures, optimize nutrition, and keep the patient medically stable and infection free. Medical management begins with the evaluation of all drugs that the patient is on and eliminating all unnecessary drugs, particularly any potential sedating ones. Major tranquilizers and other catecholamine receptor-blocking agents can impair motor recovery after TBI, as well as attention, concentration, and memory. Haloperidol can have a negative affect on motor learning and recovery after TBI. Other commonly used drugs (e.g., metoclopramide and H_2 blockers) can cause sedation and a substitute found for them or discontinued. Antispasticity medications (e.g., baclofen and tizanidine) should be discouraged because of their hypoarousal effects. Epileptic drugs, including benzodiazepines, should be discontinued, if at all possible. The next major element in the medical management of the vegetative or comatose patients is to perform "trails" of neurostimulants (**Table 45-11**). Dopaminergic agonist has been found to have some efficacy in facilitating emergence from the vegetative state. Amphetamine type stimulants (e.g., methylphenidate) and the narcolepsy drug, modafinil, can have some efficacy. Vegetative patients can have unregulated sleep-wake cycles with daytime sedation and nighttime arousal. Proper sleep hygiene is encouraged, and may be assisted short-acting hypnotics (e.g. zolpidem and choral hydrate). Environmental factors (e.g., quiet, uninterrupted time at night and sunlight early in the morning) might help to regulate the circadian rhythm.

Table 45-11. Drugs to treat hypoarousal following traumatic brain injury

Drug Name	Side Effects	Action
Amantadine	Nausea, dizziness, insomnia	Dopamine agonist
Bromocriptine	Hypotension, confusion, nausea, dizziness, Raynaud's phenomenon	Dopamine agonist
Carbidopa or levodopa	Gastrointestinal upset, dizziness	Dopamine agonist
Methylphenidate	Insomnia, hypertension, anorexia, anxiety, akathisia	Central nervous system stimulant
Modafinil	Arrhythmias, headache, nausea, insomnia	Unknown

G. The incidence of early seizures following traumatic closed head injury (CHI) is 5% and 35% to 50% with penetrating head injury. Anticonvulsant prophylaxis can successfully reduce the incidence of early seizures in CHI, but the protective effects might not extend beyond 1 week. Anticonvulsants have been shown to impair cognitive functioning and their use is discouraged in CHI beyond the first days, unless the patient develops actual seizures.

H. Patients with mild TBI comprise most of the hospitalizations for brain trauma. Mild TBI is defined as any traumatically induced disruption of brain function. Evidence of disruption could include altered mental state, GCS of 13 to 15, loss of consciousness for <30 minutes, and posttraumatic amnesia of no more than 24 hours. Most of the patients who experience mild TBI recover, but a few can become severely disabled. After mild TBI, patients can have protracted experiences of headache, neck pain, occipital neuritis, dizziness, vertigo, memory loss, difficulty concentrating, and other cognitive dysfunction. Patients with mild TBI can experience mood swings, depression, anxiety, irritability, and personality changes. Anyone who presents to a trauma center with symptoms of a concussion should be given information about the signs of posttraumatic concussion. Patients with persistent symptoms should seek the attention of a physiatrist or a neurologist familiar with mild TBI. From a rehabilitation prospective, the primary goal is arresting the symptoms of mild TBI, which often require a multidisciplinary team approach. Team members can include a physiatrist, speech cognitive therapists, psychologist, psychiatrist, and physical and occupational therapist.

I. Agitation (RLA level IV) in patients with TBI is a challenging problem. On the one hand, agitated and restless behavior is a natural stage of the recovery; on the other hand, these behaviors might disrupt medical care. From a rehabilitation point of view, it is preferred that agitation and restlessness be managed by environmental and behavior interventions rather than sedation, unless the medical stability of the patient is being threatened. The initial phase of management of these patients is to eliminate any potential irritants (e.g., catheters, unnecessary lines, nasogastric tubes, tracheal tubes, and restraints). The environment should not be overstimulating. If possible, use silent alarms, place patients in private rooms away from noise, and avoid multiple visitors, multiple simultaneous conversations, and background noise when communicating with the patient. If possible, use a veil bed and glove mitts, rather than restraints on wrist or ankle. Medical management starts by eliminating or substituting for drugs acting on the CNS that could potentially cause confusion and sedation. Neuropharmacologic agents may be required to treat agitation. In selecting the agent, consider the negative effect on functional, including cognitive, recovery. Benzodiazepines and major neuroleptics are typically not recommended because it is believed that they negatively affect recovery of the injured brain. Stimulants are among the class of drugs most commonly suggested to treat agitated patients. (**Table 45-12**). Some evidence supports the use of tricyclic antidepressants for the treatment of the agitated patient with TBI, which might work by increasing cortical arousal, thereby decreasing confusion and agitation. Buspirone is a non-benzodiazepine anxiolytic agent that can treat agitation without having a negative impact on cognitive recovery. Other classes of drugs that can be used to treat the agitated patient with TBI include beta-blockers, antiepileptics, serotonin reuptake inhibitors, and lithium.

J.   Cognitive impairment is a common consequence of TBI (**Table 45-9**), with deficits in arousal, attention, and memory. Neuropsychological testing helps the rehabilitation form a comprehensive picture of brain functioning. A variety of test batteries are available to examine various aspects of attention, memory, language, visual-spatial abilities, and executive functioning. A multimodal interdisciplinary treatment plan can be formulated. Treatment strategies include the use of neurostimulants (e.g., methylphenidate) and modafinil in conjunction with cognitive remediation therapies.

K.   The proper management of spasticity has significant functional significance. Spasticity can cause pain, increase metabolic demand, and lead to joint contracture, skin breakdown, and pain. The rationale for selecting antispasticity drugs for the patient with TBI differs from that used in managing SCI-related spasticity. Dantrolene is the preferred initial choice to manage increased tone in the patients with TBI because of its peripheral action and lack of sedating effects. As in the SCI population, aggressive ROM, early rigid casting, splinting in functional joint positions, and neuromuscular blocking agents are employed. Patients should be placed in positions that encourage the breaking up of the dominating synergistic pattern. For instance, in patients with severe trunk and lower body extension, positions that allow hip and knee flexion (e.g., sitting) are encouraged.

Table 45-12.   Medications to manage agitation in patients with traumatic brain injury

Medication
Nortriptyline
Methylphenidate
Amantadine
Buspirone
Carbamazepine
Morphine
Propranolol
Risperidone

VII. Burns: Rehabilitation Interventions and Considerations

    A. Burn injuries lead to loss of physical function because of their effect on joint, skin, and muscle mobility; on peripheral nerve injury; and on heterotopic ossification. Endurance and activity tolerance can also be affected by lung injuries and immobility related deconditioning.

    B. The emphasis on rehabilitation of the patient with burns is to preserve or restore functional joint mobility by influencing the scar tissue. Early ambulation, burned segment mobility, and static and dynamic bracing are essential to the rehabilitation effort. The major splints used in the acute phase are resting hand, dorsiflexion, and knee extension and elbow extension splints. Ambulation is sometimes delayed to allow lower extremity skins grafts to vascularize. Once wounds heal, aggressive efforts must be made to limit the amount and consistency of the scar tissue by using custom-fitted elasticized garments, silicone, and splinting.

    C. Both localized and generalized peripheral neuropathies (**Table 45-13**) occur following burn injuries, which can affect functional recovery. Some localized nerve injuries result from pressure on exposed nerves and, therefore, can be prevented.

VIII. Rehabilitation in the Intensive Care Unit

    A. Patients in the intensive care unit (ICU) present special rehabilitation challenges because of their inherent medical instability. Nevertheless, rehabilitation professionals are important part of the ICU trauma team. The

Table 45-13. Peripheral nerve injuries in patients with burns

Nerve	Mechanism	Intervention
Brachial plexus	Compressed between the clavicle and the first rib when the arm is abducted	Supine patients positioned in 15 degrees of arm horizontal adduction
Suprascapular	Stretched by hyperprotracted shoulder positions	Stabilized scapula
Radial	Compressed in spiral grove, wrist restraints	Avoid compression
Median	Aggressive hyperextension at the wrist	Caution with range of motion and splinting
Peroneal	Pressure over the fibula head, pressure from braces, dressings, body weight	Avoid pressure, trochanter roll to prevent hip external rotation, a laterally placed derotation bar on ankle splints

rehabilitation goals in the ICU are to prevent the negative effect immobility, maintain functional anatomy, and initiate functional training at the earliest possible time. Therapeutic interventions most often delivered in the ICU setting are joint ROM, positioning, and upper and lower extremity splinting. In appropriate patients, bed mobility training, sitting balance, strengthening exercises, and progressive ambulation training can be performed. Speech services can be delivered for cognitive, speech, and swallowing assessments, and interventions (e.g., instruction with communication boards in nonverbal patients). The ICU physician or the physiatrist should set strict homodynamic parameters to be followed by the therapist in the performance of therapeutic activities.

B.   Severe muscle weakness in critically ill ICU patients is a very challenging rehabilitation problem. Critical illness polyneuropathy and critical illness myopathy are two entities that have been described to explain most of these cases marked by difficulty in weaning from the ventilator.

C.   Critical illness polyneuropathy is seen in a setting of multiorgan failure typically involving sepsis and encephalopathy, flaccid paralysis, and loss of tendon reflexes. EMG findings show evidence of sensory and motor axonal loss without evidence of demyelination.

D.   Critical illness myopathy is most often seen a setting of high dose corticosteroid use, and nondepolarizing blocking agents. Small polyphasic motor unit potentials and a robust interference pattern on EMG, with normal conduction studies, might help distinguish myopathy form neuropathy. Aggressive physical and occupational therapy for strengthening and mobility training are important to functional recovery.

SELECTED READING

ASI Association. *International standards for neurological and functional classification of spinal cord injuries.* Chicago: American Spinal Injury Association, 1996.

Barohn RJ, et al. Prolonged paralysis due to nondepolarizing neuromuscular blocking agents and corticosteroids. *Muscle Nerve* 1994: 17(6):647–654.

Cardenas DD. Current concepts of rehabilitation of spinal cord injury patients. *Spine: State of the Art Review* 1999;13(3):583.

Dumitru D. Reaction of the peripheral nervous system to injury. In: Dumitru D, ed. *Electrodiagnostic medicine.* Philadelphia: Hanley & Belfus, 1994:341–383.

Feeney DM, Gonzalez A, Law WA. Amphetamine, haloperidol, and experience interact to affect rate of recovery after motor cortex injury. *Science* 1982;217(4562):855–857.

Groswasser Z, Sazbon L. Outcome in 134 patients with prolonged posttraumatic unawareness. Part 2: Functional outcome of 72 patients recovering consciousness. *J Neurosurg* 1990;72(1):81–84.

Gutmann L. Critical illness neuropathy and myopathy. *Arch Neurol* 1999;56(5): 527–528.

Helm PA, Fisher SV, Cromes Jr G F. Burn injury rehabilitation. In: Delisa A, ed. *Rehabilitation medicine principles and practice.* Philadelphia: Lippincott-Raven, 1998.

Holbrook TL, et al. Outcome after major trauma: discharge and 6-month follow-up results from the Trauma Recovery Project. *J Trauma* 1998;45(2):315–323; discussion 323–324.

Katz DI, Alexander MP. Traumatic brain injury. Predicting course of recovery and outcome for patients admitted to rehabilitation. *Arch Neurol* 1994;51(7):661–670.

Merli GJ, et al. Deep vein thrombosis: prophylaxis in acute spinal cord injured patients. *Arch Phys Med Rehabil* 1988;69(9):661–664.

The Multi-Society Task Force on PVS. Medical aspects of the persistent vegetative state (2). *N Engl J Med* 1994;330(22):1572–1579.

Nesathurai S. *The rehabilitation of people with spinal cord injury.* Malden: Blackwell Science, 2000:95–101.

Pullium GF. Splinting and positioning. In: Fisher SV, Helm PA, eds. *Comprehensive rehabilitation of burns.* Baltimore: Williams & Wilkins, 1984:64–95.

Shin DY, et al. Evoked potential assessment: utility in prognosis of chronic head injury. *Arch Phys Med Rehabil* 1989;70(3):189–193.

Siragusa S, et al. Low-molecular-weight heparins and unfractionated heparin in the treatment of patients with acute venous thromboembolism: results of a meta-analysis. *Am J Med* 1996;100(3):269–277.

Staas WE, et al. Spinal cord injury and spinal cord injury medicine. In: Delisa A, Gans BM, eds. *Rehabilitation medicine: principles and practice,* 3rd ed. Philadelphia: Lippincott-Raven, 1998:1259–1291.

Stein J. Spasticity. In: Frontera W, Sliver JK, eds. *Essentials of physical medicine and rehabilitation.* Philadelphia: Hanley & Belfus, 2002:743–752.

Temkin NR, et al. A randomized, double-blind study of phenytoin for the prevention of post-traumatic seizures. *N Engl J Med* 1990; 323(8):497–502.

Waters RL, et al. Motor and sensory recovery following incomplete paraplegia. *Arch Phys Med Rehabil* 1994;75(1):67–72.

Whyte J, et al., Effects of methylphenidate on attentional function after traumatic brain injury. A randomized, placebo-controlled trial. *Am J Phys Med Rehabil* 1997;76(6):440–450.

Young B, Rapp RP, Norton JA, et al. Early prediction of outcome in head-injured patients. *J Neurosurg* 1981;54(3):300–303.

46

Medicolegal Considerations and Duties

Brett D. Pangburn, Esq, Laura L. Stephens, Esq, Carolyn V. Wood, Esq, and Robert L. Sheridan, MD

I. Introduction

Prominent—and often complex—legal issues arise daily in the typical trauma unit. In addition to requirements imposed on emergency medicine practitioners by federal law, states also impose additional requirements that vary from jurisdiction to jurisdiction. Whereas the focus of any trauma unit, of course, should be on patient care, it is important that all emergency room healthcare providers have a basic understanding of the legal requirements underlying emergency room care, as well as when it is appropriate to consult with legal counsel.

The following is an overview of the major legal considerations facing a trauma unit, including several vignettes illustrating some of the legal concepts that are presented.

II. Treatment Issues

A. Duty to Treat in General

In general, the law assumes that people who are in need of emergency care want to be—and should be—treated. Of note, special consideration must be given to patients who are unable or unwilling to consent to treatment (see **Sections III and IV below**).

B. Emergency Medical Treatment and Active Labor Act

The Emergency Medical Treatment and Active Labor Act (EMTALA) is a federal law that was enacted to prevent hospitals from denying emergency treatment to patients who lack the means to pay for it (sometimes called "patient dumping"). EMTALA now applies to all individuals who come to a hospital's emergency department requesting an examination or treatment for a medical condition (or where the individual's representative makes such a request on his or her behalf). Legally, the request is implied when a prudent lay person observer would believe, based upon the individual's appearance or behavior, that the individual needs examination or treatment of a medical condition. EMTALA also applies to an individual who comes to other areas of the hospital requesting an examination or treatment for an emergency medical condition (or who has that request made for him or her, or where such request is legally implied if a prudent lay person observer would believe, based upon the individual's appearance or behavior, that the individual needs examination or treatment for an emergency medical condition). EMTALA is one of the most important laws regulating the behavior of physicians and hospitals treating emergency patients. It is constantly being interpreted by courts and regulators. Emergency department staff need to keep up to date on amendments to EMTALA, as well as newly issued agency interpretations.

EMTALA requires that hospitals providing emergency care (1) must provide an appropriate medical screening examination within the capability of its emergency department to patients who seek care (as described above) (or who are in active labor) to determine if the patient has an emergency medical condition, and (2) if the patient is found to have an emergency medical condition, the hospital must then treat the patient within its capabilities until the patient's condition has stabilized to the point that he or she can be discharged or transferred to another hospital. Additionally, a hospital cannot delay screening or stabilizing treatment to inquire about an individual's method of payment or insurance status or to obtain preauthorization under managed care plans. Transfers of patients with unstabilized medical conditions can take place under two conditions:

1. The patient (or representative) requests the transfer. In this case, the physician must inform the patient (or representative) of the patient's medical condition, the hospital's obligation to treat the patient, and the risks and benefits of transfer. The patient (or representative) must make the transfer request in writing and indicate that the patient is aware of the risks and benefits of the transfer.
2. The treating physician determines, based on the hospital's capacity (staffing and/or facilities), that the hospital is unable to meet the patient's needs. In this case, the physician must certify that the medical benefits reasonably expected from the medical care to be provided at the receiving hospital outweigh the risks of being transferred, including a summary of the risks and benefits on which that conclusion is based.

In all cases of transfer, the transferring hospital must first, within its capacity, provide treatment that minimizes the risks of transfer to the patient (and to the unborn child if the patient is in labor). Further, the transferring hospital must also (1) confirm that the receiving hospital has available space, personnel qualified to treat the patient, and has agreed to accept the patient; (2) send the receiving hospital all medical records that relate the patient's emergency condition; and (3) ensure that the transfer is done by qualified personnel and using appropriate equipment.

Violations of EMTALA are serious matters and can result in fines and exclusion of the hospital from the Medicare and Medicaid programs. Physicians who violate EMTALA can also be subject to fines. In addition, EMTALA provides for civil actions against hospitals by individuals who suffer personal harm as a direct result of the hospital's violation of an EMTLA requirement. The individual harmed by the EMTALA violation can sue the hospital in federal court for damages that are available for personal injury under the laws of the state in which the hospital is located. Finally, a hospital that receives a transferred patient who the hospital believes was transferred in violation of EMTALA must report the violation to the Centers for Medicare and Medicaid Services.

It should be noted that a physician who violates EMTALA does not necessarily commit malpractice nor is a failure to detect a medical condition during an appropriate screening examination a per se violation of EMTALA (although it can be malpractice). EMTALA was written to ensure access to emergency medical care; a hospital and its staff fulfill their obligations by providing the required screening examination and stabilizing treatment (or an appropriate transfer) if an emergency medical condition is found. Malpractice laws, on the other hand, address the quality of medical care (see **Section XII** below).

HYPOTHETICAL SITUATION: THE DUTY TO TREAT

Facts: A patient is brought to a hospital emergency room by ambulance after suffering a massive stroke. The emergency room physician stabilizes her condition, and on the instruction of the patient's private physician, transfers the patient to a second hospital. A receptionist at the second hospital tells the patient's family that the patient cannot be treated there because the patient's health plan calls for a different hospital. The family tells the second hospital that they will pay for the cost of care. The emergency department personnel at the second hospital subsequently refuse to treat the patient, reiterating that the patient's health insurance plan prevents them from doing so. The patient is eventually transferred to a third hospital (which is covered by the patient's health insurance plan). At the third hospital, the patient dies of a second stroke. Did the second hospital violate EMTALA?

Analysis: Yes. Although the patient's medical condition was stable when she arrived at the second hospital, she subsequently developed difficulties that her family perceived as being an emergency. When patient's family members requested the assistance of the second hospital's emergency department staff, the staff refused, saying that the patient's insurance would not cover the treatment. Because the family had requested medical assistance for the perceived emergency, the second hospital had a duty under EMTALA to provide the patient with a screening examination and appropriate treatment (or transfer).

III.   Requirement of Informed Consent
A.   Informed Consent in General

One of a patient's most basic rights is the ability to make his or her own decisions concerning medical treatment—up to and including the refusal of treatment. Ideally, informed consent requires that the physician, before treatment, perform the following:

1.   Explain the patient's condition in terms that the patient can understand.

2.   Provide the patient with relevant information about the recommended course of treatment and other treatment alternatives (including the purpose of a particular treatment, known risks, and the likelihood of success for each, as well as the consequences of no treatment).

3. Allow the patient an opportunity to ask questions, as well as sufficient time to consider the proposed treatment.

B. Obtaining Informed Consent

The responsibility of obtaining a patient's informed consent rests with the clinician performing the particular treatment or procedure, and should be documented through a consent form signed by the patient. At a minimum, the physician should make a note in the patient's medical record concerning the patient's informed consent to the proposed treatment, and include any unique circumstances of the consent.

Although obtaining informed consent can be challenging in the context of a busy trauma unit, it remains a crucial part of a patient's care. Where, however, an emergency situation exists, the patient is unconscious, or does not clearly have the capacity to give informed consent to medical treatment (and no proxy, family member, or guardian is immediately available for consultation) a trauma unit should proceed with the necessary medical treatment.

1. Determining a Patient's Ability to Give Informed Consent

To give informed consent, a patient must understand the following:

    a. The diagnosis

    b. Proposed medical treatment and alternatives

    c. Nature and consequences of his or her decision to accept or reject the proposed treatment

The treating physician must make the initial decision regarding whether a patient has the mental capacity to consent to medical treatment. If a patient's competency is unclear, and time permits, the patient should be evaluated by a specialist such as a psychologist and/or a neurologist. A trauma unit should have procedures in place, consistent with state law, addressing competency determinations for patients. Likewise, procedures must be established for handling patients who are unable to give informed consent because of an emergency situation, youth, or mental illness.

2. Incompetent Patients

A patient who is mentally incompetent cannot rationally give informed consent to medical treatment, nor can that patient rationally refuse such treatment. Because a person can be impaired temporarily by alcohol, drugs, or a physical or mental condition that dissipates over time, it is possible that a person is competent at one time but not at another. Importantly, so long as a patient understands the proposed treatment and the consequences of a personal decision, that person is considered competent—even where the reasons for the decision appear unreasonable, foolish, or irrational, and even where healthcare providers may disagree with the patient's decision. Where, however, a patient does not understand the consequences of his or her decision, that patient will usually be found to be incompetent for purposes of informed consent and, thus, will require a surrogate decision maker to make medical care decisions on that person's behalf (see **Section III. B.** below).

3.   Consent Issues Concerning Minors and "Emancipated" Minors

A minor, defined in most states as a person under 18 years of age, does not posses the same rights as an adult regarding consent to medical treatment. Consent, therefore, typically must be obtained from the child's parent or guardian. In an emergency situation where a minor requires medical care and the child's parent or guardian cannot be reached, the emergency room physician should go forward with the necessary treatment.

As a child moves closer to the age of majority, however, the child's right to make medical care decisions increases vis-à-vis the parents or guardian. Some states have determined that minors who are "emancipated" (or "mature") can make their own personal decisions, including decisions about their own medical care. A child may be considered an *emancipated minor* when that child's lifestyle and lack of parental control render him or her an adult for purposes of medical care decision making. Factors suggesting that a minor is emancipated may include the following:

   a.   If the minor is close to the age of majority, lives away from home and is managing own affairs
   b.   If the minor is a parent
   c.   If the minor is pregnant (or believes herself to be pregnant)
   d.   If the minor is married, divorced, or widowed
   e.   If the minor is serving in the armed forces or has graduated from high school

Where a minor makes credible representations to an emergency room physician that he or she is emancipated from parents, the physician, after considering the particular facts and circumstances of the child's case, may determine that it is appropriate to obtain informed consent directly from the emancipated minor. When a finding is made that that a minor is emancipated, the physician should note this, as well as the criteria supporting this determination, in the patient's chart.

C.   Decision-Making on Behalf of an Incompetent Patient

Where a determination is made that a patient is incompetent to give informed consent for medical treatment, the healthcare facility should look for written evidence expressing the patient's intent regarding healthcare and for an appropriate person to give substituted informed consent on the incompetent patient's behalf. Again, it is critical that a trauma unit establish policies and procedures for addressing situations where a person is incompetent for purposes of medical decision-making.

1.   Advanced Directives

Many states allow an adult patient or emancipated minor to give advance instructions on how he or she would like healthcare decisions to be made by others in the event that the patient is rendered incompetent. Advanced healthcare directions can be given through a *living will,* whereby the patient specifies in a signed declaration (made while that person still had capacity to make medical care decisions) what types of treatment he or she does or does not want to receive and under what circumstances. A commonly seen advanced directive is a *do not resuscitate* (DNR) order, which is an accepted practice in most states. Some states will also give consideration to less formal expressions of a patient's wishes regarding healthcare (e.g., statements about medical care expressed to family members or friends made when the patient was competent). The result of a living will, DNR or other evidence of a patient's wishes regarding medical treatment is that healthcare decisions are made by the incompetent patient based on that patient's previously expressed intentions. Additionally, most states also allow a patient to appoint a *healthcare proxy,* whereby the patient, while competent, authorizes a person or persons (in writing) as his or her agent to make medical care decisions on his or her behalf if the patient ever becomes incompetent.

In the event that a patient is determined to be incompetent and informed consent is required, the treating physician in the emergency room should confirm whether the patient has completed an advanced directive, and note this fact in the patient's medical record. If an advanced directive is present, the treating physician should follow such a document unless a court order instructs the healthcare facility to do otherwise or a reasonable basis exists for questioning the document's legitimacy.

2.   Decision-Making by a Patient's Spouse, Next of Kin, or Caretaker

Where an incompetent patient requiring emergency care has no advanced directives regarding the medical care at issue, the trauma unit should look to the patient's spouse, next of kin, primary caretaker, or legal guardian to make healthcare decisions for the patient. Generally, a spouse who is not separated or divorced from the patient is given precedence over a patient's next of kin for medical care decisions, and a person who has secured legal guardianship over the patient's medical care decisions will have decision-making authority that supersedes all others (unless a court document specifies otherwise).

Absent a healthcare proxy or guardianship, determining who has decision-making authority over an

incompetent patient's medical care can be complicated by factors such as separated spouses, children
and siblings who have been out of contact with the patient for a long time, and family members or guardians
who disagree over what is best for the patient. Dis-
putes between family members over an incompetent
patient's care often arise and it may be unclear who
has authority to make medical decisions on behalf of
the patient. It is important, therefore, that an emergency room have a person available (e.g., social
worker) who can meet with family members, obtain
the opinions of key family members who may have
been left out of the decision-making process, and
assist the family in reaching a consensus regarding
an incompetent patient's care. It may also be appropriate to suggest to those who disagree with a patient's surrogate decision-maker that such person
seek legal guardianship (as discussed in next sections). Of course, in an emergency situation where it
is unclear who has decision-making authority for an
incompetent patient, or family members disagree over
what medical care is appropriate, the trauma unit
should proceed with medically necessary treatment.

3.   Judicial Resolution

Unless an emergency exists, a trauma unit cannot
proceed to treat an incompetent patient without the
consent of an appropriate third party. Where an appropriate surrogate cannot be located to make medical
care decisions on behalf of an incompetent patient,
the hospital should have a process in place for contacting legal counsel to discuss the necessity of obtaining a legally appointed guardian for the patient.
Likewise, a party seeking control over an incompetent patient's medical treatment decisions may also
seek legal guardianship of the patient.

A guardianship proceeding involves presenting
evidence to a judge (or court-appointed investigator)
that a patient is incompetent to consent to medical
treatment, and that a guardian who can make such
medical decisions on the patient's behalf should be
appointed. Depending on the state, a court may itself
make medical decisions for the patient (which the
guardian is directed to carry out), applying either a
substituted judgment test (i.e., a subjective analysis
where the court determines what the patient, if competent, would have decided under the particular circumstances) or a *best interests* test (i.e., an objective
test where the court determines what is in the patient's
best interest). In an emergency situation wherein no
legally authorized agent or next of kin is available
and there is no time to obtain a guardianship for the
incompetent patient, the emergency room should provide the required medical treatment.

Sometimes uncertainty exists to whether the patient's need for care is emergent, yet not enough time

exists to follow the steps outlined above to obtain a legally authorized decision-maker. Common sense and good medical practice would dictate providing medical treatment if delaying treatment might result in substantial harm to the patient.

HYPOTHETICAL SITUATION: INFORMED CONSENT

Facts: A young woman claiming to be a baby sitter enters the emergency room with a 13 year-old girl, Brittany, who has severely injured the fingers on her right hand as a result of a skateboarding accident. An initial evaluation indicates that several of Brittany's fingers are beyond repair; meanwhile Brittany is screaming "DON'T TAKE MY FINGERS!" It is likely that an amputation of one or more fingers will be required. The baby sitter is visibly shaken and offers little help in locating Brittany's parents or in describing how the accident occurred.

Analysis: Here, the patient is a minor and presents no evidence of *emancipation* that would otherwise render her competent to make her own medical care decisions. If time permits, the treating physician should speak with Brittany and her baby sitter to try to locate a parent or guardian who can give consent to treat and, if necessary, amputate Brittany's fingers. If her parents cannot be contacted and Brittany's health would be seriously threatened by such a delay, the emergency room physicians should proceed with the necessary medical treatment (despite Brittany's strong objections). The treating physician should be sure to note in Brittany's medical record that she is a minor and, thus, unable to give informed consent and, if time allowed, that an attempt was made to contact a family member or guardian before proceeding with the required emergency treatment

IV. Patients Who Refuse Medical Treatment
   A. A Patient's Right to Refuse Medical Treatment
   Rooted in the right to privacy is the right of a competent adult or emancipated minor patient to refuse treatment—even if the patient will die without it, and even if the patient's decision is contrary to that of family members, the trauma unit staff, or both. If a patient refuses medical care, the treating physician should (1) confirm that the patient is competent and (2) determine the patient's reasons for refusing treatment to be sure that the decision is informed. Just as documenting informed consent is important, it is also important that a patient's refusal of medical treatment is recorded in the medical record, which, at a minimum, should include that the patient refused treatment after being advised of the consequences.

   In an emergency situation where doubt exists about the patient's mental capacity or whether the patient has had the opportunity to make an informed decision, emergency treatment should be given until the person's mental competency can be definitively determined and, if possible, informed consent can be obtained.
   B. Limits Placed on a Patient's Ability to Refuse Medical Treatment
   Courts have imposed limitations on a patient's "right to die" where another individual would be harmed by a patient's

refusal of treatment, and have ordered treatment of a patient in certain instances (e.g., ordering a patient to have a blood transfusion where the patient's minor children would be left without a caretaker and, thus, dependent on the state if the parent died). Two particular dilemmas—Jehovah's Witnesses and a parent who refuses treatment on behalf of a minor child—are discussed in further detail below.

1. Patients Refusing Blood Transfusions or Blood Products

Some patients may choose to refuse blood transfusion and any blood products based on religious grounds (e.g., Jehovah's Witnesses). It is important that an emergency room have established policies for handing such situations. Although, in general, competent adult patients can refuse medical treatment (even where death will result), exceptions to this rule have been recognized where a parent's refusal of a blood transfusion would cause minor children to become wards of the state. In such situations, it may be appropriate for healthcare providers to seek a judicial order authorizing the blood transfusion, if time permits. Of note, courts have allowed Jehovah's Witnesses who were parents to refuse blood where it was demonstrated that the children would be cared for after the parent's death.

2. Parents Refusing Medical Treatment on Behalf of Minor Children

Although parents generally have great latitude concerning the care and raising of their children, a parent (or guardian) does not posses an absolute right to refuse medical treatment on a minor's behalf. A court can find that the interests of the child and the state override the parents' ability to make medical care decisions for their child. Courts have consistently concluded that a parent cannot refuse life-sustaining treatment on behalf of a child where the refusal would be fatal to the child and where the child's prognosis with the proposed treatment is good. Likewise, courts are more likely to order that a child receive medical treatment over the parents' objections where the treatment at issue has a high likelihood of benefit and relatively low risks (e.g., a blood transfusion) and where the child at issue is young and not involved in the decision-making process. Additionally, where a parent or guardian's refusal of treatment for a child poses a danger to the child, a state's child welfare laws can be triggered, requiring the trauma unit to contact a child welfare agency to evaluate the situation (and possibly remove the child from the parent or guardian's custody).

Procedures established in advance are essential for emergency situations where a parent or guardian is refusing treatment on behalf of a child. A healthcare facility may find it necessary to obtain a court order permitting a physician to proceed with the necessary treatment or may need to seek intervention from a child welfare protection agency.

HYPOTHETICAL SITUATION:
REFUSAL OF MEDICAL TREATMENT

Facts: Steve, age 14, is brought into the emergency room by his 17-year-old sister, Andrea. Steve claims that he has severe pain in his left leg. After removing a series of bandages from Steve's leg, the treating physician observes a large wound that has become gangrenous. The physician believes that amputation of Steve's leg is required to prevent the spread of infection. Steve's parents are contacted and, on arriving at the hospital, they immediately request that the staff only change the bandages on Steve's leg, claiming, "God will take care of little Steve, not this hospital." Despite the treating physician explaining the recommended course of treatment to Steve's parents, they remain unwavering in their belief that prayer, rather than medical care, is the answer. Steve is fearful and immature, and defers to his parents' wishes. What should the hospital do?

Analysis: The issue here is whether Steve's parents have the right to refuse treatment on his behalf. Because Steve is a minor, and exhibits no signs of emancipation, his parents would normally have medical decision-making authority on his behalf. Where, however, a child's welfare is threatened, the parents' decision-making authority regarding their child can be suspended. If time permits, the treating physician should arrange a meeting with the parents (and perhaps include another physician for a second opinion) to again explain the need for the amputation, as well as the consequences to Steve of not having the operation. Moreover, in most states, healthcare providers are required to report instances of suspected child abuse and negligent child care to the state's child welfare protection agency. Despite being based on sincere spiritual beliefs, Steve's parents' denial of critical medical care to their child clearly fits under this category. Steve's parents, therefore, should be advised that their failure to authorize necessary medical treatment would result in the hospital notifying the state's child welfare protection agency (who may then seek to intervene on Steve's behalf). If the parents continue to refuse treatment, and time permits, the hospital can also contact its legal counsel to seek an emergency court order to proceed with the amputation. If, however, the amputation must take place immediately to save Steve's life, the hospital should document the circumstances of Steve's case and proceed with the surgery.

V. Autopsies

In normal circumstances, a healthcare facility must obtain the consent of a patient or the appropriate family member or guardian before undertaking an autopsy. Informed consent applies to obtaining permission for an autopsy. It, therefore, should be explained to the patient, family member, or guardian that during the autopsy photographs may be taken of the deceased patient and that organs will be kept for analysis, as well as whether any removed tissue will be used for research. Where, however, a deceased patient has suffered unexplained injuries or serious trauma, consent of the patient's family or guardian is not required for a state medical examiner to perform an autopsy. In such a situation, the physician should explain to the deceased patient's family that the trauma unit is required by law to contact a state medical examiner, and that it is then up to the medical examiner whether an autopsy will be performed.

VI.   Organ and Tissue Donation

All states have adopted some form of the Uniform Anatomical Gifts Act, which allows a person to make a gift of all or part of his or her body at death. A deceased patient's family can also make the anatomical gift, so long as the patient did not indicated an intention to the contrary prior to death. Because of federal law requirements, states typically have organ donor laws requiring healthcare facilities to (1) develop a procedure for identifying potential organ donors; (2) ask the deceased patient's family whether the patient had authorized organ donations; and (3) inform the deceased patient's family of the option to donate the patient's organs if the patient did not already do so or expressed a contrary intention. Of note, these rules generally do not apply where the deceased patient's organs are not suitable for clinical transplantation or where the request for donation would create great emotional stress on the deceased patient's family.

VII.   Confidentiality of Patient Information

A.   Duty of Confidentiality in General

Patients have rights and privileges with regard to confidentiality of medical information. Because emergency room patients often present exceptional circumstances, staff must understand the general rules of confidentiality so they can determine when to disclose information or when to keep even the fact of the patient's presence in the emergency department a secret to safeguard a patient.

The general rule is that patients have a right to confidentiality of their medical information. Communications between a patient and a medical care provider are confidential and should not be disclosed to outsiders without the patient's consent. Certain exceptions are permitted or required by law, as discussed below. Confidentiality is based on the special nature of the doctor patient relationship because confidentiality provides an underpinning that encourages full disclosure by the patient seeking medical care. The rule of confidentiality has been established in state court decisions and in state laws protecting privacy in general (or medical information in particular). Recently, the federal government has stepped into the arena: to ensure that patients in every state enjoy basic rights of privacy and access to their health information, it has enacted laws and regulations effective in April of 2003 (the Health Insurance Portability and Accountability Act [HIPAA], as discussed in **Section VII.B.** below).

1.   Privileged Information

In some states, patients enjoy a statutory privilege with regard to information they have disclosed to certain caregivers (e.g., psychiatrists, psychologists, social workers, sexual assault counselors, domestic violence counselors). This means that the patient has the right not to testify—and to keep the clinician from testifying—regarding the patient's confidential communications in judicial and administrative proceedings. Exceptions to the privilege may apply in circumstances when a judge determines that the disclosure of confidential information is more important than protecting the treatment relationship.

2. The Right of Privacy

Laws in every state protect the privacy of its citizens, and may serve as the basis for a lawsuit by a patient who feels that his or her right to privacy has been violated (e.g., a breach of confidentiality of medical information). Some states have established specific rights of privacy for patients. Massachusetts, for example, protects a patient's right to privacy "during medical treatment or other rendering of care within the capacity of the facility." This may require extra effort in the context of the emergency department, but may also be particularly applicable to the trauma unit patient. Reasonable care should always be taken. Patient's names should not be written on boards within public view or used in public areas. Voices should be lowered when discussing medical issues in an area where other patients or visitors are nearby. Curtains should be drawn when it would respect a patient's privacy dignity during an examination. Most importantly, every staff member must be educated about the duty to keep information about patients strictly private, including the fact that a person has appeared in the emergency department seeking treatment for self or for a family member. This requirement applies whether the patient is John Doe, a rock star, a baseball player, or a politician—or a drug-overdosed son or battered spouse of any of the foregoing.

B. HIPAA: Federal Privacy Requirements

1. HIPAA in General

The Department of Health and Human Services has issued regulations, effective April 2003, which protect the privacy of patient information. These regulations are required by a federal statute entitled the Health Insurance Portability and Accountability Act of 1996 (commonly known as *HIPAA*). Healthcare providers (including emergency departments), healthcare plans, and "clearing houses" are covered by HIPAA. In the spring of 2002, the Bush administration proposed modifications to the regulations, but did not delay their effective date. The final form of the regulations was announced in August 2002.

One impetus for the regulations was the fact that states vary widely in the protection of health information, and even in whether they allow patients access to their own medical records. Federal privacy regulations provide a minimal standard of privacy requirements and right of access by patients to their medical information. States can continue to enforce their own laws only if they provide more privacy protection or a greater right of access to medical records by patients.

HIPAA covers all medical information, in whatever form it is stored or communicated (e.g.., paper, electronic, or oral means). Healthcare providers must establish policies carrying out the federal requirements and inform patients at the outset of care of the provider's privacy practices with regard to medical information. This disclosure must include the following:

a. Uses and disclosures that will be made for the purpose of treatment, payment, and healthcare operations

b. Uses and disclosures the provider is permitted to make of patient information *without* patient authorization (e.g. those required by law)

c. Uses and disclosures the provider is permitted to make *only with* patient authorization

d. Uses and disclosures the provider is permitted to make, but must allow the patient an opportunity to prohibit by objection

e. Rights of the patient to inspect and obtain a copy of personal medical records, as well as to request restrictions on disclosures or amendments of health information, and to obtain an accounting of such disclosures

2. Staff Responsibilities

Every staff person associated with a hospital or direct care physician's office must be educated about the requirements of HIPAA and how it will affect their own state laws. One provision of HIPAA that is particularly applicable to the emergency department governs the disclosure of patient information for the purposes of involving others in a patient's care and for emergency notification, as discussed below.

3. Disclosure under HIPAA for Purposes of Involving Others in a Patient's Care

Under HIPAA, healthcare providers can disclose information about a patient to inform or assist in the notification of a patient's family member, personal representative, or another person responsible for the patient's care of the location, general condition, or death of the patient. If the patient is present, the provider can do so only if the patient agrees or is given the opportunity to object and does not do so. If the patient is not present (or cannot agree or object because of incapacity or an emergency circumstance), the provider, in exercising professional judgment, can determine whether the disclosure is in the patient's best interest, and then disclose only the information directly relevant to the person's involvement with the patient's health care.

4. Disclosure under HIPAA for Purposes of Emergency Notification

Under HIPAA, a provider can disclose patient information to a public or private entity authorized by law or its corporate charter to assist in disaster relief efforts to coordinate with such entities. The disclosure requirements discussed in **Section VII. B.1.** above, relative to objection, apply to the extent that they do not interfere with the provider's ability to respond to emergency circumstances.

C. Newsworthy Patients and Confidentiality

Extra care may be necessary to protect the privacy of newsworthy patients, including coordinating efforts with hospital security, public relations, and admitting and information systems departments. These are patients who are of particular interest to the public at large or to specific third parties. This could be a well-known performer or politician, or a victim of trauma who has been injured in a battering or gang-related assault. The patient may also be a more locally famous hospital officer, chief of surgery, or other staff person or employee. The emergency department should establish policies and procedures for protecting patients whose medical information is of special interest, or whose security requires secrecy of their location. Vigilance may be required, as outsiders have been known to use creative ways of seeking information: a person who appears to be a nun in religious garb may be a reporter with a hidden camera; a weapon can be concealed in a pizza box; and nefarious individuals can telephone and identify themselves as anxious family members looking for a loved one.

VIII. Required Reporting

A. Reporting in General

As noted earlier in **Section VII,** instances exist when patient health information is permitted or required to be disclosed. The hospital may be under a legal mandate to report certain patient information to specified public officials. This will depend on specific requirements, most of which are imposed by state law. Questions with regard to reporting should be addressed with hospital legal counsel. Examples of required reporting include the following:

1. Reports to police of gunshot or stab wounds
2. Reports to police of sexual assaults (may *or may not* require disclosing the victim's identity)
3. Reports to fire officials of more serious burn injuries
4. Reports to child protective authorities of child abuse
5. Reports to state protective authorities of abuse of elderly or disabled persons
6. Public Health reporting: lead poisoning
7. Public Health reporting: diseases dangerous to the public health (anthrax, tuberculosis, sexually transmitted diseases)
8. Public Health reporting: human immunodeficiency virus (HIV) infection (may *or may not* require disclosing identify of patient)
9. Public Health reporting: work-related diseases and injuries
10. Medical examiner reporting of deaths, as specified by state laws and regulations

      11.   Report of death of a patient in restraints or seclusion or related to the use of restraints or seclusion to the Centers for Medicare and Medicaid Services

B.   The USA Patriot Act of 2001

In light of the September 11, 2001 terrorist attacks, the federal government enacted the *USA Patriot Act of 2001.* With regard to hospital patients, the government can request records of visits by, and medical records of, certain foreign patients and may be more aggressive in search and seizure operations regarding patients receiving care at hospitals. Of note, HIPAA has exceptions that permit responding to government requests for patient information in certain situations (e.g., for national security).

IX.   Patients Dangerous to Themselves and/or Others

    A.   Disclosure of Confidential Patient Information and Warning Others

The emergency department is often the first stop on the route to voluntary or involuntary psychiatric hospitalization for a person who exhibits behavior that is dangerous to self or others. In caring for such patients, it may be necessary to disclose patient information that otherwise would be confidential without the patient's consent. The legal basis for this disclosure is necessity—to protect the patient or others. In general:

      1.   If it is determined that the patient needs psychiatric hospitalization, information necessary to transfer the patient to an appropriate facility may be disclosed.

      2.   If the patient has communicated a threat to a reasonably identifiable person and appears to have the ability to carry out the threat, the threat should be disclosed to the potential victim, law enforcement authorities, or both. This will not apply if the patient is being hospitalized and, thus, cannot carry out the threat, although the fact of the threat should be communicated to the receiving facility.

      3.   Documentation should include a description of the thought process in determining the necessity to disclose confidential medical information that justified the disclosure.

B.   Use of Patient Restraints and Seclusion

In emergency situations, it might be necessary to place a patient in restraint or seclusion to protect the patient and/or others from harm. A restraint can be either a physical restraint or a drug restraint. Use of seclusion and restraint is closely regulated by state and federal authorities because these interventions themselves can be harmful. Federal regulations permit restraint or seclusion in emergency situations only if needed to ensure the patient's physical safety, and only if less restrictive interventions have been determined to be ineffective. The seclusion or restraint must be in accordance with an order of a physician or other licensed independent practitioner permitted by the state and the hospital to order seclusion or restraint. It must be carried out by trained personnel. The federal regulations create a minimal standard and are superseded by more restrictive state requirements. Emergency department staff must be familiar with the laws of their particular jurisdiction.

The patient's well-being while in restraints or seclusion is of paramount importance. The patient must continually be assessed, monitored, and reevaluated. Restraint and seclusion may not be used simultaneously unless the patient is continually monitored face-to-face by an assigned staff member, or by staff in close proximity to the patient using both video and audio equipment.

All staff who have direct patient contact must have ongoing education and training in the proper and safe use of seclusion and restraint application, and techniques and alternative methods for handling behavior, symptoms, and situations that traditionally have been treated through the use of restraints or seclusion.

The hospital must report to the Centers for Medicare and Medicaid Services any death that occurs while a patient is restrained or in seclusion, or where it is reasonable to assume that a patient's death was the result of restraint or seclusion.

X. Handling Unruly Patients and Visitors

Healthcare workers in the emergency room sometimes encounter violent, threatening, or otherwise disruptive patients whose actions do not result from mental illness and who, therefore, cannot be involuntarily committed. Likewise, family members and acquaintances of a patient in a trauma unit may also become disruptive, thereby presenting security issues as well. To prevent disruptive persons from interfering with patient care, it is important that a trauma unit have policies and procedures in place that include the ability to quickly involve hospital security and/or law enforcement, if the situation so requires.

A good starting point with a disruptive person in the emergency room is to immediately set limits, if possible, which may include requiring the person to stop threatening or harassing the staff and making sure that the person is unarmed while on hospital grounds. In a serious emergency, the trauma unit must provide necessary medical care even to an unruly patient and, thus, the presence of hospital security or police may be required in some situations. For disruptive visitors, access to the patient can be restricted to certain scheduled times and to certain designated areas, with security present, if necessary. In extreme cases, a visitor who continues to threaten trauma unit staff or disrupt patient care can be banned from the trauma unit (or from the hospital grounds altogether) as a visitor.

XI. Treating Patients Involved In Criminal Activity
A. In General

Trauma units are likely to see victims of crime as well as those who have committed crimes on a regular basis. It is important, therefore, that a trauma unit has clear policies established in advance addressing its role in criminal matters, and that healthcare providers in the emergency room are familiar with them.

B. Disclosing Criminal Activity of Patients

A trauma unit generally has no legal obligation to disclose to law enforcement authorities that a patient has confessed to committing a crime or to other involvement in criminal activity. A trauma unit should remain focused on providing patient care, and allow state and federal authorities to investigate and prosecute crimes. Moreover, a healthcare provider's disclosure of information about a patient could be seen as breach of federal and state laws that require a healthcare provider to keep patient information confidential (as discussed earlier in **Section VII**). Reporting may be necessary, however, in situations involving child abuse, gunshot or stab wounds. Reporting may also be necessary where a strong public policy exists to report certain information and the healthcare provider believes that the failure to release particular information will cause harm to others (as discussed previously in **Sections VIII and IX**).

C.   Testing for Drugs and Alcohol

Law enforcement authorities, the registry of motor vehicles, or another third party may request that a trauma unit take a blood or urine sample from a patient for an alcohol or drug analysis, and may even ask for the release of medical records (e.g., laboratory results) containing such information. Without the treating physician first obtaining a patient's informed consent, neither should be done absent a court order requiring the trauma unit to perform the test or release the medical information. A patient's consent to, or refusal of, a blood or urine test requested by a third party should be documented in the patient's medical record. Additionally, the patient can also request that the trauma unit perform a blood or urine analysis to establish sobriety, contradict a test previously administered by law enforcement, or both. An emergency room should have a policy in place addressing whether it will perform such tests at a patient's request without a medical need. Of note, a trauma unit should not take blood or urine from a deceased patient at the request of law enforcement for purposes of alcohol or drug testing. Such requests should be addressed to the state medical examiner, who will determine if such a test is necessary.

D.   Patient Contraband and Evidence

A trauma unit may confiscate and destroy (or in the alternative turn over to law enforcement personnel) drugs, weapons, or other contraband brought into the emergency room by patients. Where a patient arrives in the emergency department with such contraband, the healthcare facility's security department should be contacted to handle the contraband. It is not necessary—and usually not advisable—to include the identity of the involved patient because law enforcement authorities can obtain such information by legal processes, if so required. Police can present with a search warrant to obtain anything removed from a victim of a gunshot or stabbing. Procedures should be in place to retain and properly label such items until it is determined that they are not needed. If a patient enters the trauma unit legally carrying a weapon, the weapon should be confiscated and stored securely until it can be returned to the patient on discharge.

HYPOTHETICAL SITUATION: TREATING A PATIENT INVOLVED IN CRIMINAL ACTIVITY

Facts: Lucie, age 25, is transported to the emergency room by an ambulance following a car accident. On arrival, the ambulance driver informs a trauma unit nurse that Lucie told him: "I killed two kids!" While evaluating Lucie, the treating physician notes that Lucie has suffered whiplash and a broken arm and that she is also very intoxicated. The treating physician glimpses a handgun stuffed in Lucie's pocket, as well as several baggies in her possession that appear to contain marijuana. Lucie's husband, Dickie, is telephoned by the hospital during her examination. On learning that she was in an auto accident, Dickie demands that the hospital perform a blood test to show that she was sober. Meanwhile, the police arrive in the emergency room and explain to the treating physician that Lucie just shot two teenagers while robbing a convenience store, and then caused a six-car accident as a result of a high-speed car chase when she fled the store. The police demand that the hospital hand over any contraband they may have found on Lucie, and request that the hospital immediately perform a blood alcohol test on Lucie. How should the trauma unit handle this situation?

Analysis: The treating physician should immediately require Lucie to turn the gun over to hospital security, as well as the baggies that appear to contain marijuana. Without a valid search warrant or court order, the police do not have a right to this contraband and, therefore, it is up to the hospital whether it will turn the items over to the police. Likewise, the hospital should not disclose to the police any statements that Lucie made to the ambulance driver. Where the police do not have Lucie's permission or a court order for the blood alcohol test, the hospital should not draw blood (or urine) from Lucie for such purposes. Moreover, the hospital is under no obligation to perform a blood alcohol test on Lucie at her husband's request and should follow its own internal policy in this situation. All of the facts and circumstances of Lucie's admission (e.g., her statements, the contraband found on her, and the requests made by the police and Dickie) should be documented in her medical record.

XII. **Liability for Emergency Medical Treatment**
    A. The Standard of Care and Medical Malpractice
       Generally, state laws provide that physicians are expected to render medical care—including emergency care—at the level of the average qualified physician in good standing and consistent with current medical advances. Physicians who are specialists are expected to provide medical care at the level of the average qualified physician in good standing in that particular specialty (both referred to here generally as the "standard of care"). It is important to note that a bad outcome is not malpractice unless it can be shown that the healthcare provider breached a duty to the patient and caused ascertainable damages.
    B. Overview of the Process of Medical Malpractice Litigation
       In practice, *malpractice* refers to several kinds of causes of action under state law that can be brought by patients

(or their executors) or their families against physicians or other healthcare providers. Although the most common cause of action is negligence, the term can also include claims of battery (where the patient is touched without giving permission), lack of informed consent, breach of contract, and breach of confidentiality.

As stated above, medical malpractice claims are most often allegations of negligent patient care. To prevail on a claim of negligence, the patient must prove that it was more likely than not that harm occurred from the actions or omissions of a healthcare provider who had a duty to provide (but who did not so provide) medical care meeting the relevant standard of care. A patient can bring a claim for battery where a healthcare provider fails to obtain informed consent before treatment. Even when consent is obtained, a patient can later claim that he or she was not made aware of information (typically complications or risks) that a reasonable patient would have wanted to know to make an informed treatment decision. Some jurisdictions, such as Massachusetts, require that there be a discussion of alternative treatments with the patient. Finally, in many states, it is possible to file a claim for damages resulting from a breach of patient confidentiality and, under federal law, violations of HIPPA's privacy and security provisions can result in civil fines, criminal penalties, or both, including fines of up to $250,000 and 10 years imprisonment.

Some states handle medical malpractice lawsuits differently than other types of civil cases. For example, in Massachusetts, actions against healthcare providers alleging malpractice, error, or mistake must first be screened by a medical malpractice tribunal consisting of a judge, a physician, and an attorney (the "Tribunal"). The purpose of the Tribunal is to conduct a hearing to determine whether the patient has evidence sufficient to raise a legitimate question of liability for a court proceeding. If the Tribunal determines the patient does not, the patient must file a bond before trial that will be used to defray the defendants' costs if the defendant prevails.

Medical malpractice claims usually have a time limit by which they must be filed. In Massachusetts, malpractice claims must be filed within 3 years after the patient learns, or reasonably should have learned, that harm occurred as a result of the conduct of a physician or other healthcare provider (no more than 7 years after the event in question). Generally, the 3-year period begins when the cause of action accrues, or when the patient knew or should have known that the acts or omissions of the medical provider caused the harm. The statute of limitations is slightly longer for malpractice claims on behalf of children. In many states, an exception to the statute of limitations exists wherein is a retained foreign body; in those cases, the statute of limitations is not triggered until discovery of the foreign object.

C. EMTALA Claims Versus Medical Malpractice

To date, courts have uniformly held that EMTALA is not a substitute for a medical malpractice claim. It is, therefore, not unusual to see lawsuits in which plaintiffs assert claims under both EMTALA and state medical malpractice laws. Unlike malpractice claims, which can be brought against physicians as well as the hospital where the physician was practicing, EMTALA provides for a private right of action for injured persons against only the hospital (although individual physicians can be fined under EMTALA in certain circumstances).

Negligence is *not* the standard by which an EMTALA violation is measured. Instead, when determining whether a hospital has met its EMTALA obligations, courts consider whether the hospital did an appropriate medical screening of the patient. Federal courts in different areas of the country have given varying interpretations of what is an "appropriate medical screening." In Massachusetts, for example, federal courts take into consideration (1) whether the screening examination was reasonably calculated to identify critical medical conditions and (2) whether a uniform level of screening was given to all patients presenting with similar symptoms. Moreover, a hospital is only obligated to provide a screening examination that is within the capabilities of that hospital, regardless whether another hospital with access to additional tests or specialists would have used such additional resources. Where these conditions are met, a hospital will not be found to have violated EMTALA—even where a screening examination results in a misdiagnosis.

D. "Good Samaritan" Laws

"Good Samaritan" statutes are state laws designed to protect from liability physicians (and perhaps nurses and other healthcare providers) who voluntarily offer assistance in emergencies for seriously ill or injured people who are not patients of those physicians. This usually occurs outside of the healthcare provider's place of employment, such as when a physician is walking or driving by, or in a public place, when an accident occurs or a person collapses. In Massachusetts, as in many other states, licensure laws require physicians to offer emergency care of which they are professionally capable.

HYPOTHETICAL SITUATION: LIABILITY FOR EMERGENCY MEDICAL TREATMENT

Facts: Kris enters the emergency room at City Hospital complaining of chest pain. Kris mentions to the attending physician performing his screening examination that he has a history of heartburn and that his symptoms might have been triggered by a spicy lunch. The attending tells Kris "this sounds like acid reflux" and gives him an antacid. Although City Hospital's protocol for patients with Kris's symptoms calls for an electrocardiogram and blood tests, the attending physician decides these are unnecessary and discharges Kris (despite his continued chest pains). An hour later Kris suffers a massive heart attack while at work. Kris subsequently files a lawsuit against City Hospital and the attending physician, alleging violations of EMTALA and malpractice. What is the likely result?

Analysis: City Hospital has violated EMTALA. Where Kris presented with symptoms suggesting a heart attack and City Hospital (1) failed to perform a screening examination that was reasonably calculated to identify his critical medical conditions and (2) the screening examination fell below the level of screening that City Hospital typically gave to other patients with similar symptoms, the screening examination was inadequate under EMTALA. Moreover, City Hospital also violated EMTALA when it discharged Kris without stabilizing his emergency medical condition. A jury is likely to award damages against the hospital for these EMTALA violations. Federal regulators may also impose fines against City Hospital and the attending physician, and also seek to bar City Hospital from the Medicare and Medicaid programs if City Hospital has violated EMTALA provisions. Both the attending physician and City Hospital have likely also violated state medical malpractice laws because the inadequate screening examination and hasty discharge were below the level of the average qualified physician.

XIII.   Ethical Issues in the Emergency Department
A.   Medical Care Where Treatment Is Futile

Occasionally, an emergency department must deal with a patient whose medical condition is so critical that further care seems to be medically contraindicated, as well as ethically incorrect. In such cases, emergency department staff are advised to consult with hospital legal counsel and/or the hospital's ethics committee.

In a landmark case, a hospital was faced with a request to provide emergency treatment to an infant who was born anencephalic. At birth, the treating clinicians placed the baby on a ventillator in order to evaluate her. They concluded that she would die because of respiratory problems, among other difficulties, within days, and recommended that no aggressive measures be taken. The baby's mother, however, insisted that the staff keep the baby on the ventillator. Eventually, the baby was transferred to a nursing home. Subsequently, however, the baby required multiple transfers back to the hospital for emergency treatment for her breathing difficulties. After the second transfer, the hospital and the baby's father sued the baby's mother, arguing that the hospital was not required to provide more than nutrition, hydration, and warmth. Eventually, a federal appellate court ruled that EMTALA required that the hospital to provide stabilizing treatment even though such treatment would ultimately be futile because the EMTALA statute did not allow for exceptions to the requirement of stabilizing care.

B.   When a Patient Arrives Accompanied by a DNR Order

Another situation in which emergency department staff may want to consult hospital legal counsel for advice and develop a procedure for the next steps occurs when a patient arrives accompanied by a DNR order. An example of such a situation might be a patient who is known to the staff to have a DNR in the medical record from a prior admission. Another example might be a patient who arrives with evidence of an expressed preference for DNR through a program such as the Massachusetts Comfort Care program, in which patients can obtain a form or bracelet expressing his or her wishes for the use of emergency medical services (EMS) personnel. (At the moment, this program is only binding on EMS personnel, not on hospitals.)

In such cases, a number of questions may be relevant, including why was the DNR ordered? What were the medical circumstances? How long ago? What is the condition for which the patient is being treated now? Can the patient confirm personal wishes with respect to medical care for the condition at hand; if not, is it possible that the patient might be able to discuss the DNR in the near future after proper treatment? Is there an appropriate surrogate decision-maker available who can assist in determining the treatment that the patient would (or would not) want?

XIV. Conclusion

Given the numerous legal issues that are likely to arise in a typical trauma unit, it is important that healthcare providers understand the basic legal issues surrounding emergency room care and that legal counsel familiar with the laws of the particular state are available for consultation. By developing in advance policies and procedures for handling common legal issues and maintaining a close relationship with hospital security, a trauma unit can help ensure that patient care is not compromised by healthcare providers caught unprepared to manage the legal issues typically found in an emergency room.

ACKNOWLEDGMENT

The authors would like to thank Marilyn A. McMahon, the Risk Management Attorney for the Massachusetts General Hospital, for her invaluable contributions to section XII. Of note, three of the authors of this chapter are members of the Office of the General Counsel of Partners HealthCare System, Inc., an integrated healthcare delivery system based in Massachusetts featuring several acute care hospitals (including the Massachusetts General Hospital). The authors also wish to thank Ernest M. Haddad, Esq. and Michael Broad, Esq. for the use of their excellent chapter *Legal Aspects of Emergency Medical Care.*

SELECTED REFERENCES

George Annas. The Rights of Doctors, Nurses and Allied Health Professionals 81 (1981).

Becker S. *Health care law: a practical guide,* 2nd ed. New York: Matthew Bender, 2001.

Behnke SH, Hilliard JT. *The essentials of Massachusetts mental health law.* New York: W. W. Norton and Co., 1998.

Haddad EM, Broad M. Legal aspects of emergency medical care. In: *Emergency medicine,* 4th ed. Baltimore: Williams and Wilkins, 1996.

Liang BA. *Health law and policy: a survival guide to medicolegal issues for practitioners.* 2000.

Mass. Gen. Laws ch. 111 § 70E(j) (2003).

US Department of Health and Human Services, Office for Civil Rights. *National standards to protect the privacy of personal health information* (modified April 30, 2002); available at: http://www.hhs.gov/ocr/hipaa>; accessed October, 2003.

US Department of Health and Human Services, Centers for Medicare and Medicaid Services. Clarifying policies related to the responsibilities of medicare-participating hospitals in treating individuals with emergency medical conditions; available at http://www.cms.hhs.gov/providers/emtala/cms-1063-f.pdf; accessed October, 2003.

Subject Index

Note: Page numbers followed by f indicate figures; those followed by t indicate tables.

A

Abbreviated Injury Scale (AIS), 18t
ABCDs of trauma care, 71, 75
ABCs, psychiatric, 663
Abdominal abscess, 473
Abdominal compartment syndrome,
    479–482
  etiology of, 479–480
  increased intracranial pressure
    and, 481
  intraabdominal pressure monitor-
    ing in, 480
  presentation of, 479–480
  systemic effects in, 480
Abdominal decompression, for
    increased intracranial pres-
    sure, 481
Abdominal packing, in hepatic
    injuries, 422–423, 431
Abdominal trauma
  abdominal wall injuries in,
    409–412, 564
  approach to patient in
    for stable patients, 396–401,
      397f
    for unstable patients, 394, 395f
  biliary tract injuries in, 413, 420,
    427–429
  blunt, 396
  colon injuries in, 462–464,
    468–474, 477–478
    in children, 586
    in pregnancy, 604
  damage control in, 475–479,
    481–482
  deceleration injuries in, 413, 414
  diagnosis in, 385–401
    in blunt trauma, 396–398
    computed tomography in,
      390–391, 392t, 396
    exploratory thoracoscopy in, 394
    laparoscopy in, 393–394
    local wound exploration in,
      391–392, 399f
    in penetrating trauma, 398–401,
      399f, 400f
    peritoneal lavage in, 114, 115t,
      389–390
    plain films in, 114, 386–387
    thoracoscopy in, 394
    ultrasonography in, 114,
      387–389, 388f, 396
  diaphragmatic injuries in,
    402–409. *See also* Diaphrag-
    matic injuries

duodenal injuries in, 446–448,
    455–461, 476–477
  fluid attenuation in, 634
  gastric injuries in, 462–466,
    477–478. *See also* Gastric
    injuries
    in children, 586
  gunshot wounds in, 398–401
  hemoperitoneum in, 416
  hepatic injuries in, 413–427,
    475–476. *See also* Hepatic
    injuries
    in children, 586
  historical perspective on, 385
  imaging studies in, 386–389,
    390–391, 392t, 631–640
  intraabdominal hemorrhage and
    air in, 632–634
  operative management of, 481–483
    complications in, 482–483
    mesh repair in, 424, 441,
      481–482
    reoperation in, 482
  pancreatic injuries in, 446–455,
    476–477
  pediatric, 575–578, 576t, 577t,
    585–586
  penetrating, 396–401
  physical examination in, 113–114,
    385–401
  in pregnancy, 604–605
  primary survey in, 394–401, 395f,
    397f
  reconstructive surgery for,
    481–482, 564
  rectus sheath hematomas in,
    411–412
  small bowel injuries in, 462–464,
    466–468, 477–478
    in children, 586
    in pregnancy, 604
  splenic injuries in, 433–445, 476
    in children, 585–586
  stab wounds in, 396–398, 399f,
    400f
  vascular injuries in, 351–370,
    478–479. *See also* Abdominal
    vascular injuries
Abdominal vascular injuries,
    351–370, 478–479
  aortic, 355–361, 356f
    infrarenal, 362–363
    seatbelt, 351
    supraceliac, 360
    supramesocolic, 355–360, 359f

Abdominal vascular injuries (*contd.*)
celiac access branch, 360–361
classification of, 357t-358t
common iliac artery, 368–369
diagnosis of, 352–353
epidemiology of, 351
exploratory laparotomy for,
354–355
external iliac artery, 368–369
hemostasis in, 355
hepatic artery, 369
iliac vein, 369
imaging studies in, 629–630
incidence of, 351
inferior mesenteric artery, 363
inferior vena cava, 363–366, 364f
initial management of, 353–354
internal iliac artery, 369
juxtahepatic venous, 424–427
in midline inframesocolic area,
356f, 362–366
in midline retroperitoneal area,
355–366, 356f
in midline supramesocolic area,
355–362, 356f
operative exploration of, 354–355
operative exposure for, 355, 356f
operative management of,
354–370
pathophysiology of, 351
in pelvic retroperitoneum,
367–369
in porta hepatis zone, 369–370
portal vein, 369–370
renal artery, 367
renal vein, 367
in retrohepatic area, 370, 424–427
retrohepatic vena cava, 424–427
signs and symptoms of, 352
superior mesenteric artery,
361–362
superior mesenteric vein, 362
surgical evaluation of, 353–355
thoracotomy for, 354
in upper lateral retroperitoneum,
366–367
zones of, 355, 356f
Abdominal wall herniation, 409–412
diagnosis of, 410
epidemiology of, 409–410
initial presentation of, 409–410
mechanism of injury in, 409–410
operative management of,
410–411
rectus sheath hematomas in,
411–412
Abdominopelvic aortography, 353
Abducens nerve injuries, 278–279
ABO crossmatch, 130–133
Abrasions
corneal, 266–267
facial, 253

Abscess
abdominal, 473
liver, 420
Abuse
child. *See* Child abuse
in pregnancy, 593
ACE inhibitors, in elderly, 614–615
Acetabular fractures, 641–642
Acetylcysteine, prophylactic, for
imaging studies, 125
Achilles tendon tear, 538
Acid burns, 155t, 170. *See also* Burns
ocular, 268
Acidemia, transfusion-related, 145
Acidosis, lactic, transfusion-related,
145
Acromioclavicular separation, 531,
649
Acute quadriplegic myopathy syn-
drome, 122
Acute renal failure, 125–127
continuous renal replacement
therapy in, 127
dialysis in, 127
rhabdomyolysis in, 125–126
Acute respiratory distress syndrome,
122
Acute stress disorder, 676
Adjustment disorder, 677
Adnexal injuries, 279–282
Adolescents. *See* Pediatric trauma
Adrenal injuries, imaging studies in,
638
Advanced directives, 714–715
Advanced Trauma Life Support, 71
Agitation, in head injuries, 705–706,
706t
Aird maneuver, 450f
Air transport, 43–47. *See also*
Transport
altitude and, 46–47
fixed-wing aircraft, 42, 47
helicopter, 42
indications for, 43, 45t
lighting and, 46
noise and, 44
personnel for, 30–31
preflight vs. inflight treatment
and, 47
safety of, 47
space issues and, 43–44
vibration and, 44–46
Airway
difficult
adjuncts for, 98–107
anticipated, 98
unanticipated, 98
examination of, 111
Airway classification, Samsoon-
Young, 595f
Airway evaluation, 75–77, 89–90

Airway injuries
in burns, 151, 161–162, 172t
in cervical trauma, 284–295
imaging of, 630–631
Airway management, 75–77, 89–107
in anesthesia, 176, 181–182, 190, 193
artificial airways in, 33
in burns, 151, 161–162, 172t
with cervical spine injury, 89, 90, 91, 95
in chest injuries, 297–298
in children, 571–572, 580
chin lift in, 76
common traps in, 87
complicating factors in, 89–90
cricothyroidotomy in, 34–35, 103–105, 104f, 105f
in diaphragmatic injuries, 403
in elderly, 611
emergent, 91
endotracheal intubation in, 33–35, 76–77, 93–98. See also Endotracheal intubation
equipment for, 72
esophageal obturator in, 33
evaluation in, 75–77, 89–90
in geriatric trauma, 616
initial evaluation in, 75–76
in intraoral injuries, 255
intubating laryngeal mask airway in, 102–103
jaw thrust in, 76
laryngeal mask airway in, 33, 100–103, 100t, 101f
light wand in, 103
Mallampati classification and, 90
mask ventilation in, 91–93
in maxillofacial injuries, 89, 92, 256–257
in neck injuries, 286–288, 287t
nonemergent, 91
pharyngeal lumen airway and Combitube in, 33
physical examination in, 89–91
postoperative, in cervical surgery, 285
in pregnancy, 593–595, 594f, 595f, 596t
prehospital, 32–35
Samsoon-Young classification and, 595f
in tracheobronchial injuries, 317, 319
tracheostomy in, 105–106
trauma team expert for, 51
urgent, 91
Airway obstruction
in inhalation injury, 162
signs and symptoms of, 93–94
Airways
esophageal obturator, 33

laryngeal mask, 33, 76, 93, 100–103, 100t, 101f
intubating, 102–103
with mask ventilation, 92, 93
nasopharyngeal, 72, 76, 92, 93
oropharyngeal, 72, 92, 93
pharyngeal lumen, 33
Akathisia, neuroleptics and, 670–671
Albumin, replacement, 186, 187t
Alcohol, blood level of, 199–201, 726
Alcohol abuse, 199–201, 203t–206t, 672–674
testing for, 199–201, 726
Alcohol withdrawal, 199–202, 673–674
Alkaline burns, 155t, 170. See also Burns
ocular, 267–268
Allen test, 544
Allergies, history of, 108
Altitude, during air transport, 46–47
Amantadine
for traumatic brain injury, 704t
in traumatic brain injury, for agitation, 706, 706t
Amblyopia, 282–283
Ambulance transport, 40–42. See also Transport
personnel for, 29–30
American Spinal Injury Association (ASIA) scoring system, 224–225, 226f–228f, 230
Aminocaproic acid, 141–142
Amniotic fluid embolism, 600
Amphetamines, for traumatic brain injury, 704, 704t
AMPLE mnemonic, 75, 108
Amputation
digital, 551–553
early, indications for, 379
lower extremity, 565–566
penile, 506
upper extremity, 551–553
Amylase levels, in pancreatic injuries, 447–448
Analgesia. See Pain management
Anesthesia, 174–194. See also Pain management
abdominal injuries and, 191–192
agents for, 180–183
airway evaluation for, 176
airway management in, 176, 181–182, 190, 193
cardiac injuries and, 191
drugs for, 174, 175t
electrolyte imbalances in, 191
emergence from, 192–193
equipment for, 174, 175t
fluid resuscitation in, 185–189
general, 177–178
historical perspective on, 6–7

Anesthesia, 174–194 (*contd.*)
  inadequate, 183
  inotropic therapy in, 189
  laboratory studies in, 190–191, 192
  life-threatening problems in, 193–194
  local
    for facial injuries, 253
    for hand injuries, 549–550, 549f
  monitoring in, 179–180, 184–185, 190–192
  neurologic injuries and, 192
  ocular, 258
  operating room setup for, 174
  for orotracheal intubation, 96–97
  orthopedic injuries and, 192
  planning for, 177–180
  preinduction stage of, 174–180
  premedication in, 178
  rhabdomyolysis and, 192
  team approach in, 174, 175t
  thoracic injuries and, 191
  transfusions and, 186
  vascular access for, 178–179
  vasopressors in, 188–189
  volume status assessment in, 176–177
Angiographic embolization
  in pelvic fractures, 522, 524
  renal, 488–489
  splenic, 442–443
Angiography
  in hepatic injuries, 416
  in neck injuries, 290
  in peripheral vascular injuries, 375–376
  in renal injuries, 353, 487
  in splenic injuries, 437
Angiosomes, 558
Angiotensin-converting enzyme inhibitors, in elderly, 614–615
Angle recession, 270
  glaucoma and, 271–272
Ankle injuries, 536–538
Anoxic brain injury, delirium in, 667
Antecubital venous access, 81
Anterior chamber, examination of, 262
Anterior cord syndrome, 229
Anterior segment
  examination of, 258–259, 262–263
  foreign bodies in, 273
  injuries of, 264–265, 273
Anterolateral thoracotomy, 310–311, 310f
  bilateral (clamshell), 311–312, 311f, 332f, 334
  with hilar clamping, 318, 318f
  left, 331–334, 332f, 333f
Anthrax, in biological warfare, 62–63

Antianxiety agents, 676–677
  for agitation, in traumatic brain injury, 706, 706t
Antibiotics
  for burns, 165–166
  for extremity fractures, 527
  for facial lacerations, 253–254
  for hand injuries, 549
  for intraoral lacerations, 255
  for lip lacerations, 255
  for mandibular fractures, 250
  for maxillofacial gunshot injuries, 256
  postsplenectomy, 444
  in pregnancy, 605
  for surgical site infections, 207
Anticholinergics, for dystonia, 670–671
Anticoagulation
  in elderly, 615
  extremity injuries in, 530, 690
  prophylactic, 197–198, 200t, 690
Anticonvulsants, prophylactic, in head injury, 218, 705
Antidepressants, 678
  for agitation, in traumatic brain injury, 706, 706t
Antidotes, for nerve agents, 65
Antifibrinolytic agents, 141–142
Antipsychotics, for delirium, 668–669
Antiseizure agents, prophylactic, in head injury, 218, 705
Antishock garment, 38
Antispasticity agents
  in spinal cord injuries, 699–701, 700t
  in traumatic brain injuries, 704
Anxiety, in burns, 160–161
Anxiety disorders, 676–677
Anxiolytics, 676–677
  for agitation, in traumatic brain injury, 706, 706t
Aortic arch injuries, 347–349, 347t, 348t
Aortic compression, for hemostasis, 355
Aortic injuries
  abdominal, 355–361, 356f. *See also* Abdominal vascular injuries
    infrarenal, 362–363
    seatbelt, 351
    supraceliac, 360
    supramesocolic, 355–360, 359f
  imaging of, 629
Aortic valve injuries, 338
Aortography, abdominopelvic, 353
Aprotinin, 141–142
ARDS, 122
Aripiprazole, for delirium, 669–671
Arm. *See* Upper extremity
Arousal, levels of, 662

Arrhythmias
  in anesthesia, 193–194
  in cardiac contusion, 335–336,
      337f
  neuroleptics and, 669–670, 670
Arterial blood gases
  in anesthesia, 179–180, 184
  in pregnancy, 596, 596t
Arterial injuries. *See also* Vascular
      injuries
  signs of, 372–375
Arterial line. *See* Vascular access
Arterial pseudoaneurysms, 383
Arterial thrombosis, renal artery,
      490–491
Arteriography. *See* Angiography
ASCOT Scale, 20t
ASIA, scoring system of, 224–225,
      226f-228f, 230
Asphyxia, traumatic, 307–308, 584
Assessment
  primary survey in, 71–88. *See also*
      Primary survey
  secondary survey in, 108–119. *See
      also* Secondary survey
  tertiary survey in, 118–119
Atlantoaxial dissociation, radiogra-
      phy of, 622–624, 624f
Atracurium, for anesthesia induc-
      tion, 182, 183
Atrial rupture, 335–338
Atriocaval shunt, 426
Atropine, for nerve agents, 65
Autonomic dysreflexia, in spinal cord
      injuries, 698
Autopsies, 719–720
Autotransplantation
  renal, 500
  splenic, 441–442
Avulsion injuries
  eyelid, 281
  facial, 254
  scalp, 561–562
  scrotal, 508
Axial flaps, 560. *See also* Soft tissue
      reconstruction
Axillary artery
  exposure of, 379
  injuries of, 379–381. *See also*
      Peripheral vascular injuries
Axonotmesis, 231, 693

B
Backboards, 37
Baclofen, for spasticity, in spinal
      cord injuries, 699, 700t, 701
Bacteriologic cultures, in extremity
      fractures, 527
Barbiturate coma, 219
  in children, 581
Barbiturates, for alcohol withdrawal,
      202

Barium contrast studies, in neck
      injuries, 289–290
Barrier precautions, 73
Barton, Clara, 4
Beck's triad, 338
  in pericardial tamponade, 84
Benzodiazepines
  for akathisia, 670–671
  for alcohol withdrawal, 202,
      673–674
  for anesthesia, 181, 183
  for anxiety, 676
  for delirium, 668–669, 671
Benztropine, for dystonia, 670–671
Berlin's edema, 274–275
Best interests test, 716
Beta blockers, in elderly, 614–615
Bicarbonate, for transfusions, 143
Biceps tendon rupture, 532
Bicycle injuries, 571, 578
Bilateral thoracosternotomy,
      311–312, 311f, 332f, 334
Bile duct injuries, 413, 420, 427–429
Bile leaks, 427–428, 430
Bilhaemia, 420–421
Biliary stricture, 430
Biliary tract injuries, 413, 420–421,
      427–429
Bilomas, 420
Biological warfare, 61–64
  anthrax in, 62–63
  botulism in, 63
  decontamination in, 68
  plague in, 63
  smallpox in, 64
  tularemia in, 64
Bipolar disorder, 677–679
Bites, of hand, 549
Bladder, neurogenic, 695
Bladder injuries, 500–503
  imaging studies in, 643–644,
      645–646
  urethral injuries with, 503
Blaisdell, William, 8
Blast injuries, 66–68, 67t, 152
Bleeding. *See also* Hemorrhage
  gastrointestinal, 207–209
      imaging of, 632–634
  hemorrhagic shock and, 81–83
  intraocular, 270–271
  intraoral, in neck injuries, 292
  intraperitoneal, in hepatic
      injuries, 416, 419, 420
  intrathoracic, 298–299, 304,
      306–307, 308
  in pelvic fractures, 521–523, 643
  splenic, 433, 633
      delayed, 443
Blindness. *See* Vision loss
Blistering agents, 64, 65
Blood, shed, recovery and reinfusion
      of, 134–136

Blood agents, 64, 65
Blood alcohol level, 199–201
Blood components
  comparison of, 133, 133t
  viscosity of, 133, 133t
Blood pressure. *See also* Hypertension; Hypotension
  monitoring of, in anesthesia, 179, 180
  in pregnancy, 596–597
Blood products, 186–188. *See also* Blood components; Transfusions
Blood sample
  collection of, 81
  crossmatching of, 130–133
Blood substitutes, 136
Blood transfusions. *See* Transfusions
Blood urea nitrogen, 126
Blood volume, in pregnancy, 597
Blowout fractures, 279–280, 621
Blunt trauma. *See also specific sites and types*
  questioning about, 109–110
Boari anterior bladder wall flap, 499
Boerhaave syndrome, 321–322
Botulinum toxin, for spasticity, in spinal cord injuries, 700
Bowel, neurogenic, 695
Bowel injuries, with hepatic injuries, 419–420
Brachial artery injuries, 381–382. *See also* Peripheral vascular injuries
Brachial plexus injuries, 235–237, 236f, 287, 686–687. *See also* Neck injuries
  in burns, 707t
Brachiocephalic vessels, imaging of, 630
Bradycardia, in anesthesia, 194
Brain death, diagnosis of, 655–657, 657t
Brain injury
  anoxic, delirium in, 667
  traumatic. *See* Head injuries
Breathing. *See also* Respiration; Ventilation
  in children, 572
  in elderly, 610–611
  evaluation of, 78–80, 87
  in pregnancy, 596
Bromocriptine, for traumatic brain injury, 704t
Bronchial injuries, imaging of, 630–631
Bronchitis, in inhalation injury, 162
Bronchoscopy, in tracheobronchial injuries, 316–317, 319
Bronchospasm, in inhalation injury, 162
Brooke formula, for burns, 159, 159t

Brown Séquard syndrome, 229–230
Buckle fractures, 587, 587f
Bullet wounds. *See* Gunshot wounds
Burns, 148–173
  airway management in, 151, 161–162, 172t
  anxiety in, 160–161
  carbon monoxide exposure in, 162–164
  chemical, 155t
    ocular, 267–268
  in child abuse, 157
  complications of
    late, 171–173
    systemic, 152–157, 161–165, 167t–169t
  contractures in, 171–172
  cyanide exposure in, 164
  depth of, 156–157
  electrical, 155t, 170
  extent of, 157, 158f
  first-degree, 156
  fluid resuscitation in, 151, 157–160
  follow-up in, 171–173
  history of, 110
  hypothermia in, 152
  inhalation injury in, 151, 153t, 161–162
  initial evaluation of, 151–157
  itching in, 172
  management of
    age-specific endpoints for, 160t
    immediate, 148
    monitoring of, 159–160
    overall strategy for, 148–149
    phases of, 148–149, 149t
    prehospital, 39, 40t
  multiple trauma and, 151–152, 171, 172t
  nutritional support in, 164–165
  ocular, 267–268
  pain management in, 160–161, 172
  peptic ulcers in, 164, 168t, 208–209
  peripheral nerve injuries in, 707, 707t
  physical examination in, 152–157, 153t-155t
  physiologic changes in, 149–151, 150t
  prehospital care in, 39, 40t
  primary survey in, 151–152
  rehabilitation in, 166, 707, 707t
  scarring in, 169t, 171–172, 707
  secondary survey in, 152–157, 153t-155t
  second-degree, 156–157
  surgery for, 166–169
  tar, 155t, 170
  third-degree, 157

transport in, 39, 40t
wound care in, 165–166, 165t, 166–169
wound infections in, 171
Burst fractures, 516
Buspirone, for agitation, in traumatic brain injury, 706, 706t

C

CAGE questionnaire, 673
Calcaneal fractures, 538
Calcium
  ionized, in citrate toxicity, 143–144
  supplemental, for transfusions, 143
Calcium channel blockers, in elderly, 614–615
Calcium chloride, 189
  indications for, 189
Calcium imbalance
  in spinal cord injuries, 698
  transfusion-related, 188
Canalicular lacerations, 281
Capacity, mental, 680, 713–717
Carbamazepine
  for agitation, in traumatic brain injury, 706, 706t
  for mania, 679
Carbidopa, for traumatic brain injury, 704t
Carbon monoxide exposure, in burns, 162–164
Cardiac arrest, 308
  in pregnancy, 598
  transport and, 43
Cardiac arrhythmias
  in anesthesia, 193–194
  in cardiac contusion, 335–336, 337f
  neuroleptics and, 669–670
Cardiac contusions, 335–336, 337f
Cardiac disease, drug therapy in, in elderly, 614–615
Cardiac drugs, in elderly, 614–615
Cardiac function
  in elderly, 610
  in pregnancy, 596–597
Cardiac injuries, 323–326, 328–341
  blunt, 335–338, 337f
  contusions, 335–336, 337f
  diagnosis of, 328–331, 330f
  historical perspective on, 328
  imaging of, 630
  initial evaluation in, 328
  penetrating, 328, 329f, 339–341
  physical examination in, 328–329
  in precordial box, 328, 329f
  rupture, 336–338
  surgical exposure for, 331–335, 332f, 333f
  valvular, 338

Cardiac massage, closed, in pregnancy, 598
Cardiac output
  in elderly, 610
  in pregnancy, 596–597
Cardiac rupture, 336–338
Cardiac tamponade, 308
  obstructive shock and, 84
Cardiogenic shock, 84
Cardiopulmonary resuscitation. *See* Resuscitation
Carotid artery injuries, 292–293
  blunt, 345–347
  penetrating, 342–344
Carotid–cavernous sinus fistula, 281
Carpal fractures, 534–535, 553–554
Carrel, Alexis, 5
Cataracts, 272–273
  electrical, 273
  glassblower's, 273
Catheter angiography. *See also* Angiography
  in neck injuries, 290
  in splenic injuries, 437
Catheterization
  pulmonary artery, 184
  in urethral injuries, 505–506
Catheters, intravenous, 72, 80–81
Cefazolin
  for mandibular fractures, 250
  for maxillofacial gunshot injuries, 256
Celiac access branches, injuries of, 360–361
Cellulitis, 171
Central cardiac vessel injuries, 339, 340f, 341, 347–349, 347t, 348t
Central cord syndrome, 229
Central nervous system injuries. *See* Cervical spine injuries; Head injuries; Spinal cord injuries
Central pain, in spinal cord injuries, 699
Central venous pressure monitoring, in anesthesia, 179–180, 184
Cephalexin, for lip lacerations, 256
Cerebral contusion, imaging studies in, 620
Cerebral perfusion pressure monitoring, 120–121
  in head injuries, 218
Cerebrovascular injuries
  blunt, 345–347
  penetrating, 344–345, 345f, 346f
Cervical collar, 36–37, 77
Cervical radiculopathy, 684–686, 685f
Cervical spine. *See also* Neck
  anatomy of, 512
  immobilization of, 77
    in elderly, 611
    prehospital, 36–38
  mobility of, assessment of, 91, 287t

Cervical spine clearance protocols, 287t, 510–511, 511t
  pediatric, 582
Cervical spine injuries, 224–230. *See also* Spinal cord injuries; Spinal fractures
  airway management with, 89, 90, 91, 95
  anatomic aspects of, 512
  anterior cord syndrome in, 229
  ASIA scoring system for, 224–225, 226f-228f, 230
  axial, 512–513
  Brown Séquard syndrome in, 229–230
  central cord syndrome in, 229
  cervical body fractures in, 513–514
  in children, 575, 581–582, 583t
  clearance protocols for, 287t, 510–511, 511t
    pediatric, 582
  endotracheal intubation and, 193
  epidemiology of, 224, 284
  facet joint dislocations in, 514
  hangman's fractures in, 512, 513, 622
  imaging studies in, 621–625, 623f, 624f
  incomplete, 229–230
  initial evaluation in, 224, 286–287, 287t
  instability with minimal/no bony injury in, 515
  Jefferson fractures in, 512–513, 513, 622
  lateral mass fractures in, 514
  level of, 224–225, 685t
  odontoid peg fractures in, 513
  patterns of, 512–515
  posterior cord syndrome in, 229
  radiographic evaluation in, 225, 289
  rehabilitation in, 230, 683–686
  scoring system for, 224–225, 226f-228f, 230
  spinal shock in, 225
  subaxial, 513–514
  surgery for
    anatomic landmarks in, 284–286, 285f
    indications for, 225–229
    postoperative care in, 230
Cervical strain, 683–684
Cervicothoracic vascular injuries
  anatomic landmarks for, 343f
  aortic arch and great vessel, 339–341, 340f, 347–349, 347t, 348t
  carotid artery
    blunt, 345–347, 345f, 346f, 347t
    penetrating, 342–343, 343f
  central vessel, 339–341, 340f, 347–349, 347t, 348t

  endovascular interventions for, 349–350
  vertebral artery
    blunt, 345–347, 345f, 346f, 347t
    penetrating, 344–345, 345f, 346f
Cesarean delivery, 598–599
Chance fracture, 626
Chemical burns, 155t, 170. *See also* Burns
  ocular, 267–268
Chemical warfare, 64–66
  blistering agents in, 65
  blood agents in, 65
  decontamination in, 68
  mustard agents in, 65
  nerve agents in, 64–65
  ricin in, 65
Chest. *See also under* Thoracic
  auscultation of, 112
  examination of, 112
  flail, 80, 302, 627
Chest decompression, needle, pre-hospital, 35
Chest films. *See* Radiography
Chest trauma, 296–341
  airway management in, 297–298, 302
  anterolateral thoracotomy in, 310–311, 310f
  asphyxia in, 307
  bilateral thoracosternotomy in, 311–312, 311f
  blunt, 296–297
  breathing in, 298
  cardiac and central vessel injuries in, 328–341. *See also* Cardiac injuries
  cardiac arrest in, 308
  cardiac tamponade in, 308
  chest wall injuries in, 80, 302, 563–564, 627
    imaging studies in, 626–627
  chylothorax in, 307–308
  diagnostic studies in, 300
  diaphragmatic injuries in, 307, 402
  esophageal injuries in, 320–326
  flail chest in, 80, 302
  hemothorax in, 306–307, 308
    in children, 584–585
    massive, 79–80, 308
  history in, 299
  imaging studies in, 625–631, 626–627
  initial evaluation in, 297–299
  intrathoracic bleeding in, 298–299, 306–307
  life-threatening conditions in, 78–80, 113t, 308
  mechanisms of injury in, 296–297
  median sternotomy for, 313
  needle decompression in, 310
  pediatric, 575, 576t, 584–585

penetrating, 297
physical examination in, 113–114, 299–300
pneumothorax in. *See* Pneumothorax
posterolateral thoracotomy for, 312, 312f
pulmonary contusion in, 122–123, 303–304
reconstructive surgery for, 563–564
respiratory failure in, 122
rib fractures in, 80, 300–302
secondary survey in, 299–300
shock in, 298–299
subcutaneous emphysema in, 305–306
sucking chest wound in, 304
surgery for
  patient preparation for, 309
  procedures and incisions in, 309–313, 311f-313f
  warming methods in, 309
tracheobronchial injuries in, 314–320
trap-door thoracotomy for, 312–313, 313f
tube thoracostomy in, 309–310
Chest tube
in diaphragmatic injuries, 405–406, 409
for hemothorax, 306
indications for, 298–299
placement of, 309–310
for pneumothorax, 305
Chest wall injuries, 80, 302, 563–564. *See also* Chest trauma
imaging studies in, 626–627
Chiasmal syndrome, 278
Child abuse, 579, 582–583
burns in, 157
head injuries in, 574, 582–583
reporting of, 723
rib fractures in, 584
shaken baby syndrome in, 574, 582–583
Children. *See* Pediatric trauma
Chin lift, 76
Chisolm, John Julian, 5
Chlordiazepoxide, for alcohol withdrawal, 674, 674t
Chlorine, 64
Chlorpromazine, for delirium, 669–671
Cholangiopancreatography
endoscopic retrograde, 448, 451, 453
transcholecystic, 452
Cholecystectomy, 428
Cholecystitis
acalculous, 427
traumatic, 427

Choroidal injuries, 274–276
Chronic pain. *See also* Pain
from burns, 172
Chylothorax, traumatic, 307–308
Circulation, Respiration, Abdominal/Thoracic, Motor, and Speech (CRAMS) Scale, 13t
Circulatory alterations, in pregnancy, 596–597
Circulatory evaluation, 80–86
Cis-atracurium, for anesthesia induction, 182, 183
Citrate toxicity, in transfusions, 143–144
Civil War, trauma surgery in, 4–5
Clamp stabilization, in pelvic fractures, 523
Clamshell thoracotomy, 311–312, 311f, 332f, 334
Clavicle fractures, 531, 647
Claw hand, 235
prevention of, 687–688, 688f, 689
Clindamycin
for lip lacerations, 256
for mandibular fractures, 250
for maxillofacial gunshot injuries, 256
Clonidine
for opiate withdrawal, 675
for spasticity, in spinal cord injuries, 700t
Closed cardiac massage, in pregnancy, 598
Clothesline injury, 316
Clotting factor concentrates, 142
Coagulation, in pregnancy, 597
Coagulation support, for massive hemorrhage, 136–141, 136f. *See also* Transfusions
Coagulopathy
dilutional, 188
prevention of, 137–140, 146f. *See also* Transfusions
fibrinolysis and, 140–141
hypothermia and, 141
in organ donors, 659
platelet dysfunction and, 141
Cocaine, 675
Coccyx fractures, 643
Cocoanut Grove fire, 7
Cognitive impairment
Rancho Los Amigos Scale for, 702–703, 703t
in traumatic brain injury, 702t, 706
Cold injury. *See also* Hypothermia
burn unit care for, 170
Cold toxicity, in transfusions, 141, 144–145
Collar, cervical, 36–37, 77
Colloids, 185, 187t
vs. crystalloids, for hemorrhagic shock, 83

Colon injuries, 462–464, 462–466, 468–474, 477–478
  blunt, 462–463, 464
  in children, 586
  diagnosis of, 463–464
  epidemiology of, 462
  imaging studies in, 463, 636–637
  laparoscopy in, 463–464
  mechanisms of, 462
  nonoperative management of, 464
  operative management of, 468–469
    complications of, 472–473
    indications for, 464
    postoperative care in, 472
  penetrating, 462, 464
  physical examination in, 463
  in pregnancy, 604
  presentation of, 463
Colostomy, 470–473, 471f, 472f
  postoperative complications in, 473–474
Coma. *See also* Head injuries
  barbiturate, 219
    in children, 581
  Rancho Los Amigos Scale for, 702–703, 703t
Combitube, 33
Common bile duct injuries, 413, 420, 427–429
Common iliac artery, injuries of, 368–369
Common peroneal nerve injuries, 692–693, 692t
Commotio retinae, 274–275
Communication
  between emergency department and emergency medical services, 53–54
  in transport, 42–43
Community-wide disaster systems, 40
Compartment pressure, measurement of, 527, 540
Compartment syndromes, 123–124
  abdominal, 479–482
  in burns, 154t
  in extremity injuries, 529–530
    immediate fasciotomy for, 379, 380f
  in hand injuries, 544, 557
Competency, 680, 713–717
Compression methods, for thromboembolism prophylaxis, 196–197
Computed tomography. *See also* Radiology *and specific injuries*
  in abdominal injuries, 114, 390–391, 392t, 404, 632–633
  in abdominal wall injuries, 410
  in bladder injuries, 501–502, 502f
  contrast blush in, 437, 442
  in diaphragmatic injuries, 404–405

  in duodenal injuries, 410
  in esophageal injuries, 322
  in extremity fractures, 526
  in hand injuries, 548
  of hemoperitoneum, 416
  in hepatic injuries, 415–416, 419–420
  in neck injuries, 290
  in orthopedic injuries, 646–647
  in pancreatic injuries, 410
  in pelvic trauma, 640–641
  pooled contrast in, 437, 442
  in pregnancy, safety of, 606
  of rectus sheath hematomas, 412
  in renal injuries, 486–487
  in splenic injuries, 436–437
  in thoracic injuries, 300
  in ureteral injuries, 495–496
  in vascular injuries, of abdomen, 352
Concussions, 705. *See also* Head injuries
Confidentiality, 720–723, 728
  duty to warn and, 724
  in performance improvement, 26
Conjunctiva
  examination of, 262
  injuries of, 264–265
Consciousness, 662–663
  assessment of, 12t, 86–87, 117t, 662–663
    in children, 574–575, 580–581
  level of, 662
  psychic content of, 662–663
Consent, 679–680, 712–717
  for organ donation, 660, 660t
Continuous renal replacement therapy, 127
Contraband, 726, 727
Contractures, burn, 171–172
Contrast blush, in splenic injuries, 437, 442
Contrast esophagography, 322–323
Contrast media
  adverse effects of, 289–290
  extravasation of, in splenic injuries, 437, 442
  renal injury from, 125
Contrast studies. *See also* Radiology
  in neck injuries, 289–290
Contusions
  cardiac, 335–336, 337f
  cerebral, imaging studies in, 620
  eyelid, 281
  orbital, 279
  pulmonary, 122–123, 303–304
    in children, 585
    imaging of, 627–628
Cornea
  examination of, 262
  injuries of, 266–269
    abrasion, 266–267

chemical, 267–268
exposure, 161, 168t, 268
foreign body, 267
laceration, 268–269
rupture, 268–269
thermal, 268
Coronary artery injuries, 339–341, 340f
Corpora cavernosa rupture, 504
Corticosteroids
for airway management, with intraoral injuries, 255
for preterm labor, 603
for spinal cord injury, 225
stress ulcers and, 209
Counseling, for organ donation, 660
Cowley, R. Adams, 7–8
CPR. *See* Resuscitation
CRAMS Scale, 13t
Cranial nerve injuries
in head injuries, 215, 216. *See also* Head injuries
in maxillofacial injuries, 239–240. *See also* Maxillofacial injuries
ocular motor, 278–279
Craniectomy, decompressive bifrontal, 219
Creatinine clearance, 126
Cricothyroidotomy, 77
needle, 77, 103–104, 104f
prehospital, 34–35
surgical, 77, 104–105, 105f
Crile, George, 5
Crime scenes, evidence preservation in, 32
Criminal activity, of patients, 725–727
Critical care, 120–127
compartment pressure monitoring in, 123–124
for elderly, 613
fat embolism in, 123, 123t
intracranial pressure monitoring in, 120–121
multiple organ dysfunction syndrome in, 124–125
neurologic examination in, 121
pain management in, 121
pediatric, 589–590
pulmonary contusion in, 122–123
rehabilitation in, 707–708
renal failure in, 125–127
respiratory failure in, 122
rhabdomyolysis in, 125–126
staffing for, 120
Critical care transport specialists, 31
Critical illness myopathy, 708
Critical illness polyneuropathy, 708
Crush injuries
extremity, 529
fingertip, 550–551
Cryoprecipitate, indications for, 139–140

Crystalloids, 185, 187t
vs. colloids, for hemorrhagic shock, 83
Cultures, bacteriologic, in extremity fractures, 527
Curare, 182, 183
Curling's ulcers, 164, 168t, 208
bleeding from, 208–209
Cushing's triad, 87
Cyanide, 64, 65–66
Cyanide exposure, in burns, 164
Cyanogen chloride, 64, 65–66
Cyclodialysis, 270
Cystography, 501–502, 502f

D

Dalteparin, prophylactic, 200
Dantrolene, for spasticity, in spinal cord injuries, 700t
Data collection/display, for performance improvement, 25–26
DDAVP, for transfusions, 142
Débridement, for extremity injuries, 378–380
Débridement resection, for hepatic injuries, 423
Deceleration injuries, abdominal, 413, 414
Decompressive cranial surgery, 219, 220
Decubitus ulcers, in spinal cord injuries, 701
Deep vein thrombosis, prevention of, 195–199, 200t
in alcohol withdrawal, 205t
in elderly, 616
in spinal cord injuries, 701
Delirium, 664–672, 665t
causes of, 665t, 667
vs. dementia, 664
drug-related, 667, 668t
evaluation of, 663, 665–667
restraints and, 724–725
signs of, 664
treatment of, 667–672
Delirium tremens, 674
Delivery
cesarean, 598–599
premature, 603
Dementia, 664
Dental injuries, 251
Dentition, airway management and, 89, 92
Dentoalveolar fractures, 251
Depression, 677–678
Desmopressin, for transfusions, 142
Dextroamphetamine, for depression, 678
Diabetes insipidus, in organ donors, 659
Diagnostic peritoneal lavage, 114, 115t, 389–390

Diagnostic peritoneal lavage (*contd.*)
  in diaphragmatic injury, 114, 115t,
      389–390
  in duodenal injuries, 447
  in hepatic injuries, 417, 420
  in pancreatic injuries, 447
  technique of, 389–390
  in vascular injuries, 353
Dialysis, 127
Diaphragmatic injuries, 307, 402–409
  airway management in, 403
  anatomic aspects of, 402
  diagnosis of, 404–406
      delayed, 409
  epidemiology of, 402
  hemorrhage in, 308
  imaging studies in, 404–406, 627
  initial evaluation in, 403
  mechanism of, 403–404
  nasogastric intubation in, 404
  operative management of, 407–409
  patterns of, 403
  physical examination in, 404
  signs and symptoms of, 404
  site of, 402–403
Diazepam
  for alcohol withdrawal, 674, 674t
  for delirium, 671
  for spasticity, in spinal cord
      injuries, 700t
Dicyclomine, for opiate withdrawal,
      675
Diet. *See also* Nutritional support
  for neurogenic bowel, 695
Difficult airway
  adjuncts for
      nonsurgical, 98–103
      surgical, 103–107
  anticipated, 98
  unanticipated, 98
Diffuse axonal injuries, 219–220
  imaging studies in, 620
DIGFAST mnemonic, 678
Digital endotracheal intubation, 35
Digital nerve block, 549f, 550
Digits. *See* Finger; Thumb; Toe
Dilution coagulopathy, 188
  prevention of, 137–140, 146f. *See
      also* Transfusions
Diphenhydramine, for dystonia,
      670–671
Direct laryngoscopy
  in difficult airway, 98–107
  equipment for, 72, 94–95
  glottic visualization in
      failure of, 98
      predictors of, 90
  technique for, 95–96
Disability, 682
  rehabilitation for. *See* Rehabilitation
Disability evaluation, 86–87
Disaster planning, 58–68

Disaster response, 58–68. *See also*
      Emergency medical services;
      Mass casualty management
  triage in, 39–40, 41t, 59–60
Dislocations
  elbow, 533
  extremity, 528
  facet joint, 514, 517
  hip, 535, 652–653
      central, 642
      rehabilitation in, 689–693, 689t
  knee, 536
  lens, 272
  midfoot, 538
  patellofemoral, 535–536
  shoulder, 531, 647–648
  sternoclavicular, 531, 649
  vertebral, 517
Disodium etidronate, for heterotopic
      ossification, 699
Disseminated intravascular coagula-
      tion, in massive hemorrhage,
      prevention of, 136–137, 146f
Distal humerus fractures, 532–533
Distal interphalangeal dislocations,
      554
Distal pancreatectomy, 452, 453f
Distal radius fractures, 534
Diuretics
  in elderly, 614–615
  for increased intracranial pres-
      sure, in children, 581
DNR orders
  ethical aspects of, 730, 731
  legal aspects of, 715
Dobutamine, 189
Documentation
  of physical examination, 119
  of resuscitation, 119
Domestic violence, in pregnancy, 593
Do not resuscitate orders
  ethical aspects of, 731
  legal aspects of, 715
Dopamine, 189
Drainage
  in duodenal surgery, 457–458,
      458f, 460
  of hemothorax, 306
  rectal, 470–472, 473f
  renal, 489, 493–494
Droperidol, for delirium, 669–671
Drug abuse, 672–675
  testing for, 726
Drug history, 109
  in elderly, 612–613
Drug therapy
  delirium and, 667, 668t
  preexisting, in elderly, 612–613
Duodenal decompression, 456–458,
      458f
Duodenal diverticulation, 429
Duodenal fistula, 461

Duodenal hematoma, 456t
  in children, 578
Duodenal injuries, 476–477
  epidemiology of, 446
  grading of, 456t
  imaging studies in, 447–448
  initial evaluation in, 447–448
  mechanisms of, 446
  nonoperative management of, 446,
    455
  operative management of, 446,
    455–459
    for combined pancreaticoduode-
      nal injuries, 459
    complications of, 460–461
    diversion in, 457–458, 458f
    drainage in, 457–458, 458f, 460
    duodenal decompression in,
      456–458, 458f
    duodenal diverticulation in, 458
    exposures in, 450f-451f, 455–456
    feeding jejunostomy in, 458f,
      460
    indications for, 448, 455
    nasogastric decompression in,
      460
    postoperative care in, 459–460
    pyloric exclusion in, 458, 459f
    repair in, 457
    technical aspects of, 456–459
  pancreatic injuries with, 456, 459
  physical examination in, 447
  presentation of, 455
Duodenal ulcers
  bleeding from, 207–209
  in burns, 164, 168t, 208–209
Duplex Doppler ultrasonography, of
    arterial injuries, 375
Dysrhythmias
  in anesthesia, 193–194
  in cardiac contusion, 335–336, 337f
  neuroleptics and, 669–670
Dystonia
  neuroleptics and, 670–671
  in spinal cord injuries, 699

E
Ear
  burns of, 168t
  examination of, 111
Echocardiography, transesophageal,
    184
  in cardiac injuries, 329–330
Edema, Berlin's, 274–275
Elastic compression stockings, 196
Elbow injuries, 532–533
  nerve injuries in, 687–688
  rehabilitation in, 687–688
Elderly. See Geriatric trauma
Electrical burns, 155t, 170. See also
    Burns
Electrical cataracts, 273

Electrocardiography, in anesthesia,
    179, 180
Electrocution, cataracts and, 273
Electrolyte imbalances. See also
    Fluid management
  in anesthesia, 191
Electromyography, in nerve injuries,
    693, 694t
Emancipated minors, consent of, 714
Embolism. See also Thromboembolism
  amniotic fluid, 600
  fat, 123, 123t
  pulmonary, prevention of,
    195–199, 200t
Embolization, angiographic,
    442–443, 488–489
  in pelvic fractures, 522, 524
Emergency department
  common traps and dilemmas in, 55
  coordination of care in, 53–54, 55,
    56f
  design of, 52–53, 56f
  direct patient care decisions in, 55,
    56f
  equipment in, 53, 56f, 71–73
  organization of, 50–55, 56f, 71–72
  personnel in, 50–52, 73. See also
    Trauma team
  training in, 55
  team concept in, 54. See also
    Trauma team
  trauma response activation in,
    54–55
Emergency medical services, 29–48
  access to patient in, 31–32
  activation of, 31
  airway management and, 32–35
  analgesia and, 38–39
  for burns, 39, 40t
  case presentation and, 74–75
  coordination of with emergency
    department, 53–54
  crime scenes and, 32
  extremity immobilization and, 38
  extrications and, 31, 32, 36–38
  fluid resuscitation and, 35–36, 36
  hazardous materials exposures
    and, 32
  for mass casualties, 39–40, 58–61.
    See also Mass casualty man-
    agement
  medical field care and, 32–40
  needle chest decompression and, 35
  911 system for, 31
  for pediatric trauma, 39
  personnel training and qualifica-
    tions in, 29–31
  pneumatic antishock garment and,
    38
  scene safety concerns and, 31–32
  scope of practice and, 30, 31
  specialized rescues and, 32

Emergency medical services (*contd.*)
  spinal immobilization and, 36–38
  in transition to hospital care,
      74–75
  transport and, 29–31, 40–48. *See
      also* Transport
  triage and, 39–40, 41t
  vascular access and, 35
  wound care and, 38
Emergency medical technicians, 30
Emergency Medical Treatment and
      Active Labor Act (EMTALA),
      710–712
  liability and, 729–730
Emesis, esophageal rupture in,
      321–322
Emotional issues. *See* Psychiatric
      issues
Emphysema, subcutaneous, in chest
      trauma, 305–306, 317
EMT. *See also* Emergency medical
      services
  scope of practice of, 30
EMT-basic, 30
EMT-intermediate, 30
EMT-paramedic, 30
Endocrine disorders, in organ
      donors, 659
Endoluminal devices, 349
Endoscopic retrograde cholangiopan-
      creatography, 448, 451
Endoscopy. *See also specific techniques*
  in esophageal injuries, 323
  in neck injuries, 289
Endotracheal intubation, 93–98. *See
      also* Mechanical ventilation
  anatomic variations and, 595f
  in anesthesia, 181–182
  in brain-injured patients, 87
  in burns, 151
  cervical spine injuries and, 89, 90,
      91, 95, 193
  in chest trauma, 298
  in children, 572
  complications of, 93, 98
  difficult
    nonsurgical adjuncts to, 98–103
    predictors of, 90
    surgical adjuncts to, 103–107
  digital, 35
  equipment for, 72, 94–95
  extubation in, 192–193
  fiberoptic, 98–100
  in flail chest, 302
  indications for, 76–77, 94
  induction agents for, 96–97
  intubating laryngeal mask airway
      in, 102–103
  light wand in, 103
  in maxillofacial injuries, 256–257
  nasotracheal, 34, 76, 97–98
  in neck injuries, 287–288
    neuromuscular blockade for, 34
    orotracheal, 33–34, 76, 94–97
      difficult, 90, 98–107
      induction agents for, 96–97
      technique for, 94–96
    in pregnancy, 593–595, 595f, 596t
    prehospital, 33–34
    rapid sequence, 93–94
    retrograde, 106–107
    sniffing position for, 95
    tube displacement in, 163t
    tube occlusion in, 162, 163t
    tube selection for, 72, 96, 98
Endovascular stents, 349
Enoxaparin, prophylactic, 197
Enucleation, 283
Epidemiology, trauma, 10
Epidural hematoma, 221, 222f
  in children, 581
Epigastric arterial injuries, rectus
      sheath hematomas and,
      411–412
Epinephrine, 189
  indications for, 189
Epiphyseal fractures, 578–579,
      588–589, 588f
Epistaxis, 244–246, 245f
Equipment
  emergency department, 53
  resuscitation, 71–72
Erb's palsy, 236–237
Erythrocyte transfusions, 133–134,
      133t. *See also* Transfusions
  alternatives/supplements to,
      134–136
  citrate toxicity and, 142–143
Esophageal injuries
  anatomic aspects of, 320–326, 321
  cervical, 293–294, 323–324. *See
      also* Neck injuries
  clinical presentation of, 322
  diagnosis of, 322–323
  epidemiology of, 320
  iatrogenic, 321
  intraabdominal, 325–326
  management of
    definitive, 323–324, 323–326
    initial, 323
    nonoperative, 326
    operative, 323–326
  mechanism of, 321–322
  nonpenetrating, 321–322
  penetrating, 321
  postemetic, 321–322
  thoracic, 324–325. *See also* Chest
      trauma
Esophageal leak, 289–290
Esophageal obturator airway, 33
Esophageal T-tube, 325
Ethical issues
  DNR orders, 730
  treatment futility, 730

Ethmoid sinus injuries, 249, 281
Etomidate
    for anesthesia, 180–181
    for orotracheal intubation, 97
Evacuation triage, 60. *See also*
        Triage
Evaluation
    primary survey in, 71–88. *See also*
        Primary survey
    secondary survey in, 108–119. *See
        also* Secondary survey
    tertiary survey in, 118–119
Evidence, 726, 727
    crime scene, preservation of, 32
Exposure, questioning about, 110
Exposure keratopathy, in burns,
        161, 168t, 268
Extensor tendon injuries, 555–556
External iliac artery, injuries of,
        368–369
Extraocular motility, 262
Extraocular muscles, examination
        of, 262
Extrapyramidal side effects, neu-
        roleptic, 670–671
Extremity injuries, 526–539
    ankle, 536–538
    antibiotic prophylaxis for, 527
    in anticoagulated patients, 530
    compartment syndrome in, 529–530
    crush, 529
    débridement of, 378–380
    discharge instructions for, 528
    early amputation for, 379
    elbow, 532–533
    elevation for, 528
    examination of, 526–527
    femur, 534–535
    foot, 538–539
    forearm, 533–534
    hand, 540–557
    high-energy, 529
    hip and proximal femur, 534–535
    ice application for, 528
    imaging studies for, 526–527
    immediate fasciotomy for, 379, 380f
    immobilization of, 38, 527
    knee, 535–536
    lower extremity, 534–539
    lower leg, 536–538
    mechanism of, 529–530
    muscle strength assessment in, 529
    with open fractures, 528–529
    orthopedic, 526–539. *See also*
        Fracture(s); Orthopedic
        trauma
    in osteoporosis, 530
    with severe deformities, 527
    shoulder, 531–532
    tibial, 536–537
    treatment of, 527–528
    in unconscious patients, 530
    upper extremity, 531–534. *See also*
        Hand injuries
    vascular, 372–384. *See also*
        Peripheral vascular injuries
    weightbearing with, 528
    wrist, 533–534
Extremity vascular injuries, 372–384
Extrication
    by EMTs, 31, 32
    Kendrick device for, 37–38
    spinal immobilization in, 36–38
Eye
    anatomy of, 259f, 260f
    examination of, 110–111, 259–263.
        See also Ocular examination
    in head injuries, 215
    foreign bodies in, 262, 263, 264,
        265–266. *See also* Foreign
        bodies, intraocular
    imaging of, 263–264
    injuries of, 258–283. *See also* Ocu-
        lar injuries
    red, differential diagnosis of, 269t
Eyelid
    avulsions of, 281
    contusions of, 281
    examination of, 262
    lacerations of, 261–262, 261f, 281

F

Facet joint dislocations, 514, 517
Facial abrasions, 253
Facial anatomy, 239–242
Facial bones
    examination of, 111
    radiography of, 621
Facial injuries. *See* Maxillofacial
        injuries
Facial lacerations, 252–256, 281
Facial nerve injuries, 240–241,
        254–255. *See also* Cranial
        nerve injuries
Factor VII, recombinant, 142
Fallen lung sign, 317
Fasciotomy
    in burns, 154t
    for compartment syndromes, 124
    immediate, for extremity injuries,
        379, 380f
FAST examination
    in abdominal trauma, 114, 352,
        387–389, 388f, 436, 631–632
    in chest trauma, 329
    in splenic injuries, 436
Fastrach laryngeal mask airway,
        102–103
Fat embolism, 123, 123t
Fecal incontinence, in spinal cord
        injuries, 695
Feeding tube
    in duodenal surgery, 457, 458f, 460
    in esophageal injuries, 324, 325

Feet, injuries of, 538–539
Femoral artery injuries, 382. *See also* Peripheral vascular injuries
Femoral nerve injuries, 693
Femoral venous access, 81
Femur fractures, 534–535
  head, 650
  imaging of, 650–651
  neck, 534, 650–651
  pediatric, 589
  rehabilitation in, 689–693, 689t
  shaft, 535
Femur injuries, 534–535. *See also* Hip injuries
Fetal heartbeat, evaluation of, 600
Fetal injury/demise, 592
  cesarean delivery in, 598–599
  gestational age and, 599–600
Fetal monitoring, perioperative, 602, 603
Fiberoptic intubation, 98–100
Fibrin glue
  for liver injuries, 424
  for splenic injuries, 441
Fibrinolysis, 140–141
Field triage, 59–60. *See also* Triage
Filters, vena cava, 197, 200t
Finger. *See also* Hand
  dislocations of, 554
  fractures of, 553–554
  traumatic amputation of, 551–553
Finger fracture technique, in hepatic surgery, 423
Fingertip injuries, 550
  amputation, 551
First responders, 29. *See also* Emergency medical services
Fistula
  carotid–cavernous sinus, 281
  duodenal, 461
  pancreatic, 460
Flail chest, 80, 302, 627
Flaps. *See also* Soft tissue reconstruction
  muscle, 558
  skin, 560–561
Fleming Alexander, 5
Flexor tendon injuries, 555
Fluid attenuation, in abdominal trauma, 634
Fluid management, 81–83. *See also* Resuscitation; Transfusions
  in anesthesia, 180, 185–189
  in burns, 151, 157–160
  in children, 573, 589–590
  equipment for, 72–73
  in head injuries, 218
  in organ donors, 658–659
  prehospital, 35–36, 36t
  solutions for, 83, 185–186, 187t
  vascular access for, 72, 80–81

  for anesthesia, 178–179, 184
  in children, 572–573, 573f
  equipment for, 72
  in pregnancy, 598–599
  prehospital, 35
  sites for, 81
Focused assessment with sonography for trauma (FAST)
  in abdominal trauma, 114, 352, 387–388, 388f, 436, 631–632
  in chest trauma, 329
  in hepatic injuries, 436
Folstein Mini Mental Exam, 663t, 665
Food intake, pre-injury, 109
Foot injuries, 538–539
Forearm, traumatic amputation of, 551–553
Forearm fractures, 533–534
  nerve injuries in, 688–689
Forearm injuries, reconstructive surgery for, 562–563
Foreign bodies, ocular, 262, 263, 264, 265–266, 267
  anterior segment, 273
  conjunctival, 265
  corneal, 267
  intraorbital, 279
  posterior segment, 276–277
  scleral, 265–266
Fracture(s)
  acetabular, 641–642
  ankle, 537
  blowout, 279–280, 621
  buckle, 587, 587f
  calcaneal, 538
  carpal, 553–554
  chance, 626
  in child abuse, 579, 589
  in children, 578–579
  clavicle, 531, 647
  coccyx, 643
  dentoalveolar, 251
  distal radius, 534
  elbow, nerve injuries in, 687–688
  in elderly, 612
  epiphyseal, 578–580, 588–589, 588f
  extremity, 526–539. *See also* Extremity injuries
  facial, 241–242, 621
  fat embolism and, 123, 123t
  femur
    head, 650
    imaging of, 650–651
    neck, 534, 650–651
    pediatric, 589
    shaft, 535
  foot, 538–539
  forearm, 533–534
    nerve injuries in, 688–689
  frontal sinus, 241, 251–252
  Galeazzi, 533–534

greater trochanter, 534–535, 652
greenstick, 580, 587, 587f
hand, 553–554
hangman's, 512, 513
  radiography of, 622
hip, 534–535, 649–652
  rehabilitation in, 689–693, 689t,
    691t
humerus
  distal, 532–533
  imaging of, 647
  nerve injuries in, 687
  proximal, 531–532
  shaft, 532
iliac, 641
imaging studies in, 646–650
Jefferson, 512, 513
  radiography of, 622
LeFort, 247–249, 248f, 280
lesser trochanter, 652
lower extremity, 534–539
  rehabilitation in, 689–693, 689t
mandibular, 242, 249–251
maxillary, 241, 247–249, 248f, 280
metacarpal, 553–554
metatarsal, 538–539
Monteggia, 533–534
nasal, 244–246, 245f
nasoorbital ethmoid complex, 249,
    281
odontoid peg, 513
olecranon, 533
open, tibial, 565–566, 565t
orbital, 249, 279–281, 621
patellar, 535
pediatric, 586–589, 587f, 588f
pelvic, 518–525, 640–646
  bladder injuries and, 502, 503
  imaging studies in, 640–646
penile, 506
phalangeal, 553–554
radial head, 533
rib, 300–302
  in children, 584
  in flail chest, 80, 302, 627
  imaging of, 626–627
sacrum, 642
Salter-Harris classification of,
    578–580, 588, 588f
scapula, 532, 627, 647
seatbelt, 517
skull, 220–221
skull base, 252, 621
spinal, 509–517
sternal, 302–303
supracondylar, 589
temporal bone, 252
thoracic
  imaging of, 626
  rehabilitation in, 686
tibia
  pilon, 537
  plateau, 536
  shaft, 536–537
toe, 539
torus, 587, 587f
tripod, 242
tuft, 554
wrist, 533–534, 553–554
zygomatic, 242
zygomaticomaxillary, 246, 280
Fracture-dislocations. See also Dislo-
    cations; Fracture(s)
  spinal, 517
Frank Jones test, 665–667
Freeark, Robert, 8
Free flaps, 561. See also Soft tissue
    reconstruction
Fresh frozen plasma, transfusion of,
    138–139. See also Transfusions
Fromen's sign, 235
Frontal bone
  anatomy of, 241
  fractures of, 251–252
Frostbite, burn unit care for, 170

G

Galeazzi fractures, 533–534
Gallbladder injuries, 413, 420,
    427–429
  imaging studies in, 636
Gamekeeper's thumb, 555
Gastric contents, questioning about,
    109
Gastric injuries, 462–466, 477–478
  anatomic aspects of, 464–465
  blunt, 462–463
  in children, 586
  diagnosis of, 463–464
  epidemiology of, 462
  imaging studies of, 463
  laparoscopy in, 463–464
  mechanisms of, 462
  nonoperative management of, 464
  operative management of,
    465–466, 466f
    complications of, 472–473
    indications for, 464
    postoperative care in, 472
  penetrating, 462
  physical examination in, 463
  presentation of, 463
Gastric ulcers
  bleeding from, 207–209
  in burns, 164, 168t, 208–209
Gastrointestinal bleeding, 207–209.
    See also Bleeding;
    Hemorrhage
  imaging of, 632–634
Gastrosoleus tear, 537
Gastrostomy tube
  in duodenal surgery, 457, 458f,
    460
  in esophageal injuries, 324, 325

General anesthesia. *See also* Anesthesia
historical perspective on, 6–7
vs. regional anesthesia, 177–178
Genital examination, 115
Genital injuries, 506–508
Genitourinary trauma, imaging studies in, 643–646
bladder, 500–503
epidemiology of, 484
genital, 506–508
mechanisms of injury in, 484
physical examination in, 114–115
renal, 484–494
surgical anatomy of, 484
ureteral, 494–500
urethral, 503–506
Geriatric trauma, 608–618
airway management in, 611, 616
chest injuries in, 610–611
comorbidities in, 612, 614–615, 617–618
complications of, 615–616
costs of, 609–610
critical care in, 613
demographics of, 609
discharge and, 617
epidemiology of, 609
imaging studies in, 612
immobilization in, 611
mechanism of injury in, 610–611
medical history in, 612
medication history in, 612–613, 614–615
mortality in, 615
neurologic injuries in, 610
nonoperative management in, 614
nutritional support in, 616
occult injuries in, 612, 617
operative management in, 613–614
orthopedic injuries in, 611, 612
pain management in, 616
physiologic changes and, 610–611
pitfalls in, 617–618
primary survey in, 611
quality of life and, 617
rehabilitation in, 616–617
renal injuries in, 611
secondary survey in, 611
thrombosis prophylaxis in, 616
triage and disposition in, 613
Gestational age assessment, 599–600
GF (nerve agent), 64–65
Ghost cell glaucoma, 272
Glasgow Coma Scale, 12t, 86–87, 117t, 662–663
in children, 574–575, 580–581
Glassblower's cataracts, 273
Glaucoma, 271–272
Globe injury, 262–263, 264
Glomerular filtration rate, 126
Golden hour theory, 7–8

Good Samaritan laws, 729
Gore-Tex mesh
for abdominal wall injuries, 481–482, 564
for chest wall injuries, 564
for liver injuries, 424
for splenic injuries, 441
Gould, A.A., 7
Grading, of trauma cases, 74
Grafts
greater saphenous vein, for peripheral vascular injuries, 377, 378f, 383
nerve, for hand injuries, 563
skin, 560. *See also* Soft tissue reconstruction
for burns, 707
Greater saphenous vein grafting, for peripheral vascular injuries, 377, 378f
complications of, 383
Greater trochanter fractures, 534–535, 652
Great vessel injuries, 339–341, 340f, 341, 347–349, 347t, 348t
Greenstick fractures, 580, 587, 587f
Grillo, Hermes, 6
Gross, Samuel, 5
Ground transport, 40–42. *See also* Transport
personnel for, 29–30
Growth plate injuries, 578–579, 588–589, 588f
Guardianship, 715–716
Gunshot wounds
abdominal, visceral injuries in, 413. *See also* Abdominal trauma
laparoscopy for, 393
brachial plexus, 237
cardiac, 339–341, 340f
cervical, 284
cranial, 223
maxillofacial, 256
in precordial box, 328, 329f
questioning about, 110
renal, 490
thoracic, 297
tracheobronchial, 315–316
transmediastinal, 315

H

Hallucinations, 664
Haloperidol
for agitation, 670
for alcohol withdrawal, 202
for delirium, 669–671
Hammond, William A., 4
Hand
blood supply of, 542
innervation of, 545–547, 546f
muscles of, 542–543

Hand injuries, 540–557. *See also*
        Finger; Thumb
    amputation, 551–553
    anatomic aspects of, 540, 541f,
        542–543
    anesthesia for, 549–550
    bite, 549
    clinical significance of, 540
    diagnosis of, 547–548
    dislocations, 554
    fingertip and nailbed, 549
    fractures, 553–554
    history in, 540–541
    imaging studies in, 547–548
    immediate management of,
        548–550
    ligamentous, 554–555
    mechanism of, 541
    nerve involvement in, 544,
        545–547, 546f, 563
    physical examination in, 543–547
    reconstructive surgery for, 562–563
    rehabilitation for, 686–689
    sequelae of, 556–557
    splints for, 687, 688, 688f, 689
    tendon, 555–556
    vascular involvement in, 547
Hand splints, 687, 688, 688f, 689
Hangman's fracture, 512, 513
    radiography of, 622
Harborview Assessment of Mortality
        (HARM) Scale, 21t
Hartmann's procedure, 470–473,
        472f
Hazardous materials, exposure to,
        32, 110
Head, examination of, 110–111,
        214–216
Head injuries, 213–223
    agitation in, 705–706, 706t
    in children, 574–575, 580–581
    classification of, 213
    cognitive impairment in, 702–703,
        702t, 703t, 706
    coma in, 702–703
    concussions in, 705
    decompressive surgery for, 219
    delirium in, 667
    diagnostic studies in, 216–217
    diffuse axonal injury in, 219–220
    endotracheal intubation in, 87
    epidemiology of, 213
    epidural hematoma in, 221, 222f
    functional outcome in, 702–704
    gunshot, 223
    imaging studies in, 619–621
    increased intracranial pressure in.
        See Increased intracranial
        pressure
    initial evaluation of, 213–216
    late complications of, 222
    management of, 216–223

    imaging studies in, 216–217
    in-hospital, 217–219
    mechanism of, 213, 214
    mild, 216
    minimally responsive state in, 703
    neurobehavioral impairment in,
        702t
    neurologic examination in, 214,
        215. *See also* Neurologic
        examination
      in children, 574, 580–581
      on-scene, 214
    neurostimulants for, 704, 704t
    penetrating, 222–223
    physical examination in, 110–111,
        214–216
    prognostic indicators in, 702
    Rancho Los Amigos Scale for,
        702–703, 703t
    rehabilitation in, 701–706
    secondary brain injury in, 213
    seizures in, 218, 705
    skull fractures in, 220–221
    spasticity in, 706
    stab, 223
    subdural hematoma in, 221–222,
        222f
    traumatic brain injury in,
        701–706, 702t
    vegetative state in, 703–704
Healing. *See* Wound healing
Healthcare proxy, 715
Health Insurance Portability and
        Accountability Act (HIPAAA),
        privacy provisions of,
        721–723, 728
Heart, injuries of. *See* Cardiac
        injuries
Heart disease, drug therapy in, in
        elderly, 614–615
Heart failure, inotropic agents for,
        189
Heel fractures, 538
Helicopters. *See* Air transport
Hematocrit, posthemorrhage goals
        for, 134
Hematomas
    duodenal, 456t
      in children, 578
    epidural, 221, 222f
      in children, 581
    hepatic, 635t
      grading of, 418t
    pancreatic
      grading of, 485t
      imaging of, 639
    pelvic, 367–368
    perireal, 504
    rectus sheath, 411–412
    renal, grading of, 485t
    splenic, 634–635
      grading of, 436t

Hematomas (*contd.*)
 subdural, 221–222, 222f
  in children, 581
 subungual, 550
Hemicraniectomy, decompressive,
  219
Hemobilia, 420, 428, 430
Hemodialysis, 127
Hemodynamic status, assessment of,
  134
Hemodynamic support. *See also*
  Fluid management
 prehospital, 35–36, 36t
Hemoperitoneum, 416
 nonoperative management and,
  419
Hemorrhage. *See also* Bleeding
 gastrointestinal, 207–209
  imaging of, 632–634
 in hepatic injuries, 416, 419, 420
 infradiaphragmatic, 308
 management of, 134. *See also*
  Transfusions
  coagulation support in, 136–141
 orbital, 279
 retinal, 275
 retroperitoneal, 192
 splenic, 433
 subarachnoid, imaging studies in,
  621
 subchoroidal, 276
 subconjunctival, 264–265
 subdural, imaging studies in,
  620–621
 vitreous, 274
Hemorrhagic shock, 81–83, 133–134,
  135t
Hemostasis, 134. *See also specific
  injuries and procedures*
Hemothorax, 306–307
 in children, 584–585
 imaging of, 629
 massive, 79–80, 308
Heparin
 prophylactic, 197–198, 200t
 thrombocytopenia due to, 198
Hepatic abscess, 420
Hepatic artery injuries, 369
Hepatic artery ligation, 423
Hepatic duct ligation, 429
Hepatic injuries, 413–427, 475–476
 anatomic aspects of, 414f, 417–418
 bilhaemia in, 420–421
 biliary tract injuries and, 419,
  420–421
 biliary tract injuries with, 413,
  420, 427–429
 bleeding in, 416, 419, 633
 blunt, 413
 bowel injuries with, 419–420
 in children, 575–577, 576t, 586
 delayed complications in, 430–431

 diagnosis of, 415–417, 431
 epidemiology of, 413
 grading of, 418, 418t
 hemobilia in, 420, 428, 430
 hemoperitoneum and, 416, 419
 imaging studies in, 415–417, 431,
  633, 635–636
 initial evaluation in, 413–417
 jaundice in, 430
 juxtahepatic venous injuries with,
  424–427
 laparotomy for, 415
 management of
  common traps and dilemmas in,
   430–431
  nonoperative, 418–421
  operative, 421–424
  postoperative care in, 430
 mechanisms of, 413
 penetrating, 413
 physical examination in, 413–414,
  415
 rebleeding in, 419, 420
 rehabilitation in, 430
 retrohepatic vena cava injuries
  with, 424–427
 vascular, 369, 370, 424–427
Hepatic vein injuries, 370, 424–427
Hepatorrhaphy, 423
Hepatotomy, with suture ligation, 423
Hernia
 abdominal wall, 409–412. *See also*
  Abdominal wall herniation
 diaphragmatic, 402–409. *See also*
  Diaphragmatic injuries
Hespan, 186, 187t
Heterotopic ossification, in spinal
  cord injuries, 698–699
Hextend, 186, 187t
Hilar injury, 318, 318f
Hindfoot fractures, 538–539
HIPAA, privacy provisions of,
  721–723, 728
Hip injuries. *See also* Pelvic trauma
 dislocations, 642, 652–653
 fractures, 534–535, 649–652
 imaging of, 649–653, 689t
 rehabilitation in, 689–693, 689t,
  691t
History, patient, 108–110
Homan's sign, 195
Horner's syndrome, 277
Humerus fractures
 distal, 532–533
 imaging of, 647
 nerve injuries in, 687
 proximal, 531–532, 647
 rehabilitation in, 687
 shaft, 532
Hydrogen cyanide, 64, 65–66
Hydromorphone, for delirium,
  671–672

Hydroxyethyl starch, 186, 187t
Hyperbaric oxygen, in inhalation
    injury, 164
Hypercalcemia, in spinal cord
    injuries, 698
Hyperkalemia
    succinylcholine and, 181
    transfusion-related, 145
Hypertension
    in anesthesia, 193
    intracranial. *See* Increased
        intracranial pressure
Hypertrophic scars, 567–568
Hyperventilation, for increased
    intracranial pressure, 218
    in children, 581
Hyphema, 270–271
Hypoarousal, in traumatic brain
    injury, 703–704, 704t
Hypocalcemia, transfusion-related,
    188
Hypotension
    in anesthesia, 193
    in organ donors, 658–659
    orthostatic, in spinal cord injuries,
        698
Hypothermia
    in burns, 151, 152
    in massive transfusion, 141, 144
    warming for, 185
Hypovolemic shock, 81–83
Hypoxemia, in anesthesia, 194
Hypoxia, in anesthesia, 194

I
ICISS Scale, 21t
Ileal interposition, 499
Iliac artery injuries, 368–369
Iliac fractures, 641
Iliac vein injuries, 369
Imaging studies. *See* Radiology *and
        specific techniques*
Immobilization
    extremity, 38, 527
    spinal, 36–38, 77
        in elderly, 611
        prehospital, 36–38
Immobilization hypercalcemia, 698
Immunization, postsplenectomy, 444
Incident command, 40
Incisions, thoracic, 310–313,
    310f–313f, 333f
Incompetency, 680, 713–717
Incontinence, in spinal cord injuries,
    695
Increased intraabdominal pressure,
    479–482
Increased intracranial pressure
    abdominal compartment syndrome
        and, 481
    abdominal decompression for, 481
    barbiturate coma for, 219

in children, 581
    decompressive surgery for, 218, 219
    hyperventilation for, 218
        in children, 581
    intravenous mannitol for, 218, 219
    monitoring for, 120–121, 218, 219
Increased intraocular pressure
    examination for, 262–263
    in glaucoma, 271–272
Indomethacin, as tocolytic, 603
Induction agents. *See* Anesthesia
Infants. *See* Pediatric trauma
Infections, surgical site, 202–207
Inferior mesenteric artery injuries,
    363
Inferior vena cava filters, 197, 200t
Inferior vena cava injuries, 363–366,
    364f
Informed consent, 679–680, 712–717
Infradiaphragmatic hemorrhage, 308
Inhalation injury, 151, 153t
    in burns, 161–162
Initial evaluation, 71–88
    primary survey in, 71–88. *See also*
        Primary survey
    secondary survey in, 108–119. *See
        also* Secondary survey
    tertiary survey in, 118–119
Injury Severity Scale (ISS), 18t
Injury severity scoring, 12t-13t,
    15–17, 18t-21t. *See also*
        Trauma scoring
Inotropic agents, 189
Intensive care unit (ICU), 120–127.
    See also Critical care
    rehabilitation in, 707–708
Internal carotid artery, injuries of,
    292–293
Internal iliac artery, injuries of, 369
Internal venous access, 81
International normalized ratio (INR)
    dilutional coagulopathy and,
        138–139, 139f
    target range for, 198
Interphalangeal joints. *See also*
        Finger; Hand; Thumb
    dislocations of, 554
Intertrochanteric fractures, 652
Intervertebral disc pathology
    cervical radiculopathy and,
        684–686
    definition of, 685t
Intestinal injuries. *See also* Colon
        injuries; Duodenal injuries;
        Rectal injuries; Small bowel
        injuries
    with hepatic injuries, 419–420
Intoxication, alcohol, 199–201
Intraabdominal pressure
    increased, 479–482
    monitoring of, 480
Intraaortic balloon pump, 189

Intracranial pressure. *See* Increased
    intracranial pressure
Intraocular foreign bodies, 262, 263,
    264, 265–266, 267
    anterior segment, 273
    conjunctival, 265
    corneal, 267
    posterior segment, 276–277
    scleral, 265–266
Intraocular pressure
    in glaucoma, 271–272
    measurement of, 262–263
Intraoral bleeding, in neck injuries,
    292
Intraoral lacerations, 255
Intraorbital foreign body, 279
Intraosseous vascular access. *See
    also* Vascular access
    in children, 572, 573f
Intrathoracic bleeding, 298–299,
    304, 306–307, 308
Intravenous lines, 72–73, 81–82
    access sites for, 81. *See also* Vascu-
        lar access
Intravenous pyelography, 486
    in vascular injuries, 353
Intravenous urography, 495
Intubating laryngeal mask airway,
    102–103
Intubation. *See* Tubes *and specific
    techniques*
Ionized calcium, in citrate toxicity,
    143–144
Iridodialysis, 269
Iris
    examination of, 262–263
    injuries of, 269–270
Iritis, traumatic, 271
Irrigation, of hand injuries, 548
Ischemia, in massive hemorrhage,
    prevention of, 136–137, 146f
Itching, in burns, 172

J
Jackson, Charles, 7
Jaundice, in hepatic injuries, 430
Jaw. *See* Mandible; Maxilla
Jaw thrust, 76
Jefferson fracture, 512, 513
    radiography of, 622
Jejunostomy feeding
    in duodenal surgery, 458f, 460
    in esophageal injuries, 324, 325
Joint examination, 116
Jones, Ellis, 6
Jones, John, 3
Jugular vein distention, 112
Jugular vein injuries, 292
Jugular venous access, 81
Juxtahepatic venous injuries,
    424–427

K
Kendrick extrication device, 37–38
Ketamine, 180, 183
    for orotracheal intubation, 97
Kidney. *See under* Renal
Klumpke's palsy, 237
Knee injuries, 535–536
Kocher maneuver, 450f, 455–456, 465
Korean War, trauma surgery in, 5–6
Kussmaul's sign, in cardiac rupture,
    338

L
Labor
    duty to treat in, 710–712
    preterm, 603
Lacerations
    canalicular, 281
    conjunctival, 265
    corneal, 268–269
    coronary artery, 339–341, 340f
    eyelid, 261–262, 261f, 281
    facial, 252–256, 281
    hepatic, 635
        grading of, 428t
    intraoral, 255
    pancreatic
        grading of, 449t
        imaging of, 639
    pulmonary, 304
        hemothorax and, 306
        imaging of, 628
    pulmonary artery, 340f, 341
    renal, grading of, 485t
    scalp, 254, 561–562
    scleral, 266
    splenic, 635
        grading of, 436t
    superior vena cava, 340f, 341
Lacrimal system injuries, 281–282
Lactated Ringer's solution, 185, 187t
Lactic acidosis, transfusion-related,
    145
Laparoscopy
    in abdominal injuries, 393–394, 415
    in diaphragmatic injuries, 407
    in hepatic injuries, 417
    in splenic injuries, 437
Laparotomy
    emergent, indications for, 113t
    exploratory, indications for,
        354–355, 415
    in splenic injuries, 440–442,
        444–445
Laryngeal injuries, 286–287, 294–295
    imaging of, 625
Laryngeal mask airway, 33, 76, 93,
    100–103, 100t, 101f
    intubating, 102–103
Laryngoscope
    Macintosh, 72, 94, 96
    Miller, 72, 94

Laryngoscopy, direct. *See also* Endo-
    tracheal intubation
  in difficult airway, 98–107
  equipment for, 72, 94–95
  glottic visualization in, 90, 98
  technique for, 95–96
Laryngotracheal injuries, 294–295,
    314–320. *See also* Neck
    injuries
  imaging of, 630
Lateral femoral cutaneous nerve
    injuries, 692–693, 692t
Laudanosine, 183
Lavage, diagnostic peritoneal. *See*
    Diagnostic peritoneal lavage
LeFort fractures, 247–249, 248f, 280
Left anterolateral thoracotomy,
    331–334, 332f, 333f
Legal issues, 710–731
  advanced directives, 714–715
  autopsies, 719–720
  capacity, 680
  competency, 680, 713–717
  confidentiality, 720–723, 728
  criminal activity of patients,
    725–727
  drug and alcohol testing, 726
  duty to treat, 710–712
  duty to warn, 724
  evidence, 726, 727
  Good Samaritan laws, 729
  guardianship, 715–716
  informed consent, 679–680,
    712–717
  liability for emergency treatment,
    727–730
  organ donation, 720
  patient contraband, 726, 727
  refusal of treatment, 680, 717–719
  reporting, 723–724
  restraints/seclusion, 724–725
  substituted judgment, 680
  treatment refusal, 680
  unruly patients/visitors, 725
Leg injuries, 534–539. *See also*
    Extremity injuries
  rehabilitation in, 689–693
  soft tissue reconstruction for,
    564–566
Lens
  cataracts of, 272–273
  examination of, 262
  subluxation/dislocation of, 272
Lesser trochanter fractures, 652
Levodopa, for traumatic brain
    injury, 704t
Lewisite, 64, 65
Liability, for emergency treatment,
    727–730
Lid avulsions, 281
Lid contusions, 281
Lid lacerations, 261–262, 261f, 281

Life-threatening conditions
  in anesthesia, 193–194
  in chest trauma, 78–80, 113t, 308
  recognition of, 71, 193–194
Ligament injuries, of hand, 554–555
Light wand, 103
Lip, suturing of, 255
Lipase levels, in pancreatic injuries,
    447–448
Lithium, for mania, 679
Liver. *See also under* Hepatic
  anatomy of, 414f, 417–418
  segments of, 414f, 417–418
Liver abscess, 420
Liver function tests, in hepatic
    injuries, 430
Liver trauma, 413–427. *See also*
    Hepatic injuries
Living will, 715
Long, Crawford Williamson, 6
Loop colostomy, 470–473, 471f, 472f
Lorazepam
  for akathisia, 670–671
  for alcohol withdrawal, 674, 674t
  for delirium, 671
Lower extremity injuries, 534–539.
    See also Extremity injuries
  rehabilitation in, 689–693
  soft tissue reconstruction for,
    564–566
Lung. *See under* Pulmonary

M

Macintosh blade, 72, 94, 96
Macular holes, 275–276
Mafenide acetate, for burns, 165t
Magnesium sulfate, as tocolytic, 603
Magnetic resonance cholangiopan-
    creatography, 448, 453
Magnetic resonance imaging. *See
    also* Radiology *and specific
    injuries*
  in diaphragmatic injuries, 405
  in extremity fractures, 526
  in hand injuries, 548
Major depressive disorder, 677–678
Malabsorption syndrome, postopera-
    tive, 473
Mallampati classification, 90
Malpractice, 727–730
Mandible
  anatomy of, 242
  fractures of, 242, 249–251
Mandibular nerve injuries, 240. *See
    also* Cranial nerve injuries
Mania, 677, 678–679
Mannitol, for increased intracranial
    pressure
  in children, 581
  in head injuries, 218
Mask ventilation, 91–93. *See also*
    Airways

Mass casualty management, 58–68
  ABCs of, 58–61
  for biological agents, 61–64
  for blast injuries, 66–68
  for chemical agents, 64–66
  decontamination in, 68
  definitive care in, 61
  evaluation in, 61
  initial stabilization in, 59–60
  principles of, 58
  search and rescue in, 59
  triage in, 39–40, 41t, 59–60
MAST trousers, 38
Maxilla
  anatomy of, 241
  examination of, 111
  fractures of, 241, 247–249, 248f, 280
Maxillary nerve injuries, 240. *See
    also* Cranial nerve injuries
Maxillofacial injuries, 239–257
  airway management in, 89, 92,
      256–257
  anatomic considerations in,
      239–242
  epidemiology of, 239
  evaluation of, 242–244
  gunshot, 256
  history in, 242–243
  imaging studies in, 243–244
  midface, 244–249
  physical examination in, 243
  skeletal, 244–252
  skull fractures with, 251–252
  soft tissue, 252–256
Mechanical ventilation, 122
  in chest trauma, 298, 319
  complications of, 163t
  endotracheal intubation in. *See*
      Endotracheal intubation
  for organ donors, 659
  sudden deterioration in, 162, 163t
  troubleshooting for, 162, 163t
Mechanism of injury, questioning
    about, 109–110
Median nerve block, 549f, 550
Median nerve examination, 545
Median nerve injuries, 234, 687–688
  in burns, 707t
  in forearm fractures, 688–689
Median sternotomy, 313, 332f, 334,
    348
Mediastinal injuries, 316, 317
  imaging of, 629
Medical field care, 32–40. *See also*
    Emergency medical services
Medical history, 109
Medical triage, 60. *See also* Triage
Medication. *See under* Drug
Medicolegal issues. *See* Legal issues
Mental capacity, 680, 713–717
Mental state, 663–667. *See also* Psy-
    chiatric issues

changes in, 664
  emotional state and, 663
  evaluation of, 663, 665–667
  thought state and, 663
Mental status examination, 663
  bedside, 665–667
Meperidine, for delirium, 671–672
Mesenteric bleeding, imaging of,
    633, 637
Mesh repair
  for abdominal wall injuries,
      481–482, 564
  for chest wall injuries, 564
  for liver injuries, 424
  for splenic injuries, 441
Metabolic derangements
  in anesthesia, 191
  in dilutional coagulopathy, 188
  transfusion-related, 145
Metacarpal fractures, 553–554
Metacarpophalangeal dislocations,
    554
Metatarsal fractures, 538–539
Methadone, for delirium, 671–672
Methylphenidate
  for agitation, in traumatic brain
      injury, 706, 706t
  for traumatic brain injury, 704t
METTAG system, for triage, 39–40,
    41t
Midazolam, for delirium, 671
Midline celiotomy, for diaphragmatic
    exposure, 407–408
Military antishock trousers (MAST),
    38
Military conflicts, trauma surgery in,
    3–6
Miller blade, 92, 94
Milrinone, 189
Minimally responsive state, 703
Mini Mental State Examination,
    663t, 665
Minors
  consent of, 714, 717
  parents' refusal of treatment for,
      718–719
Miosis, traumatic, 277
Missile injuries. *See* Gunshot
    wounds; Penetrating injuries
Mitral valve injuries, 338
Mivacurium, 183
Mnemonics
  ABCD, 71, 75
  AMPLE, 75, 108
  DIGFAST, 678
  SIGECAPS, 677
Modafinil, for traumatic brain
    injury, 704t
Modified Brooke formula, for burns,
    159, 159t
Modified Seldinger technique, for
    venous access, 81

Monteggia fractures, 533–534
Mood disorders, 677–679
Mood stabilizers, for delirium, 669
Morgan, John, 3
Morphine
    abuse of, 675
    for agitation, in traumatic brain
        injury, 706, 706t
    for anesthesia, 181. *See also*
        Anesthesia
    for delirium, 669, 671–672
    switch from IV to enteral, 672
Morton, William, 6, 7
Mouth
    bleeding in, in neck injuries, 292
    lacerations in, 255
    lacerations of, 255
Multiple organ dysfunction syn-
        drome, 124–125
Multiple trauma, burns and,
        151–152, 171, 172t
Muscle(s)
    extraocular, examination of, 262
    of hand, 542–543
Muscle flaps, 558. *See also* Soft tis-
        sue reconstruction
Muscle relaxants, in anesthesia
    for induction, 181–182
    for maintenance, 183
Muscle spasms, in cervical spine
        injuries, 684, 685
Muscle strength assessment, in
        extremity injuries, 529
Musculoskeletal injuries. *See*
        Extremity injuries; Orthope-
        dic trauma
Mustard agents, 64, 65
Mydriasis, traumatic, 277
Myopathy, critical illness, 708

N
Nailbed injuries, 550
Naltrexone, for opiate intoxication,
        675
Narcotics
    abuse of, 675
    for agitation, in traumatic brain
        injury, 706, 706t
    for anesthesia, 181, 183. *See also*
        Anesthesia
    for delirium, 669, 671–672
    switch from IV to enteral, 672
Nasal airways, 76, 92
Nasal anatomy, 242
Nasal endotracheal intubation, 34.
        See also Endotracheal
        intubation
Nasal examination, 111
Nasal fractures, 242, 244–246, 245f,
        281
Nasal packing, 244–245, 245f

Nasogastric intubation. *See also*
        Endotracheal intubation
    in esophageal injuries, 324, 325
    in neck injuries, 287–288
Nasolacrimal duct obstruction, 282
Nasoorbitalethmoid complex
        injuries, 249, 281
Nasopharyngeal airways, 76, 92
Nasopharyngeal intubation, fiber-
        optic, 98–100
Nasotracheal intubation, 34, 76,
        97–98. *See also* Endotracheal
        intubation
    indications for, 76
Neck. *See also* Cervical spine
    examination of, 111–112, 286–288,
        288f. *See also* Neck exploration
    surgical anatomy of, 284–286, 285f
    zones of, 112t, 284–286, 285f
Neck exploration
    anatomic landmarks for, 343f, 345f
    indications for, 291
    techniques of, 291
    vascular, 343, 343f
Neck injuries, 284–295
    blunt, 284
    epidemiology of, 284
    esophageal, 293–294
    imaging of, 288–290, 624–625
    initial evaluation in, 286–288,
        287f, 287t, 288f
    laryngotracheal, 294–295
    mechanisms of, 284
    penetrating, 284
    secondary survey in, 288, 288f
    surgery for
        indications for, 291
        postoperative care in, 295
        technique of, 291
    tracheobronchial, 314–320
    vascular, 292–293, 339–341, 340f
Needle cricothyroidotomy, 77,
        103–104, 104f
Needle decompression, for tension
        pneumothorax, 310
    prehospital, 35
Negative clinical examination, in
        spinal injuries, 287t, 511t
Negligence, 727–730
Nerve agents, 64–65
Nerve blocks. *See also* Anesthesia
    for hand injuries, 549–550, 549f
Nerve grafts, for hand injuries, 563
Nerve injuries. *See also* Neurologic
        injuries
    classification of, 693
    of hand, 68–688, 544, 545–547,
        546f, 563, 688f
    of upper extremity, 544, 545–547,
        546f, 563, 686–689
Neurapraxia, 693

Neurobehavioral impairment, in traumatic brain injury, 702t
Neurogenic bladder, 695
Neurogenic bowel, 695
Neurogenic shock, 85, 225
Neuroleptics
  for agitation, 670
  for delirium, 668–671
Neurologic examination
  in burns, 152–156
  in children, 574–575, 580–581
  Glasgow Coma Scale in, 12t, 86–87, 117t, 662–663
    in children, 574–575, 580–581
  in hand injuries, 544, 545–547, 546f
  in head injuries, 214, 215
    in children, 574, 580–581
  in ICU, 121
  in primary survey, 86–87
  in secondary survey, 116–117, 117t
Neurologic injuries. See also Nerve injuries
  in children, 574–575, 580–582
  in head trauma. See Head injuries
  ICU care in, 120–121
  peripheral nerve, 230–237
  spinal cord, 224–230. See also Cervical spine injuries; Spinal cord injuries
Neurologic monitoring, in ICU, 120–121
Neuromuscular blockade
  agents for, 121–122
  for endotracheal intubation, 34
Neuropraxia, 231
Neurostimulants
  for agitation, in traumatic brain injury, 706, 706t
  for traumatic brain injury, 704, 704t
Neurotmesis, 231–232, 693
New Injury Severity Score (NISS), 21t
911 system, 31
9/11 attack, 8–9
Nitrogen mustard, 64, 65
Nitrous oxide, in anesthesia, 182–183
Norepinephrine, 188
  indications for, 188
Nortriptyline, for agitation, in traumatic brain injury, 706, 706t
Nose. See under Nasal
Nosocomial infections, surgical site, 202–207
Nuclear weapons, 61
Nurses, trauma team, 52
Nutritional support
  in burns, 164–165
  for children, 590
  in duodenal surgery, 457, 458f, 460
  in elderly, 616
  in esophageal injuries, 324, 325

O
Obstetric evaluation, 597
Obstetric transfer, 597
Obstructive shock, 84–85
Occupational therapist, 683
Ocular anesthesia, 258
Ocular examination, 259–263
  anterior segment, 262–263
  equipment for, 258
  external, 259–262
  extraocular motility in, 262
  in head injuries, 215
  imaging studies in, 263–264
  key questions for, 258–259
  posterior segment, 263
  pupillary, 262
  visual acuity in, 259
  visual fields in, 262
Ocular injuries, 258–283. See also Eye
  adnexal, 279–282
  amblyopia and, 282–283
  anterior chamber, 270–272
  anterior segment, 264–265, 273
  burn, 161, 168t, 267–268
  choroidal, 274–276
  ciliary body, 270
  conjunctival, 264–265
  corneal, 266–269
  diagnostic studies in, 263–264
  epidemiology of, 258
  initial evaluation of, 258–263
  iris, 269–270, 271
  lacrimal system, 281–282
  lenticular, 272–273
  ophthalmologic consultation for, 264
  optic nerve, 277–279
  pediatric, 282–283
  posterior segment, 273–277
  pupillary, 277
  rehabilitation after, 283
  retinal, 274–276
  scleral, 265–266
  vitreous, 273–274
Ocular motility, assessment of, 262
Oculomotor nerve injuries, 278
Odontoid peg fractures, 513
Olanzapine, for agitation, 670
Older adults. See Geriatric trauma
Olecranon fractures, 533
On-site triage, 60. See also Triage
Open-book thoracotomy, 312–313, 313f, 332f, 334
Open fractures. See also Fracture(s)
  tibial, 565–566, 565t
  of wrist and hand, 553–554
Open globe injury, 262–263, 264
Open pneumothorax, 79, 304–305
Ophthalmic nerve injuries, 240. See also Cranial nerve injuries

Ophthalmoscopic examination, 258–259
  in head injuries, 215
Opiates
  abuse of, 675
  for agitation, in traumatic brain injury, 706, 706t
  for anesthesia, 181, 183. *See also* Anesthesia
  for delirium, 669, 671–672
  switch from IV to enteral, 672
Optic nerve injuries, 277–279
Oral airways, 72, 92, 93. *See also* Airways
Oral bleeding
  from lacerations, 255
  in neck injuries, 292
Oral lacerations, 255
Orbit
  anatomy of, 260f
  injuries of, 249, 279–281, 621
  radiography of, 621
Orchiectomy, 507
Organ donation, 655–661, 720
  brain death criteria for, 655–657
  common traps and decision dilemmas in, 660–661
  family counseling and consent for, 660, 660t
  nonbeating heart, 659–660
  organ procurement systems for, 657
  potential donors for
    exclusion of, 657
    identification of, 655–657
    referral for, 658
    supportive care for, 658–659
  steps in, 656t
  United Network for Organ Sharing and, 657–658
Oropharyngeal airways, 72, 92, 93. *See also* Airways
Oropharyngeal intubation, fiberoptic, 98–100
Oropharyngeal structures, Samsoon-Young classification of, 595f
Orotracheal intubation, 33–34, 76, 94–97. *See also* Endotracheal intubation
  difficult
    adjuncts for, 98–107
    predictors of, 90
  equipment for, 72, 94–95
  induction agents for, 96–97
  technique for, 94–96
Orthopedic trauma. *See also* Extremity injuries; Fracture(s)
  cervical spine injuries in, 224–230
  compartment pressure monitoring in, 123–124
  extremity fractures in, 526–539
  fat embolism and, 123, 123t

  geriatric, 611, 612
  hand injuries in, 540–557
  imaging studies in, 646–653
  pediatric, 578–579, 586–589
  pelvic fractures in, 518–525
  physical examination in, 115–116
  rehabilitation in, 683–693
  skull fractures in, 220–221, 251–252, 574–575, 632l
  soft tissue reconstruction in, 564–566
  spinal fractures in, 509–517
Orthosis, thoracolumbar-sacral, 516
Orthostatic hypotension, in spinal cord injuries, 698
Osmotic therapy, for increased intracranial pressure, in children, 581
Osteoporosis, extremity fractures, 530
Oxazepam, for alcohol withdrawal, 674, 674t
Oxygen administration
  in inhalation injury, 164
  by mask, 91–93

P
Packing
  abdominal, in hepatic injuries, 422–423, 431
  nasal, 244–245, 245f
  perihepatic, 423–424, 431
Pain management. *See also* Anesthesia
  in burns, 160–161, 172
  in children, 590
  in elderly, 616
  in ICU, 121
  for physical examination, 118
  postoperative, 193
  in pregnancy, 605
  prehospital, 38–39
  in rib fractures, 301
  in spinal cord injuries, 699
Pancreatectomy, distal, 452, 453f
Pancreatic bed infection, 461
Pancreatic fistula, 460
Pancreatic injuries, 446–455, 476–477
  duodenal injuries with, 456, 459
  endoscopic retrograde cholangiopancreatography in, 448, 451, 453
  epidemiology of, 446
  grading of, 448, 449t
  imaging studies in, 447–448, 638–639
  initial evaluation in, 447–448
  major duct disruption in, 451–452
  mechanisms of, 446
  nonoperative management of, 446, 448–449

Pancreatic injuries (*contd.*)
  operative management of, 446,
      449–455, 450f, 451f, 454f
    technical aspects of, 452–455,
        453f, 455f
    visualization in, 451–452
  physical examination in, 447
  serum amylase/lipase in, 447–448
Pancreaticoduodenal injuries. *See
    also* Duodenal injuries; Pan-
    creatic injuries
  operative management of, 459
Pancreaticoduodenectomy, 429
Pancreatic pseudocyst, 460
Pancreatography
  endoscopic retrograde, 448, 451,
      453
  intraoperative, 451–452, 453
Pancuronium, 183
Paralysis. *See* Spinal cord injuries
Paralytics, for endotracheal intuba-
    tion, 34
Paramedics, 29–31. *See also* Emer-
    gency medical services
Parotid duct injuries, 254
Parotid gland injuries, 241
Patella fracture, 535
Patellar tendon injuries, 536
Patellofemoral dislocation, 535–536
Patient
  criminal activity of, 725–727
  unruly, 725
Patient confidentiality. *See*
    Confidentiality
Patient history, 108–110
Patient-physician privilege, 720–721
Patient positioning, in pregnancy,
    593, 594f, 597–598, 602
Patient transfer, for definitive care,
    119
Patient transport, 40–48. *See also*
    Transport
Patriot Act, 724
PDCA cycle, 24
Pediatric trauma
  abdominal, 575–578, 576t, 577t
  airway management in, 571–572,
      580
  anatomy and physiology of,
      571–573
  bicycle injuries in, 571, 578
  blunt, 571
  central nervous system injuries in,
      574–575, 580–582
  cervical spine injuries in, 575,
      581–582, 583t
  in child abuse, 221, 579, 582–583.
      See also Child abuse
    reporting of, 723–724
  common pitfalls in, 590–591
  critical care in, 589–590
  definitive care in, 580–591

endotracheal intubation in, 572
epidemiology of, 571
evaluation in, 573–579
fluid management in, 571–573,
    589–590
head injuries in, 221, 574–575
hemothorax in, 584–585
hepatic injuries in, 586
imaging studies in, 573–574, 584
increased intracranial pressure in,
    581
management of, 580–591
mechanisms of injury in, 571
nutritional support in, 590
ocular injuries in, 282–283
orthopedic injuries in, 586–589
pain management in, 590
Pediatric Trauma Scale for, 19t
penetrating, 571
pneumothorax in, 584–585
prevention of, 571
primary survey in, 571–573
pulmonary contusion in, 585
rehabilitation in, 590
resuscitation in, 571–573, 589–590
rib fractures in, 584
shock in, 572
skull fractures in, 221
spinal injuries in, 574–575
splenic injuries in, 585–586
thoracic, 575, 576t
transfer criteria in, 580
traumatic asphyxia in, 584
types of injuries in, 571
vascular access in, 572–573, 573f
vital signs in, 572t
Pediatric Trauma Scale (PTS), 19t
Pedicle flaps, 560. *See also* Soft tis-
    sue reconstruction
Pelvic aortography, 353
Pelvic disruption, 519–521
Pelvic hematoma, 367–368
Pelvic retroperitoneum, vascular
    injuries of, 367–369
Pelvic stability, 518
Pelvic trauma, 518–525, 640–646
  acetabular, 641–642
  anatomic aspects of, 518
  angiographic embolization in, 522,
      524
  bladder injuries and, 502, 503
  bleeding in, 521–523, 521–524,
      643
  classification of, 519, 520f, 641–643
  evaluation in, 519–521
  iliac, 641
  imaging studies in, 640–646
  instability in, 518, 519, 520t, 521
  management of
    definitive, 524
    external fixation in, 522–523
    hemostatic, 521–524

initial, 521–522, 521–524
protocols for, 523, 524f
recommendations for, 523–524
sheet wrapping in, 523
mechanism of injury in, 519, 521
outside pelvic ring, 642–643
pelvic disruption in, 519–521
radiography of, 519–521
rehabilitation in, 691–692
vascular injuries in, 367–369,
521–523, 643
Penetrating injuries. *See also* Gunshot wounds; Stab wounds
of brachial plexus, 237
of head, 223
maxillofacial, 256
of neck, 284
in precordial box, 328, 329f
questioning about, 110
Penicillin, for mandibular fractures,
250
Penile injuries, 506
Penrose drain, in renal surgery,
493–494
Pentobarbital coma, 219
in children, 581
Peptic ulcers
bleeding from, 207–209edit
in burns, 164, 168t
Performance improvement, 17–22,
23–26
common problems in, 26–27
Pericardial effusion, diagnosis of,
329–330
Pericardial tamponade, obstructive
shock and, 84
Pericardiocentesis
diagnostic, 330
for pericardial tamponade, 84–85
Pericardiotomy, subxiphoid,
330–331, 330f
Perihepatic packing, 423–424, 431
Perineal hematoma, 504
Peripheral nerve injuries, 230–237
anatomic considerations in, 230,
231f
brachial plexus, 235–237, 236f
in burns, 161, 707, 707t
causes of, 230–231
diagnostic studies in, 232
electrodiagnosis of, 693, 694t
evaluation of, 232
femoral nerve, 693
in forearm fractures, 688–689
lateral femoral cutaneous nerve,
692–693, 692t
median nerve, 234, 687–688
in elbow injuries, 687
in forearm fractures, 688–689
nerve changes after, 231–232
pathophysiology of, 231–232
peroneal nerve, 235, 692–693, 692t

radial nerve, 233–234
in forearm fractures, 688–689
in humerus fractures, 687
rehabilitation in, 692–693, 693t
sciatic nerve, 235, 692–693, 692t
tibial nerve, 235, 692–693, 692t
treatment of, 232–233
ulnar nerve, 234–235
in elbow injuries, 687
in forearm fractures, 688–689
Peripheral vascular injuries,
372–384
arterial, signs of, 372–375
associated injuries in, management of, 377–379
axillary artery, 379–381, 381–382
blunt, 372
brachial artery, 381–382
diagnostic evaluation of, 375–376
early amputation for, 379
epidemiology of, 372
femoral artery, 382
immediate fasciotomy for, 379, 380f
infection of, 383
nonoperative management of, 376
operative management of,
376–383
complications of, 383
exposures in, 379–382
interposition grafting in, 377,
378f
primary repair in, 377
orthopedic stabilization for, 378
patterns of, 372, 373f
penetrating, 372
popliteal artery, 382
pseudoaneurysm and, 383
signs of, 372–375
venous injuries and, 378
Peritoneal dialysis, 127
Peritoneal fluid, imaging of, 633–634
Peritoneal lavage, diagnostic, 114,
115t, 389–390
in diaphragmatic injury, 114, 115t,
389–390
in duodenal injuries, 447
in hepatic injuries, 417, 420
in pancreatic injuries, 447
technique of, 389–390
in vascular injuries, 353
Peroneal nerve injuries, 235
in burns, 707t
Perphenazine, for delirium, 669–671
Personnel
emergency department, 50–52
emergency medical, 29–31
Phalanges. *See* Finger; Thumb; Toe
Pharyngeal injuries, imaging of, 625
Pharyngeal leak, 289–290
Pharyngeal lumen airway and Combitube, 33

Pharyngoesophageal injuries, 289, 293–294. *See also* Neck injuries
Phenergan, for opiate withdrawal, 675
Phenobarbital
  for alcohol withdrawal, 202
  in barbiturate coma, 219
  in children, 581
Phenol injections, for spasticity, in spinal cord injuries, 700
Phenylephrine, 188
  indications for, 188
Phobias, 676
Phosgene, 64
Phosgene oxime, 64, 65
Physeal injuries, 578–579, 588–589, 588f
Physical examination
  abdominal, 113–114
  cervical, 111–112
  documentation of, 119
  genitourinary, 114–115
  head in, 110–111
  musculoskeletal, 115–116
  neurologic, 116–117, 117t
  thoracic, 112–113
Physical therapist, 683
Physician-patient privilege, 720–721
Pilcher, Lewis, 5
Pilon fractures, 537
Ping-Pong ball fractures, 221
Plague, in biological warfare, 63
Plain film series, 619
Plan-Do-Check-Act (PDCA) cycle, 24
Plasmalyte, 185, 187t
Platelet dysfunction, in massive transfusion, 141
Platelet transfusion, 137–138
Pneumatic antishock garment (PASG), 38
Pneumatic compression, for thrombo-embolism prophylaxis, 196–197
Pneumomediastinum, 316, 317
  imaging of, 629
Pneumonia, in inhalation injury, 162
Pneumoperitoneum, imaging of, 634
Pneumothorax, 304–305
  in children, 584–585
  imaging of, 628
  in mechanical ventilation, 163t
  open, 79
  simple, 304–305
  subcutaneous emphysema and, 306
  tension, 78–79, 304–305, 308
    imaging of, 628–629
    needle decompression for, 35, 310
    obstructive shock and, 84
  tracheobronchial injuries and, 316, 317

Polyneuropathy, critical illness, 708
Polypharmacy, in elderly, 612–613
Polytrauma, burns and, 151–152, 171, 172t
Pond fractures, 221
Pooled contrast, in splenic injuries, 437, 442
Popliteal artery injuries, 382. *See also* Peripheral vascular injuries
Porta hepatis injuries, 369–370
Portal triad compression, 422–423, 425
  in venovenous bypass, 426
Portal vein injuries, 369–370
Positioning, maternal, 593, 594f, 597–598, 602
Positive end-expiratory pressure, 122
Positive-pressure ventilation, in tracheobronchial injuries, 319
Postemetic esophageal disruptions, 321–322
Posterior cord syndrome, 229
Posterior segment examination, 263
Posterolateral thoracotomy, 312, 312f, 332f, 334–335
  for bronchial injuries, 320
Postmortem examination, 719–720
Postoperative infections, 202–207
Posttraumatic stress disorder, 676–677
Potassium imbalance
  succinylcholine and, 181
  transfusion-related, 145
Pralidoxime, for nerve agents, 65
Precordial box, penetrating injuries in, 328, 329f
Pregnancy
  abdominal assessment in, 601
  abdominal trauma in, 604–605
  abuse in, 593
  airway management in, 593–595, 594f, 595f, 596t
  amniotic fluid embolism in, 600
  antibiotic prophylaxis in, 605
  blunt trauma in, 604
  breathing in, 596
  cardiac arrest in, 598
  cardiac assessment in, 601
  cesarean delivery in, 598–599
  drug therapy in, 605
  duty to treat in, 710–712
  extremity assessment in, 602
  fetal heartbeat documentation in, 600
  fetal injury/demise in, 592
  fetal monitoring in, 602, 603
  genitourinary assessment in, 601
  gestational age assessment in, 599–600
  hematologic assessment in, 601–602

imaging studies in, 605–606, 645
maternal respiratory rate in, 600
obstetric evaluation in, 597
obstetric transfer in, 597
pain management in, 605
patient positioning in, 593, 594f, 597–598, 602
penetrating trauma in, 604
perioperative management in, 602–603
postoperative contractions in, 603
preterm delivery in, 603
primary survey in, 593–599
radiation exposure in, 605–606
resuscitation in, 598–599
seatbelt injuries in, 604–605
secondary survey in, 599–602
tocolytics in, 603
trauma epidemiology in, 592
uterine rupture in, 604
vascular access in, 598
Prehospital care, 29–48
emergency medical services in, 29–40. *See also* Emergency medical services
transition to hospital care from, 74–75
transport in, 40–48. *See also* Transport
Preterm labor, 603
Primary survey, 75–88
airway evaluation in, 75–77
basic framework for, 75
breathing evaluation in, 78–80
cervical spine immobilization in, 77
circulatory evaluation in, 80–86
common traps in, 87–88
life-threatening conditions in, 71
neurologic examination in, 86–87
Pringle maneuver, 422–423, 425
in venovenous bypass, 426
Privacy, 720–723, 728
duty to warn and, 724
patient, in performance improvement, 26
Privileged information, 720–721
Procedural experts, on trauma team, 51
Propofol, 180
for orotracheal intubation, 96–97
Propranolol
for agitation, in traumatic brain injury, 706, 706t
for akathisia, 670–671
Prothrombin complex concentrates, 142
Prothrombin time, dilution coagulopathy and, 138–139, 139f
Proximal humerus fractures, 531–532, 647
Proximal interphalangeal dislocations, 554

Pruritus, in burns, 172
Pseudoaneurysm, arterial, 383
Pseudocyst, pancreatic, 460
Psoas hitch, 498–499
Psychiatric ABCs, 663
Psychiatric issues, 662–680
anxiety disorders, 676–677
consciousness, 662–663
delirium, 664–672
dementia, 664
legal, 679–680
mental state, 663–667
mood disorders, 677–679
psychosis, 679
substance abuse, 672–675
Psychologists, 683
Psychosis, 679
Pulmonary artery catheterization, 184
Pulmonary artery lacerations, 339, 340f, 341
Pulmonary complications, in organ donors, 659
Pulmonary contusions, 122–123, 303–304
in children, 585
imaging of, 627–628
Pulmonary embolism, prevention of, 195–199, 200t
Pulmonary function
in children, 572
in elderly, 610–611
evaluation of, 78–80
in pregnancy, 596, 596t
in spinal cord injuries, 698
Pulmonary lacerations, 304
hemothorax and, 306
imaging of, 628
Pulses
in arterial injuries, 375
evaluation of, 116
Pupils
examination of, 262
in head injuries, 214, 215
injuries of, 277
Purpura fulminans, 171
Purtscher's retinopathy, 275
Pyloric exclusion, 458, 459f

Q
QT prolongation, neuroleptics and, 669–670
Quadriceps tendon injuries, 536
Quality assurance, 23–26
Quality management, 23–24
Quetiapine, for agitation, 670
Quinine, for opiate withdrawal, 675

R
Radial collateral ligament rupture, 555
Radial nerve block, 549, 549f

Radial nerve examination, 545–546
Radial nerve injuries, 233–234
  in burns, 707t
  in forearm fractures, 688–689
  in humerus fractures, 687
Radiography. *See also* Radiology *and*
    specific injuries
  in abdominal injuries, 114,
      386–387, 404
  acetylcysteine prophylaxis in, 125
  in cardiac injuries, 329
  in diaphragmatic injuries, 404, 405f
  in esophageal injuries, 322–323
  in extremity fractures, 526–527
  in hand injuries, 547–548
  in neck injuries, 289
  in pelvic injuries, 519–521, 640, 641
  in peripheral vascular injuries, 376
  plain film series in, 619
  in pregnancy, safety of, 606
  in spinal injuries, 510–511, 511t
  in thoracic injuries, 289, 300,
      316–317, 322–323, 329
  in tracheobronchial injuries,
      316–317
Radiology. *See also specific tech-*
    niques
  in abdominal injuries, 114,
      386–389, 390–391, 392t,
      631–640
  in abdominal vascular injuries,
      629–630
  in adrenal injuries, 638
  in airway injuries, 630–631
  in bladder injuries, 643–644,
      645–646
  in bronchial injuries, 630–631
  in cardiac injuries, 630
  in cervical injuries, 621–625, 623f,
      624f
  in chest injuries, 625–631
  in chest wall injuries, 626–627
  in colon injuries, 636–637
  in diaphragmatic injuries,
      404–405, 404–406, 405f, 627
  in elderly, 612
  in gallbladder injuries, 636
  in gastrointestinal bleeding, 633
  in genitourinary trauma, 643–646
  in head injuries, 619–621
  in hepatic injuries, 415–416, 431,
      633, 635–636
  in hip dislocations, 652–653
  in hip fractures, 649–652, 653
  in mediastinal injuries, 629–631
  in neck injuries, 288–290
  in orthopedic injuries, 646–653
  in pancreatic injuries, 638–639
  in pediatric trauma, 573–574
  in pelvic injuries, 640–646
  in peripheral vascular injuries,
      375–376

  in pleural injuries, 628–629
  in pneumothorax, 628
  in pregnancy, 605–606, 645
  in pulmonary injuries, 627–628
  in renal injuries, 637–638
  in scapular injuries, 627
  in shoulder injuries, 647–649
  in small bowel injuries, 636–637
  in spinal cord injuries, 621–625,
      623f, 624f
  in spinal fractures, 510, 511t,
      622–624, 626
  in splenic injuries, 633, 634–635
  in thoracic injuries, 300
  in tracheal injuries, 630
  in urethral injuries, 644–645
Radius fractures
  distal, 534
  head, 533
Rancho Los Amigos Scale, 702–703,
    703t
Random flaps, 560. *See also* Soft tis-
    sue reconstruction
Rapacuronium, for anesthesia induc-
    tion, 182
Rapid sequence intubation, 93–94.
    See also Endotracheal
    intubation
Recombinant activated factor VII,
    142
Recombinant tissue plasminogen
    activator, for venous throm-
    boembolism, 198–199
Reconstructive ladder, 559–560
Rectal examination, 115
Rectal injuries, 469–472. *See also*
    Colon injuries
  anatomic aspects of, 469–470
  management of, 470–472
Rectus sheath hematomas, 411–412
Red cell transfusions, 133–134, 133t.
    See also Transfusions
  alternatives/supplements to,
      134–136
  citrate toxicity and, 142–143
Red eye, differential diagnosis of,
    269t
Reemstma, Keith, 6
Refusal of treatment, 680, 717–719
Refusal to treat, 710–712
Regional anesthesia. *See also* Anes-
    thesia
  vs. general anesthesia, 177–178
Rehabilitation, 682–708
  in burns, 166, 707, 707t
  in cervical spine injuries, 683–686
  in geriatric trauma, 616–617
  in head injuries, 701–706
  in hip injuries, 689–693, 689t, 691t
  in ICU, 707–708
  in lower extremity injuries,
      689–693

in orthopedic trauma, 683–693
pediatric, 590
in pelvic injuries, 691–692
in peripheral nerve injuries, 692–693, 693t
phases of, 682
in spinal cord injuries, 230, 684–686, 693–701
team approach in, 682–683
in upper extremity injuries, 686–689
visual, 283
Rehabilitation psychologist, 683
Reimplantation, fingertip/hand/forearm, 551–553
Religion, treatment refusal and, 718
Renal angiography, 487
Renal arteriography, 353
Renal artery injuries, 367, 493
Renal artery thrombosis, 490–491
Renal autotransplantation, 500
Renal failure, 125–127
    continuous renal replacement therapy in, 127
    dialysis in, 127
    rhabdomyolysis in, 125–126
Renal function tests, 126–127
Renal injuries, 484–494
    classification of, 484–485, 485t
    débridement in, 492
    diagnosis of, 485–487
    epidemiology of, 484
    grading of, 484–485, 485t
    gunshot, 490
    imaging studies in, 486–487, 637–638
    mechanism of, 484
    nonoperative management of, 487–489
        angiographic embolization in, 488–489
        percutaneous drainage and ureteral stenting in, 489
    operative management of, 489–494
        collecting system repair in, 492
        complications of, 494
        drain placement in, 493–494
        exposures in, 489–492
        hemostasis in, 492
        indications for, 489–491
        parenchymal débridement in, 492
        parenchymal repair in, 492–493
        postoperative care in, 494
        technical aspects of, 489–494
        vascular repair in, 492–493
    physical examination in, 485
    presentation of, 484–485
    urinalysis in, 485–486
    urinary extravasation in, 489
    vascular, 367, 370, 493
Renal replacement therapy, 127

Renal vein injuries, 367, 370, 493
Reporting
    of child abuse, 723
    of criminal activity, 725–727
    legal requirements for, 723–724
Respiration. See also Breathing
    in children, 572
    in elderly, 610–611
    evaluation of, 78–80, 87
    in pregnancy, 596
Respiratory failure, 122
    in inhalation injury, 162
Respiratory function, in elderly, 610–611
Respiratory rate, maternal, 600
Restraints, 724–725
Resuscitation, 71–88
    airway management in, 32–35, 75–77, 89–107. See also Airway management
    anesthesia in, 193–194
    breathing/ventilation and, 78–80
    cervical spine immobilization in, 36–38, 77
    chest trauma and, 78–80
    common traps in, 87–88
    documentation of, 119
    equipment for, 71–73
    fluid, 80–86, 81–83. See also Fluid management
        prehospital, 35–36, 36t
    immediate, 71–88. See also Primary survey
    life-threatening problems in, 193–194
    neurologic status and, 86–87
    in pediatric trauma, 571–573
    personnel for, 73. See also Trauma team
    in pregnancy, 598–599
    prehospital, 29–48. See also Emergency medical services
    preparation for patient arrival and, 73–75
    primary survey in, 75–88. See also Primary survey
    secondary survey in, 108–119
    tertiary survey in, 118–119
    transfusions in, 128–145
Retinal examination, 263
Retinal injuries, 274–276
Retrograde urethrography, 505
Retrohepatic vena cava, injuries of, 424–427
Retroperitoneal drainage, in renal surgery, 493–494
Retroperitoneal hemorrhage, 192
Revised Trauma Score, 13t
Revolutionary War, trauma surgery in, 3–4
Rhabdomyolysis, 125–126, 192
Rh crossmatch, 130–133

Rib fractures, 300–302
  in children, 584
  flail chest and, 80, 302, 627
  imaging of, 626–627
Ricin, 66
Right to die
  advance directives and, 714–715
  treatment refusal and, 717–718
Risperidone, for agitation, 670
  in traumatic brain injury, 706,
    706t
Rocuronium
  for anesthesia induction, 182
  for orotracheal intubation, 97
Rotator cuff injuries, 532, 686–687
Roux-en-Y choledochojejunostomy,
    429
Rupture. *See specific organ*

S
Sacrum fractures, 642
Saline solution, 185, 187t
Salivary gland injuries, 241, 254
Salter-Harris classification, of epi-
    physeal fractures, 578–580
Saphenous vein grafting, for periph-
    eral vascular injuries, 377,
    378f
  complications of, 383
Sarin, 64–65
Scalp injuries, 254, 561–562
  examination in, 110
  reconstructive surgery for,
    561–562
Scapula injuries, 532, 627, 647
Scars
  burn, 169t, 171–172, 707
  hypertrophic, 567–568
  revision of, 567–568
Scene report triage, 43
Sciatic nerve injuries, 235, 692–693,
    692t
Sclera, injuries of, 265–266
Scope of practice
  for air medical crew, 31
  for EMTs, 30, 31
Scopolamine, 181
Screening, for alcohol abuse, 673
Scribe, 52
Scrotal skin loss, 508
Search and rescue, 59. *See also* Mass
    casualty management
Seatbelt injuries
  aortic, 351
  bladder, 501
  in pregnancy, 604–605
  spinal, 517
  splenic, 435, 578
  thoracic, 112
Seclusion, 724–725
Secondary brain injury, 213. *See also*
    Head injuries

Secondary survey, 108–119
  analgesia in, 118
  diagnostic procedures in, 117–118
  patient history in, 108–110
  patient needs in, 118
  physical examination in, 110–117.
    See also Physical examination
Seidel test, 266
Seizures
  alcohol withdrawal, 674
  in head injuries, 218, 705
Seldinger technique, for venous
    access, 81
Selective serotonin reuptake
    inhibitors, 678
Sellick maneuver, 94
Seniors. *See* Geriatric trauma
Senior traumatologist, 52
Sensory evaluation, in hand injuries,
    544
Sentinel events, 24–25
Sepsis, postsplenectomy, 444
September 11 attack, 8–9
Septic shock, 85
Serum amylase, in pancreatic
    injuries, 447–448
Serum lipase, in pancreatic injuries,
    447–448
Shaken baby syndrome, 574,
    582–583
Sheet wrapping, in pelvic fractures,
    523
Shippen, William, 3
Shock, 80–86
  cardiogenic, 84
  in children, 572
  grading of, 134, 135t
  hemorrhagic, 81–83, 133–134,
    135t
  neurogenic, 85, 225
  obstructive, 84–85
  resuscitation in. *See* Fluid man-
    agement
  septic, 85
  spinal, 225
Shoulder injuries, 531–532, 627,
    647–648
  imaging of, 627, 647–648, 653
  nerve injuries in, 687
  rehabilitation in, 686–687
Shoulder pain, in spinal cord
    injuries, 699
Shunt, atriocaval, 426
SIGECAPS mnemonic, 677
Sigmoidoscopy, 470
Silo closure, 481
Silver nitrate, for burns, 165t
Silver sulfadiazine, for burns, 165t
Simple pneumothorax, 304–305
Skin flaps, 560–561. *See also* Soft tis-
    sue reconstruction

Skin grafts, 560. *See also* Soft tissue reconstruction
  for burns, 707
Skull base fractures, 252
Skull fractures, 220–221
  in children, 221, 574–575
  imaging of, 621
  with maxillofacial injuries, 251–252. *See also* Maxillofacial injuries
Sleep problems, for traumatic brain injury, 704
Slit lamp examination, 258–259, 262–263
Small bowel injuries, 462–464, 462–466, 466–468, 468f, 477–478. *See also* Duodenal injuries
  anatomic aspects of, 466–467
  blunt, 462–463
  in children, 586
  diagnosis of, 463–464
  epidemiology of, 462
  imaging studies in, 463, 636–637
  laparoscopy in, 463–464
  mechanisms of, 462
  nonoperative management of, 464
  operative management of, 467–468
    complications of, 472–473
    indications for, 464
    postoperative care in, 472
  penetrating, 462
  physical examination in, 463
  in pregnancy, 604
  presentation of, 463
Small bowel obstruction, postoperative, 473
Smallpox, in biological warfare, 64
Sniffing position, for orotracheal intubation, 94–95
Sodium pentothal, 180
Sodium thiopental, for orotracheal intubation, 96
Soft tissue infections, 171
Soft tissue reconstruction, 558–568
  for abdominal wall injuries, 564
  anatomic principles of, 558–559
  axial flaps in, 560
  for chest wall injuries, 563–564
  delayed complications in, 567–568
  evaluation for, 559–561
  free flaps in, 561
  healing by secondary intention in, 560, 569
  for lower extremity injuries, 564–566
  muscle flaps in, classification of, 558
  postoperative care in, 566–567
  random flaps in, 560
  reconstructive ladder in, 559–560
  rehabilitation in, 567
  for scalp injuries, 561–562
  skin grafts in, 560
  for upper extremity injuries, 562–563
  wound care in, 566–567
  wound healing and, 559
  zone of injury in, 565
Solutions, resuscitation, 83, 185–186, 187t
Soman, 64–65
Spasticity
  in head injuries, 706
  in spinal cord injuries, 684, 685, 699–701, 700t
Speech-language pathologist, 683
Spinal clearance protocols, 287t, 510–511, 511t
  pediatric, 582
Spinal cord injuries, 224–230. *See also* Cervical spine injuries; Spinal fractures
  anterior cord syndrome in, 229
  ASIA scoring system for, 224–225, 226f–228f, 230
  autonomic dysreflexia in, 698
  Brown Séquard syndrome in, 229–230
  central cord syndrome in, 229
  central pain in, 699
  in children, 575, 581–582, 583t
  classification of, 693–694
  clearance protocols for, 287t, 510–511, 511t
    pediatric, 582
  decubitus ulcers in, 701
  dystonia in, 699
  epidemiology of, 224
  functional outcome in, 694–695, 696t–697t
  heterotopic ossification in, 698–699
  hypercalcemia in, 698
  imaging studies in, 621–625, 623f, 624f
  incomplete, 229–230
  initial evaluation in, 224
  level of, 224–225
    impairment and, 695, 696t–697t
  neurogenic bladder in, 695
  neurogenic bowel in, 695
  posterior cord syndrome in, 229
  pulmonary problems in, 698
  radiographic evaluation in, 225
  rehabilitation in, 230, 684–686, 693–701
  scoring system for, 224–225, 226f–228f, 230
  spasticity in, 684, 685, 699–701, 700t
  spinal shock in, 225
  surgery for
    indications for, 225–229
    postoperative care in, 230
  venous thromboembolism in, 701

Spinal fractures, 509–517
  assessment of, 510
  burst, 516
  cervical, 512–514. *See also* Cervi-
      cal spine injuries
  chance, 517
  classification of, 509
  clearance protocols for, 287t,
      510–511, 511t
    pediatric, 582
  diagnosis of, 510
  flexion, 517
  fracture-dislocation, 517
  imaging studies in, 510, 511t,
      622–624, 626
  instability with minimal/no bony
      injury in, 515
  neurologic injuries in, 509. *See
      also* Cervical spine injuries;
      Spinal cord injuries
  operative management of
    for burst fractures, 516
    indications for, 511–512, 512t
  overview of, 509
  physical examination in, 510
  rehabilitation in, 684–686
  seatbelt, 517
  spinal clearance in, 287t, 510–511
  spinal cord injury in. *See* Spinal
      cord injuries
  thoracic, 515
    imaging of, 626
  thoracolumbar, 515–517
    rehabilitation in, 686
  wedge, 515
Spinal immobilization, 38, 77
  in elderly, 611
  prehospital, 36–38
Spinal shock, 225
Spinal stability, 509
Spine clearance protocols, 287t,
      510–511, 511t
  pediatric, 582
Spleen
  accessory, 435
  autotransplantation of, 441–442
  structure and function of, 434–435
  vascularization of, 434, 439–440,
      439f
Splenectomy, 437, 442
  antibiotic prophylaxis after, 444
  in children, 585, 586
  complications of, 443–444
  indications for, 444–445
  partial, 441
  return to activity after, 444
  sepsis after, 444
  thrombocytosis after, 443–444
  vaccination after, 444
Splenic injuries, 433–445, 476
  anatomic aspects of, 434–435,
      439–440, 439f

antibiotic prophylaxis and, 444
bleeding in, 433, 633
  delayed, 443
in children, 575, 576t, 585–586
common traps and dilemmas in,
    444–445
delayed bleeding in, 443
delayed complications in, 443–444
diagnosis of, 435–437
grading of, 436t
hilar, 635
imaging studies in, 436–437, 633,
    634–635
initial evaluation of, 435–437
nonoperative management of,
    437–438, 438t
operative management of, 439–443
  anatomic aspects of, 439–440,
      439f
  angiographic embolization in,
      442–443
  autotransplantation in, 441–442
  complications of, 443–444
  exposures in, 440
  indications for, 439, 444–445
  partial splenectomy in, 441
  postoperative care in, 443
  splenectomy in, 442
  splenic repair in, 440–442, 441f
physical examination in, 435–436
physiologic aspects of, 435
presentation of, 433–434
return to activity and, 444
vaccination and, 444
vascularization and, 434, 439–440,
    439f
Splenic pseudocyst, 444
Splints, 38
  hand, 687, 688, 688f, 689
  for spasticity, in spinal cord
      injuries, 699
Spousal abuse, in pregnancy, 593
Stab wounds
  abdominal, 396–398, 399f, 400f.
      See also Abdominal trauma
    laparoscopy for, 393
    laparoscopy of, 393
    local exploration of, 391–392
  cardiac, 339–341, 340f
  cervical, 284
  craniofacial, 223
  in precordial box, 328, 329f
  questioning about, 110
  thoracic, 297
  tracheobronchial, 315–316
Standard of care, liability and, 727
Steering wheel injuries, 302–303
Stents
  endovascular, 349
  ureteral, 489
Sternal fractures, 302–303
Sternoclavicular dislocation, 531, 649

Sternotomy, median, 313, 332f, 334
Steroids
    for airway management
        in intraoral injuries, 255
        with intraoral injuries, 255
    for preterm labor, 603
    for spinal cord injury, 225
    stress ulcers and, 209
Stillbirth. *See* Fetal injury/demise
Stimulants, for agitation, in trau-
        matic brain injury, 706, 706t
Stomach. *See under* Gastric;
        Gastrointestinal
Stool softeners, for neurogenic
        bowel, 695
Strain, cervical, 683–684
Strangulation, penile, 506
Stress ulcers
    bleeding from, 207–209
    in burns, 164, 168t, 208–209
Subarachnoid hemorrhage, imaging
        studies in, 621
Subchoroidal hemorrhage, 276
Subconjunctival hemorrhage,
        264–265
Subcutaneous emphysema, in chest
        trauma, 305–306, 317
Subdural hematoma, 221–222, 222f
    in children, 581
Subdural hemorrhage, imaging stud-
        ies in, 620–621
Sublingual gland injuries, 241
Subluxation
    atlantoaxial, imaging of, 622–624,
        624f
    lens, 272
Submandibular gland injuries, 241
Substance abuse, 672–675
    testing for, 726
Substituted judgment, 680
Substituted judgment test, 716
Subtrochanteric fractures, 652
Subungual hematoma, 550
Subxiphoid pericardiotomy, 330–331,
        330f
Succinylcholine
    for anesthesia, 181–182
    for orotracheal intubation, 97
Sucking chest wound, 304
Suicide, 678
Sulfur mustard, 64, 65
Superior mesenteric artery injuries,
        361–362
Superior mesenteric vein injuries,
        362
Superior vena cava injuries, 339,
        340f, 341
Supracondylar fractures, 589
Suprarenal vena cava, ligation of,
        366
Suprascapular nerve injuries, in
        burns, 707t

Surgery. *See also specific sites and
        procedures*
    golden hour theory for, 7–8
    history of, 3–9
        civilian, 6–9
        military, 3–6
    thoracic, 309–313, 311f-313f
Surgical anesthesia. *See* Anesthesia
Surgical site infections, 202–207
Suturing
    of facial lacerations, 253, 255
    of hand lacerations, 548–549
    of intraoral lacerations, 255
    of lip, 255
Sympathetic ophthalmia, 283

T

Tabun, 64–65
Tachycardia, in anesthesia, 193
Talar fractures, 538
Tamponade
    cardiac, 308
    for juxtahepatic venous injuries,
        426–427
    pericardial, obstructive shock and,
        84
Tar burns, 155t, 170. *See also* Burns
Tarsal tunnel syndrome, 692–693,
        692t
Teeth
    fractures of, 251
    injured/absent, airway manage-
        ment and, 89, 92
Temporal bone fractures, 252
Tendon injuries
    Achilles tendon, 538
    biceps tendon, 532
    of hand, 555–556, 563
    patellar tendon, 536
    quadriceps tendon, 536
Tension pneumothorax, 78–79,
        304–305, 308
    imaging of, 628–629
    needle decompression for, 310
    prehospital, 35
    obstructive shock and, 84
    tracheobronchial injuries and, 316,
        317
Terrorism, 61–68
    biological weapons and, 61–64. *See
        also* Biological warfare
    blast injuries and, 64–68
    chemical weapons and, 64–66. *See
        also* Chemical warfare
    nuclear weapons and, 61
Tertiary survey, 118–119
Testicular injuries, 506–507
Testicular repositioning, 508
Thacher, James, 3–4
Thiamine, for alcohol withdrawal,
        674

Thoracic fractures, 515. *See also*
Spinal fractures
imaging of, 626
rehabilitation in, 515
Thoracic outlet, anatomic landmarks
of, 345f
Thoracic trauma. *See* Chest trauma
Thoracolumbar fractures, 515–517.
See also Spinal fractures
rehabilitation in, 515–517
Thoracolumbar-sacral orthosis, 516
Thoracoscopy
in abdominal injuries, 394
in diaphragmatic injuries, 406
Thoracosternotomy, bilateral,
311–312, 311f
Thoracostomy
equipment for, 72
tube
in diaphragmatic injuries,
405–406, 409
for hemothorax, 306
indications for, 298–299
for pneumothorax, 305
technique of, 309–310
Thoracostomy tubes, 72
Thoracotomy
anterolateral, 310–311, 310f
with hilar clamping, 318, 318f
left, 331–334, 332f, 333f
clamshell, 311–312, 311f, 332f
in diaphragmatic injuries, 406–407
emergency department, 85–86
posterolateral, 312, 312f, 332f,
334–335
for bronchial injuries, 320
trap-door, 312–313, 313f, 332f,
334, 348
Thought state, 663
Three tube drainage, in duodenal
surgery, 457–458, 458f
Thrombectomy, 199
Thrombocytopenia, heparin-induced,
198
Thrombocytosis, postsplenectomy,
443–444
Thromboembolism. *See also*
Embolism
prevention of, 195–199, 200t
in alcohol withdrawal, 205t
in elderly, 616
in spinal cord injuries, 701
Thrombolytic therapy, 198–199
Thrombosis, renal artery, 490–491
Thumb. *See also* Finger; Hand
dislocation of, 554
gamekeeper's, 555
Tibial fractures
open, 565–566, 565t
pilon, 537
plateau, 536

shaft, 536–537
Tibial nerve injuries, 235, 692–693,
692t
Tissue ischemia, in massive hemor-
rhage, prevention of, 136–137,
146f
Tissue plasminogen activator, for
venous thromboembolism,
198–199
Tizanidine, for spasticity, in spinal
cord injuries, 700t
Tocolytics, 603
Toe, fractures of, 539
Tongue, lacerations of, 255
Tooth injuries, 251
Torus fractures, 587, 587f
Toxic epidermal necrolysis, 171
Tracheal injuries. *See* Laryngotracheal injuries; Tracheo-
bronchial injuries
Tracheal intubation. *See* Endotracheal intubation
Tracheobronchial injuries. *See also*
Chest trauma; Neck injuries
anatomic aspects of, 314–315, 315f
blunt, 315–316
clinical presentation of, 316–317
definitive management of,
318–320
diagnosis of, 317–318
distribution of, 315, 315f
epidemiology of, 314
hilar injury in, 318, 318f
imaging of, 630
initial management of, 317–318,
318f
mechanism of, 315–316
nonoperative management of, 320
penetrating, 315–316
surgery for, 318–320
Tracheobronchitis, in inhalation
injury, 162
Tracheostomy, 105–106
in elderly, 616
Traction, 38
Training, of trauma team, 55
Transcholecystic cholangiopancreatography, 452
Transesophageal echocardiography,
184
in cardiac injuries, 329–330
Transfer, to definitive care, 119
Transfusions, 128–145
acidemia in, 145
anesthesia and, 186
blood products for, 186–188
comparison of, 133, 133t
viscosity of, 133, 133t
blood substitutes for, 136
citrate toxicity in, 143–144
coagulation support in, 136–141

complications of, 129t
  hemostatic, 136–141, 146f
  metabolic, 129t, 142–145, 146f
  prevention of, 146f
crossmatching for, 130–133
cryoprecipitate, 139–140
dilutional coagulopathy in,
    137–140, 146f
  prevention of, 137–140
expedited, 130–133, 131t
fibrinolysis and, 140–141
fresh frozen plasma, 138–139
for hemorrhagic shock, 82–83
hyperkalemia in, 145
hypocalcemia and, 188
hypothermia in, 141, 144–145
identification procedures for,
    128–130, 130t
logistics of, 128
pharmacologic adjuncts in, 141–142
platelet, 137–138
prehospital, 36
prothrombin time and, 138–139,
    139f
red cell, 133–134, 133t
  alternatives/supplements to,
    134–136
refusal of, 718
Rh type and, 130–133
safety measures for, 128–130
shed blood recovery and reinfusion
    in, 134–136
whole blood, 133
Transport, 40–48
  air, 42, 43–47. See also Air transport
    personnel for, 30–31
    special considerations in, 43–48
  ambulance, 40–42
    personnel for, 29–30
  of burn patients, 39, 40t
  during cardiac arrest, 43
  communication in, 42–43
  to community vs. tertiary care hos-
    pital, 47–48
  critical care transport specialists
    for, 31
  delays at scene in, 47
  destination guidelines for, 43, 44t,
    47–48
  device dislodgement and, 42, 43–44
  scoop and run vs. stay and play in,
    47
Transureteroureterostomy, 499
Trap-door thoracotomy, 312–313,
    313f, 332f, 334, 348
Trauma, epidemiology of, 10
Trauma alert, 74
Trauma cases, grading of, 74
Trauma centers, 10–15. See also
    Trauma systems
  designation of, 14
  development of, 8

transport to, 40–48. See also
    Transport
  verification of, 11–14
Trauma consult, 74
Trauma executive committee, 25
Trauma Injury Severity Score
    (TRISS), 20t
Trauma management
  ABCDs of, 71, 75
  airway management in, 32–35,
    75–77, 89–107
  equipment for, 71–73
  initial evaluation in, 71–88
  personnel in, 73
  phases of, 75
  preparation for patient arrival in,
    73
  primary survey in, 75–88
  recognition of life-threatening
    injuries in, 71
  resuscitation in. See Resuscitation
  transition from prehospital to hos-
    pital care in, 74–75
Trauma program performance com-
    mittee, 25
Trauma registry, 17–23
Trauma response
  activation of, 54–55
  levels of, 54–55
Trauma Score, 12t
Trauma scoring, 15–17
  anatomic, 16, 18t–19t
  common problems in, 26–27
  criteria for, 16
  future, 17, 21t
  methods of, 16–17
  outcome, 17, 20t
  physiologic, 12t–13t, 16
  purpose of, 16
Trauma service performance
    improvement plan, 24–25
Trauma stat, 74
Trauma surgery
  golden hour theory for, 7–8
  history of, 3–9
    civilian, 6–9
    military, 3–6
Trauma systems, 10–15. See also
    Trauma centers
  cost effectiveness of, 14
  design of, 15
  development of, 10–11
  efficacy of, 14
  financing of, 15
  implementation of, 15
  performance improvement and,
    17–22, 23–26
  state oversight of, 10–11, 14
  trauma registry and, 17–23
  trauma scoring and, 12t–13t,
    15–17, 18t–21t

Trauma team
  common traps for, 55
  concept of, 54
  designated leader of, 73
  members of, 50–52, 73
  organization of, 50–56
  training of, 55
Traumatic asphyxia, 584
Traumatic brain injury, 701–706.
      See also Head injuries
  mild, 705
Traumatologist, senior, 52
Treatment
  duty to provide, 710–712
  liability for, 727–730
  refusal of, 680, 717–719
Triage, 39–40, 41t, 59–60. *See also*
      Emergency medical services;
      Mass casualty management
  algorithm for, 43, 44f
  conventional, 59
  evacuation, 60
  field, 59–60
  in geriatric trauma, 613
  medical, 60
  on-site, 60
  scene report, 43
Tricuspid valve injuries, 338
Tripod fractures, 242
Trochanter fractures, 534–535, 652
Trochlear nerve injuries, 278
T-tube, esophageal, 325
Tubes
  endotracheal, 72, 96. *See also*
      Endotracheal intubation
  esophageal T-tube, 325
  thoracostomy, 72
Tube thoracostomy
  in diaphragmatic injuries,
      405–406, 409
  for hemothorax, 306
  indications for, 298–299
  for pneumothorax, 305
  technique of, 309–310
  tubes for, 72
Tuft fractures, 554
Tularemia, in biological warfare, 64
Two-point discrimination, in hand
      injuries, 544

U
Ulcers
  Curling's, 164, 168, 208–209
  decubitus, in spinal cord injuries,
      701
  stress
    bleeding from, 207–209,
      208–209
    in burns, 164, 168, 208–209
Ulnar collateral ligament injuries,
      555

Ulnar nerve block, 549f, 550
Ulnar nerve examination, 545
Ulnar nerve injuries, 234–235, 687
  in forearm fractures, 688–689
Ultrasonography. *See also* Radiology
      and specific injuries
  abdominal, 114, 352, 387–389,
      388f, 436, 631–632
    in blunt trauma, 396
  in chest trauma, 329
  duplex Doppler, in peripheral vas-
      cular injuries, 375
  in hand injuries, 548
  in hepatic injuries, 415
  renal, 487
  scrotal, 507
United Network for Organ Sharing,
      657–658
Universal precautions, 73
Upper extremity injuries, 531–534
  nerve injuries in, 686–689
  reconstructive surgery for,
      562–563
  rehabilitation in, 686–689
  splints for, 688, 688f
  traumatic amputation in, 551–553
Ureteral injuries, 494–500
  diagnosis of, 495–496
    delayed, 496
    intraoperative, 496
  epidemiology of, 484
  grading of, 495t
  imaging studies in, 495–496
  management of, 496–498
  mechanism of, 484
  physical examination in, 495
  presentation of, 494–495
  urinalysis in, 495
Ureteral stenting, 489
Ureteroneocystostomy, 498–499
Ureteroureterostomy, 498
Urethral injuries, 503–506
  epidemiology of, 484
  imaging studies in, 644–645
  mechanism of, 484
Urethrography, 505
Urinalysis
  in bladder injuries, 501
  in renal injuries, 485–486
  in ureteral injuries, 495
Urinary catheterization, in urethral
      injuries, 505–506
Urinary extravasation, in renal
      injuries, 489
Urinary incontinence, in spinal cord
      injuries, 695
Urography, 495
USA Patriot Act, 724
Uterine rupture, in pregnancy, 604
Uterine size assessment, in preg-
      nancy, 599–600

V

Vaccination, postsplenectomy, 444
Valproic acid, for mania, 679
Valvular injuries, cardiac, 338
Vascular access, 80–81. *See also*
    Fluid management
  for anesthesia, 178–179, 184
  in children, 572–573, 573f
  equipment for, 72
  in pregnancy, 598–599
  prehospital, 35
  sites for, 81
Vascular injuries
  abdominal, 351–370. *See also*
      Abdominal vascular injuries
  aortic arch, 347–349, 347t, 348t
  arterial, signs of, 372–375
  cervicothoracic, 339–349. *See also*
      Cervicothoracic vascular
      injuries
  endoluminal devices for, 349
  examination for, 112
  extremity, 372–384. *See also*
      Peripheral vascular injuries
  great vessel, 339, 340f, 341,
      347–349, 347t, 348t
  of neck, 292–293
  peripheral, 372–384. *See also*
      Peripheral vascular injuries
  stenting for, 349
Vasopressin, 188
  indications for, 188
Vasopressors, 188–189
  for hemorrhagic shock, 82
  indications for, 188–189
Vecuronium, 183
  for anesthesia induction, 182
Vegetative state, 703–704
Vena cava
  inferior, injuries of, 363–366
    retrohepatic, injuries of, 370,
        424–427
  superior, injuries of, 339, 340f, 341
  suprarenal, ligation of, 366
Vena cava filters, 197, 200t
  for elderly, 616
Venous access. *See* Vascular access
Venous thrombectomy, 199
Venous thromboembolism, preven-
    tion of, 195–199, 200t
  in alcohol withdrawal, 205t
  in elderly, 205t
  in spinal cord injuries, 701
Venovenous bypass, 426
Ventilation
  in children, 572
  in elderly, 610–611
  evaluation of, 78–80
  mask, 91–93
  in pregnancy, 596, 596t
Ventricular rupture, 335–338
Ventricular septal defects, 338

Verdan's zones, of flexor tendon lac-
    erations, 555
Vertebral artery injuries, 292–293
  blunt, 345–347
  penetrating, 344–345, 345f, 346f
  surgical exposure for, 344, 346f
Vertebral fractures. *See* Spinal frac-
    tures
Viet Nam War, trauma surgery in, 6
Vinyl chlorine, 64
Violence, duty to warn and, 724
Violent crime scenes, evidence
    preservation in, 32
Vision assessment, in head injuries,
    215
Vision loss
  in children, 282
  differential diagnosis of, 271t
  examination for, 259
Visitors, unruly, 725
Visual acuity evaluation, 259
Visual field assessment, 262
Visual rehabilitation, 283
Vital examinations, repeat, 118–119
Vital signs, in children, 572t
Vitreous, examination of, 263
Vitreous detachment, 273–274
Vitreous hemorrhage, 274
Volume assessment, 185
Vomiting, esophageal rupture in,
    321–322
VX (nerve agent), 64–65

W

Warfarin
  in elderly, 615
  extremity injuries in, 530, 690
  prophylactic, 197–198, 198, 200t,
      690
Warming methods, 185
Warren, John, 3, 7
Warren, Joseph, 3
Wars, trauma surgery in, 3–6
Washed red cells, 134–136
Weakness, critical illness, 708
Weapons of mass destruction, 61–68
  biological, 61–64. *See also* Biologi-
      cal warfare
  blast injuries and, 66–68
  chemical, 64–66
  decontamination and, 68
  nuclear, 61
Wedge fractures, 515
Wells, Horace, 6–7
Whiplash, 683–684
Whipple procedure, 453, 454f, 457
White syndrome, 198
Whole blood, 133
Withdrawal
  alcohol, 199–202, 203t-206t,
      673–674
  opiate, 675

World Trade Center attack, 8–9
World War I, trauma surgery in, 5
World War II, trauma surgery in, 5
Wound care
  in burns, 165–166, 165t
  in hand injuries, 548–549
  prehospital, 38
Wound healing
  factors influencing, 559
  primary, 560
  by secondary intention, 560, 561
  tertiary, 560
  types of, 559
Wound infections, 202–207
Wrist fractures, 534–535, 553–554

X
X-ray films. *See* Radiography
X-ray technician, 52

Y
Young Burgess classification, of
  pelvic fractures, 519

Z
Ziprasidone, for agitation, 670
Zone of injury, 565
Zygoma, anatomy of, 242
Zygomaticomaxillary fractures, 246,
  280